Anatomy & Physiology for Health Professions

An Interactive Journey

Anatomy & Physiology for Health Professions

An Interactive Journey

Third Edition

Bruce J. Colbert
Director of Allied Health
University of Pittsburgh at Johnstown

Jeff Ankney
Director of Clinical Education
University of Pittsburgh at Johnstown

Karen T. Lee
Associate Professor of Biology
University of Pittsburgh at Johnstown

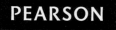

Boston   Columbus   Indianapolis   New York   San Francisco   Upper Saddle River
Amsterdam   Cape Town   Dubai   London   Madrid   Milan   Munich   Paris Montreal   Toronto
Delhi   Mexico   City   Sao Paulo   Sydney   Hong Kong   Seoul   Singapore   Taipei   Tokyo

Publisher: Julie Levin Alexander
Publisher's Assistant: Regina Bruno
Acquisitions Editor: Marlene Pratt
Program Manager: Faye Gemmellaro
Editorial Assistant: Lauren Bonilla
Development Editor: Jill Rembetski, iD8-TripleSSS Media
    Development, LLC
Marketing Manager: Brittany Hammond
Senior Marketing Coordinator: Alicia Wozniak
Marketing Specialist: Michael Sirinides
Project Management, Team Lead: Cindy Zonneveld
Project Manager: Yagnesh Jani
Full-Service Project Management: Bruce Hobart, SPi-Global
Associate Product Strategy Manager: Lee Noto
Senior Operations Specialist: Mary Ann Gloriande
Digital Program Manager: Amy Peltier
Media Project Manager: Lorena Cerisano
Creative Director: Andrea Nix
Art Director: Maria Guglielmo Walsh
Cover and Interior Designer: Studio Montage

Cover Image: Adimas/Fotolia
Composition: SPi-Global
Printing and Binding: Printed in the United States by LSC
Cover Printer: Printed in the United States by LSC
Text Font: 11/13.5 Adobe Garamond Pro

Notice: The authors and the publisher of this volume have taken care that the information and technical recommendations contained herein are based on research and expert consultation and are accurate and compatible with the standards generally accepted at the time of publication. Nevertheless, as new information becomes available, changes in clinical and technical practices become necessary. The reader is advised to carefully consult manufacturers' instructions and information material for all supplies and equipment before use, and to consult with a health care professional as necessary. This advice is especially important when using new supplies or equipment for clinical purposes. The authors and publisher disclaim all responsibility for any liability, loss, injury, or damage incurred as a consequence, directly or indirectly, of the use and application of any of the contents of this volume.

Library of Congress Cataloging-in-Publication Data
Colbert, Bruce J., author.
[Anatomy & physiology for health professions]
Anatomy & physiology for health professions / Bruce J. Colbert, Jeff Ankney, Karen T. Lee. -- Third edition.
    p. ; cm.
Preceded by Anatomy and physiology for health professions / Bruce J. Colbert, Jeff Ankney, Karen T. Lee. 2nd ed. c2011.
Includes bibliographical references and index.
ISBN 978-0-13-385111-3 — ISBN 0-13-385111-7
I. Ankney, Jeff, author. II. Lee, Karen T., author. III. Title.
[DNLM: 1. Anatomy. 2. Physiological Phenomena. QS 4]
QM23.2
612—dc23   2014043337

4 17

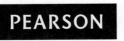

ISBN 10: 0-13-385111-7
ISBN 13: 978-0-13-385111-3

To all the future health care professionals learning anatomy and physiology: May your chosen professions be as personally rewarding as ours have been.

—*Your Travel Guides Bruce, Jeff, and Karen*

I dedicate this book to those closest to me who share this wonderful journey through life: my wife Patty, my sons Joshua and Jeremy, my daughter-in-law Ali, and my three brothers and sister. Also a special thanks to the many teachers who encouraged me to develop my writing skills. Finally, a special dedication to the memory of my Mom and Dad, who taught me the importance of education.

—*Bruce*

A special thanks to all my family for their support and understanding through this long process. Mom and Dad, thank you both for always being there no matter where my journey took me.

A sincere thank you to Mr. James McCall, who inspired me to become a teacher those many years ago. And to my past teachers and professors—here's proof that under-achievers sometimes do hit their stride!

—*Jeff*

I dedicate this book to my family, who have always supported me, no matter where life has taken me: not only my "real" family—my late father Ed, my mother Pat, brother Eddie, sister-in-law Sheila, and assorted aunts, uncles, and cousins, who really had no choice but to be part of my life—but also those members of my extended family who have inexplicably chosen to be part of my life, giving me the gift of their friendship. I couldn't have done it without them.

—*Karen*

BRIEF CONTENTS

CONTENTS

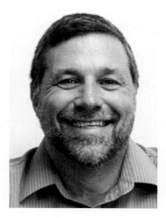

Bruce Colbert is the Director of the Allied Health Department at the University of Pittsburgh at Johnstown. He holds a master's degree in health education and administration, has authored nine books and several articles, and has given over 250 invited lectures and workshops at both the regional and national levels. Many of his workshops provide teacher training involving techniques to make the health sciences engaging and relevant to today's students. In addition, Bruce has presented workshops on developing effective critical and creative thinking, stress and time management, and study skills. He is an avid basketball player, even after three knee surgeries, which may indicate that he has some learning difficulties.

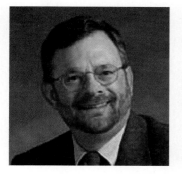

Jeff Ankney is the Director of Clinical Education for the University of Pittsburgh at Johnstown Respiratory Care program, where he is responsible for the development and evaluation of hospital clinical sites. In the past, he has served as a public school teacher, Assistant Director of Cardiopulmonary Services, and Program Coordinator of Pulmonary Rehabilitation, and has been a member of hospital utilization review, hospital policy, strategic planning, and patient safety committees. Jeff is a consultant on hospital management and pulmonary rehabilitation concerns. He was also the recipient of the American Cancer Society Public Education Award. He is a pretty fair fly fisherman and wing shot, although his springer spaniel, Rusty, would probably disagree.

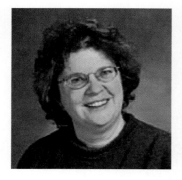

Karen Lee is an Associate Professor in the Biology Department at the University of Pittsburgh at Johnstown, where she teaches all the anatomy courses, including anatomy and physiology for nursing and allied health students. She presents regularly at scientific conferences and has published several articles on crustacean physiology and behavior. An active member of the Council on Undergraduate Research, she is also the campus Undergraduate Research Coordinator. For the last many years Karen has sung bass in women's barbershop choruses and quartets and more recently has been harmonizing with any singer or guitar player who will let her near the microphone.

Anatomy and physiology is a critical academic course one must master to succeed in the health professions. This third edition of **_Anatomy and Physiology for Health Professions: An Interactive Journey_**—is written in a manner that will enhance learning of the material versus mass memorization of facts. Too often students adopt the strategy of memorizing massive amounts of information and simply storing it in their short-term memories. Then they spew out this information during their exams, which may allow them to *survive* the course. However, memorization alone does not help learners internalize the material nor make the lasting connections that will help them *thrive* as health care practitioners.

To each student, in the course of your day as a health professional, you will be exposed to a variety of diseases involving all parts of the body; therefore, you must truly learn the workings and interrelatedness of all the body systems and functions. Imagine standing over a patient in cardiac arrest and saying to that patient's loved one, "Sorry, I memorized CPR six months ago but now I forget what to do." We think you get the picture.

New to This Edition

- New and exciting illustrations and micrographs will increase visual appeal and understanding.
- An added feature called Focus on Professions showcases a variety of allied health professions.
- Information about disease terminology and physical assessment concepts has been added.
- Data on body system disorders have been updated and expanded.
- The coverage on relevant geriatric topics has been increased.
- The Glossary has been greatly expanded.
- Updated Test Your Knowledge exercises appear within each chapter.
- A new text design makes content easier to locate.
- Amazing Facts and Clinical Application boxes have been updated with the latest research and clinical information. Some examples of new topics include three-dimensional printing, traumatic brain injury (TBI) and concussions, epidemiology, biological importance of water and hydration, drug resistance and its implications, prions and related diseases, and new theories and research on senses.

What Is NOT New to This Edition

- We haven't changed the user-friendly, conversational writing style that is rich with analogies and encourages relevant learning that has made the first and second editions so popular.

So what have we done to facilitate learning the material? First, we have placed study skills and stress management tips in a *Study Success Companion* in the back of your book to help you along your journey through this class and beyond. Second, we have strived to make anatomy and physiology "come alive" by using an engaging writing style to make it seem as if we are sitting next to you talking about the concepts. We have made every effort to put together an anatomy and physiology book that you will actually enjoy reading. We hope you consider us as assistants to the most important guide through this journey: your teacher.

Humor, where appropriate, and analogies to compare the human body to everyday things to which you can relate have been interwoven throughout the text. Finally, we have added special features in a unique fashion tailored to the visual learning styles and relevant learning that today's students require.

We have worked hard to create an even more exciting and visually appealing third edition and sincerely hope these features will help make studying anatomy and physiology a positive experience. Have a safe and happy journey!

Resources

- Textbook
- Student Workbook (available separately) contains even more practice and reinforcement opportunities and helps you prepare for quizzes and exams. Also includes concept maps and crossword puzzles.

The Instructor Package:

- Instructor's Resource Manual contains a wealth of information to help faculty plan and manage the anatomy and physiology course.
- PowerPoint Slides
- MyTest test bank

Interactive Media

Visit our new MyHealthProfessions Lab to accompany Anatomy & Physiology for Health Professions. Here you'll find a wealth of resources, including:

- A pre-/post-test homework engine, which enables students to learn and master concepts as homework, preparing them for classroom work.

- A set of highly visual animations for each of the 13 body systems, to be used in the classroom, as homework, or as an independent review.
- Additional animations that explain difficult-to-teach and -retain concepts:
  - how muscle fibers contract
  - process of kidney filtration
  - nerve impulses and how neuro-junctions work
  - oxygen transport
  - cellular and external respiration
  - how the immune system reacts to a foreign substance

- steps in the healing process of a skin wound
- electrophysiology of the heart
- blood types, matching, and cross-matching
- what happens to food in the digestive tract
- regulation of the menstrual cycle
- Animations will be housed in a media library for both instructors and students; they will be available to students through an etext.
- A series of case studies that put A&P concepts into the context of health professions practice. These can be used as either classroom or homework assignments.

We gratefully thank Jill Rembetski, who acted as an invaluable guide through the development and completion of both the first and second editions as well as this new edition of *Anatomy and Physiology for Health Professions*. We value all her hard work and attention to details that added so much to this project. To all those at Pearson who were so helpful and friendly in this monumental process, especially Yagnesh Jani, Faye Gemmellaro, and Marlene Pratt, thank you. A special thank-you to Mark Cohen for his enthusiastic belief and continued support in the vision and execution of this unique project. Also, we gratefully acknowledge a great group of reviewers who helped shape this project with their thoughtful insights. Finally, special thanks to Jan Snyder for putting up with two quirky authors and helping in so many ways.

Third Edition

Dan Bickerton, MS
Instructor – Biology
Ogeechee Technical College
Statesboro, Georgia

Deborah Rhoades, BS, NCMA, HT (ASCP)
Instructor – MA and MRT
Harrison College
Grove City, Ohio

Diane Hartel, RMA
Director of Curriculum – FCC Division
International Education Corporation
Ft. Lauderdale, Florida

James Brasiel, MD, MHA, MICP
Principal – Medical Education & Quality Improvement
Ready Enterprises
Concord, California

Maria R. Rivera, MD
Academic Chair – Allied Health
Florida Technical College
Orlando, Florida

Mindy Brown, RMA
Instructor – Medical Assisting/Administrative Assisting
Pima Medical Institute
Colorado Springs, Colorado

Paula Denise Silver, BS, PharmD
Instructor – Medical Assisting
ECPI University
Newport News, Virginia

Second Edition

Jyoti Abraham, PhD
Bacone College
Muskogee, Oklahoma

Ana T. Alvarez-Calonge,
    MLT, RMA, AHI
Keiser Career College
Miami Lakes, Florida

April Andrews, MBA
The Katharine Gibbs School
Norristown, Pennsylvania

Karen Bakuzonis, PhD, RHIA
Santa Fe College
Gainesville, Florida

Dan Bickerton
Ogeechee Technical College
Statesboro, Georgia

Joan Bonczek, BS RT(R)
Johnson College
Scranton, Pennsylvania

Tim Feltmeyer, MS, AHI
Erie Business Center
Erie, Pennsylvania

Jonathan D. French, DC
YTI Career Institute
Lancaster, Pennsylvania

Michael Giovanniello, MS, RT(R)
Broward College
Ft. Lauderdale, Florida

Jeff Kingsbury, MD
Mohave Community College
Lake Havasu City, Arizona

Lynette S. McCullough, MS, NREMT-P
Griffin Technical College
Griffin, Georgia

Don V. Plantz Jr., PhD
Mohave Community College
Bullhead City, Arizona

Robert Plick
Medical Dean
Westwood College
Denver, Colorado

Nina Pustylnik
Keiser Career College
Miami Lakes, Florida

Julie Shay, RHIA
Santa Fe College
Gainesville, Florida

Betty Sims, RN, MSN, FRE
Coastal Bend College
Beeville, Texas

Lorrie Tate, RN, BSN
Coosa Technical College
Rome, Georgia

First Edition

Margaret N. Anfinsen, RN, MSN
Southwest Florida College
Fort Myers, Florida

Nina Beaman, MS, RNC, CMA
Bryant and Stratton College
Richmond, Virginia

Dorothea Best, RN, BA, BSHS
Scranton, Pennsylvania

Jeanine Brice, RN, MSN
Pasco-Hernando Community College
New Port Richey, Florida

Minda Brown, RMA
Pima Medical Institute
Colorado Springs, Colorado

Carmen Carpenter, RN, BSN, CMA, MS
South University
West Palm Beach, Florida

Stephanie Cox, BA, LPN
York Technical Institute
Lancaster, Pennsylvania

Susan DeGirolamo, RMA, NCPT, NCICS
CHI Institute, Southampton Campus
Southampton, Pennsylvania

Kathie Folsom, MS, BSN, RN
Skagit Valley College
Oak Harbor, Washington

Nadine Forbes, MS
Johns Hopkins University
School of Medicine
Baltimore, Maryland

Shirley Jelmo, CMA
Pima Medical Institute
Colorado Springs, Colorado

Dee Ann Kerr, BA, MA
Minnesota School of Business
Waite Park, Minnesota

Jennifer A. Leach, BS
Lehigh Valley College
Center Valley, Pennsylvania

Stacey Long, BS
Miami Jacobs Career College
Dayton, Ohio

Janet M. Bohachef Martin, BA, MEd
Amarillo College
Amarillo, Texas

Andrew E. Muniz, OT, BBA, MBA
Baker College
Auburn Hills, Michigan

Ruth Ann O'Brien, MHA
Medical Assisting
Dayton, Ohio

Eddie Rhodes, Jr., MEd., MT(AMT), CPT(ASPT)
West Georgia Technical College
LaGrange, Georgia

Sharon Romine, RN, BSN, MSN
Bessemer State Technical College
Bessemer, Alabama

Mary K. Sargent, MS
Ivy Tech State College
Valparaiso, Indiana

Jaqueline T. Smith, AAS, CPhT
National College of Business and Technology
Bluefield, Virginia

Barbara Snyder, CMA
Thompson Institute
Harrisburg, Pennsylvania

Irma Villarreal, MS
DeVry University Irving, Texas and Everest
    College Dallas, Texas

Joyce A. Wilson, RN, BA
South Plains College
Levelland, Texas

1

Introduction to Anatomy and Physiology

LEARNING THE LANGUAGE

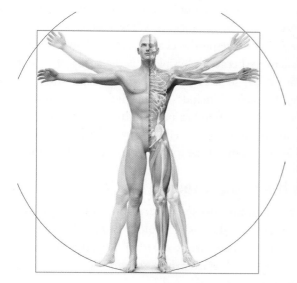

Imagine getting ready to travel to a foreign country where you do not speak the language. To maximize the success of your journey, one of the most important preparatory steps is to develop a basic understanding of the native language. Every profession has a specialized "native" language all of its own along with numerous abbreviations. Medical terminology is the professional language of medicine that one needs to master for success. This chapter lays the foundation for learning medical terminology, and future chapters will build on this foundation so that at our journey's end, not only will you understand anatomy and physiology but you will also be fluent in medical terminology.

LEARNING OUTCOMES

At the end of your journey through this chapter, you will be able to:

- Understand the terms *anatomy* and *physiology* and their various related areas.
- Construct and define medical terms using word roots, prefixes, and suffixes.
- Identify commonly used medical abbreviations.
- Contrast the metric and English systems of measures.
- Describe various signs and symptoms along with associated disease terminology.
- Explain the concepts and importance of homeostasis and metabolism.

Pronunciation Guide Pro·nun·ci·a·tion

Correct pronunciation is important in any journey so that you and others are completely understood. Here is a "see and say" Pronunciation Guide for the more difficult terms to pronounce in this chapter. Please note that even though there are standard pronunciations, regional variations of the pronunciations can occur.

anabolism (ah NAB oh lizm)
anatomy (ah NA tom ee)
catabolism (ka TAB oh lizm)
diagnosis (DYE ahg NOH sis)
etiology (EE tee ALL oh jee)
homeostasis (HOH mee oh STAY sis)
macroscopic anatomy (MAK roh SCOP ic)

metabolism (meh TAB oh lizm)
microscopic anatomy (MY kroh SCOP ic)
pathology (path ALL oh jee)
physiology (fiz ee ALL oh jee)
prognosis (prog NOH sis)
rhinoplasty (RYE noh PLASS tee)
syndrome (SIN drohm)

WHAT IS ANATOMY AND PHYSIOLOGY?

You're probably so accustomed to hearing the words *anatomy* and *physiology* used together that you may not have given much thought to what each one means and how they differ. They each have unique meanings. Let's take a closer look.

Anatomy

Anatomy is the study of the internal and external *structures* of plants, animals, or, for our focus, the human body. The human body is an amazing and complex machine that can perform an almost limitless number of tasks. To truly understand how something works, it is important to know how it is put together. The word *anatomy* is from the Greek language and literally means "to cut apart," which is exactly what you must do to see how something is put together. For example, the study of the arrangement of the bones that comprise the human skeleton, which is the anatomical framework for our bodies, is considered *skeletal anatomy*. Leonardo da Vinci, in the 1400s, correctly drew the human skeleton and could be considered one of the earliest *anatomists* (one who studies anatomy).

Just as we can subdivide biology into more specific concentrations, such as cell biology, plant biology, and animal biology, we can also broadly divide anatomy into microscopic anatomy and macroscopic anatomy. **Microscopic anatomy** is the study of structures that can be seen and examined only with magnification aids, such as a microscope. The study of cellular structures (cytology) and tissue samples (histology) are examples of microscopic anatomy.

Macroscopic anatomy, sometimes called **gross anatomy**, represents the study of the structures visible to the unaided or naked eye. For example, the study of the various bones that make up the human body is skeletal anatomy. Viewing x-ray of the arm to determine the type and location of a ken bone is considered an examination of gross anatomy.

Physiology

Physiology focuses on the *functions* and processes of the various structures that make up the human body. Physiological processes include muscle contraction, our senses of smell and sight, how we breathe, and the list goes on. We will focus on each of these processes in their respective chapters. Physiology is closely related to anatomy because physiology is the study of how a structure (anatomy) such as a cell or bone actually functions (physiology). Physiology includes all the vital processes of life; it is complex, and therefore has many subspecialties. Human physiology, animal physiology, cellular physiology, and neurophysiology are just some of the specific branches of physiology.

Putting It All Together

In summary, anatomy focuses on *structure* and how something is put together, whereas physiology is the study of how those different structures work together to make the body *function* as a whole. For example, anatomy would be the study of the structure of the red blood cells (RBCs), and physiology would be the study of how the RBCs carry vital oxygen throughout the body. FIGURE 1–1 ■ shows deformed RBCs (sickle or curved shaped) that are present in the disease sickle cell anemia. Because of the anatomical deformity, the physiological process of carrying oxygen is adversely affected, and blockages in blood flow can result.

You will notice on your journey that the design of a structure is often related to its function. For example, joint anatomy is dictated by the functions of those bones forming the joint. Hinge joints are located at the knees, where back and forth bending movement is required, whereas the ball and socket joint of the hip provides for a greater range of motion.

Therefore, it makes sense to combine these two sciences into anatomy and physiology (A&P). Human anatomy and physiology forms the foundation for all medical practice. Anything that negatively changes the normal structure or function can be called *disease*, and the study of disease is *pathophysiology*.

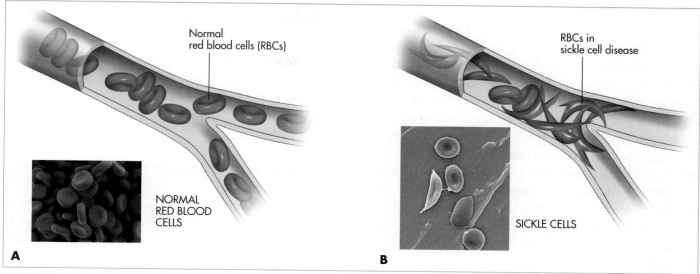

FIGURE 1–1 ■

A. Normal red blood cells (RBCs) are flexible and donut-shaped and move with ease through blood vessels. **B**. The anatomical distortion of the structure of RBCs in sickle cell anemia affects its normal function to carry oxygen. In addition, the sickle cells lose their ability to bend and pass through the small blood vessels, thereby causing blockages to blood flow.

TEST YOUR KNOWLEDGE 1–1

Indicate whether the following examples are gross anatomy or microscopic anatomy by putting a G or an M in the space provided.

1. _____ Viewing an x-ray to determine the type of bone break

2. _____ Classifying a tumor to be cancerous by cell type

3. _____ Viewing bacteria to determine what disease is present

4. _____ Examining the chest for any obvious deformities

5. _____ Working as a histotechnologist or cytotechnologist

THE LANGUAGE

Even if you're traveling to another city within your home country, you will most likely need to learn a few things about the language its citizens speak. For example, think of the many different names people use to identify a sandwich made on a long skinny roll. Your "sub" might be someone else's "grinder," "hoagie," or "hero."

Anatomy and physiology also has its own unique language that you must learn before you can converse comfortably. Some words, such as *cardiac*, *respiratory*, and *hypertension*, are already familiar to you. Others will seem strange and foreign. Let's take a closer look.

Medical Terminology

As stated earlier, the language of anatomy and physiology is primarily based on medical terminology. Understanding medical terminology may seem like an overwhelming task because, on the surface, there appears to be *so* many terms. In reality, there are only a relatively few word roots, prefixes, and suffixes, but they can be put together in a host of ways to form numerous terms.

Most of the medical terms are derived from the Greek and Latin languages because much of the science of medicine originated in ancient Greek- and Latin-speaking societies that originated in the Mediterranean region.

Each medical term has a basic structure on which to build, called the *word root*. For example, *cardi* is the word root for terms pertaining to the heart. Rarely is the word root used alone. Instead, it is combined with prefixes and suffixes that can change its meaning. Prefixes come before the word root, whereas suffixes come after the word root. The suffix *ology* means "study of," and therefore, we can combine *cardi* and *ology* to form **cardiology**, which is the study of the heart. The prefix *tachy* means "fast" and can be placed in front of the word root to form **tachycardia**, which means a fast heart rate.

Often you will be given a **combining form**, which is the word root and a connecting vowel (usually *o*), to make it easier to pronounce and combine with possible suffixes. For example, the combining form for heart is *cardi/o*. FIGURE 1–2 ■ shows the components of a medical term.

FOCUS ON PROFESSIONS

There are many medical specialties ("ologists"), and just by searching online or skimming the Yellow Pages of a phone book you can see firsthand the vast array that exists—from anesthesiologists to urologists.

Listed in TABLE 1–1 ■ are some common combining forms to get you started.

Now let's add some common prefixes that can be placed before the word roots to alter their meaning (see TABLE 1–2 ■) and some common suffixes (TABLE 1–3 ■) and see what kinds of words we can form with just these few parts.

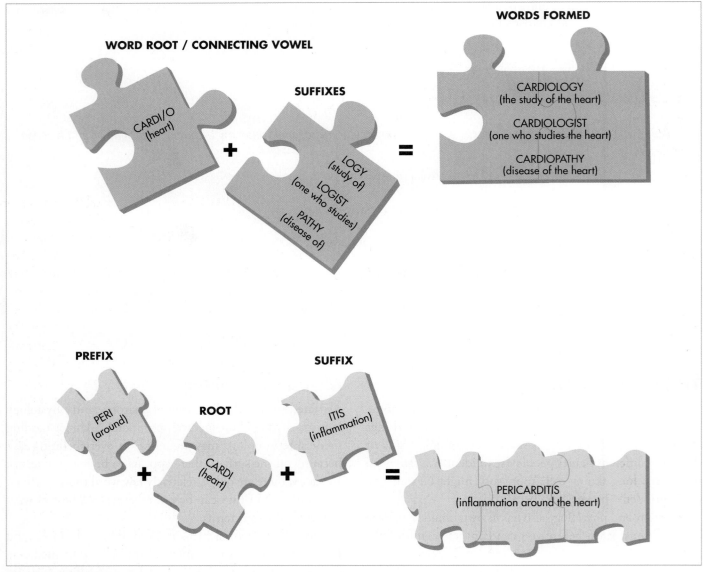

FIGURE 1–2 ■

How prefixes and suffixes can be combined with a word root to form many medical terms.

TABLE 1–1 COMMON COMBINING TERMS

WORD ROOT/ COMBINING FORM	MEANING
abdomin/o	abdomen
aden/o	gland
angi/o	vessel
arthr/o	joint
cardi/o	heart
col/o	colon
cyan/o	blue
cyt/o	cell
derm/o	skin
erythr/o	red
gastr/o	stomach
glyc/o	sugar
hemat/o, hem/o	blood
hepat/o	liver
hist/o	tissue
leuk/o	white
mamm/o	breast
nephr/o	kidney
neur/o	nerve
oste/o	bone
path/o	disease
phag/o	to swallow
pneum/o, pneumon/o	air or lung
rhin/o	nose

TABLE 1–2 COMMON PREFIXES

PREFIX	MEANING
a, an	without
acro	extremities
brady	slow
dia	through
dys	difficult
electro	electric
endo	within
epi	upon or over
hyper	above normal
hypo	below normal
macro	large
micro	small
peri	around
sub	under, below
tachy	fast

Using Tables 1–1, 1–2, and 1–3, look at all the terms you can make from just the one word root, *cardi/o*. *Cardiology* is the study of the heart, and a *cardiologist* is one who studies the heart. *Bradycardia* is a slow heart rate, *tachycardia* is a fast heart rate, and an *electrocardiogram* is an electrical recording of the heart. If your heart were enlarged due to inflammation *(carditis)*, you would have *cardiomegaly*, which would mean you have heart disease *(cardiopathy)*. The Tin Man from *The Wizard of Oz* thought he had no heart *(acardia)*, but realized that he had *cardiomegaly* all along. Disclaimer: Although having an enlarged heart, or cardiomegaly, was good for the Tin Man, it is an abnormal and serious medical condition.

LEARNING HINT

General Hints on Forming Medical Terms

Although you can learn the various word roots, prefixes, and suffixes, it gets confusing trying to put them correctly together. In most instances, the medical definition indicates the last part of the term first, especially when suffixes are used. For example, an inflammation of the stomach is *gastritis*, not *itisgastro*, and one who studies the stomach is a *gastrologist*, not an *ologistgastro*. When using prefixes, you usually put the parts together in the order you say the definition. For example, slow heart rate is *bradycardia*, not *cardiabrady*. As with all general rules, there are exceptions, but with practice, using medical terminology will become familiar to you.

TABLE 1–3 COMMON SUFFIXES

SUFFIX	MEANING
-al, ic	pertaining to or related to
-algia	pain
-cyte	cell
-ectomy	surgical removal of
-gram	a recording
-graphy	the process of recording
-ist	one who specializes
-itis	inflammation of
-megaly	enlargement of
-ologist or -logist	one who studies
-ology or -logy	study of
-oma	tumor
-osis	disease or condition of
-ostomy	surgically forming an opening
-otomy	cutting into
-pathy	disease
-penia	decrease or lack of
-phobia	fear of
-plasty	surgical repair
-scope	instrument to view or examine

LEARNING HINT

Combining and Forming Medical Terms

If a suffix begins with a vowel, drop the vowel in the combining form. For example, the combining form for stomach is *gastr/o*, and if we add the suffix for inflammation, *itis*, the medical term becomes *gastritis*. The suffixes *ology* and *logy* are both acceptable for "the study of." If you use *ology* and a combining form such as *cardi/o*, an *o* would be dropped to form *cardiology*. A general rule is that when a suffix begins with a vowel, drop the vowel in the combining form.

Abbreviations

Abbreviations are used extensively in the medical profession. They are useful in simplifying long, complicated terms for disease, diagnostic procedures, and therapies that require extensive documentation. For now, review TABLE 1–4 ■ for some common abbreviations you may have heard in a health care setting or on television.

TABLE 1–4 COMMON MEDICAL ABBREVIATIONS

ABBREVIATION	MEANING
A&P	anatomy and physiology
ACLS	advanced cardiac life support
b.i.d.	give twice a day
BP	blood pressure
CA	cancer
CAD	coronary artery disease
CBC	complete blood count
CPR	cardiopulmonary resuscitation
CXR	chest x-ray
GI	gastrointestinal
ICU	intensive care unit
IV	intravenous
NPO, npo	Latin *nil per os*, which means "nothing by mouth"
prn	whenever needed
q.i.d.	give four times a day
SOB	shortness of breath
STAT	Latin *statim*, which means "immediately"
t.i.d.	give three times a day
*ED/ER	emergency department/ emergency room

*Note: Traditionally, the hospital emergency areas were called *emergency rooms (ERs)* but those areas have expanded to where they are considered a whole department. Both abbreviations are acceptable, but many health care professionals now prefer the term *emergency department (ED)*.

TEST YOUR KNOWLEDGE 1–2

Define the medical terms:

1. acrocyanosis

_____

2. nephrologist

_____

3. cytomegaly

_____

4. dermatitis

_____

5. appendectomy

_____

Give the correct medical term:

6. removal of the stomach _____

7. disease of the bones _____

8. electrical recording of the heart _____

9. inflammation of the joints _____

10. one who studies the nervous system _____

11. abbreviation for patient not allowed to eat or drink _____

12. abbreviation for giving a drug or treatment as needed _____

Of course, you will learn many more medical terms and abbreviations as we explore the upcoming chapters and become fluent in conversational medical language. This will help you avoid using lay terms (common, everyday terms) to describe medical and anatomical concepts. Now you know that the correct term for "getting a nose job" is **rhinoplasty**.

The Metric System

Whereas medical terminology represents the written and spoken language for understanding anatomy and physiology, the metric system is the "mathematical language" of anatomy and physiology to measure weight, volume, and length. For example, blood pressure is measured in millimeters of mercury (mm Hg), and organ size is usually measured in centimeters (cm). Medications and fluids are given in milliliters (mL) or cubic centimeters (cc), and weight is often measured in kilograms (kg). What exactly does it mean when you are taught that normal cardiac output is 6 liters per minute? You can now see why you must be familiar with the metric system to truly understand anatomy and physiology and medicine. Although the metric system may seem complicated if you are not familiar with it, it really isn't if you have a basic understanding of math. In fact, once you have enough practice, using the metric system is actually easier than the measurements you are used to using.

Medical assistants must become familiar with medical terminology in their workplace. Additionally, **coders, transcriptionists**, and **health information technicians**, all of whom deal extensively with the medical charts and patient records, must master this language.

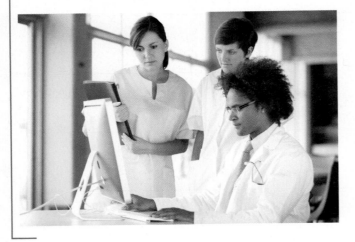

Amazing Facts

The Longest Medical Term
The longest medical term is *pneumonoultramicroscopicsilicovolcanoconiosis* of 45 letters, which is a form of pneumoconiosis (condition of the lung) caused by very fine (ultramicro) silicate or quartz dust.

Two major systems of measurement are in use today. The U.S. Customary System (USCS) is used in the United States, and the International System of Units or SI (Systéme International) is used everywhere else, and especially in health care, science, and the pharmaceutical industry. The SI system is also known as the international or **metric system** and is based on the power (or multiples) of 10.

The USCS system is based on the British Imperial System and uses several different designations for the basic units of length, weight, and volume. We commonly call this the **English system**. For example, in the English system, volumes can be expressed as ounces, pints, quarts, gallons, pecks, bushels, or cubic feet. Distance can be expressed in inches, feet, yards, and miles. Weights are measured in ounces, pounds, and tons. This may be the system you are most familiar with, but it is not the system of choice used throughout the world and within the medical profession because the English system has no common base and is

therefore very cumbersome to use. It is difficult to know the relationships between each unit of measure because they are not based in an orderly fashion according to the powers of 10 as in the metric system. For example, how many pecks are in a bushel? Just what is a peck? How many inches are in a mile? These all require extensive calculations and memorization of certain equivalent values, whereas in the metric system, you simply move the decimal point the appropriate power of 10.

This has been a brief overview of the two types of measurement systems that you will encounter in your everyday activities as a health care professional. If you want to learn more about the metric system, please refer to the Study Success Companion at the end of this text, where a simplified explanation is given on how to easily use the metric system in the health care setting. In addition, the Study Success Companion will show you a simplified method for conversions both within and between the metric and English systems. See Table 3, page 449, which gives common prefixes of the metric system and compares the metric and English systems.

Amazing Facts

Metric Emergency
In 1989, an Air Canada passenger jet ran out of fuel and the pilot had to glide the jetliner onto a runway for, thankfully, a safe emergency landing. The near disaster occurred because the fuel had been erroneously measured in pounds instead of kilograms at a time when Canada was converting to the metric system!

THE LANGUAGE OF DISEASE

This chapter is about planning for a smooth trip by learning the language used at our destination. However, even with the most careful planning, things can still go wrong. Flat tires, airport delays, and loss of money or credit cards can ruin a trip. Similarly, problems can happen to the human body. Ideally, the body works to make things function smoothly and in balance. Sometimes things happen to alter those functions. Eating habits, smoking, inherited traits, trauma, environmental factors, and even aging can alter the body's balance and lead to **disease**. Disease, which literally means "not [dis] at ease," is a condition in which the body fails to function normally.

Although this is an A&P course that focuses on *normal* function and structure, it is often helpful to reinforce the concepts with some elaboration of what can go wrong. Therefore, at the end of each system chapter, a *brief* discussion on some of the major and more common diseases associated with that system is provided. For example, a future physical therapist or massage therapist may want to spend more time exploring in-depth disease information on the muscular system, a dental hygienist may wish to learn more about the function of teeth in the digestive system, and a radiologic technologist may want to focus on the skeletal system. For now, a brief discussion of some of the unique language of disease is needed to lay the foundation for future discussions.

Signs and Symptoms of Disease

Think back to a time when you were sick. You may have had a fever, cough, nausea, dizziness, joint aches, or a generalized weakness. These are examples of **signs** and **symptoms** of disease. Although the terms *signs* and *symptoms* are often used interchangeably, each has its own specific definition. Signs are more definitive, *objective* (measurable), obvious indicators of an illness. They can actually be measured and expressed as numbers. Fever or monitoring the change in the size of a mole are good examples of signs. **Vital signs** are common, measurable indicators that help us assess the health of our patients. Vital signs are the signs essential to life and include pulse (heart rate), blood pressure, body temperature, and respiratory rate. The vital sign standard values can change according to the patient's age and sex. Pain is now being considered as the fifth vital sign due to the importance of proper pain management therapy.

Clinical Application

THE VITAL SIGN OF PULSE

Although there are several body locations where a pulse can be taken, the pulse is commonly taken by applying slight finger pressure over the radial artery located in each wrist (on the thumb side) and counting the number of beats in a 60-second period (see **FIGURE 1-3** ■). The normal heart rate for an adult is 60 to 100 beats per minute, a child's rate is approximately 70 to 120, and a newborn's rate is 90 to 170 beats per minute. If an adult has a heart rate of 165 beats per minute, what medical term would you use to describe that condition?

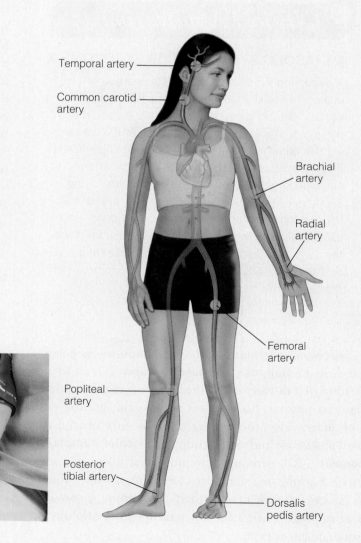

Temporal artery

Common carotid artery

Brachial artery

Radial artery

Femoral artery

Popliteal artery

Posterior tibial artery

Dorsalis pedis artery

FIGURE 1-3 ■

A health care professional taking a radial pulse and common pulse points.

Symptoms, on the other hand, are more *subjective*, based on the individual's perception and therefore more difficult to measure consistently. Although pain is now being considered the fifth vital sign, it is still a subjective evaluation very much like a symptom. For example, tolerance to pain varies among individuals, so an equal amount of pain (as in a needle stick) applied to a number of people could be perceived as a light, moderate, or intense level of pain, depending on each individual's perception. Symptoms are hard to measure. They are, however, still very important in the diagnosis of disease. Sometimes a disease exhibits a set group of signs and symptoms that may occur at about the same time. This specific grouping of signs and symptoms is known as a **syndrome**. Signs, symptoms, and syndromes are further explained throughout the textbook as they relate to the anatomy and physiology of the various body systems.

Clinical Application

METABOLIC SYNDROME, OR SYNDROME X

A disturbing syndrome that affects nearly one-quarter of the U.S. adult population is known as *metabolic syndrome*, or *syndrome X*. A patient with this syndrome exhibits at least three of the following five common conditions: high blood sugar levels (hyperglycemia), high blood pressure (hypertension), abdominal obesity, high triglycerides (a lipid substance in the blood), and low blood level of HDL (a good form of blood cholesterol). Individuals who exhibit this syndrome are at increased risk for diabetes, heart attacks, and/or strokes. Poor diet and a lack of exercise clearly contribute to the development of this syndrome.

Discovering as many signs and symptoms as possible can help to **diagnose** a disease. A *diagnosis* is an identification of a disease determined by studying the patient's signs, symptoms, history, and results of diagnostic tests. The diagnostic procedure is done by first obtaining a patient history and determining their **chief complaint/concern (CC)**. Although the individual may have many medical problems, the chief complaint is what brought them *now* to seek medical help. Obtaining a complete medical history can help in determining the **etiology**, or cause, of the disease.

It is also helpful to determine if the chief complaint was gradual or of a sudden onset. Quite often, symptoms gradually develop from a disease process that may have been there for some time. These often are **chronic conditions** as opposed to **acute conditions** that exhibit a rapid onset of signs and symptoms. One of the problems with chronic conditions is that due to their usually gradual onset, older patients often attribute them to "just getting older" and often ignore them as an indicator of disease. As these conditions worsen, these people can no longer ignore these conditions and they seek help. By that time, treating the disease may be more complicated or difficult due to its severity.

The signs and symptoms of a chronic disease may disappear at times; this period is known as **remission** of the disease. **Relapses** are recurrences of the signs and symptoms of disease. If the signs and symptoms acutely "flare up," this is known as an **exacerbation** of the disease. **Mortality** is the measure of the number of deaths attributed to a specific disease in a given population over a period of time. **Morbidity** is the measure of the disabilities and extent of problems caused by an illness. For example, although polio has a low mortality rate (few deaths associated with the disease), it does have a high morbidity rate due to the paralysis, limb deformities, and difficulty breathing later in life.

The Centers for Disease Control and Prevention (CDC) tracks disease worldwide. If a disease is continually present within a specific population or region, it is called **endemic**. If the disease occurs suddenly in large numbers over a specific region, it is called an **epidemic**. If the disease spreads country or worldwide, it is called a **pandemic**.

Diseases that have a prognosis of death are referred to as **terminal** diseases. The **prognosis** is the prediction of the outcome of a disease. Hopefully, your *prognosis* for doing well in this anatomy and physiology course is excellent.

LEARNING HINT

What's in a Word?

The word *gnosis* is Greek for "knowledge." *Dia* means "through or complete"; therefore *diagnosis* literally means "know through or completely." *Pro* is a prefix meaning "before or in front of." Perhaps you can figure out that *prognosis* literally means "the foreknowledge or predicting of the outcome of a disease."

TEST YOUR KNOWLEDGE 1–3

Answer the following questions:

1. Use a checkmark to indicate which of the following are vital signs:

   _____ a. pulse

   _____ b. cough

   _____ c. blood pressure

   _____ d. age

   _____ e. indigestion

   _____ f. respiratory rate

   _____ g. body temperature

2. Which of the following is the medical term for the cause of a disease?
   a. prognosis
   b. diagnosis
   c. etiology
   d. syndrome

3. Which of the following is the medical term for the outcome of a disease?
   a. prognosis
   b. diagnosis
   c. etiology
   d. syndrome

4. If you describe a disease as "terminal," you are describing the
   a. diagnosis.
   b. prognosis.
   c. etiology.
   d. treatment.

5. A disease that is not deadly but has a lot of disabling characteristics that impact a person's quality of life would be said to have
   a. high mortality and low morbidity.
   b. low mortality and low morbidity.
   c. high mortality and high morbidity.
   d. low mortality and high morbidity.

6. If an outbreak of a disease such as Avian flu occurs worldwide, it would be said to be
   a. pandemic.
   b. endemic.
   c. epidemic.
   d. chronic.

ANATOMY AND PHYSIOLOGY CONCEPTS YOU WILL ENCOUNTER ON YOUR JOURNEY

In this section, we take a closer look at some additional concepts related to the study of anatomy and physiology that you will learn more about as you travel through the chapters in this text. Let's begin with one of the most important concepts in maintaining normal health.

Homeostasis

For the body to function normally, it must constantly monitor both its internal and external environment and make the appropriate adjustments. For cells to thrive, they must be maintained in an environment that provides a proper temperature range, balanced oxygen levels, and adequate nutrients. Heart rate and blood pressure must also be monitored and maintained within a certain range, or **set point**, for optimal functioning. **Homeostasis** is the physiological process in which your body monitors and maintains a stable internal environment or equilibrium. Survival depends on the body's ability to maintain homeostasis. *Homeostatic regulation* refers to the adjustments made in the human organism to maintain this stable internal environment. Although the ending *stasis* literally means "standing still," as you will soon see, *homeostasis* is actually a dynamic state of equilibrium.

The thermostat in your house functions like a homeostatic mechanism. A temperature is set and then maintained by a sensor that monitors the internal environmental temperature and either heats the house if the sensor registers too cold or cools the house if the sensor registers too hot. There is a continuous feedback loop from the sensor to the thermostat to determine what action is needed. Because the feedback loop opposes the stimulus (cools down if too hot, heats up if too cold), it is referred to as a **negative feedback loop**.

The body also relies on negative feedback loops that continually sense the internal and external environment and make adjustments to maintain homeostasis (see **FIGURE 1–4** ■). The hypothalamus in the brain represents the body's temperature control. If the hypothalamus senses a very cold environment, it opposes this cold stimulus (negative feedback loop) and

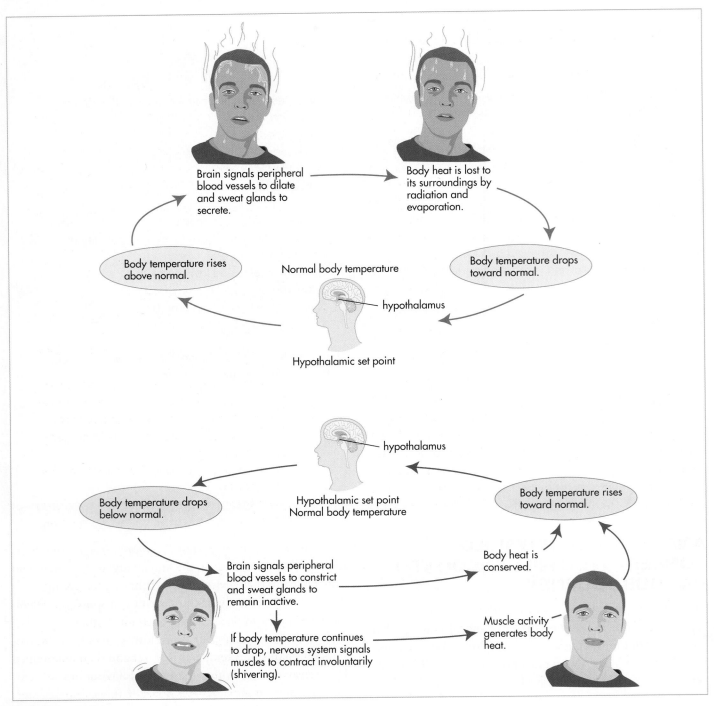

FIGURE 1–4 ◼

The homeostatic control of normal body temperature (37°C or 98.6°F).

performs physiological processes to gain heat within the body to maintain an internal temperature near 98.6°F (37°C). The body begins to shiver, and this increased muscular activity generates heat. In addition, because most heat loss is through peripheral areas (head, arms, and legs), the body decreases the size of the peripheral blood vessels (vasoconstriction), causing the blood to be deeper from the skin surface where the heat would be lost to the cold environment. This keeps the blood closer to the core of the body, where it is warmer. Of course, we can assist the body by wearing a heavy coat and hat, which would remove much of the stress of the cold environment or simply getting out of the cold to a warmer environment.

Conversely, if you are in the desert and the temperature is 120°F, the body senses this as too hot and stimulates physiological processes to cool you down. These processes include sweating (evaporation is a cooling process) and enlarging the peripheral vessels (peripheral vasodilation) to dissipate the body heat into the external environment. In health care practice, if a patient presents with a very high temperature, the person may need to be rapidly cooled with ice packs or baths to reduce his or her temperature toward the normal range. Much of health care practice is just that—assisting the body through therapy and treatments in returning it to homeostasis.

Your body is also capable of **positive feedback**, which increases the magnitude of a change. This process is also known as a *vicious cycle*. Positive feedback is not a way to regulate your body because it increases a change away from the ideal set point. Often, positive feedback is harmful if the vicious cycle cannot be broken, but sometimes positive feedback is necessary for a process to run to completion.

A good example of necessary positive feedback is the continued contraction of the uterus during childbirth. When a baby is ready to be born, a signal, not well understood at this time, tells the hypothalamus to release the hormone oxytocin from the posterior pituitary. Oxytocin increases the intensity of uterine contractions. As the uterus contracts, the pressure inside the uterus caused by the baby moving down the birth canal increases the signal to the hypothalamus. More oxytocin is released, and the uterus contracts harder. Pressure becomes higher inside the uterus, the hypothalamus is signaled to release more oxytocin, and the uterus contracts yet harder. This cycle of ever-increasing uterine contractions due to ever-increasing release of oxytocin from the hypothalamus continues until the pressure inside the uterus decreases—that is, until the baby is born.

Clinical Application

"BREAKING" A FEVER

It is believed that most fevers are the body's way of making an inhospitable environment for a pathogen. Why is it that when someone begins sweating after a prolonged fever (increase in body temperature), the fever is said to be "breaking"? A fever sets the hypothalamus to a higher set point temperature. The body increases metabolism to generate more heat to reach this now higher set temperature (just like when you turn up the thermostat in your house). Once whatever is causing the fever is gone, the temperature set by the hypothalamus is turned back down to the true normal. The body must now rapidly get rid of the excess heat by the cooling process of evaporation through sweating.

Amazing Facts

Bizarre Signs and Symptoms!

Here are some strange signs and symptoms that have been indications of diseases. To keep lawyers from making a ton of money on this text, please note that there are other signs, symptoms, and tests to determine specific diseases. Please do not use this list of oddities as a sole diagnostic tool!

1. Generalized itching skin of unknown origin can be an indication of Hodgkin's disease.
2. Sweating at night may indicate tuberculosis.
3. A desire to eat clay or starchy paste may indicate an iron deficiency in the body.
4. Breath that smells like fruity flavored chewing gum or nail polish remover may be an indication of diabetes.
5. A magenta-colored tongue may be indicative of a riboflavin deficiency.
6. A patient with profound kidney disease often doesn't have moons (lunula) on the fingernails.
7. A "hairy" tongue may mean that a patient's normal mouth flora has died from improper use of antibiotics.
8. Spoon-shaped fingernails may point to an iron deficiency in the body.
9. Brown linear streaks on the fingernails of fair-skinned people may indicate melanoma (skin cancer).
10. Having trouble smelling peanut butter from a distance? Recent studies show difficulty in smelling peanut butter from a foot away can indicate early stages of Alzheimer's disease, Parkinson's disease, or even multiple sclerosis.
11. If you have a stabbing pain in your heel and haven't stepped on a sharp object, you could have a herniated disc. This is because the sciatic nerve runs from your back to your heel.

METABOLISM

If you travel to other countries, you will see many different cultures and customs. Even though each culture is unique, they all share certain similarities. The same can be said for all of us who are unique but share certain functions in order to maintain life. All humans, for example, need food and water to produce complex chemical reactions needed for growth, reproduction, movement, and so on. On the cellular level, all humans require the process of **metabolism** in order to survive. *Metabolism* refers to all the energy and material transformations that occur within living cells.

Metabolism is further subdivided into two opposite processes. **Anabolism** is the process by which simpler compounds are built up and used to manufacture materials for growth, repair, and reproduction, such as the assembly of simple amino acids to form complex proteins. This is the building phase of metabolism. **Catabolism** is the process by which complex substances are broken down into simpler substances. For example, the breakdown of food into simpler chemical building blocks for energy use is a catabolic process. An abnormal and extreme example of catabolism is a starvation victim whose body "feeds upon itself," actually consuming the body's own tissues.

SUMMARY: Points of Interest

- Anatomy is the study of the actual internal and external structures of the body, and physiology is the study of how these structures normally function. Pathology is the study of the disease processes by which abnormal structures and abnormal body functions can occur.

- Medical terminology is the language of medicine and combines word roots, prefixes, and suffixes to construct numerous medical terms to describe conditions, locations, diagnostic tools, and so on.

- The metric system is the mathematical language of medicine based on powers of 10. If you require more practice with this system, please go to your student *Study Success Companion* at the end of this text for a simplified review.

- A change in objective measurable values such as temperature (signs) and subjective patient perceptions (symptoms) can indicate a disease is present. Vital signs are pulse, respirations, temperature, and blood pressure.

- The body tries to maintain a balanced or stable environment called homeostasis. It must constantly monitor the environment and make changes to maintain this balance. It often accomplishes homeostasis through negative feedback loops.

- Metabolism refers to all of the chemical operations going on within the body and can be broken down into two opposite processes. The building phase of metabolism is anabolism, in which simpler compounds are built up and used to manufacture materials for growth, reproduction, and repairs. The tearing down phase is catabolism, in which complex substances are broken down into simpler substances, such as food broken down for energy use.

CASE STUDY

A 45-year-old Hispanic male involved in a vehicular accident is taken to the ICU with SOB and abdominal pain. He has acrocyanosis, tachycardia, and a past medical history of cardiopathy and coronary artery disease (CAD). He weighs 150 pounds and is 5 feet 6 inches tall. His chest x-ray shows an enlarged heart. Blood pressure shows hypertension at 155/95 mmHg. His facial injuries will require future rhinoplastic surgery. An electrocardiogram and lower GI series is ordered.

a. What is his CC(s) and etiology?

_____

_____

b. Where exactly in the hospital was the patient taken?

_____

_____

c. Describe the patient's color, heart rate, and breathing.

_____

_____

d. What is the medical term for what the x-ray showed?

_____

_____

e. What future facial surgery will he need?

_____

_____

Multiple Choice

1. Which of the following is an example of microscopic anatomy?
   a. viewing an x-ray
   b. examining the shape of an organ during an autopsy
   c. classifying a type of bacterial cell
   d. watching how the pupils in the eyes react to light

2. Acromegaly means which of the following?
   a. a large stomach
   b. enlarged extremities
   c. an inflamed stomach lining
   d. a large acrobat

3. The process that prevents movement away from a normal set point is called
   a. positive feedback.
   b. negative feedback.
   c. vicious cycle.
   d. control center.

4. In the medical field, science, engineering, and pharmaceutical industries, volume is measured in
   a. kilograms.
   b. liters.
   c. meters.
   d. gallons.

5. The cause of a disease is referred to as the
   a. prognosis.
   b. diagnosis.
   c. pathology.
   d. etiology.

6. Which of the following is a sign?
   a. nausea
   b. fever
   c. dizziness
   d. fatigue

7. A man reports to the emergency department with nausea and vomiting. He has a fever and his pulse and blood pressure are elevated. After some tests, it is determined that he has a stomach virus. Which of the following is his prognosis?
   a. rest and drink plenty of fluids
   b. a viral infection
   c. you'll be fine in a few days
   d. nausea, vomiting, and fever

8. Which of the following is not a vital sign?
   a. heart rate of 76
   b. blood pressure of 135/70 mmHg
   c. temperature of 97.4 F
   d. vital capacity of 6 liters

Fill in the Blank

1. Ted injured his knee at last night's football game. Today his doctor wants to make a small incision and use a device to "look around the joint" to assess the damage. What is the term for this device? _____

2. _____ is the study of the structures of the body, and _____ is the study of the functions of these structures.

3. Bob has just been told he has hepatomegaly. This means his _____ is _____.

4. Pulse and temperature represent two _____ signs of the body.

5. Jill is badly injured in a car accident. She is bleeding excessively. Her blood pressure is dropping rapidly. Her heart beats faster to try to raise her blood pressure, yet it keeps dropping due to blood loss. This is an example of _____.

Short Answer

1. Explain the difference between diagnosis and prognosis.

   _____
   _____
   _____
   _____

2. Knowing that difficulty swallowing is called dysphagia, what is the function of a phagocyte?

   _____
   _____
   _____
   _____

3. Contrast negative and positive feedback loops.

_____

_____

_____

_____

4. Describe one example of homeostasis in your body.

_____

_____

_____

_____

5. After saving for 10 years for a ski trip to the Alps, Jose experienced a spectacular wipeout on the first run down the mountain. A broken leg is the diagnosis. List his symptoms, prognosis, etiology, and treatment.

_____

_____

_____

_____

6. Contrast the terms endemic, epidemic, and pandemic.

_____

_____

_____

_____

7. Contrast catabolism and anabolism.

_____

_____

_____

_____

Visit our new **MyHealthProfessions Lab** to accompany *Anatomy & Physiology for Health Professions*. Here you'll find a rich collection of quizzes, case studies, and animations for deeper understanding and application.

2

The Human Body

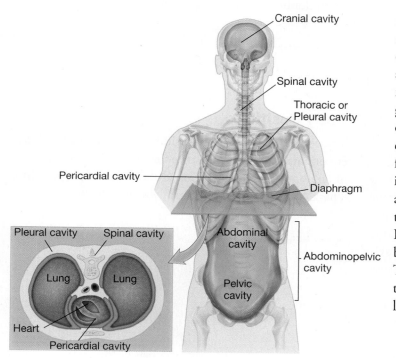

Cranial cavity

Spinal cavity

Thoracic or Pleural cavity

Pericardial cavity

Diaphragm

Pleural cavity   Spinal cavity

Lung   Lung

Heart

Pericardial cavity

Abdominal cavity

Abdominopelvic cavity

Pelvic cavity

Now that we have a basic understanding of the native language and some basic anatomy and physiology concepts, how will we successfully navigate through an unfamiliar city or country? We must, of course, study maps so we can plan our visit and know where we are going. The same effort is required to learn the "terrain" of the human body. This chapter provides the major external map of the human body that serves as a guide for future chapters, which will map the internal regions in detail. Medical directional terms and body locations are the foundations we will need as we journey together through this wondrous creation called the human body. Isn't it ironic that if there is one thing we should know better than anything else, it should be our own bodies? To borrow from an old saying, by the end of our journey through this textbook, you will know your entire body like "the back of your hand."

LEARNING OUTCOMES

At the end of your journey through this chapter, you will be able to:

- List and describe the various body positions.
- Define the body planes and associated directional terms.
- Locate and describe the body cavities and their respective organs.
- List and describe the anatomical divisions of the abdominal region.
- Identify and locate the various body regions.

Pronunciation Guide

Correct pronunciation is important in any journey so that you and others are completely understood. Here is a "see and say" Pronunciation Guide for the more difficult terms to pronounce in this chapter. Please note that even though there are standard pronunciations, regional variations of the pronunciations can occur.

abdominopelvic cavity (ab DOM ih noh PELL vik)
antecubital (an tee CUE bi tal)
buccal (BUCK al)
caudal (KAWD al)
cephalic (seh FAL ik)
coronal plane (koh ROH nal)
cranial (KRAY nee al)
distal (DISS tal)
dorsal (DOR sal)

gluteal (GLOO tee al)
mediastinum (ME dee ah STY num)
midsagittal plane (mid SAJ ih tal)
pleural cavities (PLOO ral)
superficial (SOO per FISH al)
thoracic cavity (tho RASS ik)
transverse (tranz VERS)
Trendelenburg (tren DELL in berg)

THE MAP OF THE HUMAN BODY

When reading a map, you need certain universal directional terms, such as *north, south, east,* and *west,* to help you understand and use the map. A map is often made to represent a specific region so that more details can be included about that particular area, making it easier to explore. Likewise, scientists have created standardized body directional terms and divide the body into distinct regions, sections, and cavities so that we can more clearly and rapidly locate and discuss anatomical features. Having certain anatomical landmarks on the body also provides needed points of reference for surgery, diagnostic procedures, and clinical discussions related to patient care. The spinal column is a major anatomical landmark for many structures in the center of our bodies and the specific vertebrae are often referenced for certain anatomical structure locations. For example, the bifurcation of the lung (where the main airways divide into the left and right lung) occurs at the fifth or sixth thoracic vertebrae on a chest x-ray.

If a patient states, "I have pain in my stomach," does that really tell you a lot of information? Often, patients use the word *stomach* when actually referring to the abdominal region. A more specific localization and description of the pain can help in determining what is wrong with a patient. It is helpful to know the type of pain (dull, sharp, or stabbing) and *exactly* where in that region the pain is located to help determine its cause. For example, pain in the general abdominal region can indicate a variety of problems, including ulcers, heart attack, appendicitis, indigestion, or liver problems. Knowing the exact body region can help a clinician better determine the precise problem.

Body Positions

The body can assume many positions and therefore has different orientations. To standardize the orientation for the study of anatomy, scientists developed the **anatomical position**. The anatomical position, as shown in **FIGURE 2–1** ■, is a

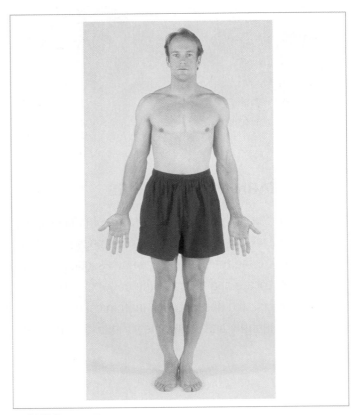

FIGURE 2–1 ■

The anatomical position.

human standing erect, face forward, with feet parallel and arms hanging at the side, with palms facing forward.

Other body positions that are important to discuss because of clinical assessments and treatments in health care are the supine, prone, Trendelenburg, and Fowler's positions. In the **supine position**, the patient is laying face *upward* (think sUPine = face UP). In the **prone position**, the patient is laying face *downward*, on the stomach (think prONe = ON stomach). When a patient is in the **Trendelenburg position**, the head of the bed is lower than the patient's feet. This position is used to help move secretions from various regions of the patient's lungs. Although this is therapeutic, certain precautions must be taken. Because the patient's head is lower than the heart, gravity increases the blood flow to the head, and therefore intracranial pressure increases. This position is contraindicated in patients with recent eye surgery or cerebral injuries or bleeding. In the **Fowler's position**, the patient is sitting in bed with the head of the bed elevated. This position is often used in the hospital to facilitate breathing and for comfort of bedridden patients while eating or talking. See **FIGURE 2–2** ■ for these body positions.

Directional Terms

Superior (**cranial** or **cephalic**) means toward the head or upper body. **Inferior** (**caudal**) means away from the head or toward the lower part of the body. **Anterior** (**ventral**) refers to body parts toward or on the front of the body, and **posterior** (**dorsal**) refers to body parts toward or on the back of the body. Remember, if during your trip you stop at the beach, you will know it is not safe to swim if you see a shark's *dorsal* fin sticking out of the water. **Medial** refers to body parts located near the middle or midline of the body. **Lateral** refers to body parts located away from midline (or on the side).

One more analogy that relates to a map is the concept of a *reference point*. If you were traveling from Colorado to Florida, for example, you would have to travel in a southeasterly direction. Colorado is your starting point and serves as your reference. However, if you were traveling from Florida to Colorado, you would travel in a northwesterly direction because Florida is now your point of reference. Any body part can be either superior or inferior depending on your reference point. For example, the knee is superior to the ankle if the ankle is the reference point. Turning this around, the ankle is inferior to the knee if the knee is the reference point.

Clinical Application

ADDITIONAL BODY POSITIONS

There are other specific positions of the human body used in medicine to facilitate diagnosis and treatment. For example the **lithotomy** position is a common position for surgical procedures and medical examination of the pelvis, lower abdomen, and reproductive organs. In the lithotomy position, patients are placed on their back with feet elevated (usually in stirrups).

This is also the traditional position for childbirth is Western nations.

The **dorsal recumbent** position has the patients lying on their back with their knees flexed and feet flat on the table or bed. This position is used for some surgical procedures and examinations of the vagina and rectum.

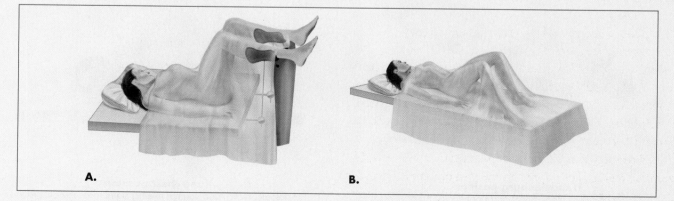

A. Lithotomy and **B.** dorsal recumbent positions.

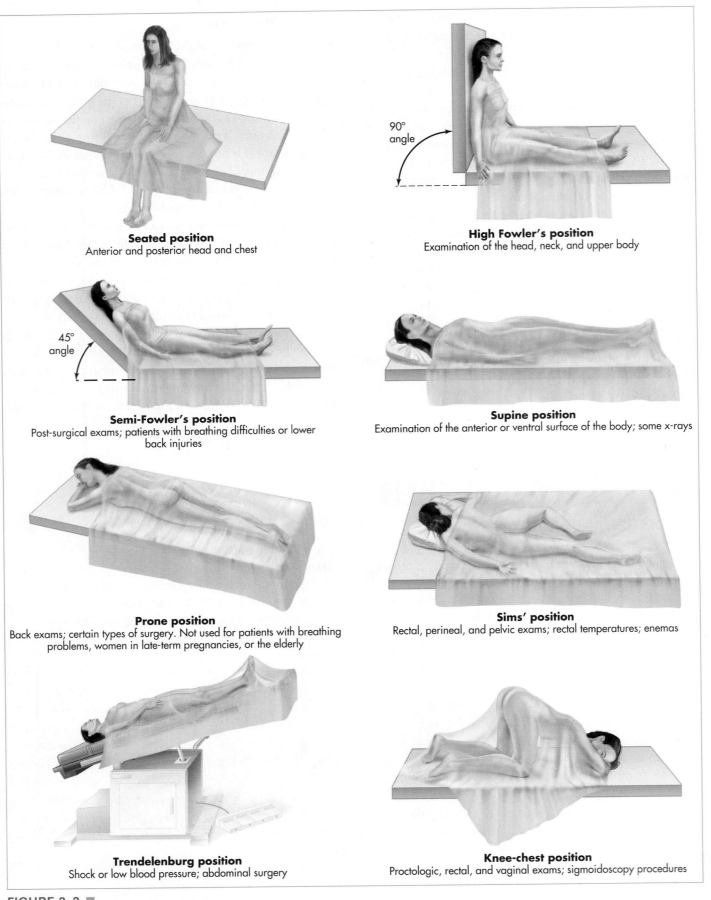

Seated position
Anterior and posterior head and chest

High Fowler's position
Examination of the head, neck, and upper body

90°
angle

Semi-Fowler's position
Post-surgical exams; patients with breathing difficulties or lower back injuries

45°
angle

Supine position
Examination of the anterior or ventral surface of the body; some x-rays

Prone position
Back exams; certain types of surgery. Not used for patients with breathing problems, women in late-term pregnancies, or the elderly

Sims' position
Rectal, perineal, and pelvic exams; rectal temperatures; enemas

Trendelenburg position
Shock or low blood pressure; abdominal surgery

Knee-chest position
Proctologic, rectal, and vaginal exams; sigmoidoscopy procedures

FIGURE 2–2 ■
Common patient positions.

Clinical Application

DO YOU KNOW YOUR LEFT FROM YOUR RIGHT?

By now, it should be clear that we need a precise, standardized language with directional terms to describe anatomy and physiology and apply it in a health care setting. Something as simple as left and right can become critical. For example, suppose you are a surgical technologist and are ordered to tag a patient's right leg to designate it as the leg to be amputated in an upcoming operation. If you approach the patient from the bottom of the bed and place the tag on the leg on YOUR right side, you have erroneously placed it on the patient's left leg, and this could have disastrous results. The take-home message is that left and right *always* refer to the patient's left and right, *not yours*. See **FIGURE 2–3** ■.

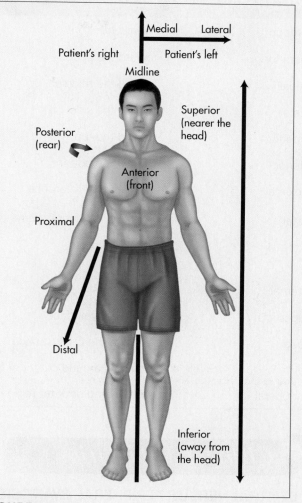

FIGURE 2–3 ■
Body directional terms.

There are other additional important directional terms. **Proximal** refers to body parts closest to a point of reference of the body. This is contrasted by **distal**, which refers to body parts furthest away from a point of reference. For example, using your shoulder as a reference point, your elbow is proximal to your shoulder, whereas your fingers are distal to your shoulder. **External** means on the outside, and **internal** refers to structures on the inside. Did you know that your skin, which is external to your entire body, is actually the body's largest organ? Most other organs are located internally within body cavities.

Superficial means toward or at the body's surface. When a clinician draws blood from you, he or she looks for superficial veins that are easy to see and access with the needle. **Deep** means away from the body's surface. The large veins in your legs are deep veins and are more protected than superficial veins because injury to them can be more critical to survival than injury to a smaller, superficial blood vessel. **Central** refers to locations near the center of the body (torso and head), and **peripheral** refers to the extremities (arms and legs) or the surrounding or outer regions of the body (see **TABLE 2–1** ■).

TABLE 2–1 DIRECTIONAL TERMS

DIRECTIONAL TERM	MEANING	USE IN A SENTENCE
anterior	toward the front	The belly button is on the *anterior* surface of the body.
posterior	toward the back	The patient had a bump on the *posterior* part of her head.
medial	toward the middle	The nose is *medial* to the eyes.
lateral	toward the side	The eyes are *lateral* to the nose.
superior	toward the top	The nose is *superior* to the mouth.
inferior	toward the bottom	The mouth is *inferior* to the nose.
proximal	near point of reference	The Recovery room is *proximal* to the Operating room.
distal	away from point of reference	The fingers are *distal* to the shoulder.
external	on the outside	The *external* defibrillator is used on the outside of the chest.
internal	on the inside	He received *internal* injuries from the accident.
superficial	at the body surface	The cut was only *superficial*.
deep	far from the body surface	The patient had *deep* wounds from the chainsaw.
central	locations around center of body	The patient had *central* chest pain.
peripheral	surrounding or outer regions	The patient had *peripheral* swelling in the feet.

Clinical Application

CENTRAL VERSUS PERIPHERAL CYANOSIS

Cyanosis is a condition of bluish-colored skin that is usually the result of low levels of oxygen in the blood. Peripheral cyanosis presents as bluish fingers and toes and may indicate the need for oxygen therapy, depending on the condition of the patient. Peripheral cyanosis is sometimes difficult to detect in people with dark skin. Central cyanosis is much more serious and presents as bluish discoloration of the torso and inside the mouth. **FIGURE 2–4** ■ illustrates central and peripheral cyanosis.

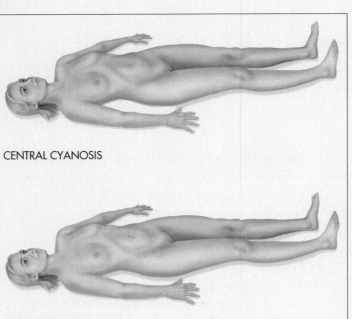

CENTRAL CYANOSIS

PERIPHERAL CYANOSIS

FIGURE 2–4 ■

Contrast of central versus peripheral cyanosis.

TEST YOUR KNOWLEDGE 2–1

Answer the following questions:

1. Try standing in the actual anatomical position.

2. Give the best body position (prone, supine, or Fowler's) for the following circumstances:
   a. getting a back massage _____
   b. eating in a hospital bed _____
   c. watching television in bed _____
   d. watching the stars at night _____

3. Give the opposite directional term:
   a. superior _____
   b. posterior _____
   c. caudal _____
   d. ventral _____
   e. distal _____

   f. external _____
   g. superficial _____
   h. peripheral _____
   i. medial _____

4. A scratch on the surface of the skin is called a(n) _____ wound.

5. The wrist is _____ to the hand and _____ to the elbow.

6. The nose is _____ to the mouth.

7. If your hands and feet are swollen with fluid (edema), you are said to have _____ edema.

8. A blue coloration of the inside of the mouth indicates _____ _____.

FOCUS ON PROFESSIONS

Surgical technologists must have a command of medical directional terms used during surgical procedures. This profession is responsible for setting up sterile fields for operations and assisting the surgeon in various duties during the operation. In addition, members of this profession work outside the operating room in emergency department and ambulatory surgery units. Learn more about this exciting profession by visiting the websites of national surgical technology organizations, such as the Association of Surgical Technologists and the National Board of Surgical Technology and Surgical Assisting.

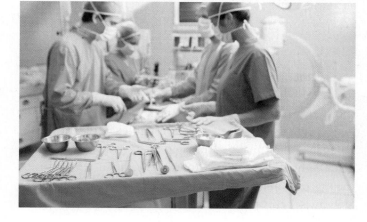

Body Planes

Sometimes it is necessary to divide the body or even an organ or tissue sample into specific sections to further examine it. A *plane* is an imaginary line drawn through the body or organ to separate it into specific sections. For example, in

FIGURE 2–5 ■, we see the **transverse plane** (or **horizontal plane**) dividing the body into superior and inferior sections. This can also be called **cross-sectioning** the body. Cross-sectioning is often done with tissue and organ samples so that internal structures can be examined.

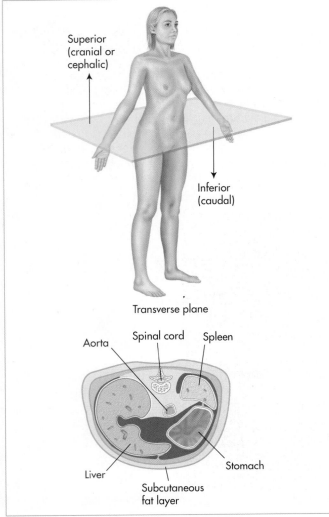

FIGURE 2–5 ■

Transverse plane and a cross-sectional view of the upper abdominal region.

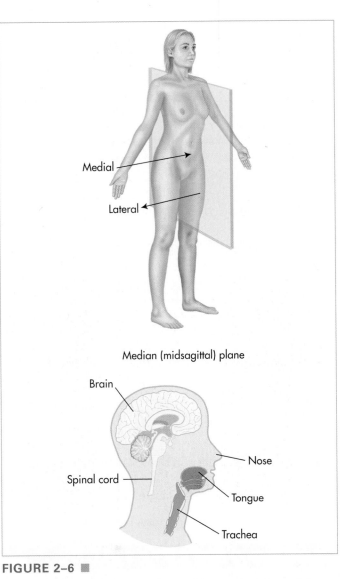

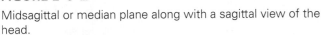

FIGURE 2–6 ■

Midsagittal or median plane along with a sagittal view of the head.

The **median plane**, also called the **midsagittal plane**, divides the body into right and left halves. **FIGURE 2–6** ■ shows this plane and the directional terms associated with it. If a technician were to section and examine an organ, he or she might make a midsagittal cut (cut the organ into equal right and left halves) to examine the internal parts of the organ or might simply make several **sagittal** (vertical or lengthwise) cuts to slice the organ into smaller sections for closer examination. Midsagittal sections are always on the midline. Sagittal sections run parallel to midsagittal sections but aren't always on the midline. Sagittal sections divide a body or organ into left and right portions.

The **frontal plane**, or **coronal plane**, divides the body into anterior (ventral) and posterior (dorsal) sections. **FIGURE 2–7** ■ demonstrates the coronal plane and associated directional terms.

X-Rays, CT Scans, and MRIs

Directional terms and positions are also important in the radiologic sciences. X-rays are a form of high-energy radiation that penetrates the body and gives a two-dimensional view of the bones, air, and tissues in the body. The standard x-ray (much like a photograph) can be enhanced with the use of computers to give much greater detail and contrast and to allow for a more realistic three-dimensional view. For example, if a golf ball–sized tumor in the lung was shown on a standard chest x-ray, you would have no idea of its actual depth because it would look flat, like a quarter. Computed tomography (CT) scanning uses a narrowly focused x-ray beam that circles rapidly around the body.

The computer constructs thin-slice images and combines them to give much greater detail and allow for a more three-dimensional view, much like a loaf of sliced bread gives a better idea of the total shape of the loaf than does a single slice. The CT scan reveals the true depth of the quarter-shaped tumor shown on the regular x-ray. A magnetic resonance imager (MRI) produces even greater detail of tissue structures, even down to individual nerve bundles. The MRI uses the body's natural magnetic properties to produce clear images of any body part. Since it relies on a powerful magnetic field, another advantage of the MRI is no radiation exposure.

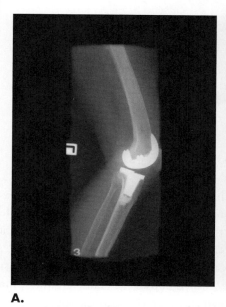

A.

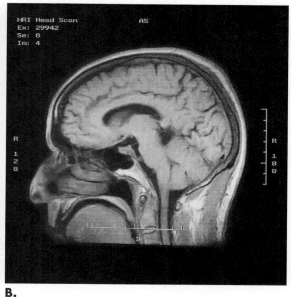

B.

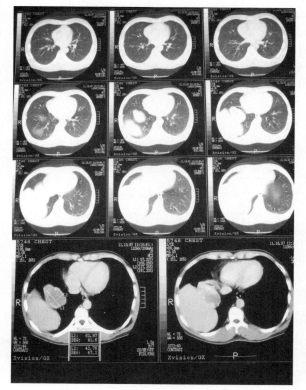

C.

Contrast of an x-ray, CT scan, and MRI. **A**. X-ray showing typical joint changes associated with knee replacement; **B**. MRI of the head; **C**. 3-D CT scan showing cross section of adult chest.

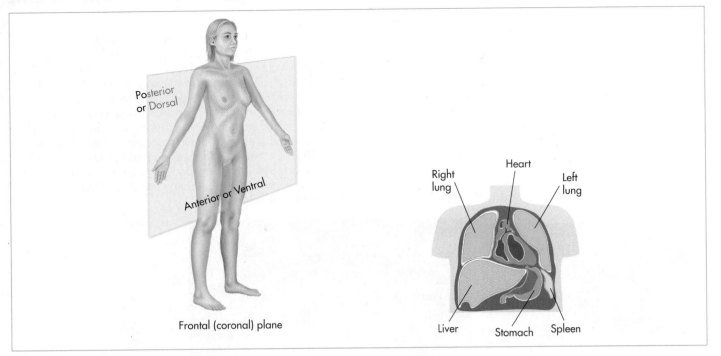

FIGURE 2–7 ■
Frontal or coronal plane along with a coronal view of the chest and stomach.

Body Cavities

The body has two large spaces or cavities that house and protect organs, the dorsal (posterior) cavity and the ventral (anterior) cavity. **FIGURE 2–8** ■ illustrates these cavities. The larger anterior cavity is subdivided into two main cavities called the *thoracic cavity* and the *abdominopelvic cavity*. These cavities are physically separated by a large, dome-shaped muscle called the *diaphragm* that is used for breathing. The **thoracic cavity** contains the heart, lungs, and large blood vessels. The heart has its own small cavity called the *pericardial cavity*. The **abdominopelvic cavity** contains the digestive organs, such as the stomach, intestines, liver, gallbladder, pancreas, and spleen in the superior or abdominal portion. The inferior portion, called the *pelvic cavity*, contains the urinary and reproductive organs and the last part of the large intestine. A *posterior cavity* is located in the back of the body and consists of the **cranial cavity**, which houses the brain, and the **spinal cavity** (**vertebral cavity**), which contains the spinal cord.

There are also smaller body cavities that are further explored in upcoming chapters. For example, the **nasal cavity** is the space behind the nose, the **oral cavity** (or **buccal cavity**) is the space within the mouth, and the **orbital cavity** houses the eyes.

TEST YOUR KNOWLEDGE 2–2

Answer the following questions:

1. The plane that divides the body into superior and inferior regions is called the _____ plane.

2. The frontal plane divides the body into _____ and _____ sections.

3. Cutting an organ into two equal halves (right and left) requires a(n) _____ incision.

4. Identify the major body cavity in which the following organs are located.
   a. heart _____
   b. spinal cord _____
   c. stomach _____
   d. lungs _____
   e. reproductive organs _____
   f. brain _____

5. The dorsal body cavities house organs from this system _____

6. The MRI creates imaging utilizing the body's natural _____ properties.

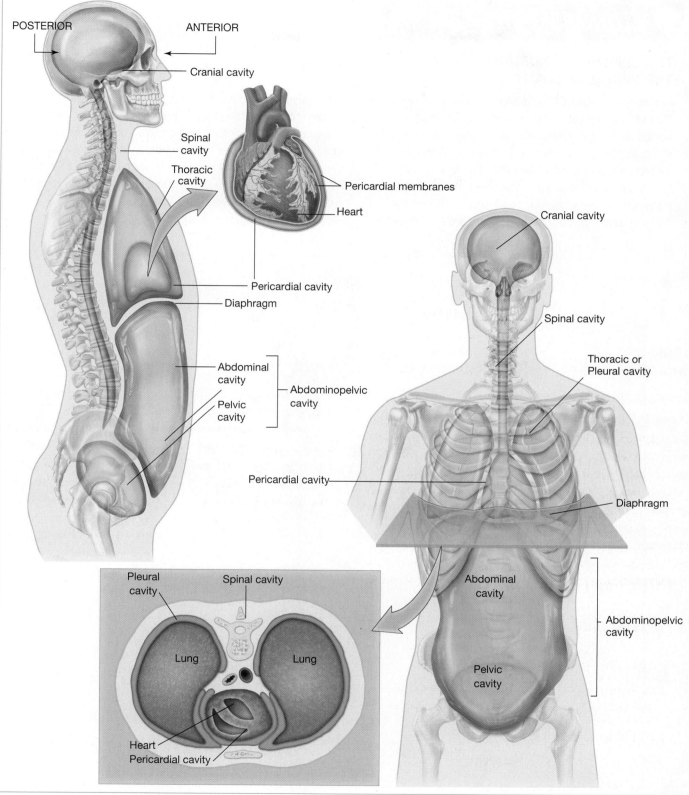

POSTERIOR ANTERIOR

Cranial cavity

Spinal cavity

Thoracic cavity

Pericardial membranes

Heart

Pericardial cavity

Diaphragm

Abdominal cavity

Pelvic cavity

Abdominopelvic cavity

Cranial cavity

Spinal cavity

Thoracic or Pleural cavity

Pericardial cavity

Diaphragm

Abdominal cavity

Abdominopelvic cavity

Pelvic cavity

Pleural cavity

Spinal cavity

Lung

Lung

Heart

Pericardial cavity

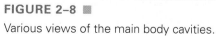

FIGURE 2–8 ◼

Various views of the main body cavities.

THE CENTRAL LANDMARK:
THE SPINAL COLUMN

The spinal or vertebral column is a major, centrally located anatomical landmark and has 5 sets of vertebrae (spinal bones) named for their location in the body (see **FIGURE 2–9** ■). The 7 cervical (C) vertebrae are located in the neck; the 12 thoracic (T) vertebrae are located in the chest; the 5 lumbar (L) vertebrae are located in the lower back; and the 5 fused sacral (S) vertebrae (sacrum) are connected to the pelvis and are located near the final coccygeal vertebra (coccyx or tailbone). The vertebral column can be used as a landmark to locate other structures. For example, the T5 vertebra is used to help locate on a chest x-ray the area where the right and left lungs begin to branch. You'll learn even more about the spinal column and cord in Chapter 6, "The Skeletal System," and Chapters 9 and 10, "The Nervous System" (Parts I and II).

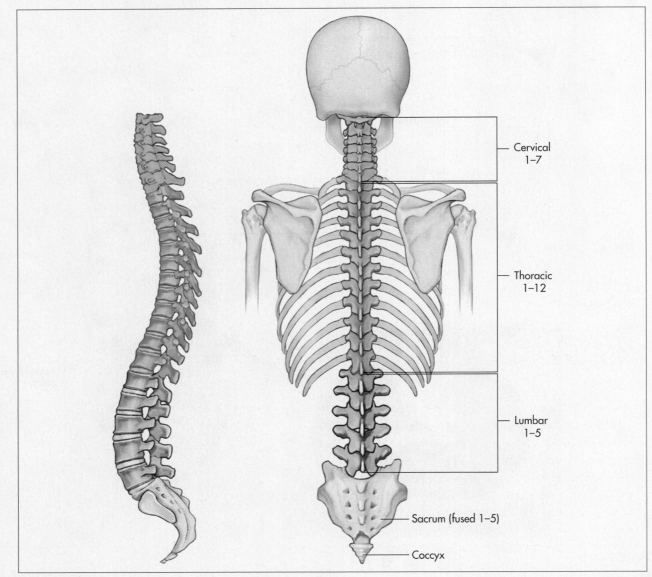

Cervical
1–7

Thoracic
1–12

Lumbar
1–5

Sacrum (fused 1–5)

Coccyx

FIGURE 2–9 ■

The spinal column.

Body Regions

The abdominal region houses a number of organs. Anatomists have divided the abdomen into nine regions (see **FIGURE 2–10** ■). Notice that understanding directional terms assists in locating the regions. For example, the **epigastric** **region** (epi, above; gastric, stomach) is located superior to the umbilical region. The right and left **hypochondriac** (hypo, below; chondro, cartilage—refers to ribcage) regions are located on either side of the epigastric region and contain the lower ribs. The centrally located **umbilical region** houses

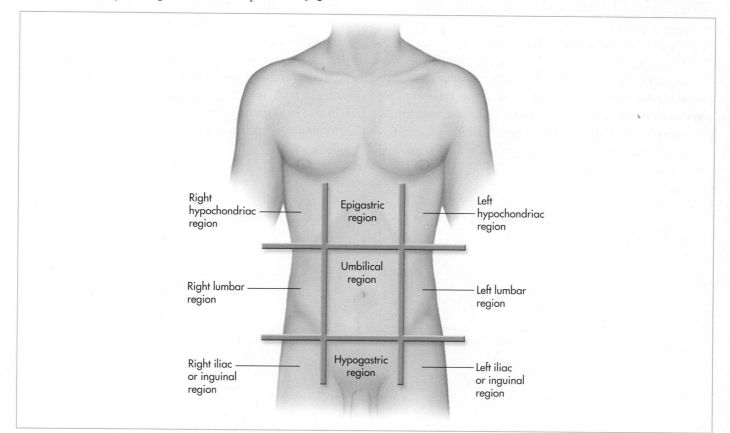

FIGURE 2–10 ■

The nine divisions of the abdominal region.

Clinical Application

HERNIAS

You may have heard of an umbilical (belly button) bulge, or an inguinal hernia, and now you know exactly where such hernias are located. Just what is a hernia? A *hernia* is a tear in the muscle wall that allows a structure (usually an organ) to protrude through it. Sometimes this can be a minor nuisance, but a hernia can also be very dangerous if the blood flow to the portion of the organ that is protruding is restricted. Restricted blood flow can lead to death of the tissue and to serious consequences. Death of tissue is called **necrosis**. **FIGURE 2–11** ■ shows an inguinal hernia with protrusion of the intestines.

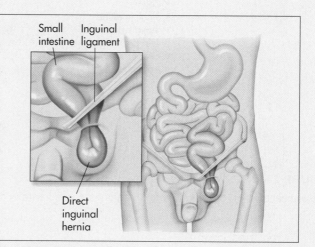

FIGURE 2–11 ■

An inguinal hernia.

the naval or belly button. You don't remember your umbilical cord being cut as a newborn, but your belly button is a reminder that you once had one. Lateral to this region are the right and left lumbar regions at the level of the **lumbar** vertebrae. The **hypogastric region** lies inferior to the umbilical region and is flanked by the right and left **iliac region**, or **inguinal region**. The inguinal region is where the thigh meets the trunk and is also called the *groin region*.

A more practical way for health professionals to compartmentalize the abdominal region is to separate it into anatomical quadrants. **FIGURE 2–12** ■ illustrates these quadrants, which are helpful in describing the location of abdominal pain. Knowing the organs located in the quadrant where the pain occurs can provide a clue to what type of problem the patient has. For example, tenderness in the right lower quadrant (RLQ) can be a symptom of appendicitis because that is where the appendix is located. Pain in the right upper quadrant (RUQ) may mean a liver or gallbladder problem.

Some additional body regions further aid in locating areas and structures. For example, what if you were asked to obtain an axillary temperature on an infant? Just where is the brachial or femoral pulse? What part of the body does carpal tunnel syndrome affect? See **FIGURE 2–13** ■ for other common body regions and parts that are discussed in later chapters. In addition, refer to **TABLE 2–2** ■ for further practical examples of the medical importance of the various body regions.

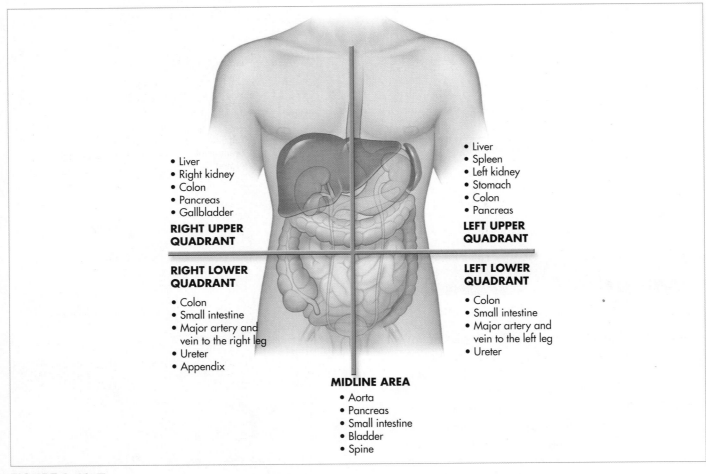

FIGURE 2–12 ■

The clinical division of the abdominal region into quadrants with related organs and structures.

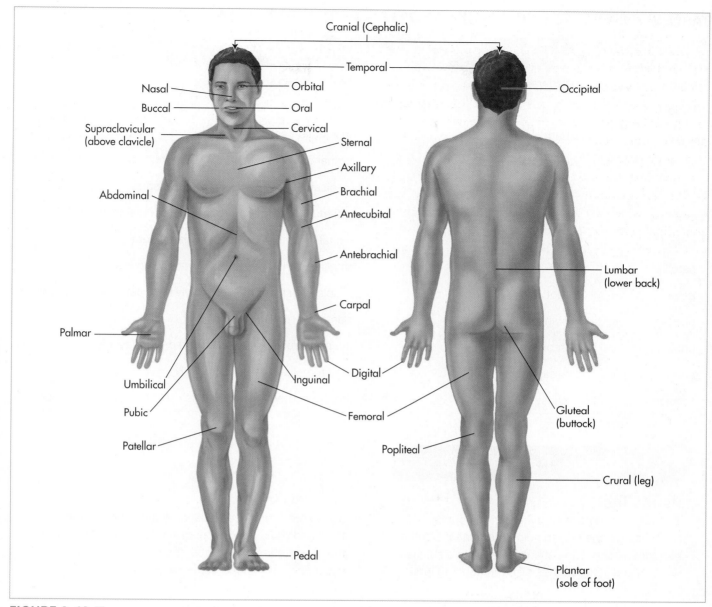

FIGURE 2–13 ■

Anterior and posterior body regions.

TABLE 2–2 EXAMPLES OF BODY REGIONS AND THEIR LOCATIONS

BODY REGION	LOCATION	MEDICAL EXAMPLE
antebrachial	forearm	between the wrist and elbow
antecubital	depressed area in front of elbow	area used to draw blood or start an IV
axillary	armpit	can be used to take temperature
brachial	upper arm	area where blood pressure is taken
buccal	cheek	checked for central cyanosis
carpal	wrist	carpal tunnel syndrome
cervical	neck	cervical collar needed for neck injuries

(continued)

TABLE 2–2 EXAMPLES OF BODY REGIONS AND THEIR LOCATIONS (*continued*)

BODY REGION	LOCATION	MEDICAL EXAMPLE
digital	fingers	digital oxygen sensors
femoral	thigh	femoral pulse checked for effective CPR
gluteal	buttocks	an injection site
lumbar	lower back	lumbar pain often occurs on long car trips
nasal	nose	medications can be given by nasal spray
oral	mouth	oral route is most common route for medications
orbital	eye area	orbital injury can cause damage to sight
patellar	knee	patellar injuries are very common in sports
pedal	foot	people with heart problems may have pedal edema (swelling)
plantar	sole of foot	plantar warts can be painful
pubic	genital region	the pubic region is often checked for body lice
sternal	breastbone area	the sternal area is used for CPR
thoracic	chest	the thoracic area is used to listen to heart and lung sounds

Amazing Facts

Psoas Test
This test—with its strange name, pronounced (SOH as)—is one way to help determine if a patient has appendicitis. The patient is placed in a supine position and instructed to raise the right leg while the practitioner places a hand on the patient's right thigh and gives a slight opposing downward force. If the patient has appendicitis, the patient will usually experience pain in the right lower quadrant.

TEST YOUR KNOWLEDGE 2–3

Fill in the blank with the appropriate medical term for the body region. These can have more than one answer.

1. People who chew smokeless tobacco or snuff are more susceptible to _____ cancer.

2. Antiperspirant sprays are usually used in the _____ region.

3. Belly button rings are usually found in the _____ region.

4. If you sit too long at your desk, you can develop _____ pain.

5. During physicals, your reflexes are checked with a little rubber hammer that taps your _____ region.

6. A patient presents with left upper quadrant pain after a car accident. This type of pain may indicate injury to the _____, a well-vascularized organ in the abdominal cavity.

7. The location point for CPR compressions is the mid _____ region.

- The body can assume many different positions. To standardize the study of anatomy, scientists often reference the anatomical position. Other positions—such as the prone, supine, Trendelenburg, lithotomy, dorsal recumbent, and Fowler's positions—are used in health care for assessments and treatments.

- The body can be divided by the use of planes into different sections, including the transverse, midsagittal, and frontal planes.

- Directional terms—such as anterior and posterior, superior and inferior, and internal and external—help us navigate the body. It is important to always remember that directions such as right and left are referenced from the *patient's* perspective and NOT yours.

- The body has several cavities that house anatomical structures (mainly organs) and specific regions that are all important to know so that health care professionals can communicate in specific terms that leave no room for confusion.

C A S E   S T U D Y

A 65-year-old female patient presents with sternal pain radiating to the left brachial area. Peripheral cyanosis is noted in the digital areas, and she exhibits pedal edema. No epigastric pain is noted. Hypertension and tachycardia are noted with slight accessory muscle use for respirations. She reports that she became dizzy and fell, bruising the right orbital region, and she received superficial cuts to the right patellar region. The physician orders an IV to be started in the left antecubital space. Please answer the following questions in common lay terms.

a. Where would you suggest placing a bandage?

_____

b. Where did her pain begin?

_____

c. Where does the pain move?

_____

d. Does she have stomach pain?

_____

e. Where will the IV be started?

_____

f. What part of her body is swollen?

_____

R E V I E W   Q U E S T I O N S

Multiple Choice

1. A massage therapist would ask you to assume which position for a back massage?
   a. prone
   b. supine
   c. Fowler's
   d. lotus

2. Which of the following is *not* in the abdominopelvic cavity?
   a. stomach
   b. liver
   c. reproductive organs
   d. heart

3. Carpal tunnel syndrome occurs in what region of the body?
   a. head
   b. cheek
   c. armpit
   d. wrist

4. The midsagittal plane divides the body into
   a. superior and inferior.
   b. anterior and posterior.
   c. cranial and caudal.
   d. left and right.

5. An organ contained in the RLQ would be:
   a. appendix.
   b. heart.
   c. lungs.
   d. brain.

6. A motorcyclist collides with a car and is bleeding profusely from a deep cut on the thigh. What artery is most likely damaged?
   a. radial
   b. brachial
   c. patellar
   d. femoral

Fill in the Blank

1. A standard position in which a human stands erect, with face forward, feet parallel, arms at sides, and palms forward is called the _____ position.

2. The _____ position is laying face upward and on your back.

3. The mouth is located _____ to the nose, whereas the nose is located _____ to the mouth.

4. The organ found in the cranial cavity is the _____.

5. _____ indicates blueness of the extremities and therefore affects the peripheral areas of the body.

6. A coroner needs to examine the third ventricle, a structure located on the midline of the brain. A(n) _____ section would be most useful.

Short Answer

1. List the organs found in the abdominal cavity.

   _____

   _____

2. Compare and contrast the prone, supine, Trendelenberg, Sims, and Fowler's positions.

   _____

   _____

   _____

   _____

   _____

   _____

3. List and describe the location of the nine abdominal regions using directional terms.

   _____

   _____

   _____

   _____

   _____

Visit our new **MyHealthProfessions** Lab to accompany *Anatomy & Physiology for Health Professions*. Here you'll find a rich collection of quizzes, case studies, and animations for deeper understanding and application.

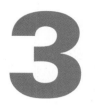

3

Biochemistry

THE BASIC INGREDIENTS OF LIFE

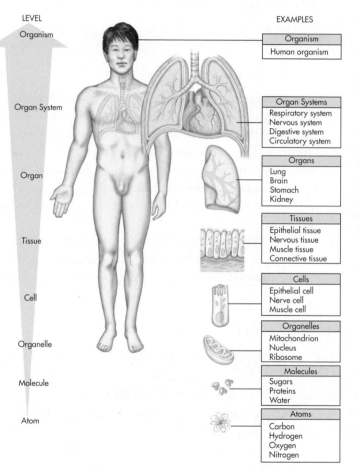

No journey would be complete without day trips to places off the beaten path that busy tourists often miss. In this chapter, we will take a day trip to chemistry. Why would we want to visit chemistry? Chemistry is the study of atoms and molecules and their interactions. Physiology, the study of how the body works, is largely about the interactions between molecules in our cells and tissues. Physiology, then, is mainly about chemistry, or, more specifically, how chemistry relates to a living organism. This special division of chemistry is known as biochemistry. To understand how the body works and to lay a foundation for the upcoming cell chapter, Chapter 4, you need at least a basic understanding of biochemistry.

LEARNING OUTCOMES

At the end of your journey through this chapter, you will be able to:

- Differentiate between atoms, elements, and ions.
- Define acids, bases, and pH and their roles in the body.
- Describe molecular bonding.
- Discuss the biological importance of water.
- Describe the properties of a solution.
- Distinguish among the types of biological molecules.
- Explain metabolism.
- Explain the role of enzymes in physiology.
- Explain cellular respiration.

Pronunciation Guide Pro·nun·ci·a·tion

Correct pronunciation is important in any journey so that you and others are completely understood. Here is a "see and say" Pronunciation Guide for the more difficult terms to pronounce in this chapter. Please note that even though there are standard pronunciations, regional variations of the pronunciations can occur.

adenosine triphosphate (uh DEN o seen)
amino (ah MEAN o)
anabolism (ah NAB oh lizm)
catabolism (ka TAB oh lizm)
covalent (coh VAY lent)
disaccharide (die SACK eh ride)
glycerol (GLIS er ol)

glycogen (GLIE koh jen)
metabolism (meh TAB oh lizm)
monosaccharide (mon oh SACK eh ride)
organelles (OR guh NELLZ)
phospholipid (FOS foh LIP id)
triphosphates (try FOSS fates)

BIOCHEMISTRY
Atoms, Elements, and Ions

All matter—whether living, such as our bodies, or nonliving, such as this textbook—is made of elements. An **element** is the smallest unit that retains the unique chemical properties of that specific type of matter. Elements cannot be broken into smaller pieces by routine chemical techniques. Elements are usually abbreviated using the letters of their chemical names. For example, the element sodium (Latin name *natrium*) is abbreviated Na, whereas the element chlorine is abbreviated Cl. **Atoms** are the smallest particles of elements

that still maintain all the characteristics of that element. Two or more atoms joined together form a **molecule**. Molecules with more than one type of element are known as *compounds*. Using our previous examples, the compound you know as table salt contains the elements of sodium and chloride, better known as sodium chloride, and is abbreviated NaCl. **TABLE 3–1** ■ shows some important trace elements found in the body.

Recall that the atom is the smallest recognizable unit of an element (see **FIGURE 3–1** ■). Atoms consist of a nucleus, containing **protons** (positively charged particles) and **neutrons**

TABLE 3–1 SOME IMPORTANT TRACE ELEMENTS IN THE BODY

ELEMENT	ADULT DAILY REQUIREMENT	MAJOR ACTIVITIES WITHIN THE BODY	DEFICIENCY SYMPTOMS	MAIN DIETARY SOURCES
Iron (Fe)	10 mg (males) 18 mg (females)	Formation of hemoglobin for oxygen delivery; enzymes	Dry skin, spoon-shaped nails; decreased hemoglobin count; anemia	Liver and other organ meats, oysters, red or dark meat, green leafy vegetables, fortified breads and cereals, egg yolk
Copper (Cu)	2.0–5.0 mg	Necessary in many enzyme systems; aids formation of red blood cells and collagen	Deficiency is uncommon; anemia; decreased white cell count; bone demineralization	Nuts, organ meats, whole grains, shellfish, eggs, poultry, green leafy vegetables
Zinc (Zn)	15 mg	Immune system health, amino acid metabolism; cellular growth; maintain enzyme systems; energy production; collagen	Retarded growth and bone formation; dwarfism; skin inflammation; impaired taste; poor healing	Oysters, crab, lamb, beef, organ meats, whole grains

ELEMENT	ADULT DAILY REQUIREMENT	MAJOR ACTIVITIES WITHIN THE BODY	DEFICIENCY SYMPTOMS	MAIN DIETARY SOURCES
Manganese (Mn)	2.5–5.0 mg	Necessary for some enzyme systems; collagen formation; central nervous system function; fat and carbohydrate metabolism; blood clotting	Abnormal skeletal growth; impairment of central nervous system	Whole grains, wheat germ, legumes, pineapple, figs
Iodine (I)	150 mcg	Necessary for activity of thyroid gland	Hypothyroidism; goiter; congenital hypothyroidism	Seafood, iodized salt
Fluorine (F)	1.5–4.0 mg	Necessary for solid tooth formation and retention of calcium in bones with aging	Dental cavities	Tea, fish, water in some areas, supplementary drops, toothpaste

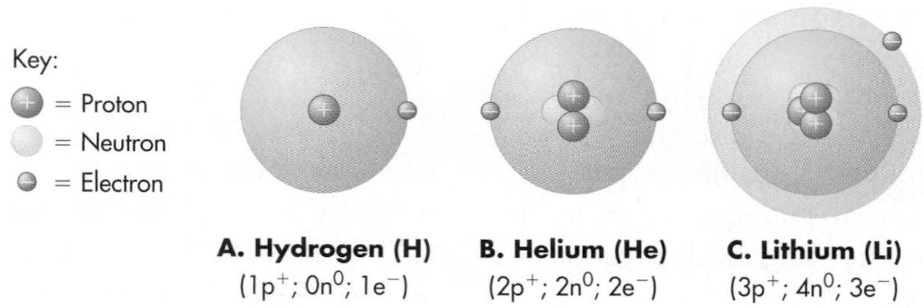

Key:
+ = Proton
 = Neutron
 = Electron

A. Hydrogen (H)
($1p^+$; $0n^0$; $1e^-$)

B. Helium (He)
($2p^+$; $2n^0$; $2e^-$)

C. Lithium (Li)
($3p^+$; $4n^0$; $3e^-$)

FIGURE 3–1 ■
The atom.

(neutral particles). The nucleus is surrounded by **electrons** (negatively charged particles). In the periodic table, all the known elements are arranged based on the number of protons in their nucleus (see **FIGURE 3–2 ■**).

In a typical atom, the number of positively charged protons (+) equals the number of negatively charged electrons (–). This balance of electrons and protons results in an atom with a neutral charge. However, under certain conditions, atoms can gain or lose electrons. These atoms are called **ions** and have either a positive or negative charge. Atoms that have lost an electron will be positively charged, whereas atoms that have gained an electron will be negatively charged. Again, we can use sodium and chlorine as examples. When NaCl (salt) is formed, it is neutral and therefore has no charge. However, if the elements are separated (ionization), sodium loses an electron, becoming Na^+, sodium ion, whereas chlorine gains an electron, thus becoming Cl^-, chloride ion. See **FIGURE 3–3 ■**. Depending on their charge, ions can repel or attract. The positively charged atom is attracted to the

negatively charged one. Conversely, negative charges repel negative charges and positive repel positive. Just remember, opposite charges attract and like charges repel.

The reason why this is important is that **electrolytes** are charged ions found within the body, and they influence the nervous system, muscle activity, and fluid balance. Important electrolytes include sodium (Na^+), potassium (K^+), calcium (Ca^{2+}), magnesium (Mg^{2+}), chloride (Cl^-), hydrogen phosphate (HPO_4^-), and bicarbonate (HCO_3^-). One of the main functions of the urinary system is to regulate electrolyte balance

LEARNING HINT

Negative Electrons

Electrons have a negative charge, so adding one makes an atom more negative$^{(-)}$. The minus sign is not an indication that the atom is smaller, but that is has gained an electron and, therefore, a negative charge.

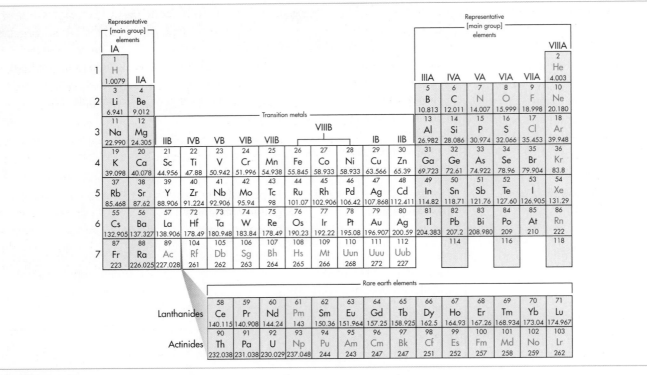

FIGURE 3–2 ■

The Periodic Table of Elements.

to maintain cardiovascular health. For example, if potassium levels get too low or too high due to improper urinary regulation, the heart rhythm can become dangerously irregular.

Acids and Bases

Acids and bases are also electrolytes because they can conduct electricity and break down (dissociate) in water. You are probably familiar with the term *acid* and know that it can be quite harmful to other substances. Acids can dissolve metals and literally burn a hole through material (don't try this at home!). The definition of an *acid* is a chemical substance that can release hydrogen ions. Acids dissolved in water release hydrogen ions that can easily react with other atoms. For example, the chemical formula for hydrochloric acid, which

is found in the stomach, is HCl, meaning one hydrogen atom combined with one chloride atom. If we break the compound HCl apart (dissociation), the released hydrogen atom can react with other atoms and potentially harm the body. This is why acids are called *hydrogen donors*—they donate hydrogen ions to the solution. Acids, such as lemon juice, taste sour.

Bases, which have a bitter taste, can accept hydrogen ions; for example, bicarbonate (HCO_3^-) can accept hydrogen ions, forming carbonic acid (H_2CO_3), which is a weak acid. Hydroxides (OH^-) are common bases, which accept hydrogen ions.

The concentration or amount of hydrogen and hydroxides are measured using the pH (potential of hydrogen) scale. The pH scale ranges from 0 to 14, where a value between 0 and 6.9 means there are more hydrogen ions (H^+) compared

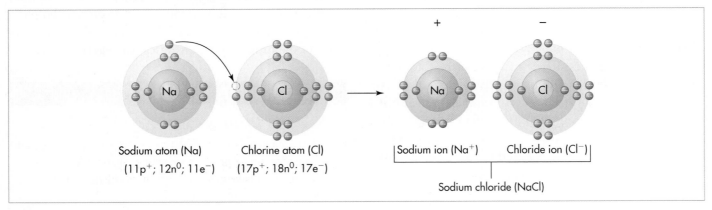

Sodium atom (Na)
($11p^+$; $12n^0$; $11e^-$)

Chlorine atom (Cl)
($17p^+$; $18n^0$; $17e^-$)

Sodium ion (Na^+)

Chloride ion (Cl^-)

Sodium chloride (NaCl)

FIGURE 3–3 ■

Formation of sodium chloride ions.

to hydroxide or hydroxyl ions (OH⁻), so the solution is said to be *acidic*. Neutral pH, in which there are the same number of hydrogen and hydroxyl ions, is 7. A pH greater than 7 indicates that there are more hydroxyl ions, and therefore it is said to be more basic, or *alkaline*. To give some examples, the pH of blood is between 7.35 and 7.45, bleach has a pH of 9.5, and grapefruit juice has a pH of 3. Since our bodies can be exposed to potentially harmful substances, we must have systems to protect the body as much as possible from changes in pH. **FIGURE 3–4** ■ shows the pH scale and where common substances rank on that scale.

The systems that help regulate the acid/base balance include the respiratory and renal systems. The role of the respiratory system (discussed in more detail in Chapter 14) is to take in air and get rid of carbon dioxide (CO_2). Carbon dioxide is a weak acid. If we do not move adequate amounts of air or even stop breathing, there is a buildup of CO_2 in the body, and this buildup of acid is detected in the brain, which gives a person an overwhelming desire to breathe. This is the simplest way of getting rid of excess acid, but if there is a problem with the respiratory system, the kidneys come to the rescue and enable the elimination of excess acid in the urine.

Molecular Bonding

Elements can be joined together to form molecules. The individual elements in molecules are held together by bonds between electrons in the atoms. If one atom *donates* electrons to the other atom, an **ionic bond** results (review Figure 3–3). Because one atom has lost electrons and the other has gained them, the atoms involved in an ionic bond are ions and carry a positive or negative charge. Using our previous example, the bond between sodium and chlorine in table salt (NaCl) is an ionic bond, and if NaCl were to dissociate (break apart), it would form Na⁺ ions and Cl⁻ ions, respectively.

If the electrons are *shared* by the atoms involved in the bond, a **covalent bond** results (see **FIGURE 3–5** ■). Covalent bonds may sometimes be unequal because one atom takes more than its share of the shared electrons. This type of covalent bond, a **polar covalent bond**, results in weak charges on the elements in the molecule. Polar covalent bonds are more polar (slight charge) than covalent bonds, but less polar than ionic bonds. For a summary of bonds and their properties, see **TABLE 3–2** ■.

Amazing Facts

An Interesting Paradox

It is interesting to note that hydrogen (H_2), a highly flammable gas, and oxygen (O_2), a gas that supports combustion, can combine to form H_2O (water) that can be used to extinguish fires.

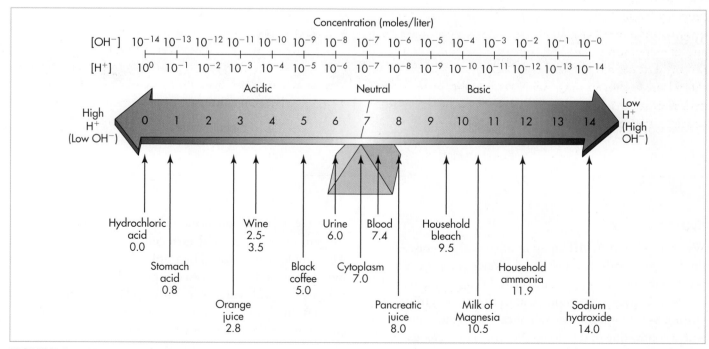

FIGURE 3–4 ■

The pH of common substances.

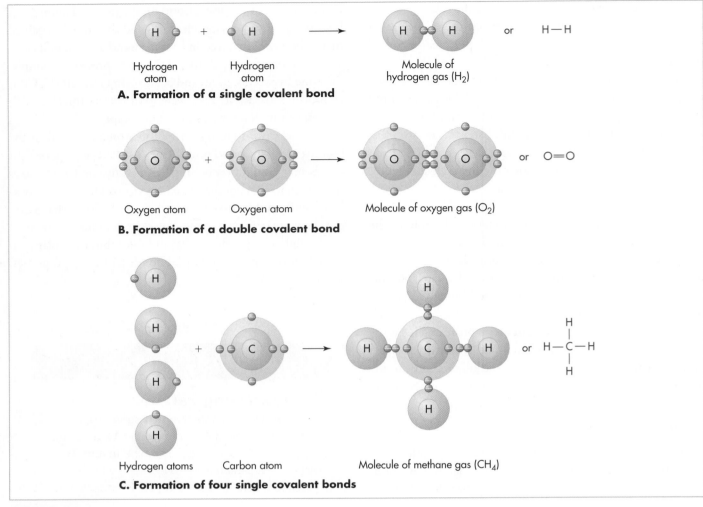

FIGURE 3–5 ■
Covalent Bonding.

TABLE 3–2 SUMMARY OF BONDS AND THEIR PROPERTIES

TYPE OF BOND	ELECTRONS SHARED?	CHARGE?	EXAMPLE
Ionic	No, electrons donated	Yes, ions formed	NaCl (salt)
Polar Covalent	Unequal sharing	Yes, molecule polar	H_2O (water)
Covalent	Equal sharing	No	CH_4 (methane)

Water

Water (H_2O) is the chief liquid in biological systems. All the fluid in your body is water based. Water is a polar solvent because the bonds between the H and O in water are polar covalent. Oxygen takes more than its share of electrons. (See **FIGURE 3–6** ■ for a comparison of carbon dioxide and water with a contrasting of the various bonds.) Thus, charged molecules will be attracted to one end or the other of a water molecule. Charged molecules containing elements such as oxygen, phosphorus, and nitrogen mix easily with water. These molecules are called **hydrophilic** (water loving). Other molecules that do not carry a charge, such as fats and oils, do not mix well with water. They are called **hydrophobic** (water fearing). In Chapter 4, we'll see how important hydrophobic and hydrophilic molecules are in regulating movement of substances across cell membranes.

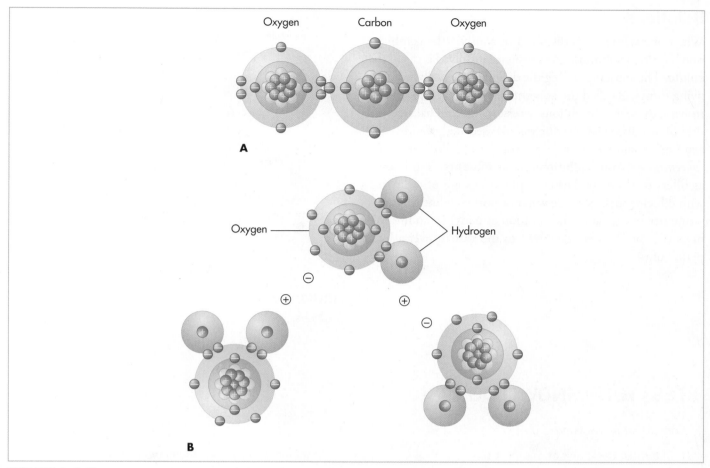

FIGURE 3–6 ■

A. Carbon dioxide. This molecule exhibits a nonpolar bond and results in a linear and symmetrical molecule. **B**. Attraction between water molecules showing polar covalent bonding.

In addition, the polarity of water causes the development of **hydrogen bonds** between water molecules. The hydrogen on one water molecule binds weakly to the oxygen on another water molecule. The bonds between the water molecules increases water's heat capacity. Water can *store* heat, meaning water heats up and cools down more slowly than air.

Water truly is an amazing molecule. The cells in our bodies are composed of 60 to 80 percent water. Water serves several purposes, including acting as a medium or solvent for other reactions to occur, helping transport material, absorbing and releasing heat (sweat) from the body to maintain core temperature, and functioning as a body lubricant.

Clinical Application

THE IMPORTANCE OF HYDRATION

Water is critical for your health, as you can surmise from all its biological functions. Proper hydration is critical for healthy skin, temperature regulation, heart function, and blood pressure to name a few vital processes. You can live for weeks or even months without food, but you would last only a few days without water.

Dehydration is defined as fluid loss of greater than 1 percent of body weight. Water is first lost from the blood and then from the body cells. A 10 to 12 percent loss of body weight due to dehydration can be fatal. This is why monitoring fluid intake and output (I's and O's) is a critical function in treating patients.

Solutions

When one substance is dissolved in another, the combination is called a **solution**. The substance dissolved is called the **solute**. The substance doing the dissolving, usually water in living things, is called the **solvent** (see FIGURE 3–7 ■). Electrolytes, those important ions necessary for fluid balance, are the solutes dissolved in your water-based body fluids. The amount of solute dissolved in a solvent is called the solute *concentration*. Some solutions act as **diluents**, also known as fillers or thinners. For example, drugs are often mixed with diluents such as sterile water or normal saline solutions (same percentage salt concentration as body) in an intravenous (IV) bottle to be delivered to the patient over a long period of time.

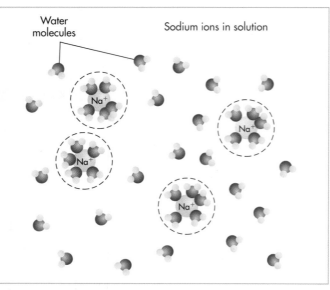

FIGURE 3–7 ■
Solutions.

TEST YOUR KNOWLEDGE 3–1

Complete the following:

1. The most basic unit of matter is the _____.

2. Atoms that can gain or lose electrons are called _____.

3. Physiologically important ions are known as _____.

4. A solution is a _____ dissolved in a _____.

5. An increase in hydrogen ions would lead to a more _____ solution and the pH would _____.

6. Solutions that act as fillers are known as _____.

7. Dehydration is fluid loss of greater than _____% of body weight.

Biological Molecules

Most of your anatomy (bones, muscles, skin, hair, etc.) is made of molecules called *biological molecules*. Biological molecules are molecules found in living systems that contain mainly the elements carbon (C) and hydrogen (H), with lesser amounts of oxygen (O), nitrogen (N), sulfur (S), phosphorous (P), and other elements. These molecules fall into four broad categories: carbohydrates, lipids, proteins, and nucleic acids.

Carbohydrates

Carbohydrates are sugars and starches. They are used as energy sources and as structural molecules. The name *carbohydrate* literally means "watered carbon." Carbohydrate molecules all have carbon, hydrogen, and oxygen in the ratio of 1 carbon to 2 hydrogens to 1 oxygen (CH_2O; see FIGURE 3–8 ■). **Monosaccharides**, or simple sugars, have 5 or 6 carbons. Glucose ($C_6H_{12}O_6$), your body's chief fuel, is a monosaccharide. If two monosaccharides are linked together, a **disaccharide** is formed. Sucrose, table sugar, consists of a glucose molecule and a fructose molecule linked together. **Polysaccharides** are made when many monosaccharides are linked together. **Glycogen**, a molecule in your liver that is used to store energy, consists of many, many glucose molecules in a long chain and therefore can be broken down to release more glucose into the blood when needed.

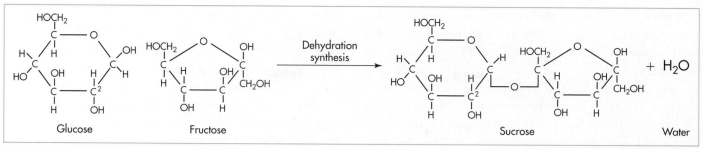

FIGURE 3–8 ■

Carbohydrates: The combining of the monosaccharides glucose and fructose to form the disaccharide sucrose.

Lipids

Lipids consist of mainly carbon and hydrogen. Because they have very little oxygen or any other ions in them, lipids are hydrophobic. Lipids are used for energy storage, communication, and protection. There are many types of lipids, as seen in **FIGURE 3–9** ■.

Fats and oils, probably the lipids most familiar to you, consist of three fatty acid chains and a glycerol molecule. They are energy storage molecules and can be broken down when needed by the body. A fat is called *saturated* if the fatty acids contain single covalent bonds. Saturated fats are solid at room temperature and can contribute to cardiovascular disease. Food examples include fatty beef, butter, and cheese. Unsaturated fats have one or more double covalent bonds and have been considered good for you. These include salmon, tree nuts, and vegetable oils.

Waxes are lipids that consist of a fatty acid chain with an alcohol molecule. They are some of the most hydrophobic substances known and are used mainly for protection, particularly waterproofing. (Why do you wax your car?)

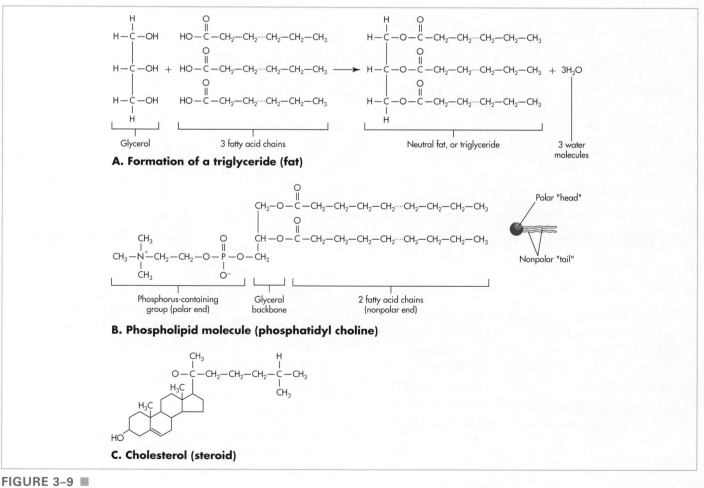

A. Formation of a triglyceride (fat)

B. Phospholipid molecule (phosphatidyl choline)

C. Cholesterol (steroid)

FIGURE 3–9 ■

Lipids.

A phospholipid molecule has two fatty acid "tails" and a phosphate (PO_4^-) "head." The tails are hydrophobic, but the head is hydrophilic. Phospholipids are key molecules in the structure and function of cell membranes. The last category of lipids is steroids. Steroids are lipids with the carbon atoms arranged in rings. They are structural molecules or are used for communication between cells. Examples of steroids are cholesterol, estrogen, and testosterone. Anabolic steroids, which have been abused by many amateur and professional athletes, are also lipids. (More will be covered on steroids in Chapter 12.)

Proteins

Proteins are molecules made of long chains of **amino acids** (see **FIGURE 3–10** ■). Because amino acids have nitrogen in them, proteins are always recognizable by the nitrogen atoms in the backbone of the molecule. A special linkage called a *peptide bond* ties the amino acids together and is unique to protein molecules. Proteins are the most versatile of all biological molecules, acting as structural molecules (collagen in tendons and ligaments), speeding up biological reactions (enzymes), storing energy (egg white albumin), moving your body (muscle protein), protecting against infection (antibodies), and allowing cells to communicate (the hormone insulin), to name just a few functions of proteins. The structure of a protein is determined by the order of amino acids in the molecule. **Denaturation** is the process by which proteins lose their structure by application of an external stress or compound such as strong acid or base, radiation, organic solvent, or heat. This loss of structural integrity disrupts the ability of the proteins to perform their intended function. A visual example is the albumin or egg whites that change from a transparent liquid to a white solid in a frying pan.

Nucleic Acids

The last category of biological molecules is **nucleic acids**. The only two nucleic acids in nature are RNA and DNA. They are involved in controlling the activities of cells and are the molecules that contain your genetic code. You will learn more about nucleic acids when we discuss cellular reproduction in Chapter 4 (see **FIGURE 3–11** ■).

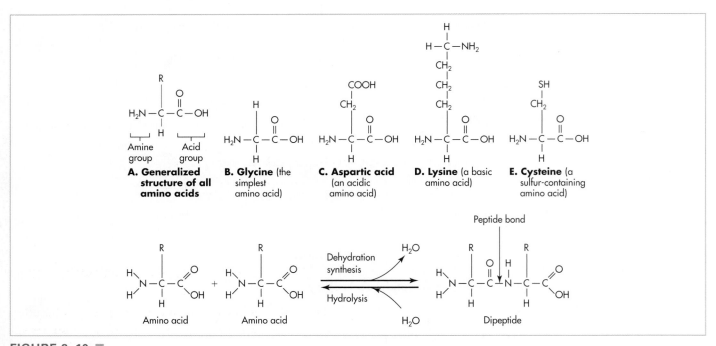

FIGURE 3–10 ■

Amino acids and proteins.

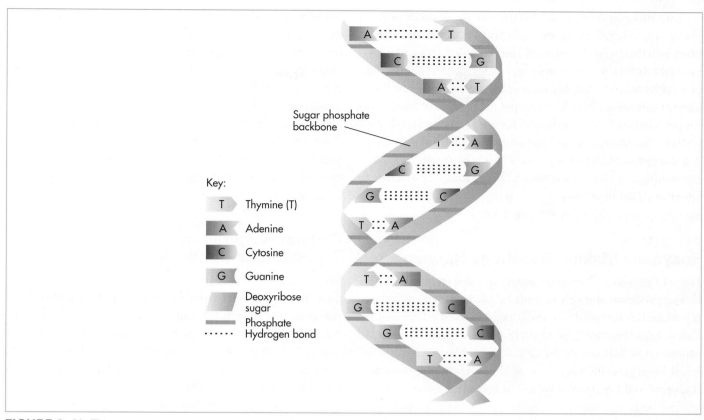

FIGURE 3–11
Nucleic acids.

TEST YOUR KNOWLEDGE 3–2

Answer the following questions:

1. _____ molecules are found in living systems.

2. The building blocks of proteins are _____.

3. $C_{27}H_{45}OH$ belongs to the _____ category of biological molecules.

4. Label each of the following molecules hydrophobic or hydrophilic.
   a. _____ $C_6H_{12}O_6$
   b. _____ wax
   c. _____ lipids

5. Carbohydrates are generally used for _____.

Metabolism

If you travel to other countries, you will see many different cultures and customs. Even though each culture is unique, they all share certain similarities. The same can be said in anatomy and physiology. We all share certain functions that are vital to survival. All humans, for example, need food to produce complex chemical reactions necessary for growth, reproduction, movement, and so on. **Metabolism** refers to all the chemical operations going on within our bodies.

Metabolism requires various nutrients or fuel to function and produces waste products much like a car consumes gas for power and produces waste, or exhaust. Metabolism, for now, can be thought of as all the life-sustaining reactions within the body.

Metabolism is further subdivided into two opposite processes. **Anabolism** is the process by which simpler compounds are *built up* and used to manufacture materials for growth, repair, and reproduction, such as the assembly of amino acids to form proteins. This is the *building* phase of metabolism. Many anabolic reactions are **dehydration synthesis reactions** in which water is removed and biological molecules are hitched together to form larger molecules. **Catabolism** is the process by which complex substances are *broken down* into simpler substances. For example, the breakdown of food into simpler chemical building blocks for energy use is a catabolic process. An abnormal and extreme example of catabolism is a starvation victim whose body "feeds on itself," actually consuming the body's own tissues. Many catabolic reactions are **hydrolysis reactions** in which water is added to break apart large molecules (see **FIGURE 3–12** ■).

Enzymes: Making Reactions Happen

For your cells to be able to do anything, some chemicals must be broken down and others must be made. You need building materials to build the small cell parts called *organelles* and to make energy. Any of these processes require chemical reactions to occur in the cell. The problem is that these reactions are usually very slow; so slow that by the time the reaction would happen, it would be too late for your cells to use the building materials. The hydrolysis and dehydration synthesis reactions used in cellular metabolism cannot happen without help. (You can't break down a piece of steak by pouring water on it!) To solve this problem, cells have special proteins called **enzymes**.

Enzymes speed up the rate of chemical reactions, making them fast enough for your cells to use the materials. Enzymes are protein molecules that have special binding sites on them. Biological molecules bind to the enzymes and are carried through the reaction, much like riders on a roller coaster (see **FIGURE 3–13** ■). When the reaction is finished, the enzyme goes back to get more molecules, called **substrates**. Because enzymes are a binding system, they are *specific*. Only certain molecules can be carried by certain enzymes. Substrates can

compete for binding sites. If all the binding sites are full, the enzymes are said to be *saturated*, and molecules must wait for an empty enzyme before going through the reaction. The enzymes can also be blocked or *inhibited*, preventing the substrate from binding. Think about filling cars on a roller coaster with people. If there are lots of people waiting in line, the people compete (line up) for seats. If one of the cars is broken, it will be blocked, perhaps by yellow tape, and people will not be able to ride on it. Like the roller coaster cars, enzymes are unchanged by their participation in the reaction.

Cellular Respiration and Adenosine Triphosphate (ATP): The Energy Molecule

We all know that we need to eat to obtain energy, but how does energy get from food to cells? In simple terms, the body takes in food and breaks it down (digestion). During this process, energy is released from the food. The problem is that cells can't use this energy directly. Only food converted to glucose can be used to make energy. Glucose can be used by your cells during a series of chemical reactions called **cellular respiration**. During cellular respiration, glucose is combined with oxygen and is transformed in your mitochondria into the high-energy molecule called **adenosine triphosphate (ATP)**. This molecule, ATP, is made of a base, a sugar, and three phosphate groups (hence, *tri*phosphate). The phosphate groups are held together by high-energy bonds. When a bond is broken, a high level of energy is released. Energy in this form can be used by the cells. When a bond is used, ATP becomes **ADP (adenosine diphosphate)**, which has only two phosphate groups. The ADP is now able to pick up another phosphate and form a high-energy bond so energy is stored and the process can begin again! Life is good (see **FIGURE 3–14** ■).

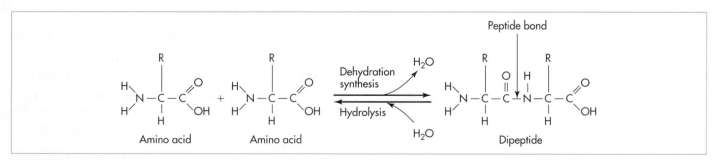

FIGURE 3–12 ■
Metabolic reactions: Dehydration synthesis builds new compounds while hydrolysis breaks down compounds.

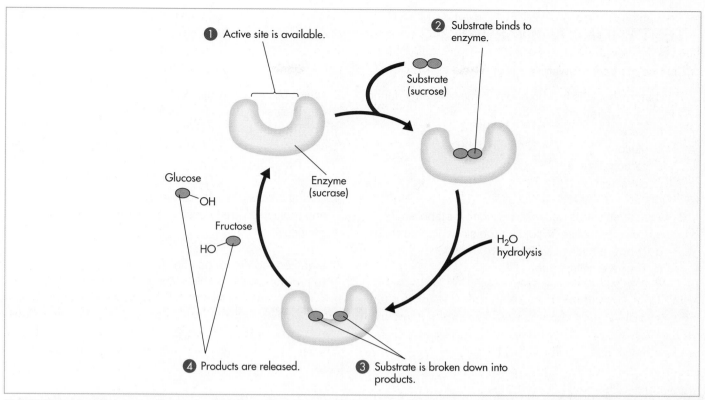

FIGURE 3-13 ■

Enzymes: Note the enzyme has the ending *ase* as in *sucrase* and the actual substrate is sucr*ose*.

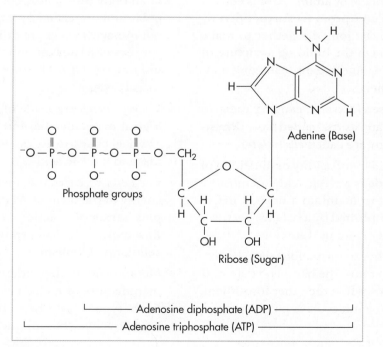

FIGURE 3-14 ■

Energy is released from the breaking of the phosphate bond in ATP when converting to ADP.

TEST YOUR KNOWLEDGE 3–3

Choose the best answer:

1. What molecule is broken down to make energy during cellular respiration?
   a. water
   b. glucose
   c. carbon dioxide
   d. citric acid

2. Why are enzymes necessary for cell metabolism?
   a. Cell metabolism would be too slow without them.
   b. They are necessary for active transport.
   c. They are cellular fuel.
   d. Our cells don't need enzymes.

3. Which of the following is true of enzymes?
   a. They slow down biological reactions.
   b. They are carbohydrates.
   c. They are not used up in the reactions.
   d. They are poisons.

4. During anabolic reactions, water is _____, and molecules are hitched together to make a larger molecule.

5. Ingested food must be converted to _____ to provide usable cellular energy.

SUMMARY: Points of Interest

- The smallest unit that is recognizable chemically is an element. Elements are made of atoms. Atoms consist of a nucleus (neutrons and protons) surrounded by electrons. Elements can be joined together to make molecules. Molecules form the building structure of cells and therefore tissues and organs. All living matter is composed of elements.

- Atoms may gain or lose electrons, causing them to have a charge. These atoms are called *ions*. Physiologically important ions are called *electrolytes*.

- The term *pH* is the measure of acidity or alkalinity of the body. Carbon dioxide is a weak acid and must be appropriately removed to maintain a normal pH in the blood. This is accomplished by a balance between the renal and respiratory systems' functions.

- Atoms are bound together to form molecules. If electrons are shared by the atoms, the bond is covalent. If one atom gains electrons while the other loses them, the bond is ionic, and the molecule is polar.

- Water is a polar covalent molecule that is the basis of all body fluids. Molecules that mix with water are polar and are called *hydrophilic*. Molecules that will not mix with water are called *hydrophobic*. A solution consists of a substance dissolved (the solute) in a liquid (the solvent). The solvent in biological systems is usually water.

- Living things are made of biological molecules. Biological molecules fall into four categories based on physical characteristics: proteins, carbohydrates, lipids, and nucleic acids.

- For cells to carry out metabolism, they must have energy in the form of ATP, which is made via a complex series of reactions called *cellular respiration*. Enzymes, biological catalysts, are also necessary for cellular metabolism.

- Metabolism is dependent on the breakdown and manufacture of molecules called *biological molecules*. Each type—carbohydrates, lipids, proteins, and nucleic acids—has unique characteristics.

Divya has always been overly concerned about her weight, even though she is considered physically attractive and fit by her peers. However, the prom is approaching, and she has resorted to the dangerous practice of using diuretics to "slim down" to fit in her gown. During gym class she suddenly became light-headed and had heart palpitations and was taken to the hospital. Her blood studies showed an electrolyte imbalance. Research diuretics and their connection to this case.

a. What electrolyte imbalance do you suspect from your research on diuretics?

_____

_____

b. What treatments would you recommend?

_____

_____

c. Do diuretics truly make you lose weight and how would you counsel Divya on the dangers of her actions?

_____

_____

Multiple Choice

1. The nucleus of an atom consists of
   a. protons.
   b. neutrons.
   c. electrons.
   d. a & b
   e. a, b, & c

2. A person loses body temperature faster in water than in air because water
   a. is hydrophilic.
   b. has a high heat capacity.
   c. is our major body fluid.
   d. is heavier than air.

3. Which of the following is not a property of enzymes?
   a. specificity
   b. saturation
   c. polarity
   d. inhibition

4. These biological molecules will not mix with water.
   a. proteins
   b. carbohydrates
   c. lipids
   d. amino acids

5. A new molecule is discovered in a deep sea cave fish. It has the following properties: hydrophilic, very large, and used for energy storage. What kind of molecule is it?
   a. lipid
   b. protein
   c. nucleic acid
   d. carbohydrate

Fill in the Blank

1. Atoms or molecules that can gain or lose an electron are called _____.

2. Unequal sharing of electrons in a bond results in a(n) _____ bond.

3. Sodium, potassium, and chloride in body fluids are known as _____.

4. NaCl can be in solution in your body. What is the solvent? _____

   What is the solute? _____

5. All the chemical reactions in your body are collectively known as _____.

6. Your cells need glucose to make this high-energy molecule: _____.

Short Answer

1. Explain the relationship between atoms, elements, molecules, and ions.

_____

_____

_____

_____

_____

2. List and explain the types of bonds between atoms.

_____

_____

_____

_____

_____

_____

3. Distinguish among the four classes of biological molecules.

_____

_____

_____

_____

_____

_____

4. Explain the chemistry of water. Why is water important in biological systems?

_____

_____

_____

_____

_____

5. Explain the functions of enzymes.

_____

_____

_____

_____

_____

6. Describe the process of cellular respiration.

_____

_____

_____

_____

_____

Visit our new **MyHealthProfessions** Lab to accompany _Anatomy & Physiology for Health Professions_. Here you'll find a rich collection of quizzes, case studies, and animations for deeper understanding and application.

4

The Cells

THE RAW MATERIALS AND BUILDING BLOCKS

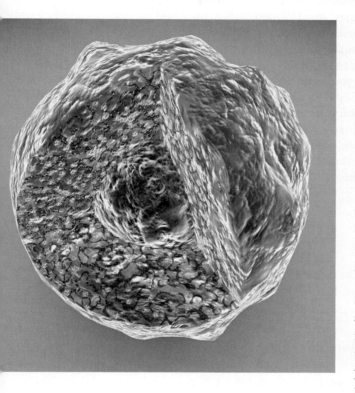

As we continue our journey, chances are that we will visit a city. A city is a complex combination of buildings and systems. A brick or cement block is a basic structure on which these buildings are constructed. The human body is also a complex combination of structures and systems, and a cell is the basic building block on which the body is built. Just as there are different types, shapes, and sizes of building blocks, there are different types, shapes, and sizes of cells. Blood cells, skin cells, nerve cells, and so on are all different from each other. We will learn more about each kind of cell in later chapters.

Although a cement block is a basic building block, it could not exist without sand, lime, and water, the components necessary to make cement. As this chapter explains, cells also consist of component parts, tiny cell structures called *organelles* that are needed to perform specific functions to keep the cell alive.

Cells of a similar type form tissue that functions to work together in an organ, whereas organs perform specific functions to create a system. For example, cardiac muscle cells form heart tissues, which form the heart, which is part of the cardiovascular system. Finally, all the systems work together to form a functioning human body! When you think about it, we are very much like a city. Cities need transportation systems, control systems, systems to import food and water, export waste, and heating and cooling systems—just like our bodies.

LEARNING OUTCOMES

At the end of your journey through this chapter, you will be able to:

- List and describe the various parts of a cell and explain their functions.
- Describe the types of active and passive transport within cells.
- Explain the process of cellular mitosis.
- Explain cellular respiration.
- Differentiate between bacteria, viruses, fungi, prions, and protozoa.

Pronunciation Guide

Correct pronunciation is important in any journey so that you and others are completely understood. Here is a "see and say" Pronunciation Guide for the more difficult terms to pronounce in this chapter. Please note that even though there are standard pronunciations, regional variations of the pronunciations can occur.

bacteria (back TEER ee ah)
benign (bee NINE)
capsid (CAP sid)
centrioles (SEN tree olz)
centrosomes (SEN troh soamz)
chromatin (CROW ma tin)
cilia (SILL ee ah)
cytokinesis (SIGH toe kih NEE sis)
cytoplasm (SIGH toe plazm)
cytoskeleton (SIGH toe SKELL eh ton)
deoxyribonucleic acid
 (dee AWK see rye bow NEW klee ick)
endocytosis (en doh sigh TOE sis)
endoplasmic reticulum
 (EN doh PLAZ mick ree TIH cue lum)
eukaryotic cell (you CARE ee AH tic)
exocytosis (EX oh sigh TOH sis)
flagella (flah JELL ah)

flora (FLOOR ah)
fungi (FUN jie)
Golgi apparatus (GAHL jee app uh RAT us)
lysosomes (LIE soh soamz)
malignant (muh LIG nant)
metastasis (meh TASS tuh sis)
mitochondria (MITE oh KAHN dree ah)
mitosis (my TOE sis)
mycelia (my SEE lee ah)
osmosis (ahss MOE sis)
pathogen (PATH oh jenn)
phagocytosis (fag oh sigh TOE sis)
pinocytosis (pie no sigh TOE sis)
prokaryotic (pro CARE ee AAH tick)
protozoa (pro tuh ZOH uh)
ribonucleic acid (RYE bow new KLEE ick)
ribosomes (RYE bow soamz)
vesicle (VESS ih kuhl)

OVERVIEW OF CELLS

Cells are the fundamental units of all living things. Some organisms are composed of only a single cell. Practically all the cells in our body are microscopic in size, ranging from about one-third to one-thirteenth the size of the dot on this exclamation point! On the other hand, certain nerve cells can be two feet in length or longer! When we refer to cells as the "building blocks" of our bodies, we immediately think of brick-shaped objects. However, cells can be flat, round, threadlike, or irregularly shaped. Although the approximately *7.5 trillion* cells found in the human body vary in size, shape, and purpose, they normally work together to allow for proper functioning of processes necessary for life, such as digestion, respiration, reproduction, movement, and production of heat and energy. FIGURE 4–1 ■ shows examples of various cell types found within the human body.

CELL STRUCTURE

Even though cells in our bodies can vary greatly in size, shape, and function, they share certain common traits. As previously stated, we consider cells the basic building

blocks of the human body. However, to better understand them, let's look at cells as miniature cities with a variety of systems, structures, and organizations that are necessary for proper function. Almost all human cells possess a nucleus (except mature red blood cells), organelles, cytoplasm, and a cell membrane. Each component of a cell has a special purpose. FIGURE 4–2 ■ represents a typical cell with its major components. We will now discuss the individual components.

Cell Membrane

We can think of the **cell membrane** as the city limits. The cell membrane is also called the *plasma membrane* because it surrounds the cyto*plasm* of the cell. This is a defined boundary that possesses a definite shape and actually holds the cell contents together. The cell membrane acts as a protective covering. For a city to thrive, people and materials must be able to travel into and out of the city. A cell membrane is responsible for allowing materials into and out of the cell. What is interesting is that the membrane allows only certain things into or out of the cell. Because the membrane selects what may pass through, it is known as a *selectively permeable* (or *semipermeable*) membrane.

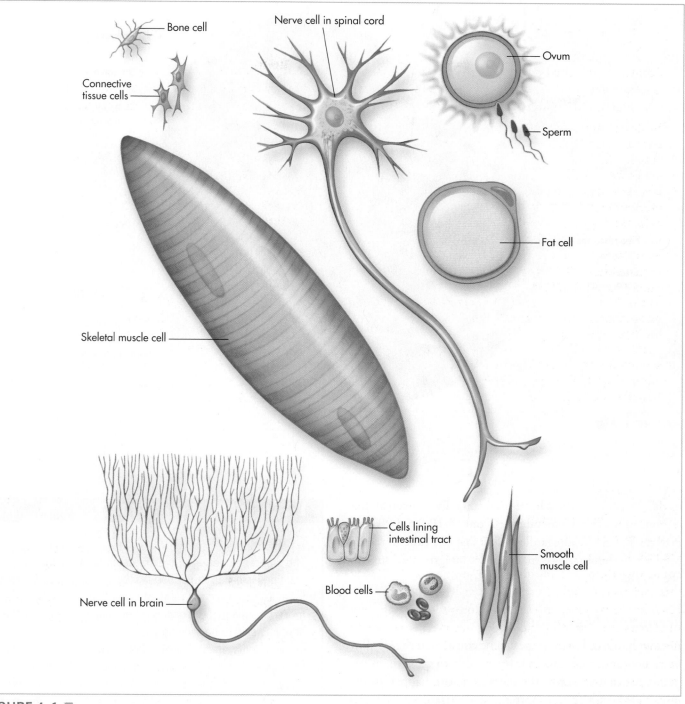

FIGURE 4–1 ■

Various types of cells within the human body.

The cell membrane is composed mainly of lipids and proteins, with some carbohydrates. The bulk of the cell membrane is composed of a double layer of phospholipids, oriented tail to tail. (Remember from Chapter 3 that phospholipids have hydrophilic heads and hydrophobic tails.) This bilayer prevents hydrophilic molecules from passing through the membrane. Hydrophobic molecules, on the other hand, can pass rather easily through the phospholipid bilayer. Cell membranes also contain abundant amounts of cholesterol.

Membrane proteins also contribute to the selective permeability of the cell membrane. Proteins may act as channels so substances can pass across the membrane or they can carry substances across the membrane. Proteins can also be identification markers showing that the cell comes from a certain person, much like PA is an "identification marker" that tells

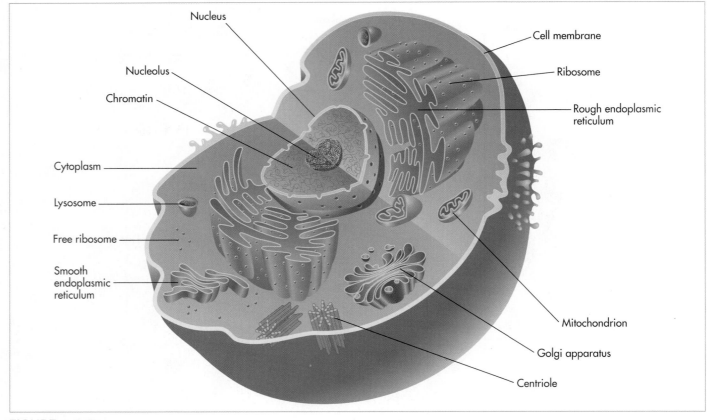

FIGURE 4–2 ■
Cellular components.

us that Pittsburgh, PA is in Pennsylvania. Even given all that responsibility, the cell membrane is only 3/10,000,000 of an inch thick. Each cell, regardless of its shape or function, must have a cell membrane to maintain its integrity and survive. See **FIGURE 4–3** ■.

Transport Methods

Although, the cell membrane can be considered the city limits or boundary, substances must be able to cross the membrane. Movement across the membrane can happen in two broad ways: passive transport and active transport. **Passive transport**, as the words suggest, requires no extra form of energy because the substance is being transported *down* its concentration gradient (see a discussion of concentration gradients in the Learning Hint). It is like riding a toboggan. You simply go down the hill. No input of energy is needed once the toboggan begins to move. (Dealing with that "starting" energy is the job of enzymes and is a separate issue from what we are discussing here.) **Active transport** requires addition of energy throughout the transport process to make it happen, because substances are being transported *up* their gradient. Climbing back up the hill is a lot more work.

LEARNING HINT

Concentration Gradient

The difference between the solute concentrations of two solutions is called the *concentration gradient* (see Chapter 3 for a discussion of the parts of a solution). If a substance moves from a higher concentration to a lower concentration, it is said to be moving *with* (down) the concentration gradient (difference). For example, if you are in a grocery store, standing in a long line "concentrated" with people and three new lanes open up, the people will quickly move from the highly concentrated line to the lower concentrated areas (the new open lanes). Soon, you will notice, all lines will equalize, demonstrating that even people move with a concentration gradient and reach equilibrium. Moving from a low concentration to a high concentration, on the other hand, is said to be going *against* (up) the gradient.

Passive Transport

Passive transport can be further divided into four types: diffusion, osmosis, filtration, and facilitated diffusion.

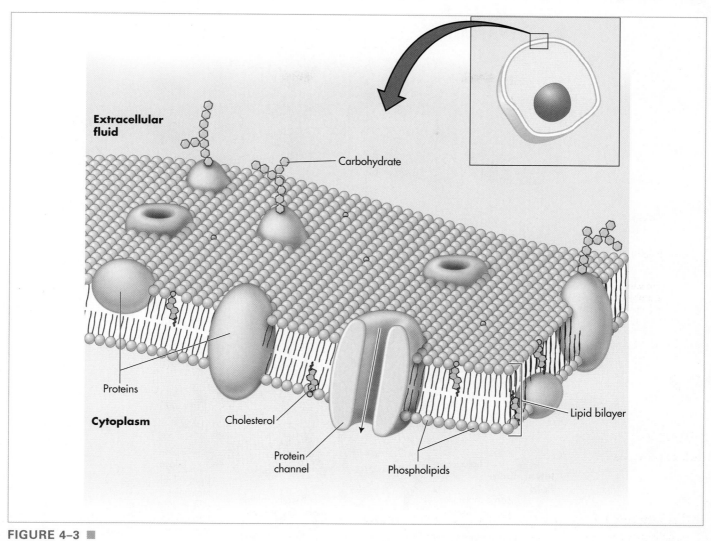

Extracellular fluid

Carbohydrate

Proteins

Cytoplasm

Cholesterol

Protein channel

Phospholipids

Lipid bilayer

FIGURE 4–3 ■

The cell membrane.

Diffusion **Diffusion** is our most common means of passive transport by which a solute travels from an area of higher concentration to an area of lesser concentration, with the gradient. This is like dumping a packet of powdered drink mix into a pitcher of water. The water gradually assumes the color and flavor of the powder until the entire contents of the container are the same color and taste (nature likes a nice, equal balance!). Another example may be one of your classmates overusing perfume or cologne. Once in the classroom, the smell diffuses from high concentration on the individual to low concentration throughout the classroom. He or she may need to be reminded of the old saying that perfume should never announce your presence before your arrival.

Diffusion is necessary in the transportation of oxygen from the lungs and into the blood. It is also needed to transport the waste (carbon dioxide) from the blood to the lungs and eventually out into the air. This vital process is further discussed in Chapter 14, "The Respiratory System." See **FIGURE 4–4** ■ for examples of diffusion.

Osmosis **Osmosis** is another form of passive transport in which water travels through a selectively permeable membrane when a concentration gradient is present. Water tends to travel across a membrane from areas that have a low concentration of a solute to areas that have a higher concentration of the solute until the concentration is the same on both sides of the membrane. Keep in mind that the water is moving *with its* gradient. See **FIGURE 4–5** ■ for a visual description. This ability of a substance to "pull" water toward an area of higher concentration of the solute is called **osmotic pressure**. The greater the concentration of the solute, the greater the osmotic pressure it exerts to bring in water.

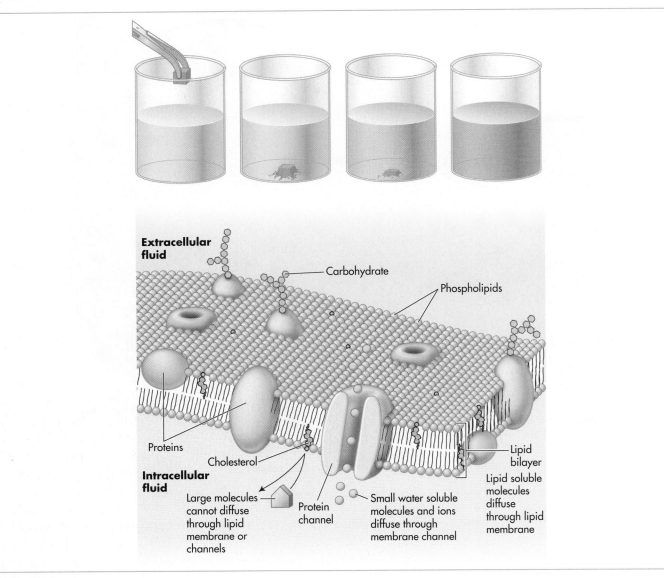

FIGURE 4–4 ■

Two examples of diffusion.

You may be wondering how water, a polar solvent, can pass through the phospholipid bilayer. Water cannot actually pass through the phospholipid bilayer. However, there are special passages in the membrane for water, so water moves across the membrane through these passages.

Filtration In **filtration**, pressure is applied to force water and its dissolved materials across a membrane. Filtration caused by pressure is similar to a rush of people being pushed through the turnstiles during rush hour or the effect you get when you squeeze the trigger on a squirt gun. The major supplier of force in the body is the pumping of the heart, which forces blood flow into the kidneys, where filtration takes place. This concept is expanded in Chapter 17,

"The Urinary System." For now, see **FIGURE 4-6** ■, which illustrates the process of filtration. Filtration is a selective process in that only solutes that can fit through channels and other openings in the membrane will filter across it.

Facilitated Diffusion (Carrier-Mediated Passive Transport) **Facilitated diffusion** is a variation of diffusion in which a carrier molecule helps a substance move across the membrane. Imagine a revolving door. Each person entering the door is a molecule binding to a carrier (see **FIGURE 4-7** ■). Glucose is the substance that is often transported this way. You may wonder, if it is helped, how can it be considered *passive* transport? It can best be thought of as a situation in which the glucose was already

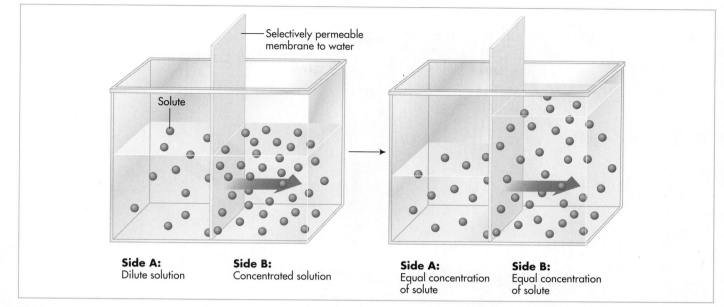

Side A: Dilute solution Side B: Concentrated solution Side A: Equal concentration of solute Side B: Equal concentration of solute

FIGURE 4–5 ■

Osmosis: Water moves from an area of low solute concentration to an area of higher solute concentration.

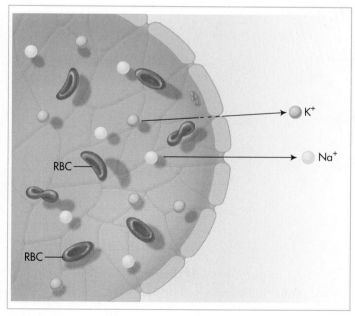

FIGURE 4–6 ■

The process of filtration in the kidneys, where smaller solutes, such as the electrolytes sodium and potassium, pass through the membrane, whereas the larger blood proteins and cells normally do not.

moving in an attempt to cross the membrane and conveniently encounters an already revolving door. Once it steps into the door, it is quickly "pushed" along until it comes out on the other side of the membrane. As long as glucose is moving *down* its concentration gradient, the transport is considered passive transport.

Because a carrier is used to transport the substance, this kind of transport is a binding system and has some of the same characteristics as enzymes (see Chapter 3). This kind of transport is also highly specific. A carrier may only be able to carry one type of molecule. Carriers may also be subject to saturation (too many substances and/or not enough carriers) and inhibition (carriers are blocked from working). Think again of the revolving door: Only some things will fit through it, only so many at a time, and if it's blocked, you can't go through it. Again, Figure 4–7 illustrates facilitated diffusion.

Active Transport

Active transport can be broken down into three types: active transport pumps, endocytosis, and exocytosis.

Active Transport Pumps (Carrier-Mediated Active Transport) Active transport pumps work in the same way as facilitated diffusion except that active transport pumps require the addition of energy in the form of an energy molecule called *adenosine triphosphate*, or *ATP* (see Chapter 3) to move a substance. Energy is needed because the cell is trying to move a substance into an area that already has a high concentration of that substance (*against* the concentration gradient). It's kind of like trying to put six pounds of sugar into a five-pound bag! It can be done, but you have to apply a lot of energy. A common example in our cells is the need to transport potassium (K^+). Cells contain a good amount of

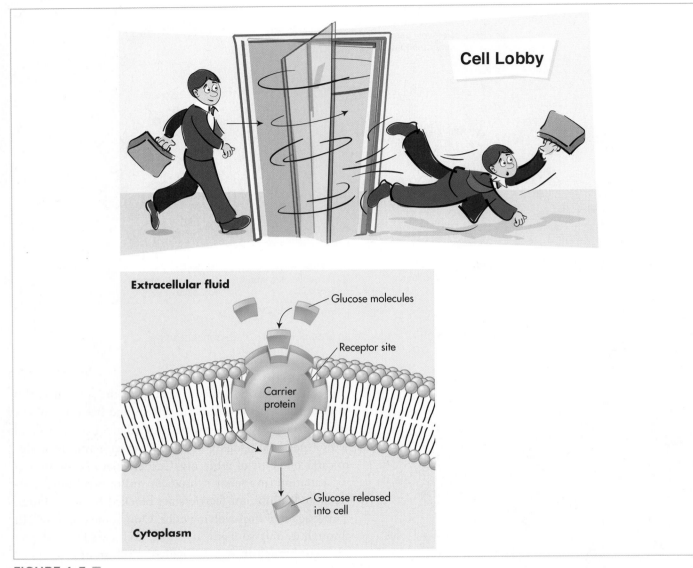

Cell Lobby

Extracellular fluid

Glucose molecules

Receptor site

Carrier protein

Glucose released into cell

Cytoplasm

FIGURE 4–7 ■
Facilitated diffusion.

potassium. The only way to get more into a cell is to apply energy to "push" it in, using a carrier molecule and expending energy.

Endocytosis Endocytosis (*endo* = within, *cyt* = cell, *osis* = condition) is utilized by the cells for the *intake* of liquid and solid particles when the substance is too large to diffuse across the cell membrane. The cell membrane actually surrounds the substance with a small portion of its membrane, forming a **vesicle** (bladder or sac), which then separates from the membrane and moves into the cell. If a solid particle is being transported, we call the transport **phagocytosis** (*phago* = eat). White blood cells do this to bacteria to prevent infections in our bodies. If the intake involves water, it is called **pinocytosis** (*pino* = to drink).

Exocytosis In some situations, the cell needs to transport substances *out of* itself using a vesicle. This is called **exocytosis** (*exo* = outside). Some cells may produce a substance needed outside the cell. Once this substance is made, it is surrounded by a membrane forming a vesicle and moves to the cell membrane. This vesicle becomes a part of the cell membrane and expels its load out of the cell. For further explanation of active transport, see **FIGURE 4–8** ■.

TABLE 4–1 ■ serves as a concise summary of all the methods of transport that have been discussed.

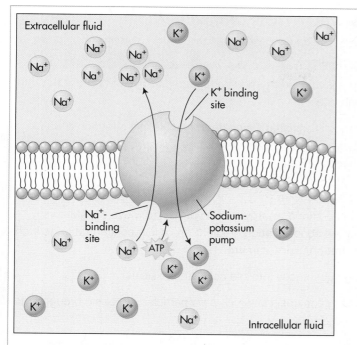

ACTIVE TRANSPORT PUMP

PHAGOCYTOSIS

PINOCYTOSIS

EXOCYTOSIS

FIGURE 4–8 ▨

Types of active transport into and out of cells.

TABLE 4–1 METHODS OF CELLULAR TRANSPORTATION

CELLULAR TRANSPORTATION METHODS	DESCRIPTION
Passive Transportation (no energy required)	
Diffusion	Moving a substance from an area of high concentration to an area of low concentration.
Osmosis	Water travels across a membrane from areas that have a low concentration of a solute to areas that have a higher concentration of solute until the concentration is the same on both sides of the membrane.

(continued)

TABLE 4–1 METHODS OF CELLULAR TRANSPORTATION (*continued*)

CELLULAR TRANSPORTATION METHODS	DESCRIPTION
Filtration	Pressure is applied to force water and dissolved materials through a membrane.
Facilitated diffusion	Substance is assisted via carrier molecule in a direction it was already traveling from an area of high concentration to an area of low concentration.
Active Transport (energy required)	
Active transport pumps	Require additional energy in form of ATP to move substances against the concentration gradient (from low concentration to high concentration) using carriers.
Endocytosis	Moving substances into the cell using vesicles.
Phagocytosis	Form of endocytosis in which *solid* particles are being brought into the cell.
Pinocytosis	Form of endocytosis in which *liquid* is being brought into the cell.
Exocytosis	Transportation of material to the outside of the cell using vesicles.

TEST YOUR KNOWLEDGE 4–1

Fill in the blanks:

1. This form of passive transportation is like combining drink mix and a pitcher of water:
   _____.

2. During osmosis, water travels across a semipermeable membrane from an area of _____ concentration of solute to an area of _____ concentration of solute.

3. _____ allows only certain sizes of particles to pass through.

4. The act of removing carbon dioxide from the blood to the lungs is achieved through _____.

5. Glucose is often transported by _____.

6. Tell whether the following processes are active or passive:
   a. endocytosis _____
   b. facilitated diffusion _____
   c. osmosis _____
   d. phagocytosis _____
   e. filtration _____
   f. pinocytosis _____

FOCUS ON PROFESSIONS

Cytology is a general term used to describe the study of cells. For example, this is especially important in determining if a patient has cancer. Here, tissue samples must be obtained and prepared on slides by a **histotechnologist** for analysis. In health care, the study of cells can be subdivided into several different specializations. Learn more about these specialties within the field of **laboratory technology** by visiting the websites of national associations such as the National Society for Histotechnology, the American Medical Technologists (AMT), and the American Society for Clinical Laboratory Science (ASCLS).

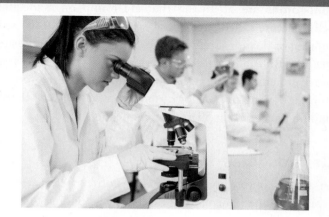

Cytoplasm

Living organisms require balanced environments in which to thrive. Humans require the right mixture of oxygen and nitrogen; sea creatures require the right balance of salt and water; a chick embryo requires albumen, or "egg white," in which to develop. Likewise, the internal parts of a cell require a special environment, called **cytoplasm**, to survive. The cytoplasm is a watery solution of organic (proteins, carbohydrates, and lipids) and inorganic chemicals such as minerals and gases.

Nucleus and Nucleolus

The **nucleus** has been described as the "brain of the cell." In our case, we will consider it to be City Hall: a control center. City Hall dictates the activity of the city departments much as the nucleus dictates the activities of the organelles in the cell. Because City Hall is crucial to the city's function, security is important to protect it from attack or damage. That is why metal detectors are installed at the doors. The function of the nucleus of a cell is similar. It is surrounded by a double-walled nuclear membrane. Even though this membrane is composed of two layers, it has large pores that allow certain materials to pass into and out of the nucleus.

Somewhere in City Hall are blueprints of the city showing the buildings, streets, water and gas lines, and so forth. The nucleus also contains "blueprints"—and "building codes" too. **Chromatin** is the material found in the nucleus that contains **deoxyribonucleic acid (DNA)**. The specifications (blueprints) for the creation of new cells are contained in DNA. Chromatin eventually forms

chromosomes, which contain **genes**. The genes determine our inherited characteristics. (Remember when you were a kid and Aunt Pearl saying how much you look like your Uncle Elmer?)

A spherical body made up of dense fibers called the **nucleolus** is found within the cell nucleus. Its major function is to synthesize the **ribonucleic acid (RNA)** that forms ribosomes. Now we have the blueprints, but what about the materials that we need? Who's in charge of getting these materials together? That's where ribosomes and centrosomes come into play. FIGURE 4–9 ■ shows the cell membrane, cytoplasm, nucleus, and nucleolus. We will continue to rebuild the cell's infrastructure as we discuss their specific functions.

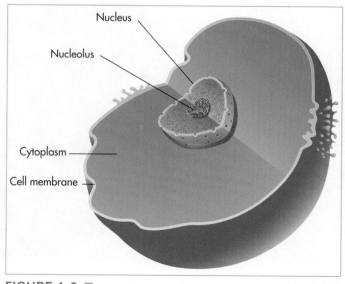

FIGURE 4–9 ■

The cell membrane, cytoplasm, nucleus, and nucleolus.

Ribosomes

Ribosomes are organelles that are found on a specific cell structure called the endoplasmic reticulum (discussed shortly) or floating around in the cytoplasm. Ribosomes are made of RNA and assist in the production of enzymes and other proteins that are needed for cell repair and reproduction. Following our analogy, ribosomes can be considered building material suppliers for remodeling and repair.

Centrosomes

In a city, completely new structures often are needed to replace old ones. Therefore, the cell needs a building contractor to build new structures. The **centrosomes** are specialized regions within the cell that fill this need. Centrosomes contain **centrioles** that are involved in the division of the cell. Cellular division, or reproduction, will be discussed once we cover all the cell parts. Centrioles are tubular shaped and usually found in pairs. See **FIGURE 4–10** ■, which now adds the ribosomes and centrioles to the cell, as well as the mitrochondira, which are discussed next.

Mitochondria

Could you possibly imagine what it would be like if we had no electricity in our city? Things would come to a stand-still. The **mitochondria**, tiny bean-shaped organelles, act as power plants to provide up to 95 percent of the body's energy needs for cellular repair, movement, and reproduction. Our cell's energy molecule, ATP, is made in the mitochondria. As a city's need for power increases, more power plants are built. Similarly, if a given cell type is very active and needs more power, there are a larger number of mitochondria in that cell. Liver cells, which are quite active, can have up to 2,000 mitochondria in each cell. Sperm cells "swim" with a tail (flagellum), so they need only a single mitochondrion coiled around the tail for energy. Special enzymes in the mitochondria help to take in oxygen and use it to produce energy. Whereas our city uses electricity for most of its power, the cell uses adenosine triphosphate (ATP), which is created by the mitochondria (again, please see Figure 4–10).

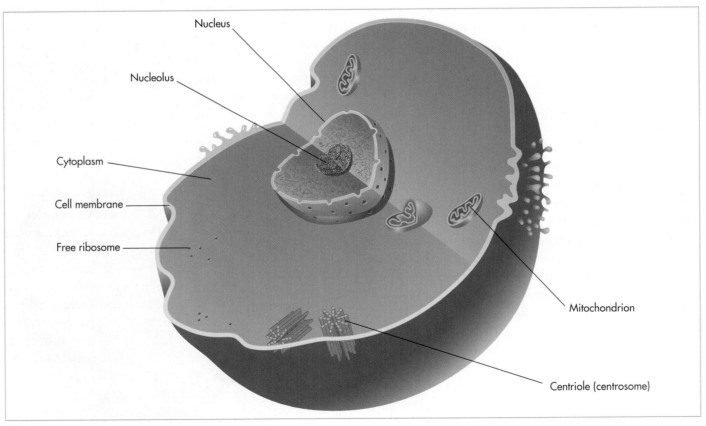

FIGURE 4–10 ■

The cell membrane, cytoplasm, nucleus, nucleolus, ribosomes, centrioles, and mitochondria.

Endoplasmic Reticulum

Although there are paths, walkways, and sidewalks in our city, the main structure for travel is a road system. The **endoplasmic reticulum** is a series of channels set up in the cytoplasm that are formed from folded membranes. The endoplasmic reticulum has two distinct forms. One has a surface much like sandpaper, the result of ribosomes on its surface, which is termed *rough* endoplasmic reticulum. It is responsible for the production or synthesis of protein. Once the protein is synthesized, it is sent to the Golgi apparatus for processing. The second form has no ribosomes on its surface, making it appear smooth, so it is called the *smooth* endoplasmic reticulum (complex stuff, huh?). The smooth endoplasmic reticulum synthesizes lipids (fats) and steroids. Think of both as a series of dirt and paved roads with butcher shops and food-processing plants along the way (see FIGURE 4–11 ■).

Golgi Apparatus

Cities have factories with their own fleet of trucks. The **Golgi apparatus** is very similar to these factories. This organelle looks like a bunch of flattened, membranous sacs. Once the Golgi apparatus receives protein from the endoplasmic reticulum, it further processes and stores it as a shippable product, much like a packaging plant does. Not only does it prepare the protein for shipping, but also a part of the Golgi apparatus surrounds the protein with a vesicle that then separates itself from the main body of this organelle. That portion, with its load, then travels to the cell membrane, where it releases (secretes) the protein! This is an actual example of exocytosis. Cells in organs with a high level of secretion or storage (like the digestive system) contain higher numbers of the Golgi apparatus. Salivary glands and pancreatic glands, for example, are made of cells containing many Golgi apparati. Some proteins made in the Golgi apparatus stay in the cell and end up in lysosomes.

Lysosomes

All cities create waste that must be removed. Cells are no different. **Lysosomes** (*lysis* = to break down) are vesicles containing powerful hydrolytic enzymes that take care of cleaning up intracellular debris and other waste. (Hydrolytic enzymes speed up the hydrolysis reactions described in Chapter 3.) Lysosomes are multitalented. They also aid in maintaining health by destroying unwanted bacteria through the process of phagocytosis. Again, see Figure 4–11, which contains all the organelles.

Other Interesting Parts

Similar in some ways to the bony skeleton, the **cytoskeleton** is a network of microtubules and interconnected filaments that provide shape to the cell and allow the cell and its contents to be mobile. Suppose we could build cities that float on large bodies of water. How would we propel them to new locations? Certain cells can solve this problem through the use of flagella. **Flagella** are whip-shaped tails that move some cells in a fashion similar to that of a tadpole.

The future may offer new ways of transporting people and materials. For example, perhaps cities will install moving sidewalks, similar to those in some airports. Certain cells have solved such transport problems already through the use of cilia. **Cilia** are short, microscopic, hairlike projections located on the outer surface of some cells. They move in a wavelike motion that carries particles in a given direction. The action is comparable to when a band member jumps into a crowd and is moved by the wave action of the audience's arms. (This is something NOT recommended by the authors.) Ciliary action is one way our lungs stay clean from the dust particles and germs that we inhale every day.

Mitosis

Cellular reproduction is the process of making a new cell. Cellular reproduction is also known as **cell division** because one cell divides into two cells when it reproduces. Cells can only come from other cells. When cells make *identical* copies of themselves *without the involvement* of another cell, that is called **asexual reproduction**. Most cells are able to reproduce themselves asexually whether they are animal cells, plant cells, or bacteria.

The cells that make up the human body are a type of cell known as an eukaryotic cell. **Eukaryotic cells** have a nucleus, cellular organelles, and usually several chromosomes in the nucleus. (*Reminder:* The genetic material of the cell, DNA, is bundled into "packages" of chromatin known as chromosomes.) Because chromosomes carry all the instructions for the cells, all cells must have a complete set after reproduction. These instructions include how the cell is to function within the body and blueprints for reproduction. No matter whether a cell has one chromosome, like bacteria, or 46 chromosomes, like humans, all the chromosomes must be copied before the cell can divide.

Let's start with the simple cellular division of a bacterium. Bacterial cells are classified as *prokaryotic* organisms; they do not have a true nucleus or nuclear membrane.

CHAPTER 4

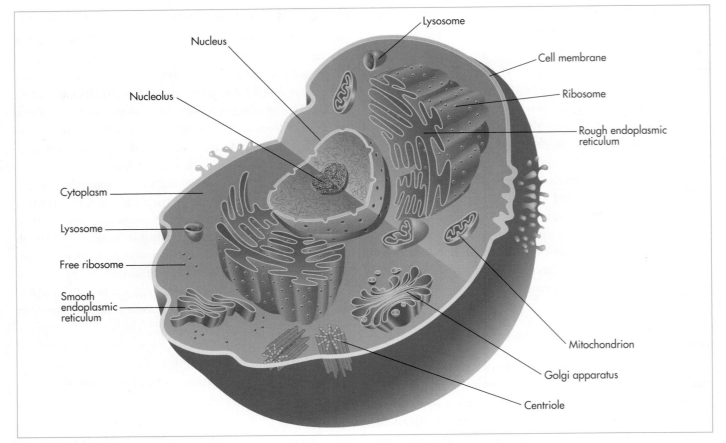

FIGURE 4–11 ■

The cell membrane, cytoplasm, nucleus, nucleolus, ribosomes, centrioles, mitochondria, endoplasmic reticulum, Golgi apparatus, and lysosomes.

TEST YOUR KNOWLEDGE 4–2

Complete the following:

1. What organelle is described in each of the following statements?

_____ a. contains genetic material

_____ b. transport for protein and lipids

_____ c. makes ATP

_____ d. puts proteins into vesicles

_____ e. responsible for sperm swimming ability

_____ f. controls the cell

_____ g. removes waste

_____ h. moves mucus within lungs

Bacteria reproduce very easily through a process known as *binary fission*. Bacterial cells simply copy their DNA, divide up the cytoplasm, and split in half!

Now let's go to the more complex cellular reproduction. Eukaryotic cells, like yours, must go through a more complicated set of maneuvers to reproduce. Not only do your cells have to duplicate all 46 of their chromosomes, but they also have to make sure that each cell gets all the chromosomes and all the right organelles. The process of sorting the chromosomes, so that each new cell gets the right number of copies of all the genetic material, is called **mitosis**. Mitosis is the only way that eukaryotic cells can reproduce asexually.

The Cell Cycle

Every minute approximately 300 million body cells die; this is referred to as *apoptosis*. Not all cells have the same life span. Certain blood cells live for only a few hours, the intestinal cells last two to three days, and muscles cells can last for up to 15 years, whereas nerve cells live a lifetime.

During its life span, a cell can divide many times. The total life of a eukaryotic cell can therefore be divided into two major phases known as the **cell cycle**. Most of the cell cycle is devoted to a phase known as **interphase**. During interphase, a cell is not dividing, but is performing its normal functions along with stockpiling needed materials and preparing for division by also copying DNA and making new organelles. Only a brief portion of the cell cycle, the **mitotic phase**, is devoted to actual cell division. The mitotic phase is divided into two major portions. Mitosis is the division and sorting of the *genetic material*, whereas **cytokinesis** is the division of the *cytoplasm*.

Mitosis, the division of the genetic material, is the most complicated part of cell division for a eukaryotic cell. What further complicates mitosis is that the process is further divided into four specific phases. As you'll soon see, the four phases are based on the position of the chromosomes relative to the new cells. They are prophase, metaphase, anaphase,

and telophase. To put all these processes and phases in perspective, please refer to the flowchart in FIGURE 4–12 ■.

The Phases of Mitosis

Let's proceed step by step through the four phases of mitosis using FIGURE 4–13 ■ as a reference.

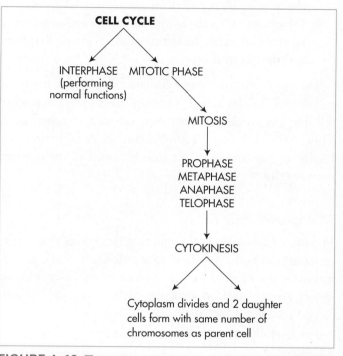

FIGURE 4–12 ■

Flowchart of the cell cycle.

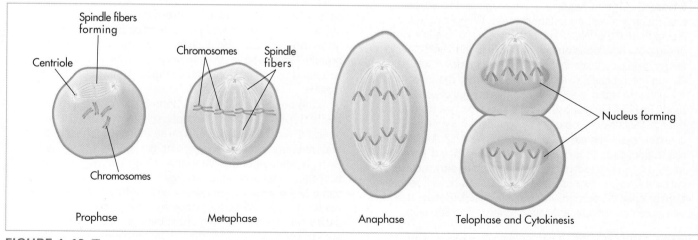

FIGURE 4–13 ■

Phases of mitosis.

1. **Prophase** (*pro* = before): The nucleus disappears, the chromosomes become visible, and a set of chromosomal anchor lines or guide wires, called the *spindle fibers*, forms.
2. **Metaphase** (*meta* = between): The chromosomes line up in the center of the cell.
3. **Anaphase** (*an* = without): The chromosomes split, and the spindle fibers pull them apart.
4. **Telophase** (*telo* = the end): The chromosomes go to the far end of the cell, the spindle fibers begin to disappear, and the nuclei reappear.

During or directly after telophase, cytokinesis happens, and the cell divides in half. The original cell was the mother cell that has divided into two new identical daughter cells. Thus, mitosis, asexual reproduction in eukaryotic cells, results in two new daughter cells identical to the original mother cell.

Mitosis in Your Body

Mitosis, or asexual cellular reproduction, serves many purposes in your body. Any time your cells need to be replaced, mitosis is the method used to replace them. Many of your tissues are replaced on a regular basis. Bone, epithelium, skin, and blood cells all replace themselves on a regular basis. Repair and regeneration of damaged tissue is accomplished by mitosis as well. If you cut your hand, the skin is replaced, first by collagen, but eventually by the original tissue. Mitosis increases the number of cells near the injury so that the damaged or destroyed cells can be replaced. A broken bone is repaired in much the same way.

Growth is also accomplished by mitosis. Lengthening of bones as you grow, increases in organ size—indeed, most ways that tissue gets bigger—are due to mitosis of cells in the tissues or organs. Without mitosis, your body would not be able to grow or replace old or damaged cells.

LEARNING HINT

Mitosis versus Meiosis

The words *mitosis* and *meiosis* sound and look alike and are therefore often confused. Remember, meiosis produces gametes or sexual cells, which contain half the chromosomes because the sexual union of male and female will contribute the other half. Mitosis (I reproduce myself) is asexual and produces exact copies of the cell and the full complement of chromosomes because no union is needed.

APPLIED SCIENCE

Cell Energy and ATP: The Energy Molecule

In Chapter 3, we introduced the process of cellular respiration, the way your cells make ATP. Here, we will expand on the introduction from Chapter 3, increasing the details. Cellular respiration is a very important process. Without it, your cells would quickly die. We all know that we need to eat to obtain energy, but how does energy get from food to cells? In simple terms, the body takes in food and breaks it down (digestion). During this process, energy is released from the food. Now, the problem is that cells can't use this energy directly. Only food converted to glucose (simple sugar) can be used to make energy. Glucose can be used by your cells during a series of chemical reactions called *cellular respiration*. During cellular respiration, glucose is combined with oxygen and is transformed in your mitochondria into the high-energy molecule called *adenosine triphosphate (ATP)*. During cellular respiration, glucose is "burned" in the presence of oxygen, making water, carbon dioxide, and lots of energy. The equation can be used to represent cellular respiration. Once the glucose is used up and energy is made, carbon dioxide and water are made as by-products. To make energy for your cells, you must have glucose (from food) and abundant oxygen. You make energy and you must be able to get rid of the waste carbon dioxide. Now you know why you breathe! You need to bring in oxygen to make energy, and you need to exhale to get rid of the waste product carbon dioxide.

The point of cellular respiration is to make energy in the form of ATP. Adenosine triphosphate or ATP, is composed of a base, a sugar, and three (hence, *tri*phosphate) phosphate groups. The phosphate groups are held together by high-energy bonds. When these high energy bonds are broken, a large amount of energy is released. This energy can now be used by the cell for cellular functions.. When a bond is broken, ATP now becomes *adenosine diphosphate (ADP)*, which has only two phosphate groups. ADP now is able to combine with another phosphate and form a high-energy bond so energy is stored and the process can begin again!

Glucose + oxygen → carbon dioxide + water + energy

(specific chemical equation)

$C_6H_{12}O_6 + 6O_2 \rightarrow 6CO_2 + 6H_2O + ATP$ (large amounts)

TEST YOUR KNOWLEDGE 4–3

Choose the best answer:

1. Cells are reproducing themselves during this portion of the cell cycle.
   a. metaphase
   b. mitotic phase
   c. meiotic phase
   d. manic phase

2. During this phase of mitosis, the nucleus disappears and the spindle appears.
   a. prophase
   b. metaphase
   c. anaphase
   d. telophase

3. During this phase of mitosis, the chromosomes begin to pull apart.
   a. prophase
   b. metaphase
   c. anaphase
   d. telophase

4. Which of the following is not a function of asexual reproduction?
   a. tissue repair
   b. replacement of cells
   c. tissue growth
   d. cloning humans

5. Meiosis produces sexual cells with _____ the number of chromosomes of the parent cell.
   a. the same amount
   b. twice
   c. one-fourth
   d. one-half

Clinical Application

MITOSIS RUN AMOK

When the body is healthy, cells grow in an orderly fashion. They grow at the appropriate rate in the appropriate number, shape, and alignment. Sometimes conditions are altered in the body (either internally or externally) that trigger changes in the way the cells grow. Cell growth can become wild and uncontrolled, leading to too many cells being produced and resulting in a lump, or tumor. Generally, tumors are classified as either benign or malignant. **Benign** tumors typically grow slowly and push healthy cells out of the way. Usually, benign tumors are not life threatening. **Malignant**, or cancerous, tumors grow rapidly and invade, rather than push aside, healthy cell tissue. Cancer actually means "crab" (remember your Zodiac signs?) and is a good description of cancer cells in that they spread out into healthy tissue like the legs and pincers of a crab. Cancerous tumors also differ from benign tumors in that parts of a cancerous tumor can break off and travel through the blood system or the lymphatic network and start new tumors in other parts of the body. This breaking off and spreading of malignant cells is called **metastasis**. One reason that lung cancer is so deadly (more women die from it than from breast cancer) is that it can metastasize for a fairly long time before it is even diagnosed in the lungs. By the time it is discovered, tumors may be growing in the liver, bones, brain, and other parts of the body, making long-term survival very difficult.

Sexual reproduction is different from mitosis because sperm and egg must have only half the number of chromosomes as other cells. **Meiosis** is the term for the division of cells necessary for sexual reproduction to occur. This process will be discussed in Chapter 18, "The Reproductive System."

MICROORGANISMS

As in any city, you have a large and diverse population. Although the vast majority of the population are good citizens who provide positive contributions to the city, some can cause problems. The same can be said for the world of microorganisms. The following "microcitizens" of our city will now be discussed: bacteria, viruses, fungi, protozoa, and prions.

Bacteria

When you hear the word **bacteria**, you probably first think of an organism that produces disease, or what is called a **pathogen** (*path/o* = disease, *gen* = producing). You are somewhat correct in assuming so because bacteria make up the largest group of pathogens. Some bacterial pathogens even release toxic substances in your body. Bacteria grow rapidly and reproduce by splitting in half, sometimes doubling as rapidly as every 30 minutes!

You will also learn throughout this book that bacteria are often harmless and, in fact, essential for life. These bacteria live within or on us and are part of what is known as our **normal flora**. For example, certain bacteria in your intestine help in digesting food, and some help in synthesizing vitamin K, which helps clot blood so we don't bleed to death when we get a cut or scrape. See **FIGURE 4–14** ■, which shows examples of various types of bacteria.

Amazing Facts

Bacterial Reproduction

Bacteria can reproduce so rapidly that an individual cell can become two cells in minutes! These two cells can now become four cells and so on and so on. No wonder a bacterial infection can get out of hand so fast.

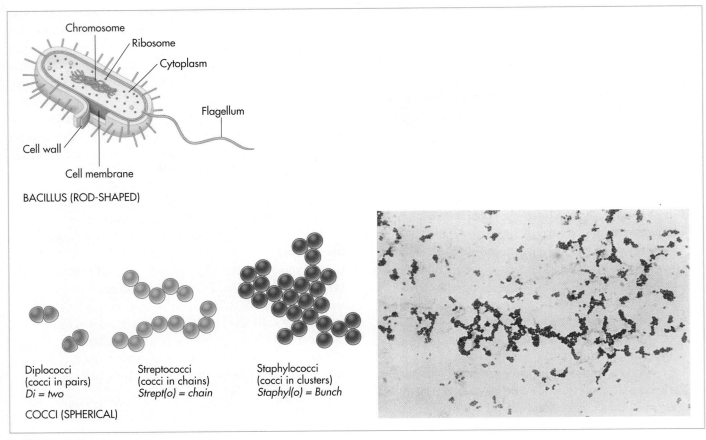

FIGURE 4–14 ■

Types of bacteria.

Viruses

An even more basic pathogen is a **virus** (see **FIGURE 4–15 ■**). Viruses (from a Latin term meaning "poison") are infectious particles that have a core containing genetic material (codes to replicate) surrounded by a protective protein coat called a **capsid**. Some viruses have an additional layer, or membrane, surrounding the capsid. Viruses are interesting because they cannot grow, "eat," or reproduce by themselves. They must enter another cell (host cell) and hijack that cell's parts, energy supply, and materials to do all the aforementioned activities. In addition, each virus must target specific cells in the body to claim as hosts. For example, the viruses that cause a cold target the cells found in the respiratory system, and the viruses that cause polio target cells that are found in the tissues of your nervous system. Most of the upper respiratory infections that people get are caused by viruses, and like all viral infections, they do not respond to antibiotics.

It is interesting to note (or disturbing for those of you who worry about everything) that viruses can stay dormant in the body and become active once again later in life. This is true for all of us who have had chicken pox. Those viruses stay in the body and may later become active and cause a potentially painful skin condition called *shingles*, caused by the *herpes zoster* virus. It is also interesting to note that the actual virus is relatively easy to kill by itself, but once it becomes part of a cell, it is hard to kill without harming the individual cell.

Fungi

Fungi, which is the plural form of **fungus**, can be either one-celled or multicelled organisms. These plantlike organisms have tiny filaments, called **mycelia**, that travel out from the cell to find and absorb nutrients. Like bacteria, fungi, such

Amazing Facts

Magnetotaxis: Some Bacteria Respond to Magnetic Fields

Believe it or not, some bacteria can sense and respond to a magnetic field. These types of bacteria are sensitive to Earth's magnetic field and orient themselves to this force! This ability to move in response to magnetic forces is called *magnetotaxis*. This discovery was made by Richard Blakemore as he observed bacteria living in sulfide-rich mud from a lake. As he changed the position of the mud, the bacteria would reorient themselves to Earth's magnetic field. After further examination, Blakemore determined that these bacteria possessed particles of iron oxide, a magnetic metal compound that is stored in a cell structure called the *magnetosome*.

as edible mushrooms, can be good, but in certain situations they can also cause problems (see **FIGURE 4–16 ■**). Fungi also can spread through the release of **spores**. Normally, we are not affected by fungi, but if the body has a problem with its immune system, then fungi have a chance to cause an infection. If tissue becomes damaged, fungi can more easily create an infection. Wind may pick up and carry spores that can be inhaled, potentially causing lung infections. Interestingly, you can inhale fungi spores and still not develop an infection. It is estimated that in certain regions of the United States up to 80 percent of the population have tested positive for the inhalation of certain fungi! Examples of fungal infections are athlete's foot and a mouth fungus called *thrush* or *candidiasis*.

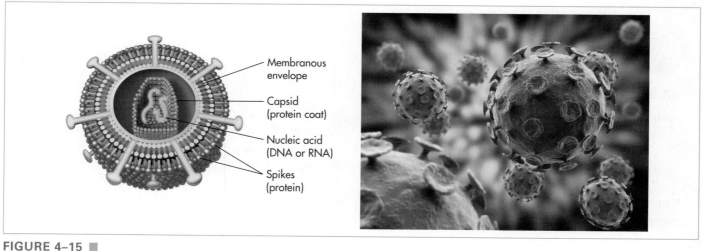

FIGURE 4–15 ■

A virus.

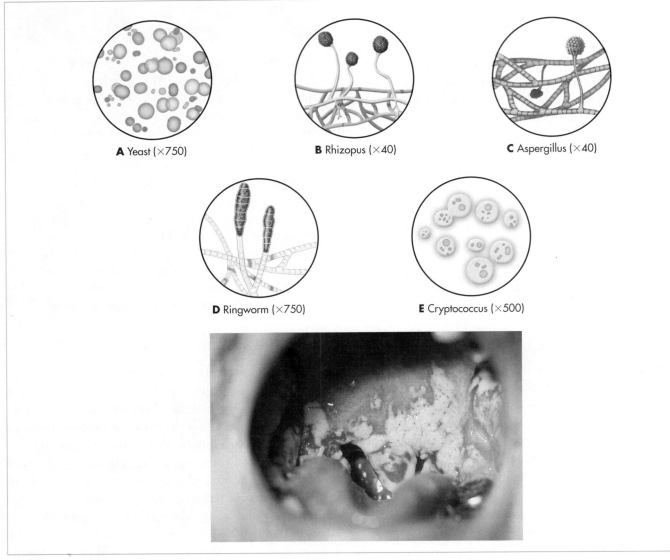

A Yeast (×750) B Rhizopus (×40) C Aspergillus (×40)

D Ringworm (×750) E Cryptococcus (×500)

FIGURE 4–16 ■

Types of fungi and a fungal infection of the palate.

Clinical Application

CLARIFYING A CONFUSING TERM

Although *antibiotic* technically means "against all life," it usually refers only to antibacterial agents and is therefore used to treat bacterial infections. There are specific antiviral agents for viral infections, and antibiotics should NOT be used to treat viral infections. The term anti-infectives can include antibiotics to treat bacterial infections, antiviral agents, antifungal agents and antiprotozoal agents. The misuse of antibiotics to treat nonbacterial infections and the poor patient compliance in taking the antibiotics have led to resistant strains being developed. One such strain is Methicillin Resistance *Staphylococcus Aureus* (MRSA) and has led to severe infectious outbreaks and death.

Protozoa

Protozoa are one-celled animal-like organisms that can be found in water, such as ponds, and in soil. Disease caused by these microorganisms can result from swallowing them (such as by drinking contaminated water) or from being bitten by insects that carry them in their bodies (such as malaria-carrying mosquitoes). See **FIGURE 4–17** ■.

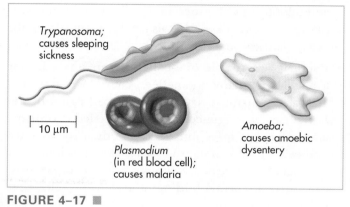

FIGURE 4–17 ■

Protozoa.

Prions

Although prions are not true organisms, they are abnormal pathogenic agents and have been included here with the other pathogens because you might hear this term in related discussions. First hypothesized in the 1960s and later isolated in the mid 1980s, this agent is able to cause an abnormal folding of specific normal cellular proteins. Tissue that is affected by the prions is full of microscopic holes causing the tissue to exhibit a spongy architecture. See **FIGURE 4–18** ■ for an example.

Since a vast amount of these proteins is found in the brain, prions have been recognized as the causative agent in certain brain diseases that exhibit neuronal loss and brain inflammation. Although rare in occurrence, these conditions are rapidly progressive and are also always fatal. In humans, Creutzfeldt-Jakob Disease (CJD) is one example, as are the diseases Chronic Wasting Disease (CWD) and Scrappie in animals.

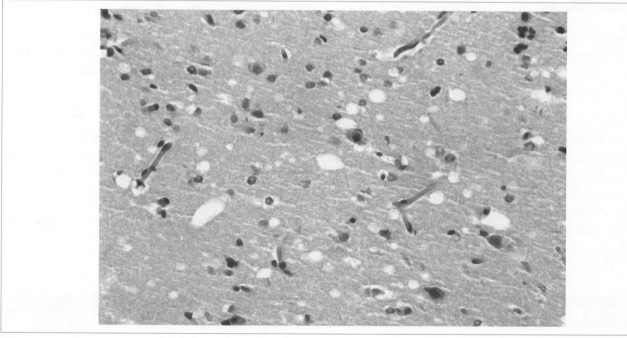

FIGURE 4–18 ■

A histologic slide showing the sponge-like architecture of a patient with Creutzfeldt-Jakob Disease.

- All living organisms are made of one or more cells. Cells are the fundamental units of living organisms. Even though cells are the fundamental units, they are composed of a variety of parts that are necessary for proper cellular function. These small parts are called *organelles*.

- Substances can cross the cell membrane via passive or active transport. Passive transport can occur through diffusion, facilitated diffusion, osmosis, or filtration. Active transport can occur through active transport pumps, endocytosis, or exocytosis.

- For cells to carry out metabolism, they must have energy in the form of ATP, which is made via a complex series of reactions called *cellular respiration*.

- Cells and tissues grow, are replaced, and are repaired by asexual reproduction. Cells make identical copies of themselves. This takes place all over your body whenever tissues grow or are repaired. Asexual reproduction in eukaryotic cells is accomplished by a relatively complex process called *mitosis* and *cytokinesis*. Mitosis, the division of the genetic material, takes place in four phases: prophase, metaphase, anaphase, and telophase. Cytokinesis is the division of the cytoplasm and organelles. Mitosis produces two daughter cells, identical to each other.

- Bacteria are simple one-celled organisms without a nucleus or many organelles. A virus is not a one-celled organism; it needs another cell to replicate. Fungi can be single-celled or multicelled organisms and can cause infections in the body. Protozoa are one-celled and can cause disease through ingestion or insect bites. Prions, although not true organisms, can cause abnormal folding of certain proteins that can lead to disease.

CASE STUDY

Given the following scenarios, identify what type of microorganism may be the causative agent.

a. Two young boys complain of a stomach ache and severe diarrhea after drinking pond water.

_____

b. Julia is a 13-year-old with a compromised immune system due to an inherited disease. Two days after returning home from a school field trip to a mushroom factory, Julia complains of shortness of breath and is diagnosed with a respiratory infection.

_____

c. Dylan has had a stubborn cold for three days and is given an antibacterial agent. However, he doesn't respond to the treatment, and the cold persists.

_____

d. Maria stepped on piece of broken glass and cut the bottom of her foot. Two days later the wound became red and swollen with pus oozing from the center.

_____

REVIEW QUESTIONS

Multiple Choice

1. The cell membrane can best be described as
   a. permeable to all materials.
   b. nonpermeable.
   c. rigid.
   d. selectively permeable.

2. All the following are passive forms of transport *except*
   a. facilitated diffusion.
   b. exocytosis.
   c. osmosis.
   d. filtration.

3. With a greater concentration of a solute, what will happen to osmotic pressure?
   a. It will become less.
   b. It will become greater.
   c. It will remain the same.
   d. There is no relation between osmotic pressure and the concentration of solute.

4. Which molecule is broken down during cellular respiration?
   a. oxygen
   b. water
   c. carbon dioxide
   d. glucose

5. Which microorganism can cause disease?
   a. bacteria
   b. fungi
   c. virus
   d. all the above

Matching

Match the following parts of the cell with their function:

_____ nucleus
_____ cell membrane
_____ Golgi apparatus
_____ mitochondria
_____ cytoplasm
_____ lysosome

a. makes ATP
b. processing, packaging, and shipping of materials
c. separates the cell from the environment
d. contains genetic material and cell instructions
e. the internal liquid environment inside the cell
f. contains hydrolytic enzymes to dissolve cellular materials

Short Answer

1. List and describe the four methods of passive transport.

_____

_____

_____

_____

2. Why do viruses need cells?

_____

_____

3. How does passive transport differ from active transport?

_____

_____

_____

_____

4. Explain the molecules used and produced during cellular respiration.

_____

_____

5. List and describe the types of microorganisms.

_____

_____

_____

_____

6. Describe prions and their relationship to disease.

_____

_____

_____

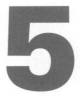

5

Tissues and Systems

THE INSIDE STORY

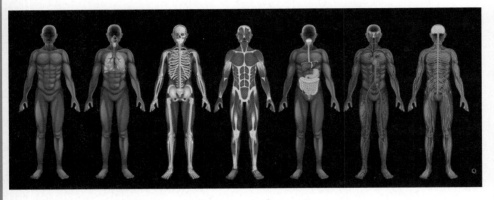

Previously, we discussed cells as the basic building blocks of the body. In this chapter, we explore tissues, which are collections of similar cells. To give a health-related analogy, we can consider cells to be individual health facility employees. At the next level, we can think of tissue as a group of those employees who have the same or similar educational background and perform similar functions, such as radiologic technicians, at a hospital. A combination of tissues designed to perform a specific function or several functions is called an **organ**. This could be compared to an x-ray department in the hospital, where specific functions such as x-rays, CT scans, MRIs, and barium swallows (a procedure, not a bird!) are performed. Organs that work together to perform specific activities, often with the help of accessory structures, form **systems**. We can compare a system to a hospital that provides a service (health care) to the citizens of our city through the combination of all the departments: laboratory, nursing, respiratory care, physical therapy, dietetics, housekeeping, and so on. This chapter provides an overview of tissues, organs, and systems, which will be expanded on in later chapters.

LEARNING OUTCOMES

At the end of your journey through this chapter, you will be able to:

- Explain the relationship between cells, tissues, organs, and organ systems.
- List and describe the four main types of tissues and variations within each type.
- Identify and describe the various body membranes.
- Differentiate the three main types of muscle tissue.
- Describe the main components of nervous tissue.
- List and describe the main functions of the body systems.

Pronunciation Guide Pro·nun·ci·a·tion

Correct pronunciation is important in any journey so that you and others are completely understood. Here is a "see and say" Pronunciation Guide for the more difficult terms to pronounce in this chapter. Please note that even though there are standard pronunciations, regional variations of the pronunciations can occur.

cuboidal (cue BOYD al)
cutaneous membranes (cue TAY nee us)
epithelial tissue (ep ih THEE lee al)
genitourinary (JEN eh toe YUR ih nair ee)
glia (GLEE ah)
lacunae (luh KOO nay)
meninges (men IN jeez)
neuroglia (noo ROG lee uh)
neuron (NOO ron)

parietal (pah RYE eh tal)
serous membrane (SEER us)
squamous (SKWAY mus)
stratified (STRAT ih fied)
striated muscle (STRY ate ed)
synovial membrane (sin OH vee al)
transitional (tran ZISH un al)
visceral (VISS er al)

OVERVIEW OF TISSUES

Just as there are many different types of cells with various functions and responsibilities, tissues come in different shapes and sizes, with their structure dependent on their function(s) and vice versa. Let's begin to explore the different tissue types.

Tissue Types

Tissue is a collection of similar cells that act together to perform a function. Imagine individual cells as bricks. Placing these bricks (cells) in a specific pattern creates the functional wall (tissue) of a building. There are many different types of tissues, depending on the required function. The four main types of tissues are

- Epithelial
- Connective
- Muscle
- Nervous

Let's take a closer look at these major types of tissue and their subdivisions.

Epithelial Tissue

Similar in purpose to the plastic wrap we use to keep food fresh or to cover bowls in the refrigerator, epithelial tissue (or epithelium) not only covers and lines much of the body but also covers many of the parts found in the body. The cells of epithelial tissue are packed tightly together, forming a sheet that usually contains no blood vessels.

The epithelium in the gastrointestinal tract is an exception, where capillaries do exist.

We can classify epithelial cells by their shape and arrangement. These cells can be flat or scalelike (**squamous**), cube-shaped (**cuboidal**), columnlike (**columnar**), or stretchy and variably shaped (**transitional**). If these cells are arranged in a single layer, we classify them as *simple*. If they are arranged in several layers, we say they are **stratified**, and they are named by the type of cell that is on the *outer layer* (such as stratified columnar). There is even a type of epithelium that looks stratified but isn't. It is called **pseudostratified**. The function required of the tissue dictates which type of cell formation is used. For example, simple squamous cells are utilized in the lungs because of their flat, thin design, which makes for easy transfer of oxygen from the lungs to the blood. Transitional epithelium is made of multiple layers of cells that can expand and contract, and therefore is used in the urinary bladder and urethra, both of which require their ability to expand and stretch with fluid. **FIGURE 5–1** ■ shows the types and locations of epithelial tissues. These are further discussed in later chapters.

Membranes Generally, *membranes* are sheetlike structures found throughout the body that perform special functions. Although membranes can be classified as organs, we discuss them along with tissues for ease of explanation. Membranes classified as *epithelial* membranes possess a layer of epithelial tissue and a thin bottom layer of a specialized connective tissue. Epithelial membranes are classified into

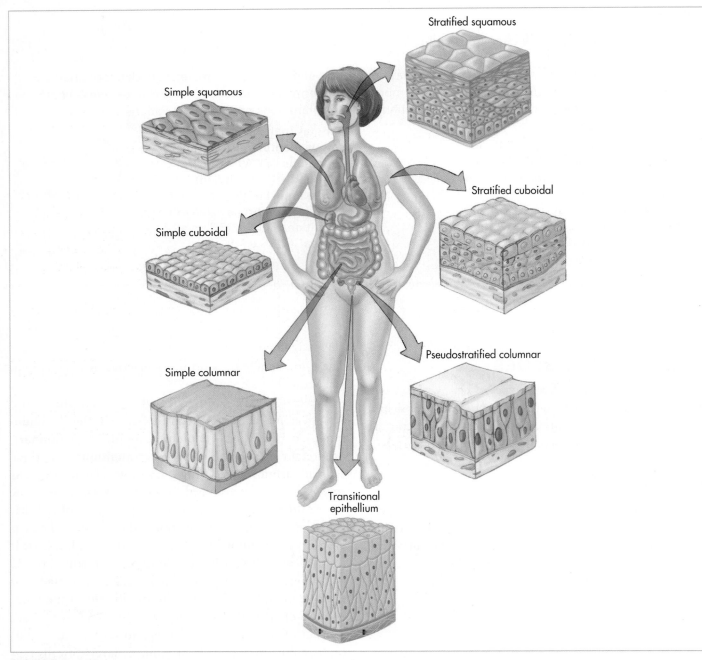

FIGURE 5–1 ■

Types and locations of epithelial tissues.

three general categories, as you can see in **TABLE 5–1** ■. **FIGURE 5–2** ■ shows the location of the serous and mucous membranes of the body.

Connective Tissue

Connective tissue, the most common tissue, is found throughout the body. That is because it is found in organs, bones, muscles, membranes, and skin. Connective tissue's functions include holding things together, providing structure and support, storing fluids and nutrients, and defending against infection. Connective tissue is structurally different from epithelial tissue because it has relatively fewer cells, and these cells are embedded in an extracellular *matrix* that gives each type of connective tissue its particular properties. A matrix is noncellular material in which cells can be embedded. (Think of a gelatin mold with gelatin and fruit inside.) Connective tissue can be divided into four subcategories: connective tissue proper, cartilage, bone, and blood/lymph fluid.

TABLE 5–1 TYPES OF EPITHELIAL MEMBRANES

1. Cutaneous	The main organ of the integumentary system, commonly known as your skin.
	Functions like a tarp placed over a boat.
	Makes up approximately 16 percent of total body weight.
	Skin is the largest organ.

2. Serous	A two-layered membrane with a potential (fluid-filled) space in between.
	Comprised of the parietal and visceral layers.
Parietal	Parietal means "wall"; this membrane lines the wall of the ventral body cavities in which organs reside.
	Produces serous fluid, which reduces friction between different tissues and organs. (Without this friction-reducing fluid, each heart beat and every breath would be uncomfortable. The effect is similar to running water over a sheet of plastic placed on the grass. You can run, jump onto the plastic, and slide. Imagine how that would feel without the water running over the plastic!) Also effectively adheres the layers together like a wet glass on a coaster.
Visceral	The combining form *viscer/o* refers to organs, therefore this membrane wraps around the individual organs
	Also produces serous fluid, which reduces friction between different tissues and organs.

| 3. Mucous | Lines openings to the outside world, such as your digestive tract, respiratory system, and urinary and reproductive tracts. |
| | Called mucous membranes because they contain specialized cells that produce mucus. Mucus can act as a lubricant, like the oil in a car. Mucus also serves several other important purposes besides grossing you out, as you will see in future chapters. |

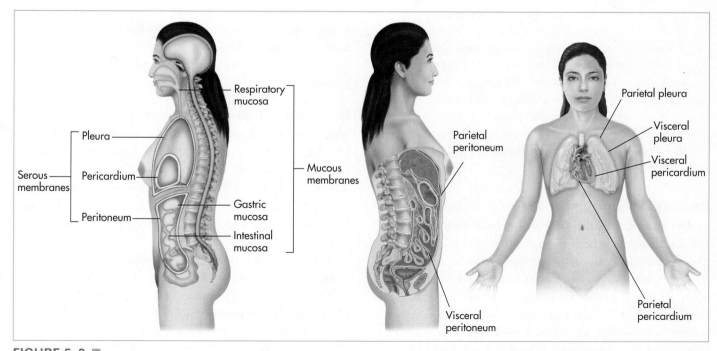

FIGURE 5–2 ■

Location of serous and mucous membranes.

Amazing Facts

Mucociliary Escalator

Keep in mind that the tissue structure determines its function. You will see stratified tissue where structural integrity is important due to its many layers. Simple squamous is found in the alveoli of the lung where gas exchange takes place and therefore is only one-cell layer thick. It is critical to keep the airways of the respiratory system free of debris. The specialized epithelium that serves this purpose is called *ciliated pseudostratified columnar*. The cilia beat at an amazing rate of approximately 1,500 per minute to help "sweep" the airways clean by moving secretions and foreign bodies up and out of the airways. Notice in the micrograph (photograph of an object seen through a microscope) the cilia at the top of the long single layer of columns. The epithelium falsely appears to be several layers due to the nuclei being staggered inside the individual columns.

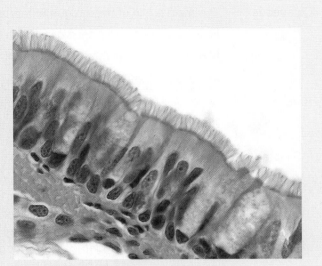

Pseudostratified ciliated columnar epithelium of the airways.

Amazing Facts

Skin and Vitamin Production

You know that you get vitamins and minerals from the foods you eat and the supplements you take, but did you know that your skin produces the specific vitamin D_3 when you are exposed to sunlight? Recently there has been some controversy regarding the excessive use of sunscreen which may significantly reduce the skin's ability to produce vitamin D_3. Current research indicates that under normal condition that sunscreens do not significantly result in vitamin D deficiency.

Connective Tissue Proper Examples of connective tissue proper include fine, delicate webs of loose connective tissue (*areolar tissue*) that hold tissues and organs together. Fat is also a loose connective tissue proper known as *adipose tissue*. Although we always seem to want to lose fat, we truly need some fat in our bodies for proper functioning because it is used for energy storage and cushioning. Connective tissue proper can also be more densely packed (dense connective tissue) and form strong cordlike structures similar to wire cables on suspension bridges. Tendons and ligaments are composed of dense connective tissue.

Cartilage and Bone Cartilage has its cells (chondrocytes) embedded in tiny holes (**lacunae**) in a gelatinous matrix. Cartilage is a much firmer tissue than connective tissue proper and is able to withstand pressure. Bone is the hardest of your body's tissues. Bone cells (osteocytes), like cartilage cells, live in lacunae. Bone matrix, however, is made mainly of calcium and phosphate and thus is very hard. Cartilage and bone are the main tissues of your skeleton, which supports your body and stores nutrients and minerals.

Blood and Lymph as Connective Tissues Even though blood and lymph are fluid, they are considered to be connective tissue because they are a liquid mixture comprised of a group of cells that have specialized functions. These fluid connective tissues contain specialized cells and dissolved proteins suspended in a watery substance. We expand on these two very important tissues in later chapters.

FIGURE 5–3 ■ illustrates the various types of connective tissues and shows some of the places they are found.

The membrane type associated with connective tissue is the **synovial membrane**. This important membrane type is found in the spaces between joints and produces a slippery substance called *synovial fluid*, which greatly reduces friction when joints move. FIGURE 5–4 ■ shows a synovial joint and membrane.

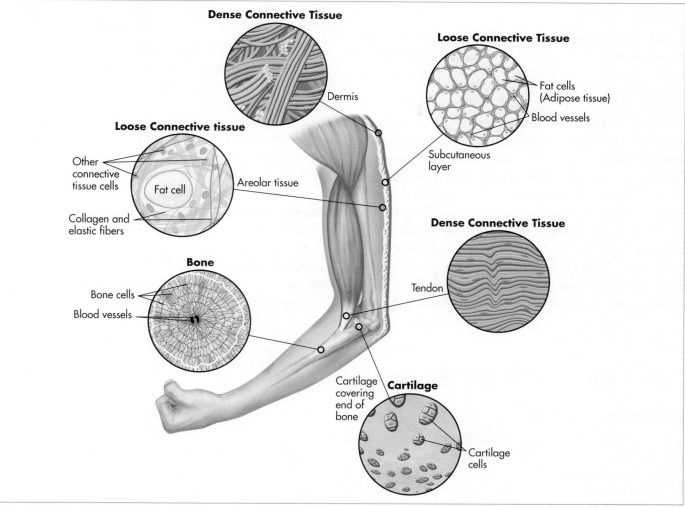

FIGURE 5–3 ■

Types and locations of connective tissues.

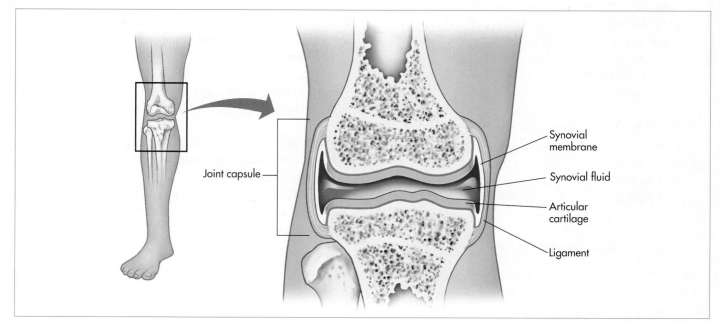

FIGURE 5–4 ■

The synovial joint and membrane.

Muscle Tissue

Muscle tissue provides the means for movement by and within the body. This form of tissue has the ability to shorten itself (contractility). There are three types of muscle tissue: skeletal, cardiac, and smooth.

Skeletal Muscle Skeletal muscle (often described as **striated muscle** because of its striped appearance) is attached to bones and causes movement by contracting and relaxing. It also surrounds certain openings of the body, such as the mouth, and controls the size of the opening. Unless you are a ventriloquist, it is very hard to speak clearly without moving your lips. The cells that make up this tissue type are long and fiberlike, with many nuclei in each cell. Your brain thinks about moving or speaking and causes the correct muscle to contract. Because this is a conscious effort, we call these muscles *voluntary* muscles.

Cardiac Muscle Cardiac muscle, which is found in the walls of the heart, is *involuntary* muscle because the heart beats without conscious input. We cannot think about our heartbeat and change it at will. Like skeletal muscle, cardiac muscle is striated, but the cells are branched and have a single nucleus in each cell. The cells in this tissue type interlock

TEST YOUR KNOWLEDGE 5–1

Choose the best answer:

1. An epithelial tissue with cells of many different shapes is called
   a. pseudostratified.
   b. columnar.
   c. transitional.
   d. cuboidal.

2. In which of these places would you find a serous membrane?
   a. joint cavity
   b. thoracic cavity
   c. vertebral cavity
   d. orbital cavity

3. A torn ligament indicates damage to what kind of tissue?
   a. dense
   b. cuboidal
   c. areolar
   d. mucus

4. Epithelial cells are named for their
   a. size.
   b. matrix type.
   c. shape.
   d. function.

5. Given that your mouth must be protected from heat, cold, and abrasion from food, which type of epithelium most likely lines your mouth?
   a. simple squamous
   b. stratified squamous
   c. simple columnar
   d. pseudostratified columnar

6. The heart is surrounded by a membrane. What kind of membrane would surround the heart?
   a. cutaneous
   b. synovial
   c. mucous
   d. serous

7. What type of tissue is utilized in the urinary bladder and urethra due to its elastic properties?
   a. transportation
   b. pseudostratified columnar
   c. transitional
   d. mucous

with each other, promoting more efficient contraction, as you will learn in Chapter 13, "The Cardiovascular System."

Smooth Muscle **Smooth muscle** tissue forms the walls of hollow organs, such as in our digestive system (which is why it is often called *visceral* muscle) and blood vessels. Because we don't have to consciously think about digesting food, it should be no surprise that this type of muscle is also *involuntary*. The ability to move food through the esophagus is a result of a series of smooth muscle contractions called *peristalsis*. Smooth muscle also controls and maintains a certain diameter or opening in your blood vessels and airways and can therefore affect your blood pressure and ability to breathe. Cells forming this tissue are not as long and fibrous as skeletal muscle, and each cell has only one nucleus. Smooth muscle is so named because it has no striations. FIGURE 5–5 ■ shows the various types of muscle tissue.

Nervous Tissue

Nervous tissue acts as a rapid messenger service for the body, and its messages can cause actions to occur. There are two types of nerve cells. **Neurons** are the conductors of information, and **neuroglia** (sometimes called **glia**) cells function as support cells. *Glia* literally means "glue," hence the name for cells that hold nerve cells together. The combining form *dendr/o* means "tree" and the branchlike formations that make up part of the neuron, called **dendrites**, receive sensory information. The trunk-shaped structure, called the **axon**, transports information *away* from the cell body. There are membranes associated with nervous tissue, covering the brain and spinal cord, called **meninges**. Nervous tissue will be discussed in detail in Chapters 9 and 10 "The Nervous System, Parts One and Two." FIGURE 5–6 ■ shows the two types of nerve cells.

Tissue Repair

Just as the structure of a building can be damaged by fire, flood, insects, or simple wear and tear, tissues also can sustain damage. As a result, the body has developed ways to repair itself when tissues lose their ability to function. Right after an injury, if blood vessels are damaged, the wound fills with blood. Blood contains substances that cause it to clot. If the clot is exposed to air, it hardens to form a scab.

At the same time, inflammation occurs, with the symptoms of redness, swelling, heat, and pain. During inflammation, white blood cells enter to destroy any pathogens that

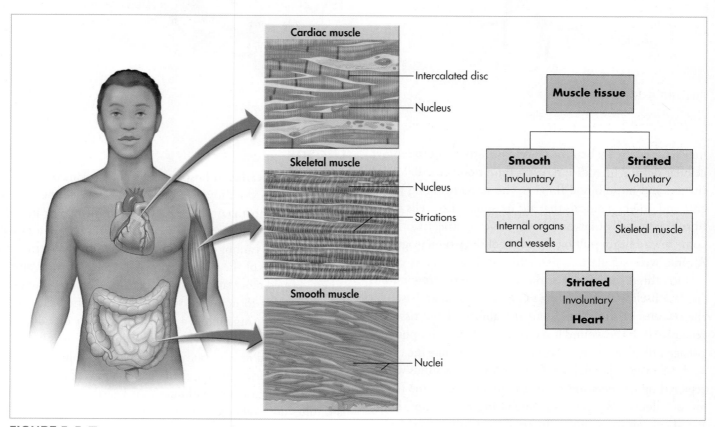

FIGURE 5–5 ■
Labeled diagram and flowchart of the three muscle tissue types.

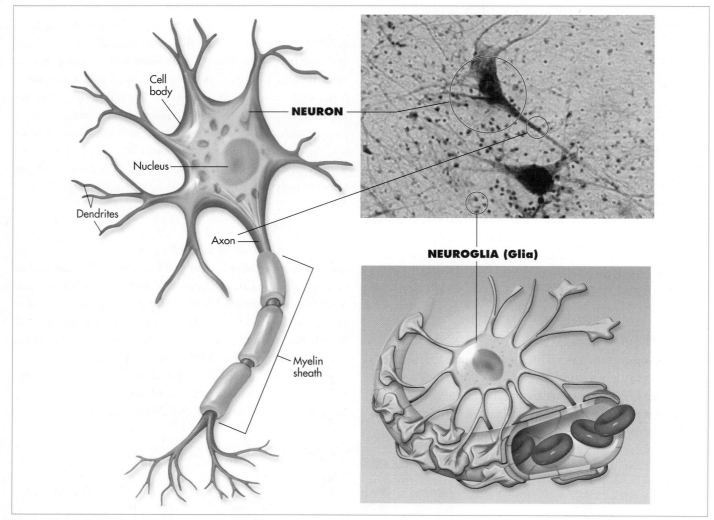

FIGURE 5–6 ■

The two main types of nerve cells.

may have entered when the wound occurred and to remove cellular debris. In addition, extra fluid floods the damaged tissues, and more blood flows to the scene bringing nutrients and other chemicals that aid healing. Next, cells called **fibroblasts** (cells that can develop into connective tissue) come in and begin pulling the edges of the wound together. A pink, well-vascularized tissue fills in the space.

After this tissue is in place, the tissue will either **regenerate** (replace itself with exactly the same tissue) or **scar**, based on the severity of the wound and the ability of the tissue to repair itself. If the wound is severe, a tough scar composed of collagen fibers may form. Scars can't function like the tissue, so the damage is permanent. Some less-severe wounds will be repaired by regeneration of the original tissue. Some tissues are excellent at regeneration, including epithelium, bone, blood, areolar tissue, and adipose tissue. Cardiac muscle and nervous tissue are basically unable to regenerate, even if damage is minor. Most other tissues are somewhere in between.

Organs

As mentioned earlier, a hospital department is made up of employees who work together to perform specific functions, much like an organ. An organ is the result of two or more types of tissues organized in a way that accomplishes a task that the tissues cannot do on their own. Some organs, those on the midline of the body, occur singly, such as the heart; others, located more laterally, occur in pairs, such as the lungs. It is interesting to note that we can survive quite well with only one healthy organ from a pair (such as a lung or kidney). Your heart, lungs, stomach, liver, and kidneys are all examples of organs found in your body. It is important to understand that not all your organs are *vital* organs. Vital organs are the ones that you can't live without. Your heart, brain, kidneys and lungs are vital organs. Organs that you can live without include your appendix, spleen, and gallbladder. TABLE 5–2 ■ is a quick reference to the various organs of the body.

Clinical Application

STEM CELLS

Stem cells are undifferentiated or unspecialized cells that can be induced to become tissue or organ specific cells. Because they have the ability for cell division, they can actually grow new healthy tissue. Therefore, stem cells can serve as an internal repair system for certain tissues. Stem cells can be harvested from both adult and embryonic sources. A recent type of stem cell is produced from genetically reprogrammed adult cells to assume a stem cell state (induced pluripotent stem cells or iPSCs). *Pluripotent* means the ability of a cell to differentiate into a variety of cell types. Research on stem cells continues to advance and evolve and provide great potential for cell-based therapies to treat disease in the emerging realm of **regenerative medicine**.

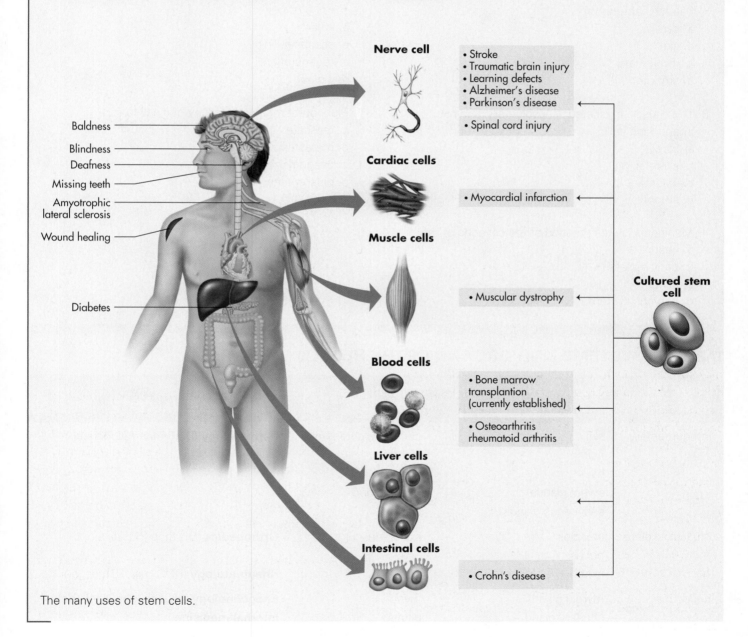

Baldness
Blindness
Deafness
Missing teeth
Amyotrophic lateral sclerosis
Wound healing
Diabetes

Nerve cell

- Stroke
- Traumatic brain injury
- Learning defects
- Alzheimer's disease
- Parkinson's disease
- Spinal cord injury

Cardiac cells

- Myocardial infarction

Muscle cells

- Muscular dystrophy

Blood cells

- Bone marrow transplantion (currently established)
- Osteoarthritis rheumatoid arthritis

Liver cells

Intestinal cells

- Crohn's disease

Cultured stem cell

The many uses of stem cells.

TEST YOUR KNOWLEDGE 5–2

Choose the best answer:

1. Which of the following cells are found only in the nervous system?
   a. transitional
   b. neurons
   c. cartilage
   d. bone

2. Which muscle allows you to walk around the mall on a Saturday afternoon?
   a. cardiac
   b. skeletal
   c. involuntary
   d. smooth

3. This muscle is striated, is involuntary, and has interlocking cells.
   a. cardiac
   b. skeletal
   c. voluntary
   d. smooth

4. Meningitis is inflammation of the covering of the
   a. heart.
   b. body surface.
   c. joints.
   d. nervous system.

5. The blood clot that forms in a wound that is exposed to air becomes a
   a. scar.
   b. scab.
   c. hematoma.
   d. keloid.

6. Wound healing can be accomplished by either scarring or
   a. inflammation.
   b. scabbing.
   c. regeneration.
   d. clotting.

7. Pluripotent means the ability of a cell to
   a. replicate.
   b. metastasize.
   c. phagocytize.
   d. differentiate.

TABLE 5–2 SYSTEMS AND ORGANS OF THE HUMAN BODY

BODY SYSTEM	ORGANS/STRUCTURES IN THE SYSTEM	COMBINING FORM	MEDICAL SPECIALTY
Integumentary	skin	dermat/o, cutane/o	**Dermatology** (DUR mah TOL oh jee)
	hair	trich/o	
	nails	ung/o	
	sweat glands	sud/o, hidr/o	
	sebaceous glands	seb/o	
Musculoskeletal	muscles	my/o, muscul/o	**Orthopedics** (OR thoh PEE diks)
	bones	oste/o	
	joints	arthr/o	**Rheumatology** (ROO mah TOL oh jee)
Endocrine	thyroid gland	thyr/o	**Endocrinology** (EN doh krin OL oh jee)
	pituitary gland	pituit/o	**Internal medicine**
	testes	test/o, orchi/o	
	ovaries	ovari/o, oophor/o	**Gynecology** (GUY neh KOL oh jee)
	adrenal glands	adren/o	
	pancreas	pancreat/o	

BODY SYSTEM	ORGANS/STRUCTURES IN THE SYSTEM	COMBINING FORM	MEDICAL SPECIALTY
	parathyroid glands	parathyroid/o	
	pineal gland	pineal/o	
	thymus gland	thym/o	
Cardiovascular	heart	cardi/o	**Cardiology** (car dee OL oh jee)
	blood	hemat/o, hem/o	**Hematology** (HEE mah TOL oh jee)
	arteries	arteri/o	**Internal medicine**
	veins	phleb/o, ven/o, veni/o	
Lymphatic and immune	spleen	splen/o	**Immunology** (IM yoo NOL oh jee)
	lymph vessels/nodes	lymph/o	
	thymus gland	thym/o	
Respiratory	nose	nas/o, rhin/o	**Otorhinolaryngology** (OH toh RYE noh LAHR in gol oh jee)
	pharynx	pharyng/o	**Thoracic** (thoh RASS ik) **surgery**
	larynx	laryng/o	
	trachea	trache/o	
	lungs	pneum/o	**Pulmonology** (pull mon OL oh jee)
	bronchial tubes	bronch/o	**Internal medicine**
Gastrointestinal	mouth	or/o	**Gastroenterology** (GAS troh EN ter OL oh jee)
	pharynx	pharyng/o	**Internal medicine**
	esophagus	esophag/o	
	stomach	gastr/o	
	small intestine	enter/o	
	colon	col/o, colon/o	**Proctology** (prok TOL oh jee) procto = anus
	liver	hepat/o	
	gallbladder	cholecyst/o	
	pancreas	pancreat/o	
Urinary	kidneys	nephr/o, ren/o	**Nephrology** (neh FROL oh jee)
	ureters	ureter/o	**Urology** (yoo ROL oh jee) uro = urine
	bladder	cyst/o, vesic/o	
	urethra	urethr/o	
Reproductive	ovaries	oophor/o	**Gynecology** gynec/o = woman
	uterus	uter/o, hyster/o	**Obstetrics** (ob STET riks)
	fallopian tubes	salping/o	
	vagina	vagin/o	
	mammary glands	mamm/o	
	testes	orchid/o	
	prostate	prostat/o	
	urethra	urethr/o	
Nervous	brain	encephal/o	**Neurology** (noo ROL oh jee)
	spinal cord	myel/o, spin/o	**Neurosurgery** (NUR oh SIR jeh ree)
	nerves	neur/o	
Senses	eyes	ocul/o, ophthalm/o	**Ophthalmology** (off thal MOL oh jee)
	ears	ot/o	**Otolaryngology** (OH toh LAHR in GOL oh jee)

SYSTEMS

A body system is formed by organs and other structures that work together to accomplish something more complex than what a single organ can do on its own. Take the heart, for example. Even if your heart is functioning perfectly, you would still die without all the other parts that make up the cardiovascular system. Much like a road system in the city, you need the arteries, veins, and blood to get vital oxygen and nutrients to the cells and to remove the waste products produced by those cells.

Although we discuss the body systems separately, it is extremely important that you understand that all the body systems are interrelated, often depending on each other for proper functioning.

Skeletal System

Throughout your journey, you will see many different kinds of buildings. The one thing all the buildings have in common is some sort of skeletal structure for support. Most people think that the skeleton's only job is to provide support and structure to the body, much like the framework of a house, but it does much more. The skeleton protects organs such as the brain; in combination with muscles, it provides movement; it acts as a storage vault for a variety of minerals, such as calcium and phosphorus; *and* it also produces blood cells! That's pretty impressive stuff! The main components of this system are bones, joints, ligaments, and cartilage. Refer to **FIGURE 5–7** ■, which shows the main components of the skeletal system.

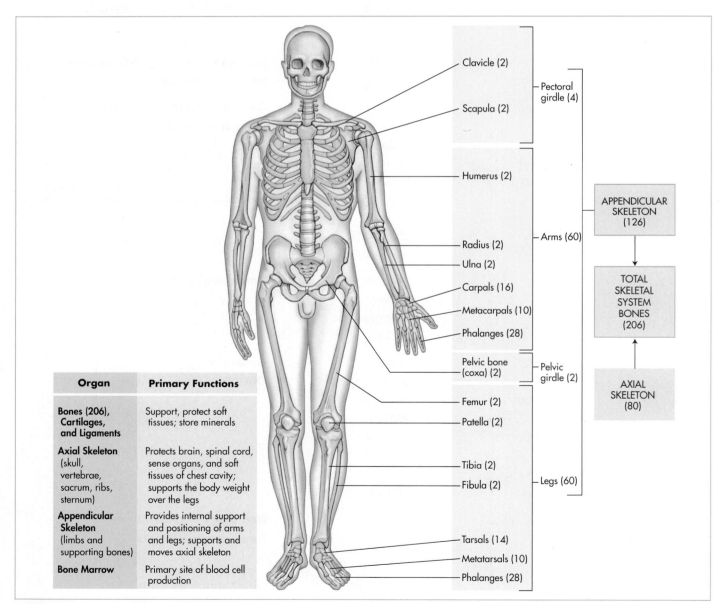

Organ	Primary Functions
Bones (206), Cartilages, and Ligaments	Support, protect soft tissues; store minerals
Axial Skeleton (skull, vertebrae, sacrum, ribs, sternum)	Protects brain, spinal cord, sense organs, and soft tissues of chest cavity; supports the body weight over the legs
Appendicular Skeleton (limbs and supporting bones)	Provides internal support and positioning of arms and legs; supports and moves axial skeleton
Bone Marrow	Primary site of blood cell production

FIGURE 5–7 ■

The skeletal system.

Muscular System

"All of this dry reading makes me thirsty. I think I'll go get something to drink." The muscular system is responsible for getting you up and over to that refrigerator (see **FIGURE 5–8** ■). This voluntary action is made possible by skeletal muscles that are attached to your bones. Two general classifications of muscle are *voluntary* (of which we just had an example) and *involuntary*. Involuntary muscles perform without consciously being told to do so. The smooth muscle found in the walls of organs, often called *visceral muscle*, and the muscle found in the heart, called *cardiac muscle*, are examples of involuntary muscles. Smooth muscle is also found in blood vessels and airways, where it helps control the diameter of passageways. So, the main parts of the muscle system are skeletal, smooth, and cardiac muscles. By the way, we were just kidding about the "dry" reading and know you're anxious to "move" on to the next system.

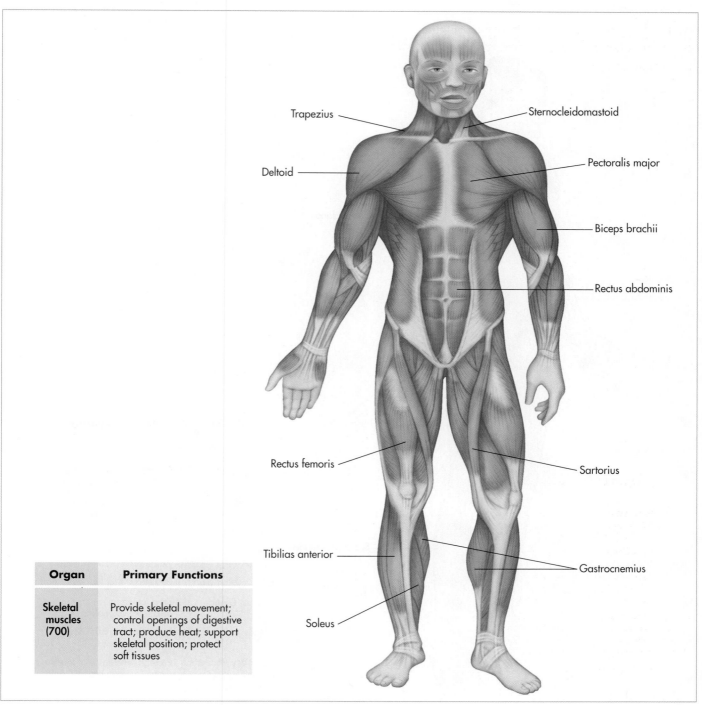

Organ	Primary Functions
Skeletal muscles (700)	Provide skeletal movement; control openings of digestive tract; produce heat; support skeletal position; protect soft tissues

FIGURE 5–8 ■

The muscular system.

Integumentary System

The body's first line of protection is your skin. Skin is the main part of the integumentary system. Besides protecting your body from invasion, the integumentary system also helps regulate body temperature through sweating, shivering, and changes in the diameter of blood vessels in the skin. Much of the sensory information received from the outside world (heat, cold, pain, pressure, etc.) comes from sensors in the skin. Glands in the skin help to lubricate and waterproof the skin and also inhibit the growth of unwanted bacteria. The main components of this system include skin, hair, sweat glands, sebaceous glands, and nails (see **FIGURE 5–9** ■).

Nervous System

Much like the activities of city hall, the nervous system is the rapid messenger system of the body that both receives and sends messages for activities to occur. The messages conducted by the

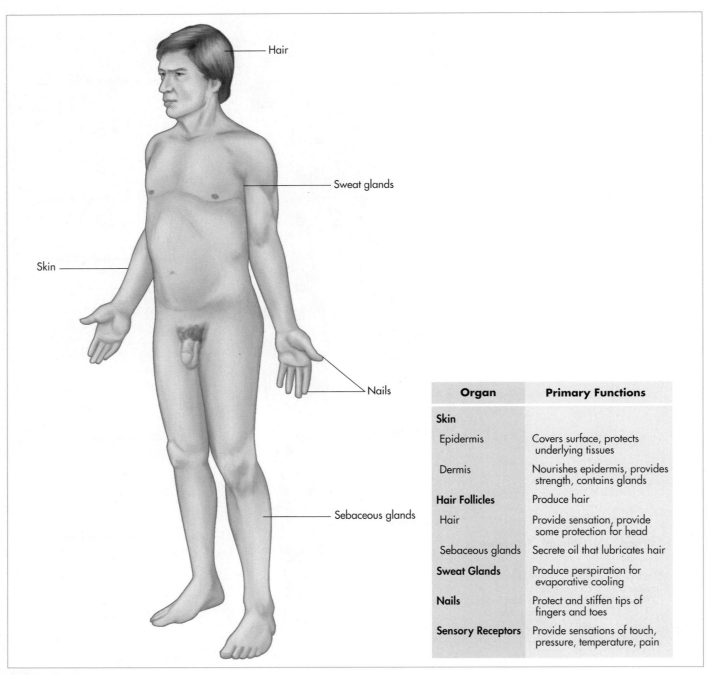

Organ	Primary Functions
Skin	
Epidermis	Covers surface, protects underlying tissues
Dermis	Nourishes epidermis, provides strength, contains glands
Hair Follicles	Produce hair
Hair	Provide sensation, provide some protection for head
Sebaceous glands	Secrete oil that lubricates hair
Sweat Glands	Produce perspiration for evaporative cooling
Nails	Protect and stiffen tips of fingers and toes
Sensory Receptors	Provide sensations of touch, pressure, temperature, pain

FIGURE 5–9 ■

The integumentary system.

nervous system are stimulated by the body's internal and external environments. This is important not only so we may experience the world around us but also to protect us from harm. Additionally, the nervous system monitors what is going on inside the body. How do we know when we are hungry or when we have had enough to eat? This information is obtained through **sensations**, which are measurements of conditions that occur inside and outside the body. These sensations are caused by stimulation of our sensory receptors. So, then, the three main functions of

the nervous system are sensory (receiving messages), processing and interpreting messages, and motor (acting on those messages). The main parts of the nervous system are the nerve cells (glial cells and neurons), the spinal cord with its spinal fluid, peripheral nerves, and of course, the brain. Because we are dealing with sensations, our special sensory organs include the eyes (sight), nose (smell), tongue (taste), and ears (for hearing *and* balance). We will place the senses in their own chapter later in this book. FIGURE 5–10 ■ depicts the nervous system.

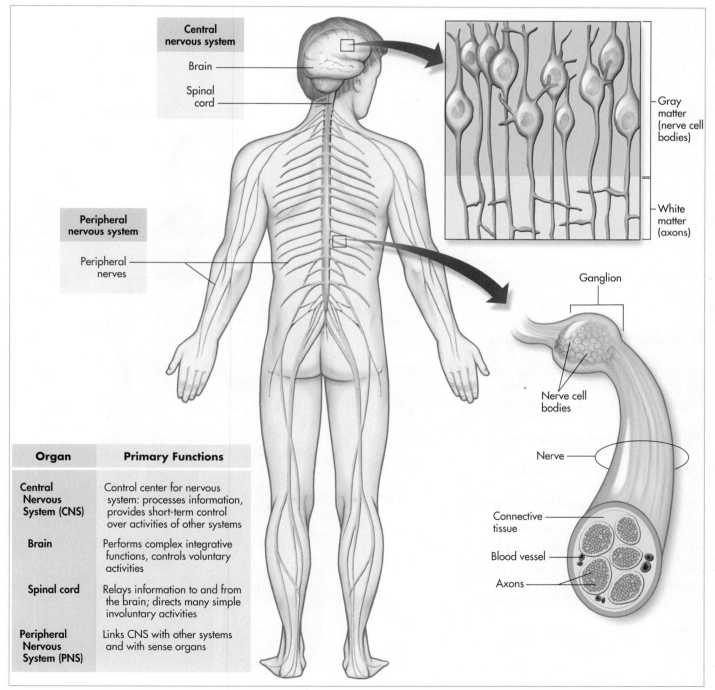

Organ	Primary Functions
Central Nervous System (CNS)	Control center for nervous system: processes information, provides short-term control over activities of other systems
Brain	Performs complex integrative functions, controls voluntary activities
Spinal cord	Relays information to and from the brain; directs many simple involuntary activities
Peripheral Nervous System (PNS)	Links CNS with other systems and with sense organs

FIGURE 5–10 ■

The nervous system.

Endocrine System

Although not as quick acting as the nervous system, the endocrine system also acts as a control center for virtually all the body's organs (see **FIGURE 5–11** ■). This control is accomplished through endocrine glands that release chemical substances called *hormones* that are circulated through the cardiovascular system. The endocrine system helps regulate the body's metabolic processes that utilize carbohydrates, fats, and proteins, and plays an important role in the rate of growth and reproduction. In addition, the endocrine system helps regulate the fluid and electrolyte balances of the body. If that weren't enough, the hormones produced by the endocrine system help you deal with general stress and the stresses produced by infection and trauma. The main parts of the endocrine system include the hypothalamus; pineal, pituitary, thyroid, parathyroid, thymus, and adrenal glands; the pancreas; and the gonads (testes in males and ovaries in females), plus a variety of hormones.

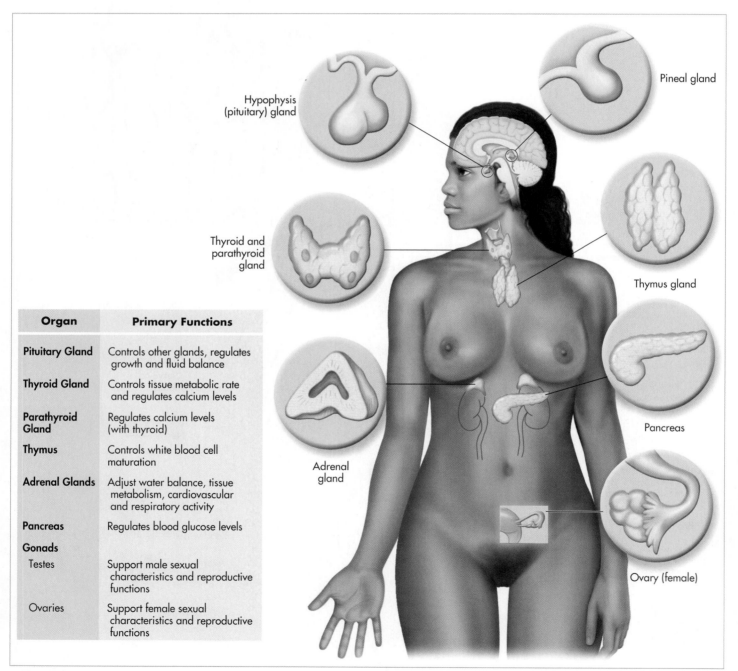

Organ	Primary Functions
Pituitary Gland	Controls other glands, regulates growth and fluid balance
Thyroid Gland	Controls tissue metabolic rate and regulates calcium levels
Parathyroid Gland	Regulates calcium levels (with thyroid)
Thymus	Controls white blood cell maturation
Adrenal Glands	Adjust water balance, tissue metabolism, cardiovascular and respiratory activity
Pancreas	Regulates blood glucose levels
Gonads	
Testes	Support male sexual characteristics and reproductive functions
Ovaries	Support female sexual characteristics and reproductive functions

FIGURE 5–11 ■

The endocrine system.

Cardiovascular System

Often referred to as the *circulatory system*, the cardiovascular system is the main transportation system to each cell of our body, much like the roads, sidewalks, and subways of our city. Please see **FIGURE 5–12** ■. Through this system, water, oxygen, and a variety of nutrients and other substances necessary for life are transported to the cells, and waste products are transported away from the cells. Also like our city, these routes can become clogged or blocked, causing major problems. Imagine what would happen to a busy four-lane highway if two of the lanes are shut down because of construction or an accident. The traffic would slow, and the pressure would build up because of the congestion, much like the blood flow does when arteries become partially obstructed. The buildup of pressure (hypertension) can be very dangerous. The main components of this system are the heart, arteries, veins, capillaries, and of course, the blood.

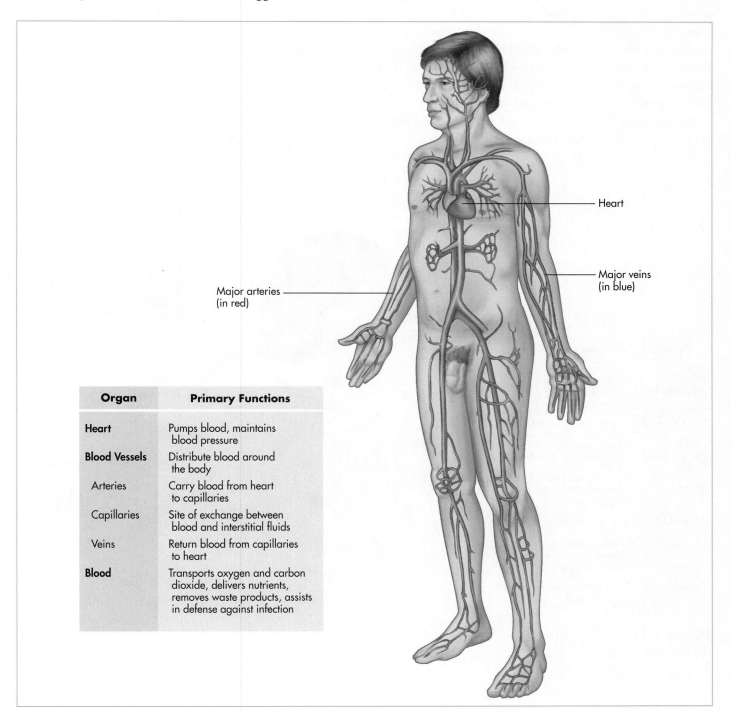

Organ	Primary Functions
Heart	Pumps blood, maintains blood pressure
Blood Vessels	Distribute blood around the body
Arteries	Carry blood from heart to capillaries
Capillaries	Site of exchange between blood and interstitial fluids
Veins	Return blood from capillaries to heart
Blood	Transports oxygen and carbon dioxide, delivers nutrients, removes waste products, assists in defense against infection

FIGURE 5–12 ▨

The cardiovascular system.

Respiratory System

Think about a time you went swimming and stayed a little too long underwater, and you will realize how important our respiratory system is! We all know the old concept of being able to live weeks without food and days without water, but think about how long you would last without oxygen. Without conscious effort, your lungs move approximately 12,000 quarts of air a day. Our respiratory system, much like the ventilation system in an office building, not only supplies us with fresh oxygen but performs several other important functions as well. Our lungs eliminate the carbon dioxide created as a result of cellular metabolism. The respiratory system filters, warms, and moistens air as it is inhaled. The mucous lining of the airway helps trap foreign particles and microorganisms. This system also helps to maintain the proper acid/base balance of the blood and aids in the elimination of ingested alcohol. The main parts of the respiratory system are the pharynx, larynx, trachea, bronchial tubes, and lungs (see **FIGURE 5–13** ■).

Lymphatic and Immune System

Much like the storm drain system of our city, the lymphatic system is a very important, but often forgotten, system. It is responsible for helping to maintain proper fluid balance in your body and for protecting it from infection. Excess body fluid that may collect in places it shouldn't is brought back into the lymphatic system, cleaned and processed, and then recirculated. Special structures called *lymph nodes* act as filters to capture unwanted infective agents. Lymph vessels and ducts, lymph nodes, the thymus gland, tonsils, and the spleen are the major parts of the immune system. In addition, the immune portion of the lymphatic system produces specialized infection-fighting white blood cells called *lymphocytes*. The immune system is

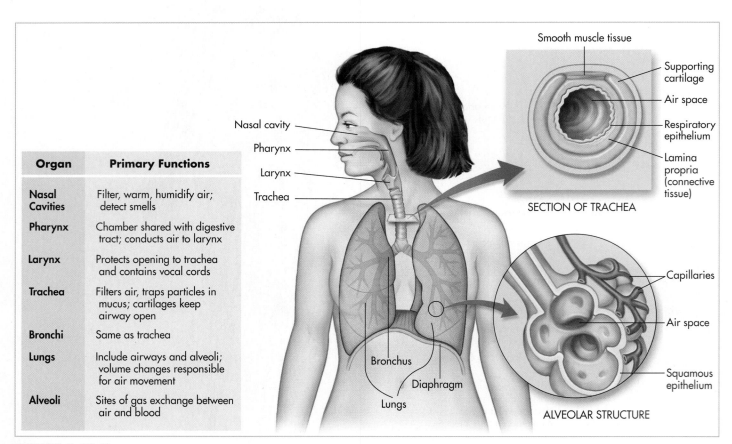

Organ	Primary Functions
Nasal Cavities	Filter, warm, humidify air; detect smells
Pharynx	Chamber shared with digestive tract; conducts air to larynx
Larynx	Protects opening to trachea and contains vocal cords
Trachea	Filters air, traps particles in mucus; cartilages keep airway open
Bronchi	Same as trachea
Lungs	Include airways and alveoli; volume changes responsible for air movement
Alveoli	Sites of gas exchange between air and blood

FIGURE 5–13

The respiratory system.

the police force of the human body, patrolling for harmful invaders (see **FIGURE 5–14** ■).

Gastrointestinal, or Digestive, System

The digestive system (often called the GI system by health care professionals) breaks down raw materials (food), both mechanically and chemically, into usable substances (see **FIGURE 5–15** ■). Once these usable substances are created, this system absorbs them for transportation to the cells of the body. Materials that aren't used, as well as cellular waste, are transported out of the body by this system, much like

the waste disposal and sewage system of our city. The main parts of the digestive system are the mouth, pharynx, esophagus, stomach, intestines, accessory organs, and anal canal.

Urinary System

Although the digestive system plays a large role in the elimination of certain digested waste, the urinary system plays an important role in the filtration of blood and the elimination of waste products such as forms of nitrogen. In addition, electrolytes, drugs and other toxins, and excessive water are removed.

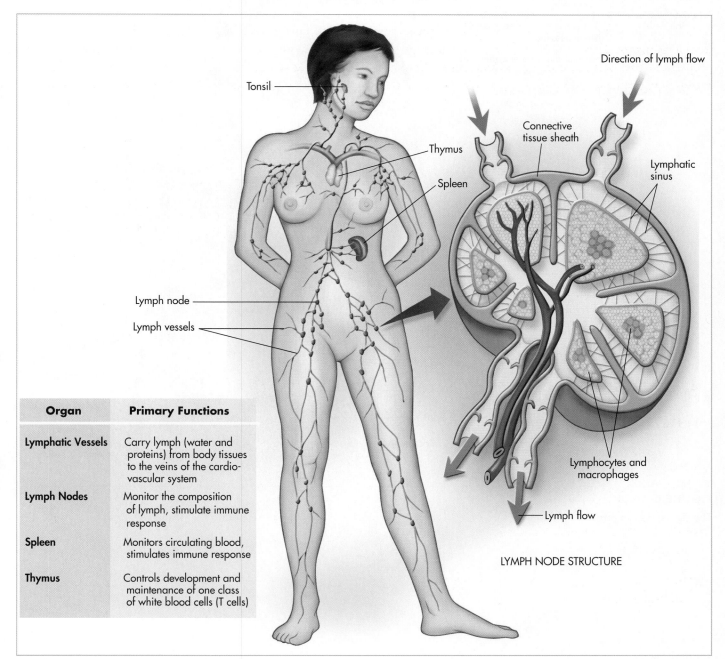

Organ	Primary Functions
Lymphatic Vessels	Carry lymph (water and proteins) from body tissues to the veins of the cardio-vascular system
Lymph Nodes	Monitor the composition of lymph, stimulate immune response
Spleen	Monitors circulating blood, stimulates immune response
Thymus	Controls development and maintenance of one class of white blood cells (T cells)

FIGURE 5–14 ■

The lymphatic system.

Organ	Primary Functions
Salivary Glands	Provide lubrication, produce buffers and the enzymes that begin digestion
Pharynx	Passageway connected to esophagus
Esophagus	Delivers food to stomach
Stomach	Secretes acids and enzymes
Small Intestine	Secretes digestive enzymes, absorbs nutrients
Liver	Secretes bile, regulates blood chemistry
Gallbladder	Stores bile for release into small intestine
Pancreas	Secretes digestive enzymes and buffers; contains endocrine cells
Large Intestine	Removes water from fecal material, stores waste

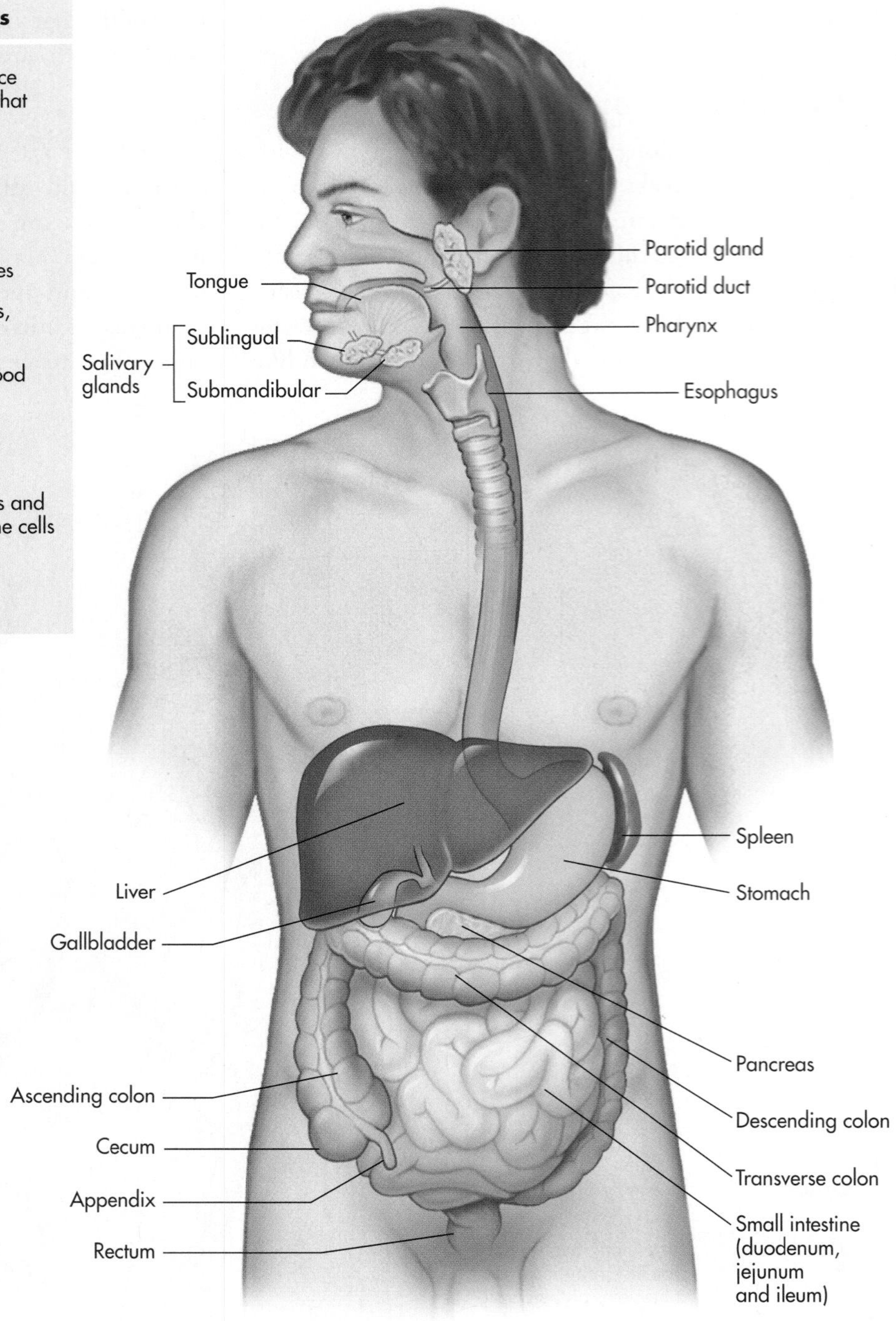

FIGURE 5–15 ■

The digestive system.

This system is crucial for maintaining the proper balance of water you have in your body and regulating your blood pressure. The urinary system helps regulate the number of red blood cells and the acid/base and electrolyte balance of blood. The main parts of the urinary system are the kidneys, ureters, urinary bladder, and urethra (see **FIGURE 5–16 ■**).

Reproductive System

We build new cities or new buildings to accommodate growing needs or to replace worn out structures. The reproductive system does the same thing. Quite simply,

without this system, we would not exist. The reproductive system is often combined with the urinary system to create the **genitourinary system** (or *GU system*). Humans require a male and female to produce offspring. The male is needed to provide sperm that contains certain genetic traits of that individual, whereas the female provides an egg with her traits and a place for the fertilized egg to grow to maturity. The main female parts of this system are the ovaries, eggs, fallopian tubes, uterus, and vagina. For men, the main parts are the testes, sperm, and penis (see **FIGURE 5–17 ■**).

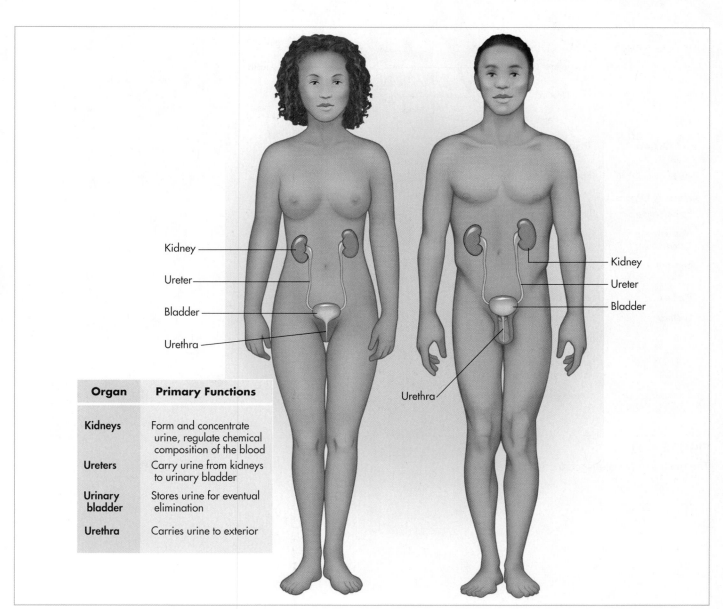

Organ	Primary Functions
Kidneys	Form and concentrate urine, regulate chemical composition of the blood
Ureters	Carry urine from kidneys to urinary bladder
Urinary bladder	Stores urine for eventual elimination
Urethra	Carries urine to exterior

FIGURE 5–16 ■

The female and male urinary systems.

Organ	Primary Functions (female)
Ovaries	Produce ova (eggs) and hormones
Uterine Tubes	Deliver ova or embryo to uterus; normal site of fertilization
Uterus	Site of development of offspring
Vagina	Site of sperm deposition; birth canal at delivery; provides passage of fluids during menstruation
Clitoris	Erectile organ, produces pleasurable sensations during sexual act
Labia	Contain glands that lubricate entrance to vagina
Mammary Glands	Produce milk that nourishes newborn infant

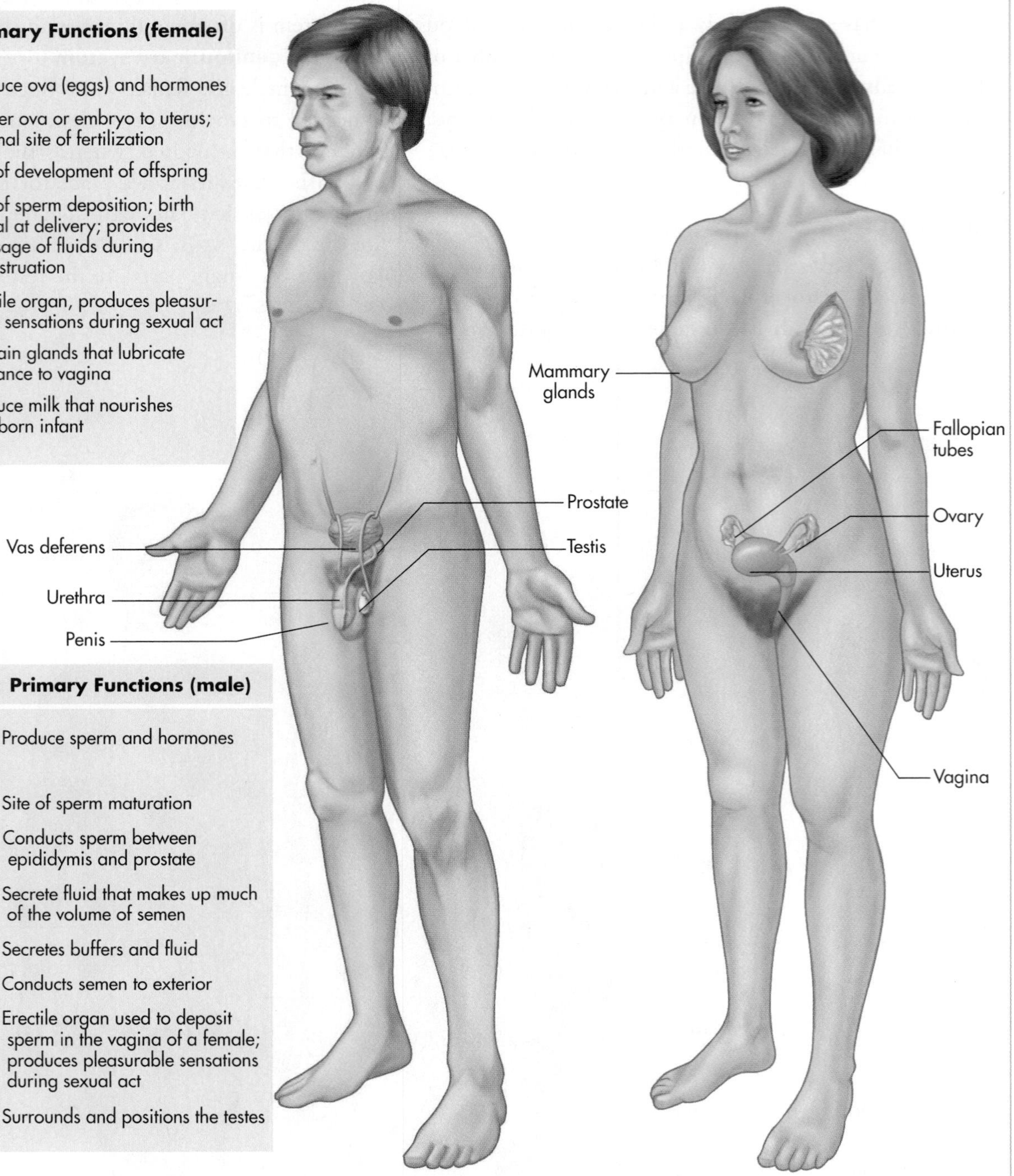

Organ	Primary Functions (male)
Testes	Produce sperm and hormones
Accessory Organs	
Epididymis	Site of sperm maturation
Vas deferens (sperm duct)	Conducts sperm between epididymis and prostate
Seminal vesicles	Secrete fluid that makes up much of the volume of semen
Prostate	Secretes buffers and fluid
Urethra	Conducts semen to exterior
Penis	Erectile organ used to deposit sperm in the vagina of a female; produces pleasurable sensations during sexual act
Scrotum	Surrounds and positions the testes

FIGURE 5–17 ■

The male and female reproductive systems.

TEST YOUR KNOWLEDGE 5–3

List the correct system for the following activities

1. Exchanges carbon dioxide for oxygen

_____

2. Eliminates nitrogen, drugs, and excessive water from the body

_____

3. Main storage for calcium

_____

4. Provides much of the sensory information from the external world

_____

5. Protects the body from invading pathogens

_____

6. Moves blood through the body

_____

7. Converts food to energy

_____

8. With the help of the sun, produces vitamin D

_____

9. Shares some structures with the urinary system

_____

SUMMARY: Points of Interest

- Cells are the basic building blocks of the body.
- Tissue is a collection of similar cells that act together to perform a function. The four main types of tissues are epithelial, connective, muscle, and nervous.
- Membranes are sheetlike structures found throughout the body; they perform specific functions. The four major membrane types are cutaneous, serous, mucous, and synovial.
- Tissues that combine to perform a specific function or functions are called an organ.
- Organs that work together, often with the help of accessory structures, to perform specific activities create a system.
- There are 11 major body systems: skeletal, muscular, integumentary, nervous, endocrine, cardiovascular, respiratory, lymphatic/immune, gastrointestinal, urinary, and reproductive. Even though these are distinct systems, they are interrelated, and their relationships are highlighted in upcoming chapters.

Mr. Harold Jenkins, a 73-year-old male presents to an emergency department of a local hospital. Initial assessment reveals the following:

- Afebrile
- Mild tachypnea with mild shortness of breath
- Acrocyanosis
- Mild tachycardia
- History of smoking
- History of diabetes
- Moderately overweight
- Family history of coronary artery disease

This problem is best worked on by a group of students. Based on the information given, have members of the group identify which system or systems of the body they would want to further investigate to determine why this individual has come to the emergency department. You have learned some medical terminology already but may need additional help from the text, medical dictionary, or website. Compile a list of specialists or health care professionals to whom you might refer this patient, and explain why.

REVIEW QUESTIONS

Multiple Choice

1. Blood can be classified as which type of tissue?
   a. connective
   b. cardiac
   c. nervous
   d. muscle

2. This membrane lines body cavities and covers the organs found in those cavities.
   a. cutaneous
   b. serous
   c. mucous
   d. mucus

3. This muscle type has interlocking cells for more efficient contraction.
   a. skeletal
   b. neuroglial
   c. cardiac
   d. smooth

4. The acid/base balance in your body is mainly controlled by the following system:
   a. skeletal
   b. urinary
   c. endocrine
   d. none of the above

5. Which of the following organs belong to the digestive system: (I) urethra, (II) gallbladder, (III) spleen, (IV) small intestine?
   a. I, II
   b. I, III, IV
   c. III, IV
   d. II, IV

6. You are given a sample of tissue. It has pink cells in a firm purple matrix. The cells are nestled in little holes. What kind of tissue is it?
   a. epithelium
   b. cartilage
   c. cardiac muscle
   d. nervous

7. A young ball player is hit in the head by a pitch and knocked unconscious. At the hospital he is seen by a specialist. Which specialist?
   a. optometrist
   b. rheumatologist
   c. neurologist
   d. gastroenterologist

Fill in the Blank

1. The system that coordinates all the body's functions is the _____ system.

2. The _____ system allows body movement.

3. Cartilage is a specific type of _____ tissue.

4. The layer of serous membrane that covers specific organs is called the _____ layer.

5. This system produces hormones: _____.

6. Which system stores calcium? _____

Short Answer

1. List in order from simplest to most complex the following: organs, cells, systems, tissues.

_____

_____

_____

_____

2. List the differences between epithelial tissue and connective tissues.

_____

_____

_____

_____

_____

3. Compare and contrast the different types of membranes.

_____

_____

_____

_____

_____

4. Contrast the three types of muscle tissues and identify where they are found.

_____

_____

_____

_____

_____

5. For the following disorders, list the primary system involved: arthritis, hepatitis, pneumonia, osteoporosis, and urinary tract infection.

_____

_____

_____

_____

_____

_____

6. Describe the potential use of stem cells

_____

_____

_____

_____

_____

The Skeletal System

THE FRAMEWORK

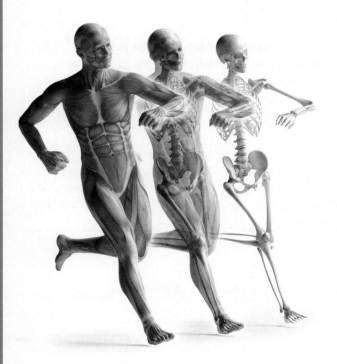

As we continue our journey, we may stop to visit friends or relatives and perhaps stay overnight. Their house will protect us from the elements and provide a safe place to sleep. Our hosts will offer us a good breakfast in the morning from the stored goods within. Although we cannot see the framework that holds up the house, without it everything would fall apart. We can think of the human body as a house. The wood framework is the skeleton, composed of bones that provide shape and strength. That is why we are beginning the system chapters with the body's own framework, on which the muscles and skin are layered much like stone or siding. Mounted on the framework are hinges that allow doors to swing open and shut and windows that glide open or closed. These are analogous to the joints and muscles attached to the skeleton that allow for body movement.

What's the first thing you think of when someone asks about the function of the skeleton? From our analogy, you would probably say, "to provide support and allow us to move." The skeleton does much more than provide support; the bones of your skeleton also protect the soft body parts, produce blood cells, and act as a storage unit for minerals and fat. In this chapter, we will also discuss the makeup and importance of the 206 bones in the adult skeleton as well as cartilage, ligaments, and joints. And now it's time to "bone up" on the skeletal system.

LEARNING OUTCOMES

At the end of your journey through this chapter, you will be able to:

- Describe the functions of the skeletal system.
- Discuss the general classification of bone based on shape.
- Identify and describe the anatomy and physiology of bone.
- Describe the process of bone growth and repair.
- Discuss the process of bone healing and aging.
- Differentiate between bone, cartilage, joints, ligaments, and tendons.
- Locate and describe the various joints and types of movement of the body.
- Locate and describe the various bones within the axial and appendicular skeleton.
- List the specific bones contained within special regions of the body.
- Describe common disorders of the skeletal system.

Pronunciation Guide Pro·nun·ci·a·tion

Correct pronunciation is important in any journey so that you and others are completely understood. Here is a "see and say" Pronunciation Guide for the more difficult terms to pronounce in this chapter. Please note that even though there are standard pronunciations, regional variations of the pronunciations can occur.

appendicular skeleton (app en DIK yoo lahr)
arthritis (ahr THRYE tiss)
articulation (ahr TICK you LAY shun)
axial (AK see al)
callus (KAL us)
diaphysis (dye AFF ih sis)
epiphyseal plate (ep ih FEEZ ee al)
epiphysis (eh PIFF ih sis)
haversian systems (haa VER zhin)
hemopoiesis (HEE moh poy EE sis)
ischium (IS kee um)

medullary cavity (MED uh LAIR ee)
osseous tissue (OSS see us)
ossification (OSS ih fih KAY shun)
osteoarthritis (OSS tee oh ahr THRYE tiss)
osteocyte (OSS tee oh site)
osteons (OSS tee ons)
periosteum (pair ee OSS tee um)
sternum (STER num)
synovial fluid (sin OH vee al)
trabeculae (tra BECK you lay)
vertebrae (VER teh bray)

SYSTEM OVERVIEW: MORE THAN THE "BARE BONES" ABOUT BONES

The skeleton has many more uses than just to scare people on Halloween. It is a wondrous structure that serves more functions than simply providing a framework for the human body. It also produces blood cells, provides protection for organs, helps us breathe, acts as a warehouse for mineral storage and, along with the muscular system, allows for movement.

General Bone Classification

Bones are the primary components of the skeleton. Although they may seem lifeless and are composed of nonliving minerals, such as calcium and phosphorus, they are very much alive, constantly building and repairing themselves. This is kind of ironic because the word *skeleton* is derived from the Greek word meaning "dried-up body."

We can classify bone types according to their shape:

- Long bones
- Short bones
- Flat bones
- Irregular bones

Long bones are longer than they are wide and are found in your arms and legs. *Short bones* are fairly equal in width and length, similar to a cube, and are mostly found in your wrists and ankles. *Flat bones* are thinner bones that can be either flat or curved and are platelike in nature. Examples of flat bones are in the skull, ribs, and breastbone (**sternum**).

Irregular bones are like the parts of a jigsaw puzzle. These are the odd-shaped bones needed to connect to other bones. Some examples of irregular bones are the hip bones and the **vertebrae** that make up your spine. See **FIGURE 6–1** ■ for a view of the various bone shapes.

Basic Bone Anatomy

Let's look at the overall construction of a bone by examining a long bone in **FIGURE 6–2** ■. Bone is covered with **periosteum** (*peri* = around, *osteum* = bone), a tough and fibrous connective tissue containing blood vessels that transport blood and nutrients into the bone to nurture the bone cells. It also contains lymph vessels, nerves, and cells that tear down and rebuild bone. In addition, the periosteum acts as an anchor point for ligaments and tendons, which we discuss later. Note in Figure 6–2 that both ends of the bone are wider than the area between the ends of the bone. Each bone end is called an **epiphysis** (*epi* = over or upon). The region between or "running through" the two ends is called the **diaphysis** (*dia* = through).

From the figure, you can see that the diaphysis is hollow. This hollow region is called the **medullary cavity** and acts as a storage area for bone marrow, much like a kitchen cabinet that contains food is hollow but well stocked. There are two kinds of bone marrow: yellow and red. *Yellow marrow* has a high fat content. *Red marrow* makes blood cells. In emergencies—for instance, in the event of massive blood loss—when you need more red blood cells, some of the yellow marrow can convert to red bone marrow to help in red blood cell production.

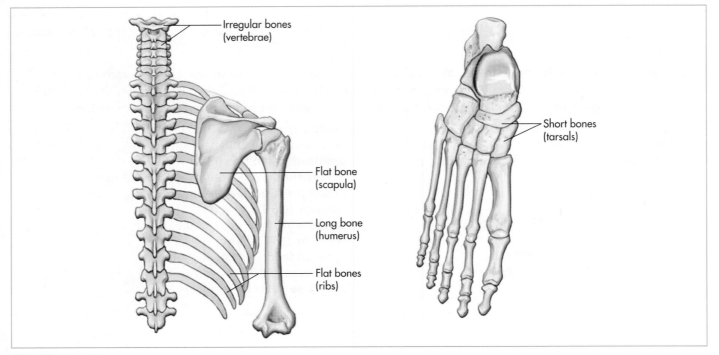

FIGURE 6–1 ■

Various bone shapes.

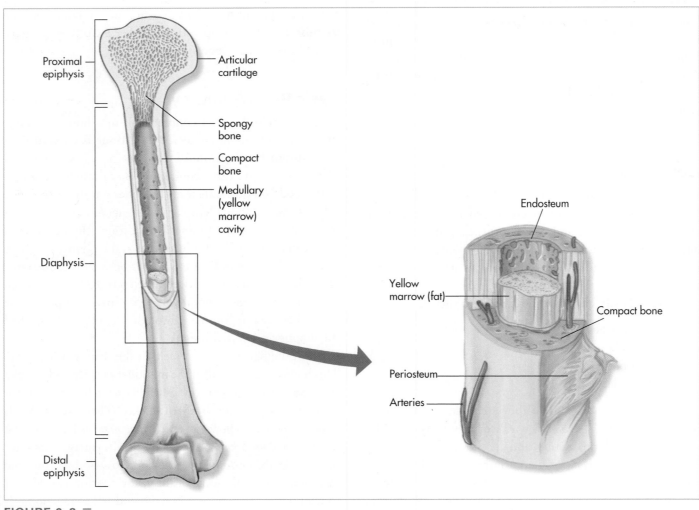

FIGURE 6–2 ■

Basic bone anatomy.

Bone Tissue

There are two types of bone tissue: compact and spongy. **Compact bone** is a dense, hard tissue normally found in the shafts of long bones and the outer layer of other bones. Microscopic examination reveals that the material of compact bone is tightly packed. This makes for a dense and strong structure. Compact bone contains microscopic cylindrical-shaped units called **osteons**, or **haversian systems**. Each unit has mature bone cells (**osteocytes**) forming concentric circles around a **central** (or *haversian*) **canal** containing blood vessels. The area around the osteocytes is filled with protein fibers, calcium, and other minerals. The osteons run parallel to each other, whereas other blood vessels run laterally, connecting with them through **perforating canals** to ensure there is sufficient oxygen and nutrients for the bone cells.

Spongy bone is different from compact bone. Instead of osteons, spongy bone tissue is arranged in bars and plates called **trabeculae**. Irregular holes between the trabeculae give the bone a spongy (porous) appearance. Spongy bone is lined with **endosteum**, a tissue similar to periosteum. Spongy bone serves two purposes: It helps make the bones lighter in weight and it provides a space for red bone marrow (see **FIGURE 6–3** ■).

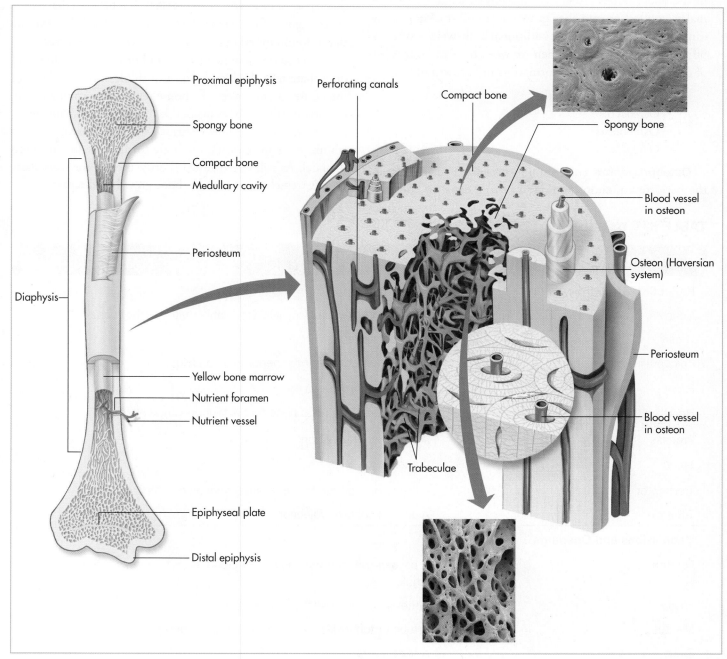

FIGURE 6–3 ■

Comparison of compact and spongy bone.

Surface Structures of Bones

Bones are not perfectly smooth. If you examine one closely, you will find a variety of projections, bumps, and depressions. Generally, projecting structures act as points of attachment for muscles, ligaments, or tendons, whereas grooves and depressions act as pathways for nerves and blood vessels. Both projecting structures and depressions can work together as joining or **articulation** points to form joints such as the ball and socket joint in the hip. TABLE 6–1 ■ lists many of these bone features.

Bone Growth

Ossification, or **osteogenesis**, is the formation of bone in the body. Bones grow *longitudinally* to lengthen (which makes you taller), and they grow wider and thicker so they can more efficiently support additional body weight and any other weight we support when we work or play. Four types of cells are involved in the formation and growth of bone:

- Osteoprogenitor cells
- Osteocytes
- Osteoblasts
- Osteoclasts

Osteoprogenitor cells are nonspecialized cells found in the periosteum, endosteum, and central canal of compact bones. Nonspecialized cells can turn into other types of cells as needed. **Osteoblasts** are the cells that actually form bones. They arise from the nonspecialized osteoprogenitor cells and secrete a matrix of calcium with other minerals that give bone its typical characteristics. **Osteocytes** are considered mature bone cells that were originally osteoblasts. In other words, osteoblasts surround themselves with a matrix of calcium to then become the mature osteocytes. Thus, bone is built up or formed by osteoprogenitor cells becoming osteoblasts, which surround themselves with a mineral matrix to become actual osteocytes (bone cells).

Not only does the body constantly build bone, but it must also constantly be able to tear down old bone. The tearing down part is the job of the **osteoclast**. It is believed that osteoclasts originate from a type of white blood cell called a *monocyte* that is found in red bone marrow. Amazingly, the osteoclasts' job is to tear down bone material and help move calcium and phosphate into the blood. You can think of osteoblasts and osteoclasts as employees of a house remodeling company: the osteo**b**lasts (think "b" as in "builder") are masons laying down brickwork to make new exterior walls, and the osteo**c**lasts (think "c" as in "clearing out") are tearing out the inside to remodel. As will be explained shortly, the job the osteoclasts do is extremely important for bone growth and repair.

TABLE 6–1 BONE FEATURES

BONE SURFACE STRUCTURES	DESCRIPTIONS
Projecting Structures	
Condyle	A large, rounded knob, usually articulating with another bone
Crest	A narrow ridge
Epicondyle	An enlargement near or superior to a condyle
Facet	A small, flattened area
Head	An articulating end of a bone that is rounded and enlarged
Process	A prominent projection
Spine	A sharp projection
Trochanter	Located only on the femur; a larger version of a tubercle
Tubercle	A small, knoblike projection
Depressions and Openings	
Foramen	A passageway through a bone for blood vessels, nerves, and ligaments; a hole
Fossa	Either a groove or shallow depression
Meatus	A tube or tunnel-like passageway through bone
Sinus	A hollow area

TEST YOUR KNOWLEDGE 6–1

Complete the following:

1. Label the diagram to the right:
   a. diaphysis
   b. proximal and distal
      epiphysis
   c. periosteum
   d. spongy bone
   e. compact bone
   f. medullary cavity
   g. epiphyseal plate

2. What is the function of red bone marrow and where is it located throughout the body?

   _____

   _____

3. List three functions of bone in your body.

   _____

   _____

4. Mature bone cells in compact bone are called
   a. marrowcytes.
   b. osteocytes.
   c. osteoblasts.
   d. monocytes.

5. The end of a long bone is called the
   a. epiphysis.
   b. periosteum.
   c. diaphysis.
   d. knob.

6. Osteocytes are found in _____ connected to each other by _____.
   a. medullary cavities; central canals
   b. osteons; perforating canals
   c. lacunae; canaliculi
   d. medullary cavities; canaliculi

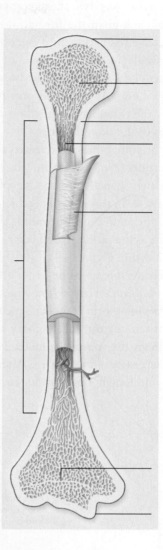

Amazing Facts

Red Bone Marrow and Red Blood Cells

Red bone marrow, which produces red blood cells, is found in the skull, clavicles (collarbones), vertebrae of the spinal column, sternum, ribs, and pelvis and in the spongy bone that makes up the epiphysis of the long bones. The production of red blood cells, known as **hemopoiesis** (also called **hematopoiesis**), is truly an incredible process. Because red blood cells last only about 120 days, their production is a constant job to maintain the 25,000,000,000,000 (give or take a few) red blood cells present in the human body. As a result, it has been calculated that approximately 3 million new red blood cells are created *every second*. What's more, your body can step up production to 10 times that rate in cases of severe blood loss. If the red marrow can't maintain the needed production, some of the yellow marrow can be converted to red marrow to assist.

Bone development and growth begins when you are growing in the womb through intramembranous and endochondral ossification. **Intramembranous ossification** occurs when bone develops between two sheets composed of fibrous connective tissue, such as in the formation of your skull. Cells from connective tissue turn into osteoblasts and form a matrix that is similar to the trabeculae of spongy bone, whereas other osteoblasts create compact bone over the surface of the spongy bone. As discussed previously, once the matrix surrounds the osteoblasts, they become osteocytes. This is how bones of the skull develop.

The majority of your bones are created through **endochondral ossification** (*endo* = within, *chondral* = referring to cartilage) in which shaped cartilage is replaced by bone. Refer to **FIGURE 6–4** ■. In this situation, which begins several months before birth, periosteum surrounds the diaphysis of the "cartilage" bone as the cartilage itself begins to break down (drawings 1 and 2 within Figure 6–4). Osteoblasts come into this region and create spongy bone in an area that is then called the *primary ossification center* (drawing 3). Meanwhile, other osteoblasts begin to form compact bone under the periosteum. Here is where the osteoclasts come into play. Their job is to break down the spongy bone of the diaphysis to create the medullary cavity (drawing 4). After you are born, the epiphyses on your long bones continue to grow. However,

shortly after birth, secondary ossification of this area begins with spongy bone forming and not breaking down. A thin band of cartilage forms an **epiphyseal plate** (often called the *growth plate*) between the primary and secondary ossification centers (drawing 5). This plate is important because, as long as it exists, the bone will continue growing (drawing 6). As will be explained in Chapter 12, "The Endocrine System," hormones control the growth of bones, which means that eventually the plates become ossified, thereby stopping bone growth.

Bone Repair

When a bone is fractured, it must be repaired. Bone repair is accomplished by the same process as bone growth, endochondral ossification. Bone tissue is very good at repairing itself, but for a bone fracture to heal, the ends of broken bone must be touching. If they are not, then a medical procedure called **reduction** (setting) must be performed. Then the bone must be immobilized so the ends will stay touching. The first stage of bone repair is *hematoma formation* and *inflammation*. Bone has lots of blood vessels, so bleeding is associated with a bone fracture. The blood collects around the fracture in a hematoma. The injured tissues release chemicals that trigger **inflammation** (for more details on inflammation,

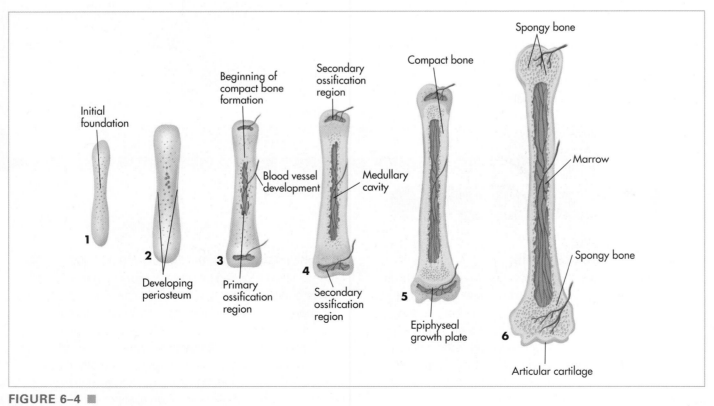

FIGURE 6–4 ■

Endochondral ossification of long bone.

see the wound healing section of Chapter 5, "Integumentary System"). The second stage of bone repair is *soft (fibrocartilage) callus formation*. During soft callus formation, cartilage fills in the space between the bones, and blood vessels begin to grow into the area. In stage three, *hard (bony) callus formation*, bone replaces the cartilage via endochondral ossification, and in stage four, the bone is *remodeled* via the activity of osteoblasts and osteoclasts until the fracture is nearly undetectable. See **FIGURE 6–5** ■ to better understand how bones heal.

Not all bone fractures are the same. Here are some of the more common fractures you may encounter throughout your career. A **hairline fracture**, which looks like a piece of hair on the x-ray, is a fine fracture that does not completely break or displace the bone. A **simple** or **closed fracture** is a break without a puncture to the skin. An individual in an accident who has a bone that is severely twisted may receive a **spiral fracture**. **Greenstick fractures** are incomplete breaks, which more often occur in children because they have softer, more pliable bones (like sapling branches) than adults (like seasoned twigs). If a bone is crushed to the point that it becomes fragmented or splintered, that is classified as a **comminuted fracture**. A fracture in which the bone is pushed through the skin is referred to as a **compound** or **open fracture**. These fractures are particularly nasty because deep tissue has the potential to be exposed to bacteria once the bone is set into place, and, hence, the chance for infection in addition to the break is increased. See **FIGURE 6–6** ■ for examples of common fractures.

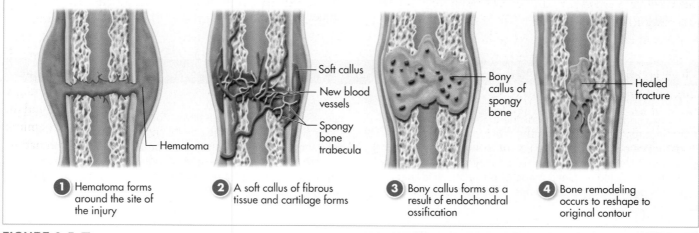

1 Hematoma forms around the site of the injury — Hematoma

2 A soft callus of fibrous tissue and cartilage forms — Soft callus, New blood vessels, Spongy bone trabecula

3 Bony callus forms as a result of endochondral ossification — Bony callus of spongy bone

4 Bone remodeling occurs to reshape to original contour — Healed fracture

FIGURE 6–5 ■

The healing process of a bone.

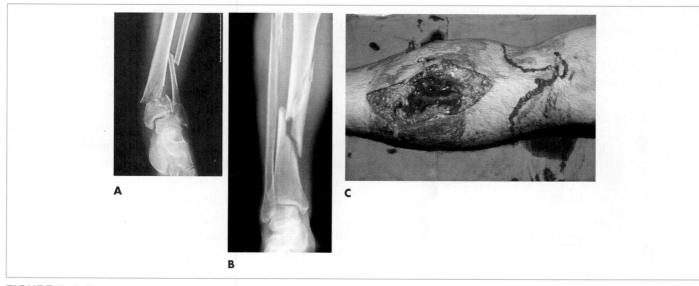

FIGURE 6–6 ■

(A) Fibula and tibia communited fracture. (B) Simple, tranverse fracture. (C) Open fracture of the lower left leg.

Amazing Facts

Aging and Bone Building

Even in adults, bone continues to be broken down and rebuilt. In fact, about 10 percent of the body's bone is torn down and rebuilt each year. Your bones continue to increase in mass well into your twenties. The osteoclasts break down and remove worn-out bone cells and deposit calcium into the blood. They last for approximately three weeks. Osteoblasts then pull the calcium out of the blood, form and surround themselves with that mineralized matrix we discussed, and mature into osteocytes. Because of this continual breakdown of old and creation of new bone, adults actually need more calcium in their diets than do children. The process of breaking down and rebuilding bone continues well into a person's forties, so there normally is no net gain or loss of bone mass.

This continuing process allows your body to sculpt bone into shapes that accommodate the body's activity. For example, exercise, such as running or weight lifting, causes calcium to stay in the bone, making it thicker, denser, and stronger than those of a sedentary person (couch or mouse potato) or an astronaut during space flight. Continuous or repeated actions or postures tend to cause bone to be resculpted. For example, due to constant squatting, a certain pattern of bumps forms on the bones of the hips, shins, and knees. As a result of this pattern, it was determined that Neanderthal man squatted rather than sat.

APPLIED SCIENCE

Copying Bones

An exciting new area of medicine is the "growing" of exact patient replicas of bone for the replacement of damaged or defective bone through the use of three-dimensional (3D) printers. Using a 3D bioprinter, a "scaffold or framework" is created using an "ink" made of polylactic acid that creates a bonelike structure, while a substance (similar to gel) called *alginate* is used as a base for the patient's stem cells to be placed to grow. The scaffolding degrades as the stem cells form actual bone and new blood vessels, creating a custom, living replacement. Although this is all new and evolving technology, it appears to have a very promising future!

FOCUS ON PROFESSIONS

Learn more about **Radiologic Technologists,** the health care professionals who use radiation to make images of bones and other body parts by visiting the websites of national organizations, such as the American Society of Radiologic Technicians (ASRT), the American Registry of Radiologic Technologists (ARRT), and the International Society of Radiology (ISR). They prepare patients for x-rays, take the "picture," and prepare the x-ray image so physicians can read (analyze) them.

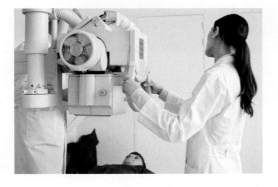

Cartilage

Cartilage is a form of connective tissue (see Chapter 5) that can withstand a fair amount of flexing, tension, and pressure. Cartilage plays many roles throughout the body. The flexible parts of your nose and ears are cartilage. Think about how much you can bend your ears without breaking them off. The cartilage found in your nose and ears will always remain cartilage, so it is called *permanent cartilage*. As some individuals age, their ears and noses can become larger because permanent cartilage has the capability to continue growing!

Cartilage also makes a flexible connection between bones. For example, the cartilage between the breastbone and ribs allows your chest to flex and give so you decrease the chance of breaking your ribs when you run into things or collide with another player during a football game. This amazing tissue also acts as a cushion between the bones. As you can see in **FIGURE 6–7** ■, *articular cartilage* is located on the ends of bones and acts as a shock absorber, preventing the bone ends from grinding together as they move. In addition, at this location, a small sac, called the **bursa**, contains a lubricant called **synovial fluid**. Even with cartilage and synovial fluid

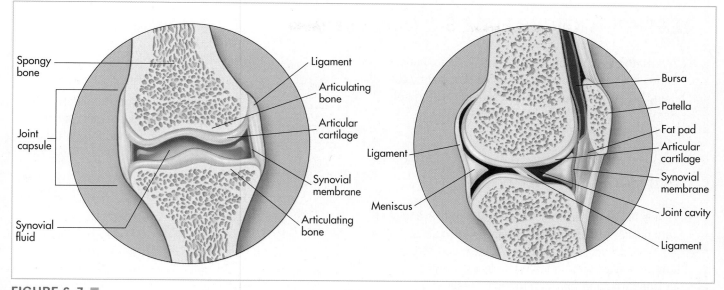

FIGURE 6–7 ■

Articular cartilage and synovial joint.

protecting the area between bones, joints can wear out and become inflamed, resulting in a condition called **arthritis**, or **osteoarthritis**.

Joints and Ligaments

Without **joints**, the body could not move. When two or more bones *join* together, a joint, or an **articulation**, is formed. Freely moving joints must be held together and yet still be movable. This is accomplished through the use of another specialized connective tissue called a **ligament**. (Again, see Figure 6–7.) Ligaments are very tough, whitish bands that connect one bone to another bone and can

withstand pretty heavy stress. Do not confuse ligaments with **tendons**. Whereas ligaments hold bone to bone, tendons are cordlike structures that attach muscle to bone. There are several types of joints, and each works in a specific way.

Joints are classified either by function or structure. In terms of function, joints can be immobile, can move a little, or can move freely. For example, skull sutures are immobile, the pubic symphysis between your pelvic bones moves a little, and your elbow moves freely. If we characterize joints by structure, we divide them based on the type of connective tissue that links the bones together.

TEST YOUR KNOWLEDGE 6–2

Choose the best answer:

1. A term that can be used to describe the formation of bone is
   a. ossification.
   b. periosteum.
   c. bonafide.
   d. osteoclasts.

2. These cells actually form bones:
   a. osteoclasts
   b. pericytes
   c. generator cells
   d. osteoblasts

3. Another name for the "growth plate" is
   a. tectonic plate.
   b. epiphyseal plate.
   c. upper palate.
   d. periostium plate.

4. This connective tissue forms a cushion in joints:
   a. tendons
   b. ligaments
   c. cartilage
   d. cartridge

(continued)

TEST YOUR KNOWLEDGE 6–2 *(continued)*

5. A skeleton is found buried in a landfill. Examination shows that the epiphysial plates are completely calcified. What was the age of the skeleton at time of death?
   a. 5 years old
   b. 10 years old
   c. 15 years old
   d. 25 years old

6. Riding his all-terrain vehicle one day, Jim falls and shatters his tibia, breaking it into many small pieces. At the hospital the surgeons use pins, plates, and screws to put the pieces back in the right places. Why?
   a. Bone must be touching to repair itself.
   b. Bone cannot repair itself.
   c. Inflammation is reduced by surgery.
   d. The bone will never be strong enough to support weight after injury.

7. Give the type of fracture:
   _____ fragmented or splintered break
   _____ incomplete break due to pliable bones
   _____ broken bone is pushed through skin

Fibrous joints are held together by short connective tissue strands. They are either immobile or slightly movable. The sutures in your skull are fibrous joints. **Cartilaginous joints** are held together by cartilage. The pubic symphysis and the joints between your ribs and sternum are cartilaginous joints. Cartilaginous joints are either immobile or slightly movable. Finally, **synovial joints** are joined by a joint cavity lined with a synovial membrane and filled with synovial fluid. All synovial joints are freely moving. Synovial joints are constructed in various ways that determine how they can move:

- *Gliding joints* are the flat, or slightly curved, plate-like bones found in your wrists and ankles. Gliding joints slide back and forth.
- *Hinge joints* are found in your knees and elbows. Typically one bone is in the shape of a cylinder and the other a trough. They can either open or close.
- *Saddle joints* have a bone shaped just like a saddle and another bone similar to a horse's back. This joint type is found in the base of your thumb. Saddle joints rock up and down and side to side.
- *Ellipsoidal* (also known as *condyloid*) *joints* are formed by oval-shaped bone fitted into a depression and provide two axes of movement, like the joint formed at the wrist with both the radius and ulna.

- *Pivot joints* (which act like a turnstile) have a circular portion of one bone that spins inside a ring-shaped portion of the other. Pivot joints are the type of joint found in your neck and forearm. They can only partially rotate.
- *Ball-and-socket joints* usually consist of a spherical articulation with a cup-shaped socket on the other bone. Ball-and-socket joints are located in your hips and shoulders and can perform all types of movement, including rotation.

To better visualize these various joints, examine **FIGURE 6–8** ■.

Movement Classification

Because joints allow various types of movement, these individualized movements can also be classified, as you can see in the examples in **FIGURE 6–9** ■. **Flexion** occurs when a joint is bent, decreasing the angle between the involved bones, as when the leg is bent at the knee. **Extension** is a result of straightening a joint so the angle between the involved bones increases, as occurs with a kicking motion. Ballerinas utilize **plantar flexion** when they dance on their toes. **Dorsiflexion** occurs when the foot is bent up toward the leg. If the joint is forced to straighten beyond its normal limits, *hyperextension* occurs.

Abduction and **adduction** can be confusing. *Abduction* means to move *away* from the body's midline (think, "**B**e gone!"

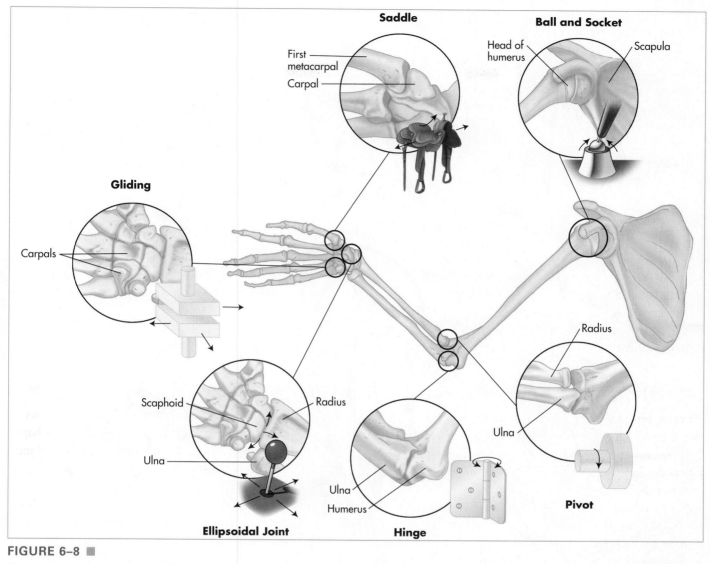

Saddle

First metacarpal

Carpal

Ball and Socket

Head of humerus

Scapula

Gliding

Carpals

Scaphoid

Radius

Ulna

Ellipsoidal Joint

Radius

Ulna

Pivot

Ulna

Humerus

Hinge

FIGURE 6–8 ■

Types of joints.

as you move your arm up and away to swat at a <u>bee</u>). *Adduction* means to move *toward* the midline of the body. To remember adduction, think of your a**dd**ress, where packages and mail come *to* you. Then when you move your arm back toward yourself *after* swatting at a bee, you are a**dd**ucting your arm.

Inversion results when the sole of one foot is turned inward so it points to the other foot, whereas **eversion** is the opposite: The foot is turned outward, pointing away from the opposite foot. **Supination** occurs when the hand is turned to the point where the palm faces upward; **pronation** turns the palm downward.

Protraction is the motion of drawing a part forward. **Retraction** is the motion of drawing backward. Figure 6–9 shows the protraction and retraction of the jaw. The movements are analogous to a turtle sticking its head out (protracting) and drawing it back in (retracting) to the shell.

Finally, **rotation** is when a bone "turns" on its axis. An example is when your head rotates (looking left and right) before you cross the street. Although you may not have heard of **circumduction**, you have seen this combination of movements in the circular arm movement that a softball pitcher utilizes. Circumduction is the movement of the end of a limb in a circle.

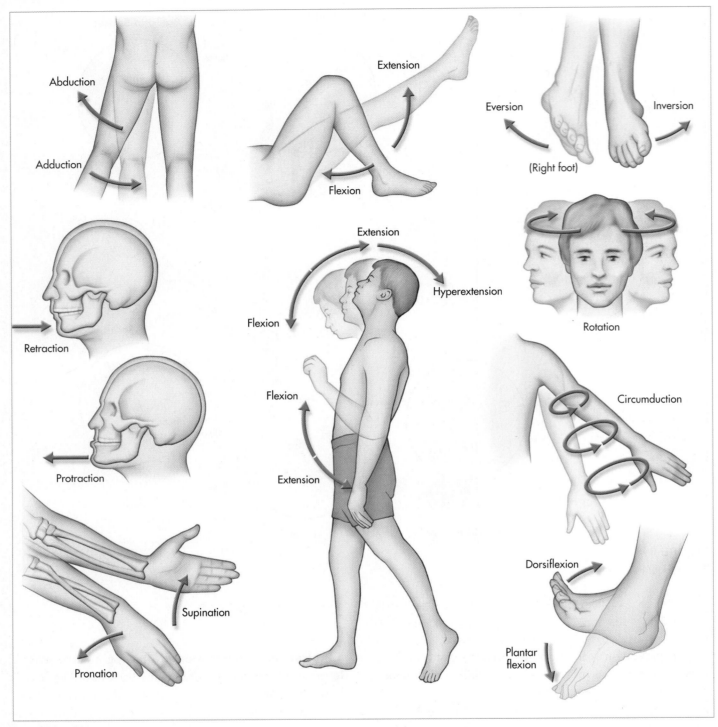

FIGURE 6–9 ■

Classification of joint movements.

TEST YOUR KNOWLEDGE 6–3

Answer the following:

1. A movement that increases the angle of a joint is known as
   a. flexion.
   b. abduction.
   c. rotation.
   d. extension.

2. A joint in which bones are connected by short connective tissue strands is known as a
   a. cartilaginous joint.
   b. fibrous joint.
   c. synovial joint.
   d. freely moving joint.

3. A joint in which flat bone surfaces move side to side past each other is known as a
   a. condyloid joint.
   b. hinge joint.
   c. saddle joint.
   d. gliding joint.

4. This lubricant helps to prevent wear in joints:
   a. pleural fluid
   b. synovial fluid
   c. mucus
   d. petroleum jelly

5. These structures attach bone to bone:
   a. ligaments
   b. tendons
   c. cords
   d. articulations

6. A young gymnast falls from the balance beam, rotating her knee. This is a problem because
   a. the knee is a hinge joint and should not rotate.
   b. the knee should only rotate when standing.
   c. the knee joint is not a freely moving joint.
   d. there is no problem; knees are supposed to rotate.

7. What head movement should you perform before crossing a busy street?
   a. circumduction
   b. flexion
   c. rotation
   d. protraction

Clinical Applications

JOINT REPLACEMENT

Sometimes joints wear out from repeated trauma, as in sports or work-related injuries, repetitive motion(s) over time, disease, or just plain wearing out due to the aging process. When previous corrective surgery or nonsurgical interventions such as muscle strengthening, weight loss, nonsteroidal anti-inflammatory drugs or steroid injections no longer are effective, an orthopedic surgeon may be consulted for a replacement of the affected joint with an artificial one. The problem may arise from bone degradation or a wearing away of the protective layer of cartilage.

Joint replacement procedures may involve the total or partial removal of the affected joint and adding an artificial replacement. The intention of this procedure is to eliminate pain and restore movement of that joint, thus improving activities of daily living (ADL). Just about any joint may be replaced—hips, knees, shoulders, and even fingers joints. Recovery time varies with the age and previous condition of the patient, extent and severity of the procedure, as well as the level of follow-up rehabilitation.

Our technology is improving, but artificial joints still aren't as good as the originals (which have had over 100,000 years to be perfected). Generally speaking, an artificial joint lasts for 10 to 15 years before it wears out.

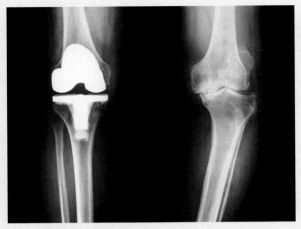

Titanium hinge joint replacement and knee

THE SKELETON

Anatomically, the skeleton can be divided into two main sections. The **axial skeleton** includes bones of the bony thorax, spinal column, hyoid bone, bones of the middle ear, and skull. This part of the skeletal system protects the organs of the body and is composed of 80 bones. The **appendicular skeleton** is, as its name implies, the region of your appendages (arms and legs), as well as the connecting bone structures of the hips and shoulder girdles, and contains 126 bones (see **FIGURE 6–10** ■). Interestingly, nearly half the total number of your bones can be found in your hands and feet.

Special Regions of the Skeletal System

The skeleton consists of many different special regions. These distinctions make it easier to locate and discuss the hundreds of bones and associated components in this system. In this section, we make a quick tour of each region, beginning at the top.

The Human Skull

The cranial portion of the skull protects and houses the brain and has openings needed for our sensory organs, such as the eyes, nose, and ears. It also forms the oral cavity, which is a common passageway for both the digestive and respiratory systems. The skull contains fibrous connective tissue joints called *suture lines* that hold the bony plates of the skull together. Although the suture lines are not truly movable, they do provide a bit of flexibility that aids in absorbing some shock from a blow to the head, thus decreasing the possibility of a skull fracture. **FIGURE 6–11** ■ shows the bones of the skull in greater detail.

The Bony Thorax

The bones of the chest form a thoracic "cage" that provides support and protection for the heart, lungs, and great blood vessels (see **FIGURE 6–12** ■). This cage is flexible because of cartilaginous connections that allow for movement during

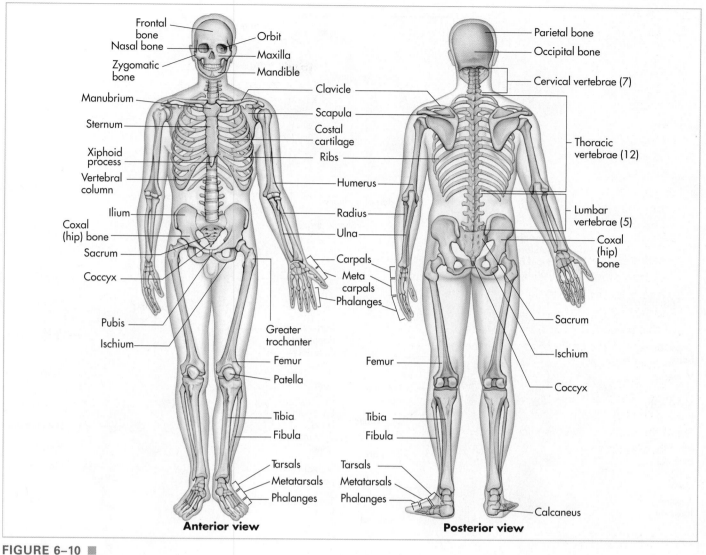

FIGURE 6–10 ■

The anterior and posterior human skeleton.

the process of breathing. The sternum, or breastbone, is the anatomical structure for conducting compressions of the heart during cardiopulmonary resuscitation (CPR). During cardiac compressions, the heart is compressed anteriorly by the body of the sternum and posteriorly by the bones of the vertebral column. The sternum is composed of three distinct structures. The *manubrium* is the superior portion, and the *body* is the largest, central portion. The *xiphoid process* is the final and inferior portion that ossifies (hardens) by age 25 and can be broken off if CPR is improperly performed.

The thoracic cage consists of 12 pairs of elastic arches of bone called *ribs*. The ribs are attached by cartilage to allow for their movement when we breathe. The true ribs

are pairs 1 to 7 and are called *vertebrosternal* because they connect anteriorly to the sternum and posteriorly to the thoracic vertebrae of the spinal column. Pairs 8 to 10 are called the false, or *vertebrocostal*, ribs because they connect to the costal cartilage of the superior rib and again posteriorly to the thoracic vertebrae. Rib pairs 11 and 12 are called the floating ribs because they have no anterior attachment.

The Spinal Column

The spinal, or vertebral, column protects the spinal cord, which is the superhighway for information coming to and from the central nervous system. The individual bones, or

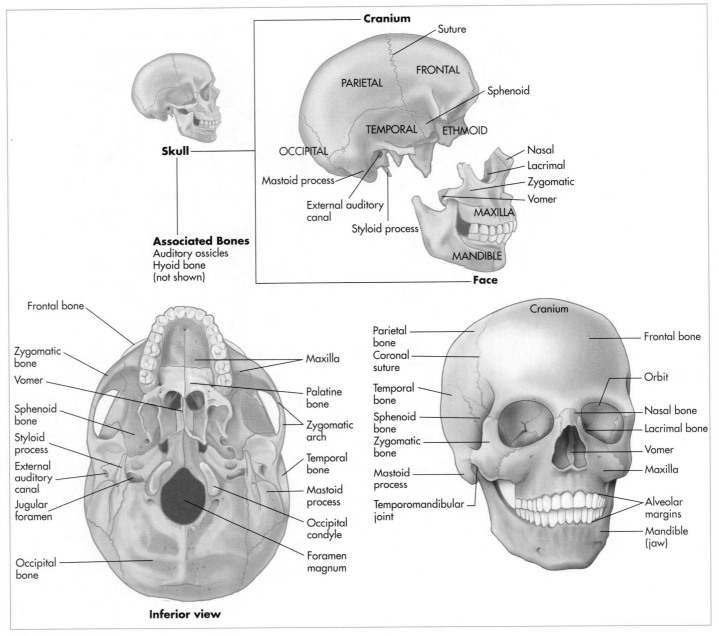

FIGURE 6–11 ■

Bones of the skull.

vertebrae, are numbered and classified according to the body region where they are located (see **FIGURE 6–13** ■). For example, seven vertebrae are found in the cervical or neck region, and they are numbered C-1 though C-7, respectively.

As seen in Figure 6–13, there are 7 vertebrae in the cervical (neck) region, 12 in the upper back (thoracic), 5 in the lower back (lumbar), 5 fused vertebrae in the

LEARNING HINT

Number of Vertebrae

To remember the number of vertebrae in each region, think of 7 days in a week for cervical and 12 months in a year for thoracic. Finally, the lumbar region has the same number of vertebrae as digits on your hand (5).

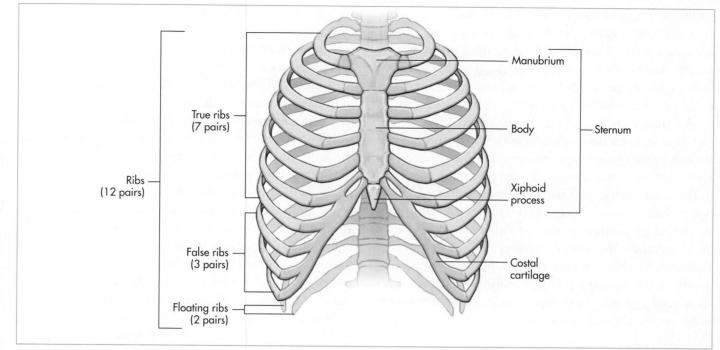

FIGURE 6–12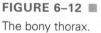

The bony thorax.

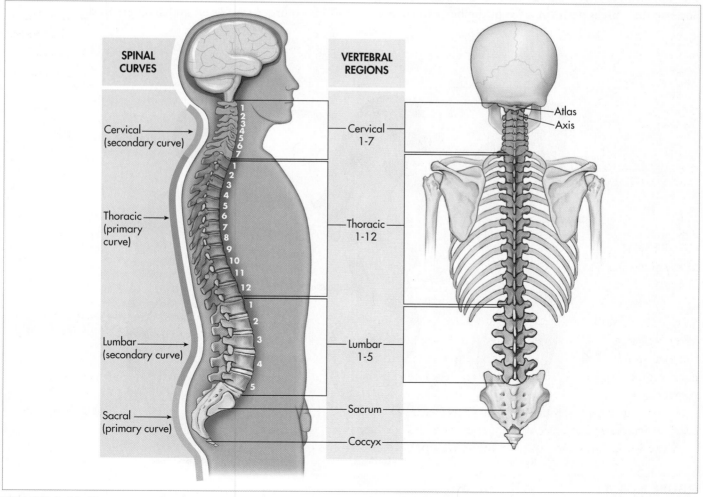

FIGURE 6–13 ■

The spinal column.

midbuttock region (sacral), and 3 to 5 small bones at the very end (tailbone, coccyx). At birth, the vertebral column is concave to the front, like a fetal position (primary curvature), but bends in the opposite direction occur as the infant starts to rise, holds her or his head up, and starts to walk. In other words, there will be secondary curvatures by the time a child is age 2. From 2 years onward, the vertebral column develops a secondary curvature in the neck, a primary curvature in the upper back, a secondary curvature in the lower back, and a primary curvature in the midbuttocks and tailbone regions. If the body is not in balance—whether due to congenital deformity, trauma, poor posture, or disease—these curvatures may be exaggerated. Abnormal curvatures can include kyphosis (humpback, usually in the thorax), lordosis (swayback, usually in the lumbar region), or scoliosis which is a sideways bend and sway in the spinal column. **FIGURE 6–14** illustrates these conditions.

Upper and Lower Extremities

The appendicular region consists of the arms and legs. Because these areas perform most of the body movement,

the greatest number of sport-related injuries occur here. The arms and legs are of similar construction, with one large bone (**humerus** in the arms; **femur** in the legs); two smaller bones in the forelimb (**radius** and **ulna** in the arms; **tibia** and **fibula** in the legs), multiple bones (**carpals** in the wrist; **tarsals** in the ankle); followed by five single bones (**metacarpals** in the hand; **metatarsals** in the foot) and digits made of multiple bones called **phalanges**. Both the arms and legs are attached to the axial skeleton via the **pectoral** and **pelvic** girdles, respectively. The pectoral girdle consists of the **clavicle** and **scapula**, whereas the pelvic girdle consists of the pelvic bones (**ischium**, **ilium**, and **pubis**). Please see **FIGURE 6–15** , which shows the bones of the upper and lower extremities. These figures show the bony landmarks of the limbs and girdles, which will be beneficial in learning and understanding where the muscles discussed in Chapter 7 will attach.

Notice in Figure 6–15 that the pelvic girdle in women is different than in men. Women have a greater pubic angle that facilitates childbirth and also a relatively broad girdle to support the extra weight of the child. This difference can be used to identify the sex of a skeleton, such as in a murder case or an archaeologic find.

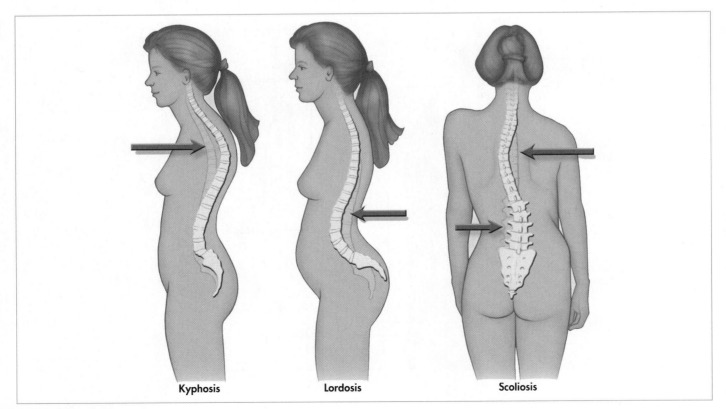

Kyphosis   Lordosis   Scoliosis

FIGURE 6–14

Common spinal disfigurements.

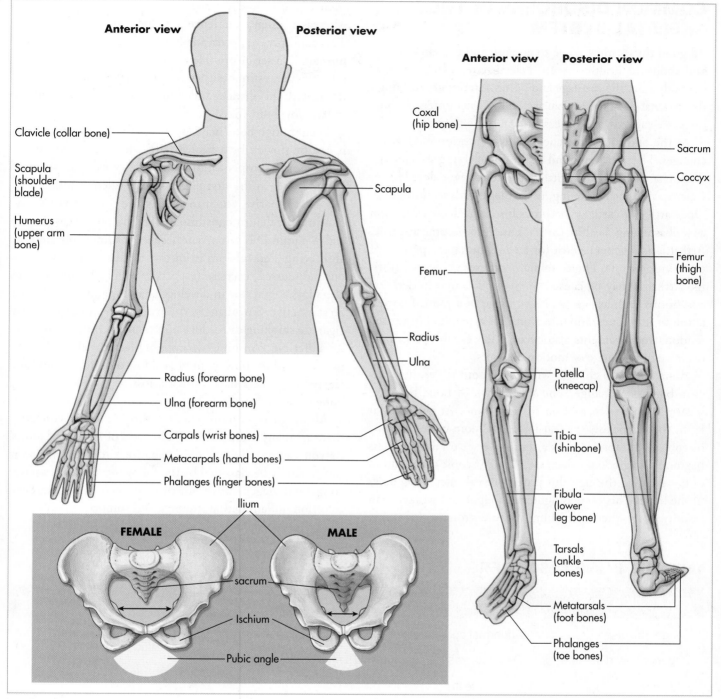

Anterior view

Posterior view

Anterior view

Posterior view

Clavicle (collar bone)

Scapula (shoulder blade)

Humerus (upper arm bone)

Radius (forearm bone)

Ulna (forearm bone)

Carpals (wrist bones)

Metacarpals (hand bones)

Phalanges (finger bones)

Scapula

Radius

Ulna

Coxal (hip bone)

Femur

Sacrum

Coccyx

Femur (thigh bone)

Patella (kneecap)

Tibia (shinbone)

Fibula (lower leg bone)

Tarsals (ankle bones)

Metatarsals (foot bones)

Phalanges (toe bones)

Ilium

FEMALE

MALE

sacrum

Ischium

Pubic angle

FIGURE 6–15 ■

Bones of the upper and lower extremities.

COMMON DISORDERS OF THE SKELETAL SYSTEM

All good things must come to an end, and the same can be said about the health of your skeletal system. In general, as the body ages, the cartilage and bones deteriorate. Although this is a natural process that we will all encounter, in some cases, we can slow the process down.

As the body ages, the chemical composition of cartilage changes. The bluish tint and flexibility of young skeletal cartilage change to a more brittle, opaque yellow-colored form. Calcification, or hardening, of cartilage leads to brittleness. Once articular cartilage becomes brittle, it doesn't function as well as young, healthy cartilage and can become arthritic. **Arthritis** is a general term for an inflammatory process of the joint or joints. There are many different types of arthritis. Arthritis may be caused by many different underlying conditions such as age, excessive usage of a joint, injuries, autoimmune issues, and infections, for example. The related tendons and ligaments also become less flexible, causing a decrease in the range of motion in joints.

Bone mass also changes with age. In our fifties, the skeleton begins to change. The breakdown of bone becomes greater than the formation of new bone. At the cellular level, the osteoclasts are tearing down more bone than the osteoblasts are forming. As a result, we see total bone mass beginning to gradually decrease. A microscopic examination of bones going through this process reveals increasing holes in the bone. This bone is lighter in weight and weaker than healthy bone, thereby making it more prone to breakage.

Men appear to lose less than 25 percent of their bone mass, whereas women experience a 35 percent loss on average. This condition of decreasing bone density, known as **osteoporosis**, is a serious problem. The National Foundation of Osteoporosis estimates there are 10 *million* Americans suffering with this disease, and almost 34 *million* are estimated to have low bone mass.

Even though bone mass loss is a natural process of aging, it can be slowed by a healthy lifestyle. It is important to consume the proper amount of dietary calcium to build strong bones in the first place. Proper calcium intake during the formative years, including the teenage years, and continued calcium consumption as the body ages, is crucial. Vitamin D is important because it allows your body to absorb ingested calcium from the digestive tract. As previously discussed, exercise (especially weight-bearing forms) also plays a vital role in developing and maintaining bones. So stay active. Surprisingly, the excessive use of caffeine and cigarette smoking can reduce bone density. Individuals who, for a lifetime, consume two cups of black caffeinated coffee per day tend to show an increased loss of bone density, and cigarette smokers have shown a loss of 5 to 8 percent of bone mineral density.

Although osteoporosis and arthritis are big concerns, there are many more potential disorders of bones and joints. As you can see in TABLES 6–2 ■ and 6–3 ■, these disorders can generally be classified by the following causative agents: congenital, degenerative, nutritional, secondary disorders, infection, inflammation, trauma, and tumors.

TABLE 6–2 BONE DISORDERS

CLASSIFICATION	EXAMPLE(S)
Congenital disorders	Abnormal curvature of the spine (kyphosis, lordosis, scoliosis), cleft palate, clubfoot
Degenerative disorders	Osteoporosis
Infection	Osteomyelitis
Nutritional disorders	Osteomalacia (vitamin D deficiency), rickets (vitamin D deficiency), scurvy (vitamin C deficiency)
Secondary disorders	Endocrine system dysfunction: gigantism, pituitary dwarfism
Trauma	Bruises, fractures
Tumors	Chondrosarcomas, myelomas, osteosarcomas

TABLE 6–3 JOINT DISORDERS

CLASSIFICATION	EXAMPLE(S)
Degenerative disorders	Osteoarthritis
Infection	Gonococcal arthritis, rheumatic fever, septic arthritis, viral arthritis
Inflammation	Bursitis, arthritis
Secondary disorders	Immune system dysfunction: rheumatoid arthritis; metabolic dysfunction: gout
Trauma	Ankle and foot injuries, dislocations, hip fractures, knee injuries

TEST YOUR KNOWLEDGE 6–4

Answer the following:

1. Which of the following bones is considered to be part of the axial skeleton?
   a. humerus
   b. patella
   c. femur
   d. sternum

2. The number of vertebra in the thoracic region is
   a. 5.
   b. 7.
   c. 12.
   d. 120.

3. The posterior skull bone is the
   a. parietal.
   b. cervical.
   c. occipital.
   d. zygomatic.

4. The last two pairs of ribs are
   a. vertebrosternal.
   b. vertebrocostal.
   c. vertebroclavical.
   d. none of the above

5. The shoulder blade is more technically known as the
   a. clavicle.
   b. scapula.
   c. sternum.
   d. pelvis.

6. Beth has fractured her humerus. What is in the cast?
   a. her leg
   b. her arm
   c. her neck is in a brace
   d. her entire body

7. A cleft palate would be classified as which type of disorder?
   a. infection
   b. tumor
   c. trauma
   d. congenital

SUMMARY: Points of Interest

- In addition to providing support and protection for the body, the skeleton also produces blood cells and acts as a storage unit for minerals and fat.

- The 206 bones of the skeleton can be classified according to their shapes—long bones, short bones, flat bones, and irregular bones—and are covered with periosteum, a tough, fibrous connective tissue.

- In long bones, each bone end is called an *epiphysis*, and the shaft is called the *diaphysis*. The hollow region within the diaphysis is called the *medullary cavity* and stores yellow marrow.

- Compact bone is a dense, hard tissue that is normally found in the shafts of long bones or is found as the outer layer of the other bone types. Spongy bone is different in that it contains irregular holes that make it lighter in weight and provides a space for red bone marrow, which produces red blood cells.

- Ossification is the formation of bone in the body. *Osteoprogenitor* cells are nonspecialized bone cells that can turn into *osteoblasts*, which are the cells that actually form bones. *Osteocytes* are considered mature bone cells that were originally osteoblasts. Osteoclasts originate from a type of white blood cell called a *monocyte*, found in red bone marrow. Osteoclasts break down bone material and help move calcium and phosphate into the blood.

- A thin band of cartilage forms an epiphyseal plate (often referred to as the *growth plate*), and as long as it exists, bone growth will continue.

- Cartilage is a form of connective tissue that can withstand a fair amount of flexing, tension, and pressure and makes a flexible connection between bones, as between the breastbone and ribs. It also acts as a cushion between bones.

- Various types of joints join two or more bones and provide various types of movement. The point at which they join is called an articulation. Ligaments are very tough, whitish bands that connect from bone to bone to hold the joint together and can withstand heavy stress.

- The skeleton can be divided into two main sections. The axial skeleton includes bones of the bony thorax, spinal column, hyoid bone, bones of the middle ear, and skull. The appendicular skeleton is the region of your appendages (arms and legs) as well as the connecting bone structures of the hip and shoulder girdles.

- As we age, the chemical composition of cartilage changes, causing it to become more brittle. Articular cartilage that ages or becomes injured can lead to arthritis, an inflammatory process of the joint or joints. Bone mass also gradually decreases with age, beginning in a person's fifties. Even though this is a natural process of aging, it can be slowed by a healthy lifestyle.

CASE STUDY

Rosemary deAngelo, a somewhat frail 62-year-old female, visits her physician's office for an annual checkup. Her social history shows she smokes a pack of cigarettes a day, claims she is a social drinker, and reports she is a heavy coffee drinker. Rosemary is on hypertension medication that includes diuretics. She has had several fractured bones in the last five years that required medical attention. During initial examination, measurements show that the patient has lost approximately an inch of height over the past year. She has also lost several pounds but states she still wears the same size clothes.

a. What bone disease does Rosemary have?

_____

_____

b. Describe the bone changes in this condition on a macro and cellular level.

_____

_____

c. What treatments and/or lifestyle changes would you suggest?

_____

_____

Multiple Choice

1. Your elbow is an example of which type of joint?
   a. hinge joint
   b. ball-and-socket joint
   c. gliding joint
   d. fibrous joint

2. The sternum is the correct medical term for which bone?
   a. shin bone
   b. breastbone
   c. shoulder blade
   d. collarbone

3. The end of a long bone is the
   a. diplodicus.
   b. epiphysis.
   c. condylcorn.
   d. perla.

4. The presence of a(n) _____ in skeletal remains indicates the skeleton is a teenager or child.
   a. Torger center
   b. ossifier
   c. Mantoux membrane
   d. epiphyseal plate

5. The aging process, excessive caffeine, and cigarette smoking can each contribute to this bone disease:
   a. ligamental stenosis
   b. osteoporosis
   c. cartilentious dementia
   d. ossification

6. Joel injured his elbow as a child and now, as an adult, his injured arm is much shorter than the other arm. Why?
   a. Fractured bone is always shorter.
   b. His epiphyseal plate was damaged, and the bone didn't grow.
   c. He has arthritis in the joint, which decreases bone growth.
   d. He has a congenital problem that caused both the injury and the shorter bone.

7. A bone fracture that pierces through skin is called a(an) _____ fracture.
   a. open
   b. spiral
   c. closed
   d. comminuted

Fill in the Blank

1. Name three large appendicular bones:
   _____, _____, and _____.

2. List three places where cartilage is found in the body: _____, _____, and _____.

3. _____ is a liquid found in joints that keeps them lubricated.

4. The specialized cells that constantly rebuild bone are called _____.

5. These specialized cells are needed to tear down bone: _____.

6. Bone must be _____ to heal after fracture.

7. The superior portion of the sternum is called the _____.

Short Answer

1. Describe the difference in function between tendons and ligaments.

_____

_____

_____

_____

2. Explain the process of endochondral ossification.

_____

_____

_____

_____

3. Explain the structural and functional classification of joints.

_____

_____

_____

_____

4. List and define the types of movements possible in freely moving joints.

_____

_____

_____

_____

5. Skeletons have a number of characteristics that allow forensic professionals to tell age, sex, health, and other characteristics of a person's life or lifestyle. List several of them.

_____

_____

_____

_____

Visit our new **MyHealthProfessions Lab** to accompany *Anatomy & Physiology for Health Professions.* Here you'll find a rich collection of quizzes, case studies, and animations for deeper understanding and application.

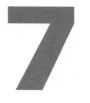

7

The Muscular System

MOVEMENT FOR THE JOURNEY

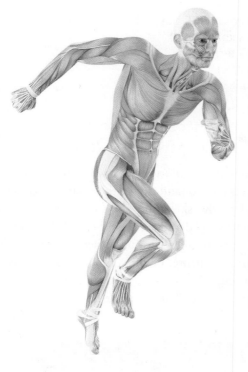

As we continue our journey of exploration, we obviously need a transportation method so that we may reach our destination. We can go by plane, train, or car. However, no matter what transportation system we use, we must utilize the body's muscular system to get to the vehicle. Although the skeletal system provides the framework for the human body, the body also needs a system that allows movement, or locomotion, which is the job of the muscular system. The movement we are most familiar with is the use of our external muscles to walk, run, or lift objects. This external movement allows us to explore all the wonderful sites throughout our journey and, yes, even to turn the pages as we journey through this book. However, movement is also required within the body. This internal movement occurs when food, air, waste products, and body fluids such as blood must all be transported within our bodies. For example, if you drink some bad water on your journey, the smooth muscles in your digestive tract will rapidly pass it through your system to be expelled in the form of urgent diarrhea. Different types of specialized muscles within the muscular system allow for both external and internal movement. This chapter defines and contrasts the different muscle types needed for both external and internal body movement.

LEARNING OUTCOMES

At the completion of your journey through this chapter, you will be able to:

- Differentiate the three major muscle types.
- Explain the difference between voluntary and involuntary muscles.
- Explain the types of skeletal muscle movement and the relationship between muscles.
- Review movement terminology.
- Identify and explain the components of a muscle cell.
- Describe the cellular activities required for muscle movement.
- Discuss how muscles receive the fuel they need to function.
- Identify specific skeletal muscles in different body regions.
- Define function and location of visceral or smooth muscle.
- Describe the function and actions of cardiac muscle.
- Name common disorders of the musculoskeletal system.

Pronunciation Guide Pro·nun·ci·a·tion

Correct pronunciation is important in any journey so that you and others are completely understood. Here is a "see and say" Pronunciation Guide for the more difficult terms to pronounce in this chapter. Please note that even though there are standard pronunciations, regional variations of the pronunciations can occur.

acetylcholine (ah SEET ul KOH leen)
actin (ak TIN)
adenosine triphosphate
  (ah DEN oh sin try FOSS fate)
aponeurosis (APP oh new ROH sis)
ataxia (ah TAK see uh)
atrophy (AT roh fee)
biceps brachii (BRA key eye)
diaphragm (DYE ah fram)
electromyography (ee LEK troh my OG rah fee)
fibromyalgia (FIE broh my AL jee uh)
flaccid (FLAS sid)
flexion (FLEK shun)
glycogen (GLIE koh jen)

Guillain-Barré syndrome (GEY yan bar RAY)
hypertrophy (high PER troh fee)
intercalated discs (in TER kuh LATE ed)
muscular dystrophy (MUS kyoo lahr DIS troh fee)
myalgia (my AL jee uh)
myasthenia gravis (my as THEE nee uh GRAV iss)
myofibril (my oh FIE bril)
myosin (MY oh sin)
rigor mortis (RIG or MORE tiss)
sarcomeres (SAR koh meerz)
sphincter (SFING ter)
tetanus (TET ah nus)
tonus (TONE us)

OVERVIEW OF THE MUSCULAR SYSTEM

Because of the numerous functions they must perform, muscles come in many shapes and sizes. The structure of the muscle matches its function, as you will see shortly.

Types of Muscles

Muscle is a general term for all contractile tissue. The term *muscle* comes from the Latin word *mus*, which means "mouse," because the movement of muscles looks like mice running around under our skin. The contractile property of muscle tissue allows it to become short and thick in response to a nerve impulse. Muscles then relax back to their original length once that impulse is removed. When contracting, the muscles do not simply shorten, but exert a force as they become shorter. This alternate contraction and relaxation is what causes movement. Muscle cells are elongated and resemble strands of metal such as those found in cables. Muscle tissue is constructed of bundles of these strands that are referred to as *muscle fibers*. These fibers are approximately the diameter of human hair. Under the direction of the nervous system, all the muscles provide for motion of some type for your body.

The body has three major types of muscles: skeletal, smooth, and cardiac. We begin with a general description and comparison of these three muscle types and then get more specific about each type.

Skeletal muscles are *voluntary muscles*, which means they are under conscious control and derive their name because they are attached to the skeleton. The fibers in skeletal muscles appear to be striped and are therefore called *striated* (striped) muscle. These muscles allow us to perform external movements—running, lifting, or scratching, for example. These are the muscles we try to develop through exercise and sports and also so we look good at the beach.

Amazing Facts

Muscles

- Muscles make up almost half the weight of the body.
- There are 650 different muscles in the human body.
- The size of your muscles is influenced by how much you use them. This is why speed skaters have large leg muscles.
- Individual elongated muscle cells can be up to 12 inches, or 30 centimeters, in length.
- At about the age of 40, the number and diameter of muscle fibers begin to decrease, and by age 80, up to 50 percent of the muscle mass may be lost. Exercise and good nutrition help to minimize this loss.

Unlike skeletal muscle, smooth muscle is *involuntary* and not under our conscious control. It is also called **smooth muscle** because it does not have the striped appearance of skeletal muscles. This involuntary muscle is found within certain organs, blood vessels, and airways. Because it is the muscle of organs, it is sometimes called *visceral muscle*. Smooth muscle allows for the internal movement of food (*peristalsis*) in the case of the stomach and other digestive organs. In addition, smooth muscle facilitates the movement of blood by changing the diameter of the blood vessels (vasoconstriction and vasodilation) and also the movement of air by changing the diameter of the airways found in our lungs.

The third type of muscle is the specialized **cardiac muscle**, which is striated like skeletal muscle. This muscle type is found solely in the heart. It makes up the walls of the heart and causes it to contract. These contractions cause the internal movement (circulation) of blood within the body. Fortunately, cardiac muscle, like smooth muscle, is an involuntary muscle. Imagine if we had to think each time for our heart to beat.

All muscles share certain characteristics such as the ability to stretch, called *extensibility*. For example, if you would swallow a large bolus of food, the smooth muscle in your esophagus must be able to stretch and allow it to pass or it would become painfully stuck. In addition they all share *contractility*, which is the ability to contract or shorten muscle fibers forcefully. All muscles exhibit *excitability*, which is muscle response to stimulation by either nerves or hormones. Finally, all muscles show some level of *elasticity*, which is the ability to return to original resting length after being stretched. **FIGURE 7–1** ■ contrasts the three types of muscles found within the body. We will now explore each of these types in further depth.

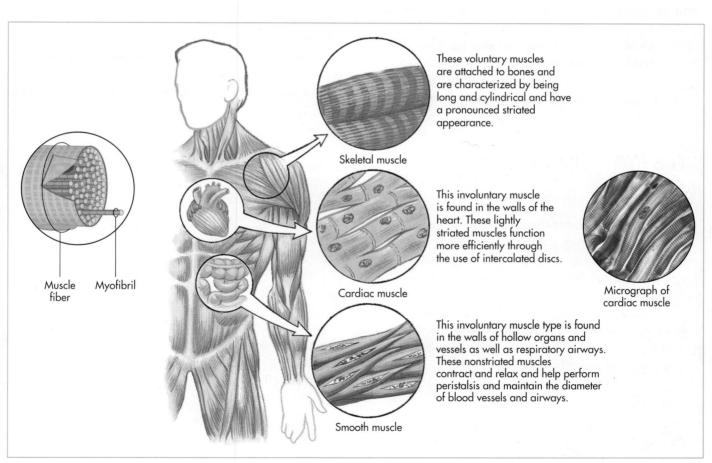

These voluntary muscles are attached to bones and are characterized by being long and cylindrical and have a pronounced striated appearance.

Skeletal muscle

This involuntary muscle is found in the walls of the heart. These lightly striated muscles function more efficiently through the use of intercalated discs.

Cardiac muscle

Micrograph of cardiac muscle

This involuntary muscle type is found in the walls of hollow organs and vessels as well as respiratory airways. These nonstriated muscles contract and relax and help perform peristalsis and maintain the diameter of blood vessels and airways.

Smooth muscle

Muscle fiber   Myofibril

FIGURE 7–1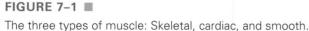

The three types of muscle: Skeletal, cardiac, and smooth.

⬤ *Clinical Application*

MUSCLE TONE

Have you ever had a cast on for an extended period of time? When it is removed, the arm or leg is much smaller and weaker than the limb without the cast. Why does this occur? Normally, all muscles exhibit muscle tone (tonus). **Tonus** is the partial contraction of a muscle with a resistance to stretching. Athletes who exercise regularly have increased muscle tone, making their muscles more pronounced. The muscle fibers in an athlete increase in diameter (*hypertrophy*) and become stronger. **Hypertrophy** refers to increased growth or development. When muscles are not used, they begin to lose their tone and become flaccid (soft and flabby). For example, if a patient is required to remain in bed (bedfast) for an extended period of time, his or her muscles waste away (**atrophy**) from the lack of use. One of the reasons patients are encouraged to get out of bed as soon as possible is to prevent atrophy from occurring. If skeletal muscle is damaged, it can regenerate itself, though not as well as bone or epithelium. However, if the damage is extensive, then a scar forms.

SKELETAL MUSCLES

Skeletal muscles are attached to bones and provide movement for your body. Remember from Chapter 6, "The Skeletal System," that **tendons** are fibrous tissues that usually attach skeletal muscle to bones and that **ligaments** attach bone to bone? Note that some muscles can attach to a bone or soft tissue without a tendon. Such muscles use broad sheets of connective tissue called **aponeuroses**. This type of connection is found, for example, in some facial and abdominal muscles.

As mentioned earlier, skeletal muscle is known as voluntary muscle; this is because its movement can be controlled by conscious thought. The numerous skeletal muscles found throughout the body are responsible for movement, maintaining our body posture, and heat generation. **FIGURE 7–2** ■ shows some of the major skeletal muscles found in the human body.

TEST YOUR KNOWLEDGE 7–1

Choose the best answer:

1. Muscle contraction is the ability of a muscle to
   a. relax when there is no nerve impulse.
   b. get smaller.
   c. shorten with force.
   d. recoil.

2. Smooth muscle is found in all the following *except* the
   a. airways.
   b. digestive system.
   c. blood vessels.
   d. heart.

3. Which types of muscles are striated?
   a. smooth and cardiac
   b. cardiac and skeletal
   c. skeletal and smooth
   d. smooth only

4. Striations are
   a. collagen strands that strengthen the muscle matrix.
   b. tendons.
   c. muscle cells.
   d. stripes on muscles.

5. Which characteristics are shared by all muscle types?
   a. contractility
   b. excitability
   c. extensibility
   d. all the above

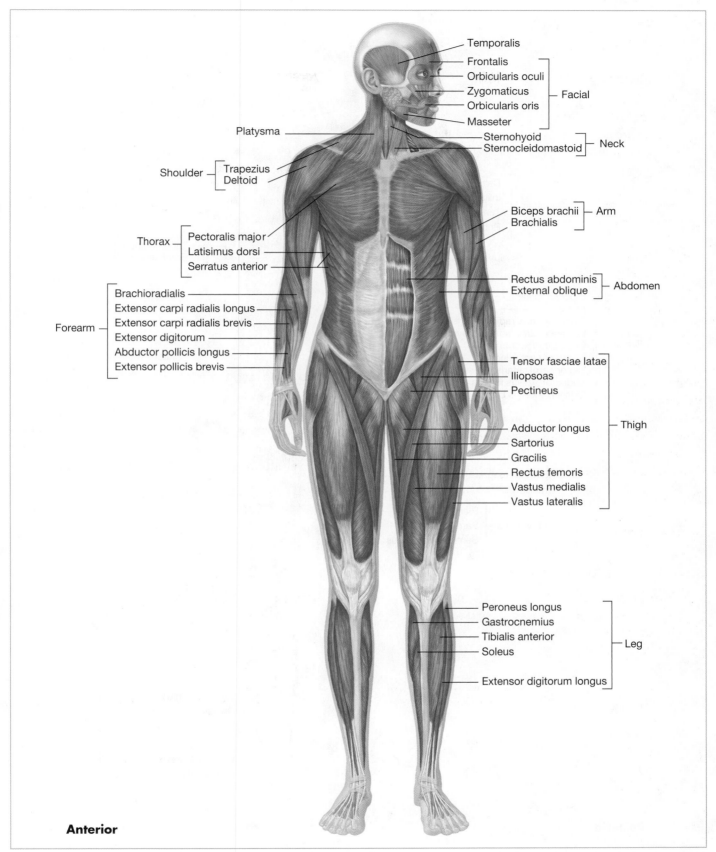

Anterior

FIGURE 7–2 ■

Anterior and posterior view of major muscles.

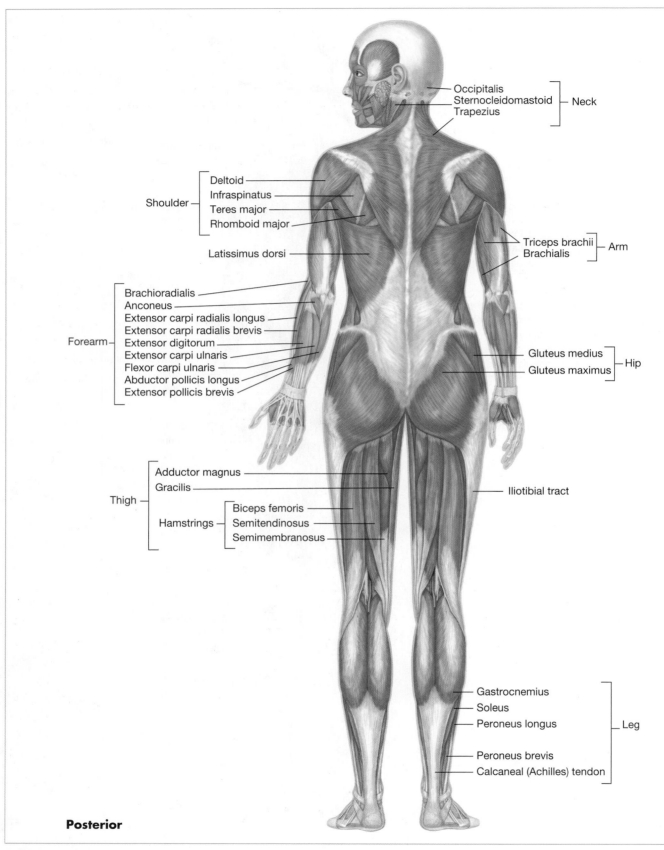

Occipitalis
Sternocleidomastoid — Neck
Trapezius

Shoulder
Deltoid
Infraspinatus
Teres major
Rhomboid major

Triceps brachii — Arm
Brachialis

Latissimus dorsi

Forearm
Brachioradialis
Anconeus
Extensor carpi radialis longus
Extensor carpi radialis brevis
Extensor digitorum
Extensor carpi ulnaris
Flexor carpi ulnaris
Abductor pollicis longus
Extensor pollicis brevis

Gluteus medius — Hip
Gluteus maximus

Thigh
Adductor magnus
Gracilis

Iliotibial tract

Hamstrings
Biceps femoris
Semitendinosus
Semimembranosus

Gastrocnemius
Soleus
Peroneus longus — Leg

Peroneus brevis
Calcaneal (Achilles) tendon

Posterior

FIGURE 7–2 ■ (*continued*)

Skeletal Muscle Movement

The body requires several different types of movement to perform various tasks. This movement is accomplished through the coordination of the contraction and relaxation of different muscles.

Contraction and Relaxation

Body movement is a result of the contraction (shortening of the muscle fibers) of certain muscles, and the relaxation of others. Consider the act of bending your arm so your fingers touch your shoulder. To really learn the concept, actually bend your arm and touch your fingers to your shoulder while resting your other hand on your biceps muscle. To do this, your forearm is drawn to your shoulder as a result of the contraction of your biceps brachii. Did you feel the shortening and bulging of the biceps brachii? Muscles, either by themselves or in muscle groups that cause movement, are known as **agonists**, or **primary movers**.

The chief muscle causing the movement is the primary mover—in this example, the biceps muscle. Typically, as your muscle contracts, one of the bones will move (lower forearm) while the other (humerus) will remain stationary. The end of the muscle that is attached to the stationary bone is the **point of origin**, and in this example, it is at the shoulder area. The muscle end that is attached to the moving bone is the **point of insertion**. It is near the elbow (see **FIGURE 7–3** ■). The action of the primary mover is to move the point of insertion toward the point of origin as the muscle contracts.

Other muscles can assist this movement, such as some of the muscles in the hands and wrist. These are called **synergistic** muscles because they assist the primary mover. (The brachioradialis muscle is a synergist to the biceps brachii because it also flexes the elbow.) To straighten that same arm requires you to relax your biceps muscle and to contract your triceps muscles. Because these muscles cause movement in the opposite direction when they contract, they are called **antagonists**. This brings us to an important concept. All movement is a result of contraction of primary movers and relaxation of *opposing* muscles. In our example, you cannot forcefully contract the biceps muscles and straighten your arm. Try it.

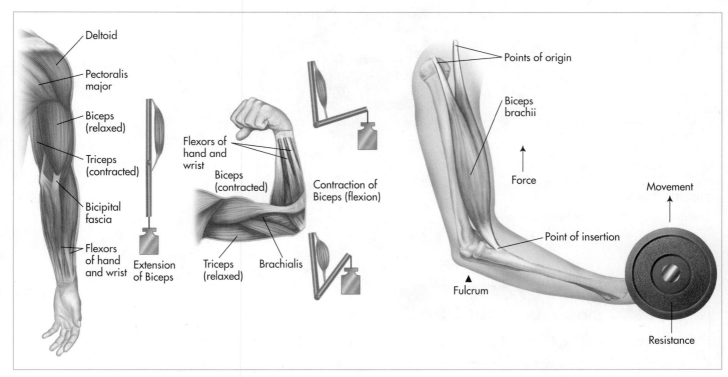

FIGURE 7–3 ■

Coordination of antagonist muscles to perform movement.

One very important skeletal muscle that controls our breathing is the **diaphragm**. This dome-shaped muscle separates the abdominal and thoracic cavities and is responsible for performing the major work of bringing air into our lungs. Exactly how this process occurs is discussed in detail in Chapter 14, "The Respiratory System." The diaphragm is unique in that it is under both voluntary and involuntary control. You don't have to think each time you breathe, but you can voluntarily change the way you breathe. **FIGURE 7–4** ■ shows the major muscle of breathing.

Movement Terminology

Certain terms are utilized to describe the direction of body movement. In Chapter 6, we discussed movement as it relates to joints in the skeletal system. In this chapter, we briefly discuss movement as it relates to muscles. (Because muscles move joints, the movement terminology is the same, but it's worth reviewing it again.) **Rotation** describes circular movement that occurs around an axis. Rotation occurs, for example, when you turn your head from left to right or right to left. **Circumduction** is the movement of a limb in a circle. Making arm circles is an example of circumduction. **Abduction** means to move *away* from the midline of the body.

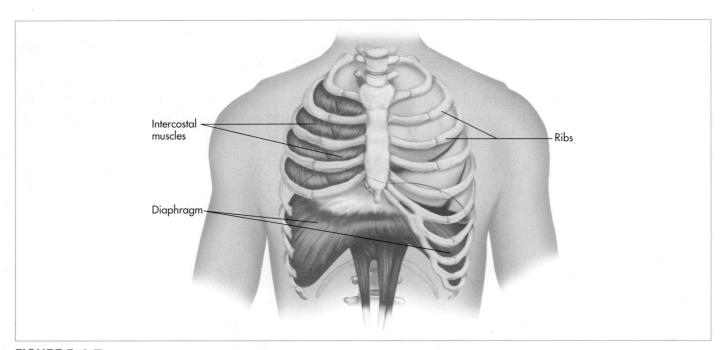

Intercostal muscles

Ribs

Diaphragm

FIGURE 7–4 ■

The diaphragm: The major muscle of breathing.

Clinical Application

LAUGHING UNTIL IT HURTS

Why is it you can get a pain in your side from hard laughing or running too long? This is because when you are breathing in deeply, your lungs push down on your diaphragm while your abdominal muscles are contracting and pushing up on the diaphragm at the same time. The repeated compression on your diaphragm is what causes a muscle spasm known in lay terms as a "runner's stitch."

FOCUS ON PROFESSIONS

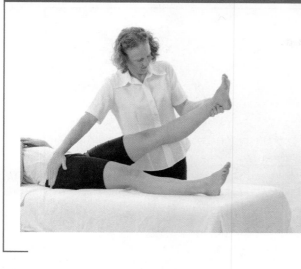

Kinesiology is the study of muscles and movement. A **kinesiologist** is one who studies movement and can perform therapeutic treatment (kinesiotherapy) utilizing specific movements or exercises. Learn more about these specialties within the field of kinesiology by visiting the websites of national associations such as the American Kinesiology Association (AKA) and the National Association of Kinesiology and Physical Education in Higher Education (NAKPEHE).

When you raise your arm to point when giving directions, you are performing abduction. **Adduction** occurs when you produce a movement that moves *toward* the midline of the body. When you bring your arm back down to your side from pointing, you are performing adduction.

Extension is a term used for *increasing* the angle between two bones connected at a joint. Extension is needed when you kick a football. In this situation, extension occurs when your leg straightens during the kick. The muscle that straightens the joint is called the **extensor muscle. Flexion** is the opposite of extension. In this situation, you *decrease* the angle between two bones. Flexion occurs when you bend your legs to sit down. Flexion and rotation occur when you get your arm into position to arm wrestle. The muscle that bends the joint is called the **flexor muscle**. In this case, a picture is worth a thousand words or at least the 124 words used to explain these concepts. **FIGURE 7–5** ■ illustrates these movements.

TEST YOUR KNOWLEDGE 7–2

Give the correct body movement term for the following activities:

1. Looking right and left at a stop sign _____

2. The first movement in curling a weight _____

3. Returning the weight from the curled position to your side _____

Complete the following:

4. The muscle that causes a movement is the _____.

5. The muscle attachment that does not move during muscle action is the _____.

6. The science of muscles and their movement is termed _____.

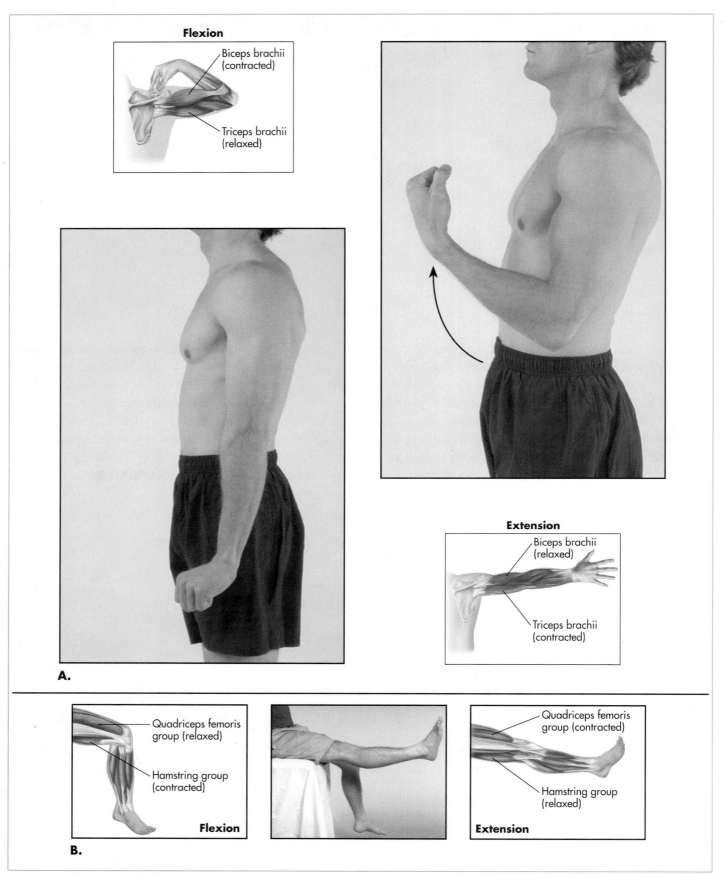

Flexion

Biceps brachii
(contracted)

Triceps brachii
(relaxed)

Extension

Biceps brachii
(relaxed)

Triceps brachii
(contracted)

A.

Quadriceps femoris
group (relaxed)

Hamstring group
(contracted)

Flexion

Quadriceps femoris
group (contracted)

Hamstring group
(relaxed)

Extension

B.

FIGURE 7–5 ■

The types of skeletal movement. (A) Flexion and extension of left forearm. (B) Flexion and extension of the leg.

MUSCULAR MOVEMENT AT THE CELLULAR LEVEL

Exactly how are muscular contraction and relaxation accomplished? How does the muscle tissue cause a coordinated and smooth contraction? Let's look in more detail at how muscles work.

The Functional Unit of the Muscle

Skeletal muscles look very simple if you examine only their macroanatomy. However, if you look deep into a skeletal muscle, it is divided into several layers of cylinders packed inside each other.

The typical muscle, like the biceps brachii, is surrounded by connective tissue, continuous with the tendon, called **epimysium**. Inside the muscle are bundles of muscle fibers (cells) surrounded by **perimysium**. The bundles are called **fascicles**.

The muscle fibers themselves are elongated cells up to 12 inches, or 30 centimeters, in length. Each muscle fiber is encased in a connective tissue sheath called **endomysium** and is filled with cylinders called **myofibrils**. The myofibrils are like a strand of metal, and these strands of metal can be put together to form a cable, which would be a muscle segment (see **FIGURE 7–6A** ■).

For contraction to take place, each fiber must possess many functional contractile units called **sarcomeres**, which are

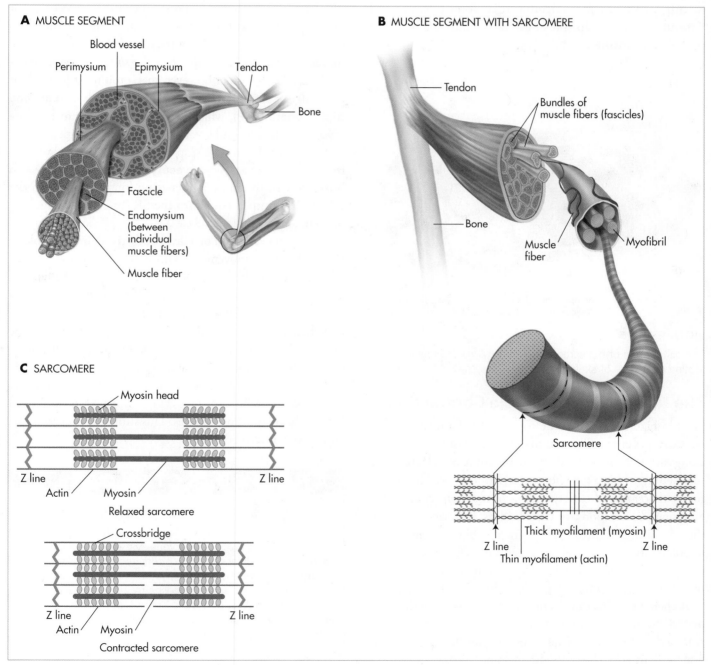

A MUSCLE SEGMENT

- Blood vessel
- Perimysium
- Epimysium
- Tendon
- Bone
- Fascicle
- Endomysium (between individual muscle fibers)
- Muscle fiber

B MUSCLE SEGMENT WITH SARCOMERE

- Tendon
- Bundles of muscle fibers (fascicles)
- Bone
- Muscle fiber
- Myofibril
- Sarcomere
- Thick myofilament (myosin)
- Z line
- Thin myofilament (actin)
- Z line

C SARCOMERE

- Myosin head
- Z line
- Actin
- Myosin
- Z line

Relaxed sarcomere

- Crossbridge
- Z line
- Actin
- Myosin
- Z line

Contracted sarcomere

FIGURE 7–6 ■

(A) The muscle segment. (B) The muscle segment with sarcomere. (C) Relaxed and contracted sarcomeres.

subunits of the myofibrils. Each fiber has the ability to contract because of the makeup of the sarcomere. Each sarcomere unit has two types of threadlike structures called thick and thin *myofilaments*. The thick myofilaments are made up of the protein **myosin**, and the thin ones are primarily made up of the protein **actin**. The sarcomere has the actin and myosin filaments arranged in repeating units separated from each other by bands called **Z lines**, which give the striated appearance to skeletal muscle. The arrangement of the myofilaments cause the striations on skeletal muscle (see Figure 7–6B and C).

In addition, muscle fibers have several other modifications for contraction, including the **sarcolemma**, a specialized cell membrane; the **sarcoplasmic reticulum (SR)**, which is a modified endoplasmic reticulum that stores calcium; and **T-tubules**, which help spread excitation into the inside of the cell (see **FIGURE 7–7** ■).

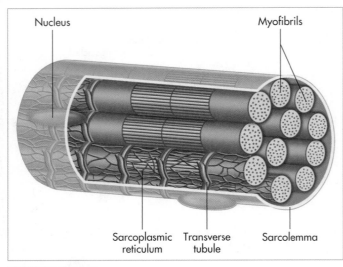

FIGURE 7–7 ■

The distribution of the sarcoplasmic reticulum and tubules around myofibrils of skeletal muscle.

The Mechanism of Muscle Contraction

Note in Figure 7–6C that the contraction of a muscle causes the two types of myofilaments to slide toward each other, shortening each sarcomere and therefore the entire muscle. Picture a tube sliding within a tube, such as on a trombone. This sliding filament action and corresponding contraction requires that temporary connections, or cross-bridges, be formed between the thick filament (myosin) heads and the thin filaments (actin) to pull the sarcomere together. When a muscle is relaxed, these cross-bridges do not form. In order for muscle to contract, the muscle must be stimulated. Just how does that happen?

A chemical signal called a **neurotransmitter**—in this case, **acetylcholine**—is released from the nervous system. (This will be discussed in more detail in Chapter 9, "The Nervous System (Part I)".) The acetylcholine binds to specialized areas

on the sarcolemma and opens channels that let sodium ions enter the muscle cell. This excites the muscle. When the muscle is excited, calcium is released from the sarcoplasmic reticulum (SR) and flows into the cytoplasm of the muscle fiber.

Remember that the relaxed muscle has no cross-bridges? The calcium released allows these cross-bridges to form so the muscle can contract. When the cross-bridges form, the myosin heads rotate and pull the actin toward the center of the sarcomere. But the myosin doesn't make cross-bridges only once; it does it repeatedly, binding and unbinding until the actin filaments overlap (see Figure 7–6C). The whole sarcomere is shorter.

When the sarcomere relaxes, the filaments return to their resting or relaxed position. Visualize a raised drawbridge, where cars cannot pass. To be functional, the cross-connection—or lowering of the drawbridge—must occur, similar to the cross-bridges needed for a muscle contraction. This model of skeletal muscle contraction is aptly called the *sliding filament–cross-bridge* model. Consider however, that a toll must be paid for the bridge to lower and connect. The body's toll is **adenosine triphosphate (ATP)**, which provides the energy to help the myosin heads form and break the cross-bridges with actin.

How does the muscle stop contracting? Acetylcholine is broken down by an enzyme **acetylcholinesterase** (*ase* = to break down), the muscle fiber is no longer excited, so the calcium is pumped back into the SR, the cross-bridges are broken, and the muscle relaxes.

Have you ever heard of a dead body rising from a table or showing signs of movement? This may sound like the opening for a movie about zombies or the "undead." Actually, it is a normal physiologic process called **rigor mortis** that can be explained by science and not by science fiction.

When a body dies, all the stored calcium cannot be pumped back into the sarcoplasmic reticulum. Therefore, excess calcium remains in the muscles throughout the body and causes the muscle fibers to shorten (contract) and stiffen the whole body. In addition, ATP is not present in a dead body to break the cross-bridges. This stiffening process of the entire body is termed *rigor mortis*.

APPLIED SCIENCE

Interrelatedness of Neuromuscular System

Contraction of a skeletal muscle requires the coordination of both the muscular and nervous systems. The initiation of a skeletal muscular contraction requires an impulse from a motor neuron of the nervous system to trigger a release of the neurotransmitter acetylcholine (ACh), which opens the sodium channels and sets the process of muscle contraction into motion. This all occurs at the neuromuscular junction. The nervous system's role in this action and the neuromuscular connection are fully explored in Chapters 9 and 10.

LEARNING HINT

Muscle Contraction Step by Step

1. Acetylcholine, a neurotransmitter, is released from a neuron.
2. Acetylcholine binds to muscle and causes sodium channels to open. Sodium flows into the muscle fiber, and the fiber becomes excited.
3. The excitement of the muscle fiber causes calcium to be released into the cytoplasm from the sarcoplasmic reticulum.
4. The calcium allows the forming of cross-bridges between myosin heads and actin myofilaments.

5. Adenosine triphosphate (ATP) is used up, allowing cross-bridges to break and reform, pulling the actin myofilaments closer together as they slide along the myosin myofilaments. The sarcomere shortens.
6. Many shortened sarcomeres result in shortening of many muscle fibers. This is muscle contraction.
7. Acetylcholinesterase degrades acetylcholine so the muscle can relax.

TEST YOUR KNOWLEDGE 7–3

Fill in the blank.

1. The thin myofilament needed for muscle contraction is composed of _____.

2. The two ingredients needed for cross-bridges to form and break are _____ and _____.

3. The fundamental unit of muscle contraction is the _____.

4. Sodium flowing into muscle fibers is triggered by the binding of _____ released from neurons.

5. During contraction _____ heads bind to _____ myofilaments.

6. The neurotransmitter substance responsible for skeletal muscle contraction is _____.

FOCUS ON PROFESSIONS

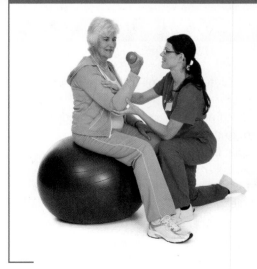

Not only do the skeletal muscles facilitate movement but, integrated with the nervous system, they provide support for posture while standing or sitting. Promoting balance and posture, along with proper muscle function, is one of the responsibilities of **physical therapists**. These professionals, referred to as PTs, perform many therapies, such as range of motion (ROM) exercises, to ensure full muscle movement. **Occupational therapists** (OTs) assist clients in using and adapting their muscle function to perform activities of daily living and improving their quality of life. Learn more about these professions by visiting the websites of national associations such as the American Physical Therapy Association (APTA) and the American Occupational Therapy Association (AOTA).

MUSCULAR FUEL

Muscle, like all tissue, needs fuel in the form of nutrients and oxygen to survive and function. The body stores a carbohydrate called **glycogen** in the muscle. Glycogen is always on reserve waiting to be converted to a usable energy source. When needed, the muscle can convert glycogen to **glucose**, which releases energy for the muscle to function. Remember cellular respiration from Chapters 3 and 4? Your cells must have glucose to make adenosine triphosphate (ATP) efficiently. Muscles with very high demands (such as leg muscles) also store fat and use it as energy. The release of energy also produces heat, and this is why strenuous or prolonged exercises can overheat our bodies.

The higher-demand muscles not only use fat as an energy source, but they also have a much richer blood supply than do less demanding muscles. These muscles are needed for endurance, such as required by long-distance running. The richer blood supply carries extra oxygen to hardworking muscles, giving those muscles a darker color.

Some muscles, such as those in the hand, have fewer heavy demands placed on them and need only a small supply of blood. They therefore have a lighter color. These muscles are faster but do not have the endurance capabilities that heavily used muscles have. Next time you take a long walk, keep pumping your hand. Although the muscles in the hand can move faster than the leg muscles, they will tire more quickly.

Another example can be found in birds. Chickens, because the breast and wing muscles are not heavily used, have white meat breasts and wings. The legs, however, endure constant use, and the meat is therefore dark. By contrast, a woodcock, a migratory bird that must fly long distances (endurance), has dark breast meat. Now you know why a chicken's breast meat is white. When is the last time you saw a chicken flying overhead?

APPLIED SCIENCE

Maintaining a Core Body Temperature

Not only do muscles produce movement, but they also help maintain posture, stabilize joints, and produce heat. Producing heat is important in maintaining the body core temperature. As the energy-rich ATP is used for muscle contraction, three-fourths of its energy escapes as heat. This process helps maintain body temperature by producing heat when muscles are utilized. This is why your temperature rises when exercising and also why you shiver when you are very cold. Shivering is your body's way of saying it is too cold, and it needs to generate a lot of heat via many muscle contractions (shivering). In turn, this increases the body temperature.

SKELETAL MUSCLES OF SPECIFIC BODY REGIONS

Many times on a journey, we need a road map for reference. These road maps are often big maps of an entire state. However, there are also inserts of specific cities that give much greater detail. Think of Figure 7–2 as our "state map" of the anterior and posterior major muscles. The following series of "city maps" will provide you with greater detail. See TABLE 7–1 ■ for specific information about selected muscles.

LEARNING HINT

Muscle Names

There are several ways to name muscles. If you remember these examples, you will have an easier time remembering the muscles. Muscles can be named based on any of the following criteria:

1. Muscle location (Example: Biceps brachii is in the arm. Brachii = arm.)
2. Number of origins (Example: Biceps brachii has two origins. Biceps = two heads.)
3. Action (Example: Adductor longus adducts the thigh.)
4. Size (Example: Gluteus maximus. Maximus = biggest.)
5. Location of attachments (Example: Brachioradialis. Radialis refers to the radius.)
6. Shape (Example: Deltoid is triangular. Delta = triangle.)
7. Direction of fibers (Example: External oblique. Oblique = angled.)
8. Combination (Example: Pectoralis major. Pectoral = chest, major = big.)

TABLE 7–1 MAJOR MUSCLES: ORIGINS, INSERTIONS, AND ACTIONS

MUSCLE NAME	MUSCLE LOCATION	MUSCLE ORIGIN	MUSCLE INSERTION	MUSCLE ACTION
Biceps brachii	anterior upper arm	scapula	radius	flexes arm at the elbow
Triceps brachii	posterior upper arm	proximal humerus & scapula	posterior ulna (proximal)	extends arm at the elbow
Orbicularis oculi	encircles eye	frontal, maxilla, and orbit	eyelid	closes eyelid
Masseter	jaw or mandible	zygomatic arch	mandible	closes jaw
Sternocleidomastoid	anterolateral neck	sternum & clavicle	mastoid process	flexes and rotates head
Pectoralis major	chest	clavicle, ribs, sternum	proximal humerus	flexes, rotates, and adducts arm
Deltoid	shoulder	clavicle & scapula	proximal humerus	abducts arm
Intercostals:	between ribs			assist in ventilation
external		inferior rib	superior rib	elevate rib cage
internal		superior rib	inferior rib	depress rib cage
Diaphragm	floor of thoracic cavity	inferior rib cage & sternum	central tendon	prime mover of inspiration
Gluteus maximus	buttocks	ilium, sacrum, & coccyx	proximal femur	extends thigh
Hamstring group	posterior portion of thigh	ischium	tibia	flexes leg at knee
Quadriceps group	anterior portion of thigh	pelvis	patella & tibia	extends leg at knee
Tibialis anterior	anterior of lower leg	proximal tibia	metatarsals	dorsiflexes foot
Gastrocnemius	main muscle of calf (posterior lower leg)	distal femur	calcaneus via calcaneal (Achilles) tendon	plantar flexes foot
Vastus lateralis	anterior thigh	femur	tibia	extends the leg; also used as site for injections

TEST YOUR KNOWLEDGE 7–4

Fill in the blank.

1. The _____ are the primary knee flexors.

2. The _____, knee extensors, originate on the _____ and insert on the _____ and _____.

(continued)

TEST YOUR KNOWLEDGE 7–4 *(continued)*

3. The _____ originates on the sternum and clavicle and inserts on the mastoid process.

4. This muscle inserts via the Achilles tendon _____.

5. The _____, an elbow flexor, is the antagonist of the _____, an elbow extensor.

6. Ben is in the middle of the Olympic trials for the 400-meter hurdles when he falls to the ground, clutching his leg. Upon examination he has pain in the posterior thigh and cannot flex his knee. Which muscles are injured? _____

7. The muscle in the leg used for an injection site is _____.

Facial Skeletal Muscles

Please see **FIGURE 7–8** ■, which shows the facial skeletal muscles.

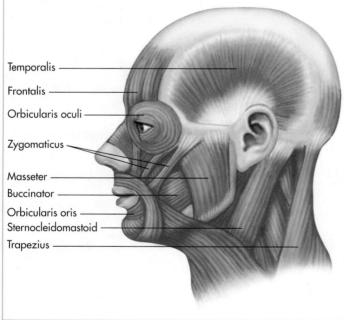

Temporalis
Frontalis
Orbicularis oculi
Zygomaticus
Masseter
Buccinator
Orbicularis oris
Sternocleidomastoid
Trapezius

FIGURE 7–8 ■
Skeletal facial muscles.

Anterior and Posterior Trunk Skeletal Muscles

Now, take an in-depth look at the muscles of the anterior and posterior trunk of the body in **FIGURE 7–9** ■.

Skeletal Muscles of the Arm and Shoulder

Moving out to the peripheral area of the body, we now zoom in on the skeletal muscles of the hand, arm, and shoulder in **FIGURE 7–10** ■.

Skeletal Muscles of the Legs

We finish our tour with the skeletal muscles of the hip and leg in **FIGURE 7–11** ■.

FOCUS ON PROFESSIONS

With physical activity and the daily stress of life, muscles often become sore and fatigued. **Massage therapists** work directly on the muscles to aid in their relaxation and optimal functioning. Massaging techniques help stimulate blood flow and relax tense muscles. Learn more about this profession by visiting the website of national organizations, such as the National Association of Massage Therapists (NAMT), the American Massage Therapy Associations (AMTA), and the National Association of Nurse Massage Therapists (NANMT).

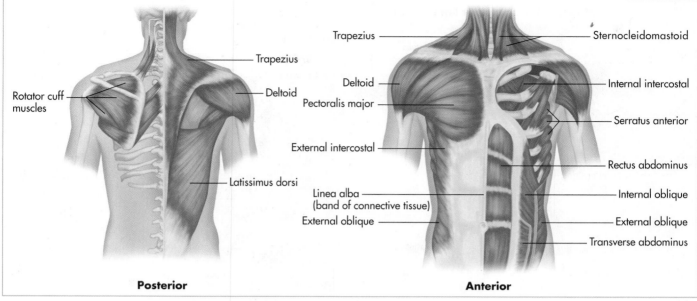

FIGURE 7–9 ■

Skeletal muscles of the posterior and anterior trunk.

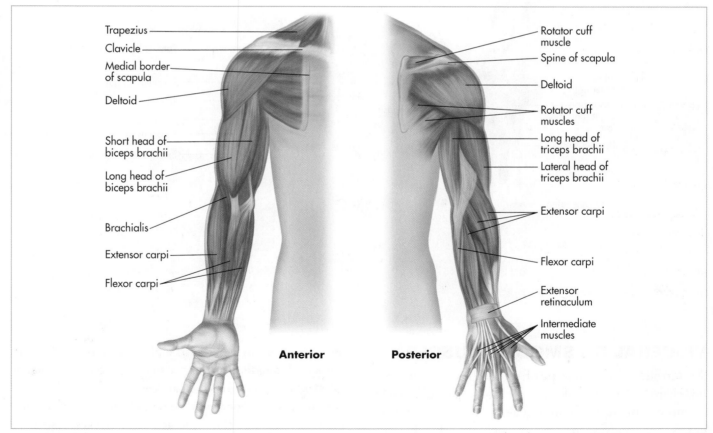

FIGURE 7–10 ■

Skeletal muscles of the shoulder, arm, and hand.

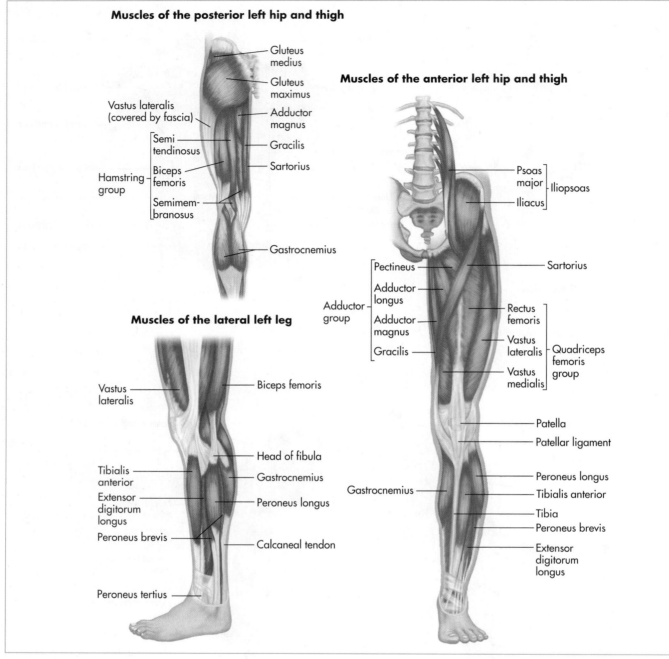

Muscles of the posterior left hip and thigh

- Gluteus medius
- Gluteus maximus
- Vastus lateralis (covered by fascia)
- Adductor magnus
- Semitendinosus
- Gracilis
- Biceps femoris
- Sartorius
- Hamstring group
- Semimembranosus
- Gastrocnemius

Muscles of the anterior left hip and thigh

- Psoas major
- Iliacus
- Iliopsoas
- Pectineus
- Sartorius
- Adductor longus
- Rectus femoris
- Adductor group
- Adductor magnus
- Vastus lateralis
- Gracilis
- Quadriceps femoris group
- Vastus medialis
- Patella
- Patellar ligament
- Peroneus longus
- Gastrocnemius
- Tibialis anterior
- Tibia
- Peroneus brevis
- Extensor digitorum longus

Muscles of the lateral left leg

- Vastus lateralis
- Biceps femoris
- Head of fibula
- Tibialis anterior
- Gastrocnemius
- Extensor digitorum longus
- Peroneus longus
- Peroneus brevis
- Calcaneal tendon
- Peroneus tertius

FIGURE 7–11 ■

Skeletal muscles of the hip and leg.

VISCERAL OR SMOOTH MUSCLE

We introduced the concept of smooth muscle earlier in this chapter; now let's take a closer look. **Visceral muscle**, or **smooth muscle**, is found in all the organs (except the heart) of the body, such as the stomach and other digestive organs, the uterus, and the blood vessels and bronchial airways. Smooth muscle's ability to contract and return to a relaxed state plays a vital role in many of the body's internal workings. For example, the vital sign blood pressure can be affected by whether the blood vessels get larger in diameter (**vasodilation**) or get smaller in diameter (**vasoconstriction**). Vasodilation can lead to decreases in blood pressure due to smooth muscle relaxation in the vessel that allows it to enlarge. The enlarged vessel has less resistance to flow, and the blood pressure therefore goes down. Conversely, vasoconstriction can cause increased blood pressure due to the smooth muscle contraction that restricts the blood vessel.

As another example, during an asthma attack, smooth muscles in the airways of the lungs constrict, making it difficult to get air into and out of the lungs. This is what causes the wheezing sound heard during an attack.

Special structures composed of smooth muscle, called **sphincters**, are found throughout your digestive system. These donut-shaped muscles act as doorways to let materials in and out by alternately contracting and relaxing. For example, two sphincters in the stomach act like doors. One opens to allow food in from the esophagus, and another opens to allow food into the small intestine. Have you ever swallowed a large amount of bread or stuffing and had it get stuck on the way down to your stomach? This is a painful reminder that there is a sphincter that must relax and open to allow food to enter your stomach. The muscles of the digestive system are discussed in greater depth in Chapter 16, "The Gastrointestinal System."

LEARNING HINT

Smooth Muscle Regulation of Blood Pressure

In considering blood pressure, visualize a large highway. If one lane is taken away (vasoconstriction), the same number of cars must now fit through one less lane, leading to traffic congestion (increase in pressure). If you open up another lane (vasodilate), you relieve some of this pressure.

Smooth, or visceral, muscles are involuntary muscles and do not contract as rapidly as skeletal muscles. Skeletal muscles, once stimulated, can contract 50 times faster than smooth muscle. Because of their slower activity and lower metabolic rate, smooth muscles receive only moderate amounts of blood. Once injured, smooth muscle rarely repairs itself and, instead, forms a scar.

CARDIAC MUSCLE

Cardiac muscle forms the walls of the heart. The rhythmic contraction of cardiac muscle squeezes blood out of the chambers of the heart, causing the blood to circulate through your body. Cardiac muscle is an involuntary muscle. Remember, this means that we don't have to consciously think about making our heart contract every time we need a heartbeat. Cardiac muscle fibers are somewhat shorter than the other muscle types, but they are striated like skeletal muscle. Because the heart must work constantly until you die, the cardiac muscles must receive a generous blood supply via the coronary arteries to get enough oxygen and nutrition, as well as to get rid of waste. In fact, cardiac muscle has a richer supply of blood than any other muscle in the body. The cardiac muscle fibers are connected to each other by **intercalated discs**. Because of this connection, as one fiber contracts, the adjacent one contracts, and so on. This is similar to the domino effect or the human wave at a football stadium if done correctly. A wave of contraction occurs, allowing blood to be squeezed out of the heart and into the body. This directed wave is important for a full and effective emptying of the blood within the heart. Imagine if everyone squeezed the tube of toothpaste in the middle: Think of all the wasted toothpaste that would be left in the tube and how happy the toothpaste manufacturers would be. See **FIGURE 7–12** ■.

Cardiac muscle does not regenerate after severe damage; this leads to tissue death known as **necrosis**, such as what occurs in a severe heart attack. If the blood supply going

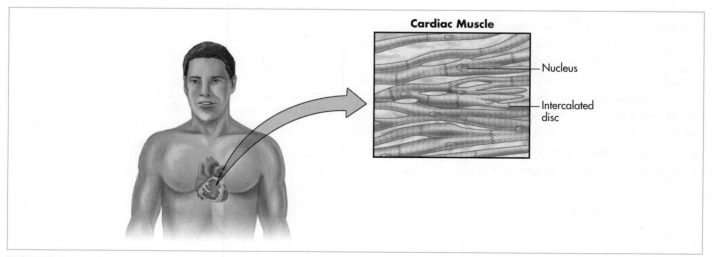

FIGURE 7–12 ■

Heart and intercalated discs.

to the heart from the coronary arteries is blocked, cardiac muscle damage can occur, causing scarring of the heart. Scar tissue does not help the healthy muscles of the heart to contract. If the scarred area is extensive, the remaining cardiac muscle may not be sufficient to pump blood efficiently. An individual with scarred cardiac muscle may have a severely diminished cardiac output, which could lead to severe disability or even death.

COMMON DISORDERS OF THE MUSCULAR SYSTEM

Because there are so many muscles covering the entire body and they are constantly being used, many disorders can occur within this system. Here are just a few examples. **Myalgia** means pain or tenderness in a muscle. **Fibromyalgia** may be one of the most common musculoskeletal disorders affecting women under age 40, but it is still not fully understood. Symptoms include aches, pains, and muscle stiffness with specific tender points on anatomical regions of the body. The exact cause is unknown, but evidence suggests that hypersensitivity to pain by the nervous system may be involved.

Ataxia is a condition in which the muscles are irregular in their actions or there is a lack of coordination. **Paralysis** is the partial or total loss of the ability of voluntary muscles to move. Sometimes it might be temporary; other times it might be permanent. A muscle that contracts involuntarily suddenly and violently for a prolonged period of time is said to have a **spasm**, or **cramp**. A spasm can occur in a single muscle or in a muscle group. **Sprains** are tears or, in severe cases, breaks in ligaments, whereas **strains** are tears or injury in muscles and tendons. A common running-related inflammatory condition of the connective muscles surrounding the tibia is called *medial tibial stress syndrome*, or, in lay terms, **shin splints**.

A **hernia** occurs when an organ or structure protrudes through the wall that normally contains it. For example, in an abdominal hernia a portion of an intestine may protrude through the muscle of the abdominal wall and become strangulated. **Tendonitis** is an inflammatory condition in which tendons may become damaged. **Muscular dystrophy** is an inherited muscular disease in which muscle fibers degenerate and there is progressive muscular weakness. Muscular disorders can be quantified by **electromyography (EMG)**, a test in which a muscle or group of muscles are stimulated with an electrical impulse. This impulse causes a muscle contraction. The strength of that muscle contraction is then recorded. Certain diseases can alter the strength of muscles.

Due to the close integration of the two systems, several diseases involve both the *nervous* system and the *muscular* system—hence, the term **neuromuscular** disease. **Myasthenia gravis** is a neuromuscular disease in which the patient exhibits gradually increasing profound muscle weakness. The first symptom of this disease is often the drooping of one or both of the upper eyelids. There is also progressive paralysis. Interestingly, tendon reflexes almost always remain. **Guillain-Barré syndrome** is a disorder of the *peripheral* nervous system that causes *flaccid* paralysis (limp muscles) and the loss of reflexes. Interestingly, the paralysis is usually *ascending*, meaning that it starts in the feet or lower extremities and progresses toward the head. Paralysis usually peaks within 10 to 14 days. Eventually, most patients return to normal, although it may take several weeks or months.

Tetanus, on the other hand, creates rigid paralysis. With this disease, any type of minor stimulus can cause muscles to go into major spasm. The stimulus can be something as simple as a loud noise or turning on a light in a room. Tetanus is a result of toxins produced by the bacteria *Clostridium tetani* found in the ground and can be spread by any type of skin puncture, not just the "rusty nail" many were warned about when they were kids. Smooth and cardiac muscle conditions are discussed in upcoming chapters.

APPLIED SCIENCE

A Useful Application of a Deadly Toxin

Botulism is a potentially deadly disease caused by food poisoning with the *Clostridium botulinum* bacteria. The toxin decreases the release of acetylcholine, thereby decreasing stimulation of skeletal muscles. Science has found a way to utilize the poison generated by this bacteria for medical and cosmetic treatment. Small amounts of botulinum toxin are used to treat wrinkles without the use of surgery. The treatment is known as Botox. In addition to cosmetic applications, botulinum toxin injections are also used to treat several other disorders, including overactive bladder, migraines, chronic muscle spasms, cerebral palsy, excessive sweating (hyperhidrosis), and strabismus (eye misalignment).

- The three main types of muscles are skeletal, smooth, and cardiac. Skeletal muscle is a striated, or striped, voluntary muscle that allows movement, stabilizes joints, and helps maintain body temperature. Smooth muscle is a nonstriated involuntary muscle found in the organs of the body and linings of vessels; it facilitates internal movement within the body. Cardiac muscle is an involuntary, striated muscle found only in the heart.

- All movement is a result of contraction of primary movers and relaxation of opposing muscles.

- Large muscles consist of many single muscle fibers comprised of myofibrils. The smallest functional contractile unit is called a sarcomere. Each sarcomere unit contains the two threadlike contractile proteins myosin and actin.

- Muscles contract as the actin and myosin protein filaments, in the presence of ATP and calcium, form cross-bridges that cause the filaments to slide past each other, thereby causing the muscle to contract or shorten. There is a relationship between the nervous and muscular systems in which the motor neuron of the nervous system initiates the activity of muscle contraction through the release of a neurotransmitter.

- There are many common diseases and conditions of the muscles, and because the nervous system is so closely related, there are also many common neuromuscular diseases.

CASE STUDY

A 30-year-old patient complains of ascending flaccid paralysis that began with tingling in the toes and muscle weakness. He had just recovered from a viral flu. This individual presented to the emergency department after the leg weakness became so profound that he could barely walk, and now he notices his arms weakening. Loss of reflexes was also noted.

a. What disease do you think this is?

_____

_____

b. Knowing that this patient is losing the ability to use skeletal muscles, what life-threatening condition could occur?

_____

_____

c. What vital signs must you monitor?

_____

_____

d. Why is muscle atrophy a problem?

_____

_____

e. What areas of patient care must be addressed?

_____

_____

f. What is the likely prognosis?

_____

_____

Multiple Choice

1. Another name for voluntary muscle is
   a. skeletal.
   b. smooth.
   c. cardiac.
   d. nonstriated.

2. Which structure does *not* contain smooth muscle?
   a. blood vessels
   b. heart
   c. digestive tract
   d. bronchi

3. Most skeletal muscles attach to bones via
   a. ligaments.
   b. joints.
   c. flexors.
   d. tendons.

4. The state of partial skeletal muscle contraction is known as
   a. homeostasis.
   b. muscle tone.
   c. partialus contractus.
   d. flexerus.

5. Cardiac muscle
   I. is a voluntary muscle.
   II. has intercalated discs to assist contraction.
   III. regenerates after injury.
   IV. lines the blood vessels.
      a. I only
      b. I and II
      c. II only
      d. I, II, III, IV

6. Jill falls and twists her ankle. Later she cannot point her toes. Her doctor tells her she has torn a tendon and must have surgery. Which tendon?
   a. patellar
   b. calcaneal
   c. rotator cuff
   d. anterior cruciate

7. Sam wakes up one morning unable to move his toes. Within a few hours he can't move his legs and calls 911. Within a week he is completely paralyzed. What disease most likely caused this?
   a. tetanus
   b. Guillain Barré
   c. muscular dystrophy
   d. muscular atrophy

Fill in the Blank

1. A sudden or violent muscle contraction is a(n) _____.

2. Partial or total loss of voluntary muscle use is _____.

3. A tear in the muscle wall through which an organ can protrude is a(n) _____.

4. The body stores a carbohydrate called _____ in the muscle; it can be converted to a usable energy source.

5. _____ means pain or tenderness in the muscle.

6. Elbow flexion is the action of the _____ muscle.

Short Answer

1. List the three major muscle types and give an example of each.

   _____

   _____

   _____

   _____

2. Explain the relationship between origin, insertion, and action of skeletal muscles.

   _____

   _____

   _____

   _____

3. List criteria for naming skeletal muscles and give examples.

_____

_____

_____

_____

4. Explain the steps needed in a skeletal muscle contraction.

_____

_____

_____

_____

5. Considering the knee, list the major muscles involved in control of the joint, their attachments, and their actions.

_____

_____

_____

_____

Visit our new **MyHealthProfessions Lab** to accompany *Anatomy & Physiology for Health Professions*. Here you'll find a rich collection of quizzes, case studies, and animations for deeper understanding and application.

The Integumentary System

THE PROTECTIVE COVERING

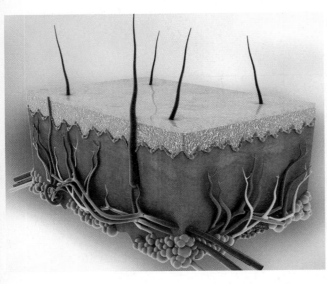

You learned in Chapter 6 that the skeletal system is like the framework of a building or house. But the framework is just one part of a building; the integrity of a house wouldn't last very long without shingles on its roof, siding of some sort, and windows, all of which help prevent the environment from damaging the main structures and inner workings. Like a house, the human body must be sheltered from the environment and that is the job of the integumentary system. Your skin forms a protective barrier to shield your body from the elements, guard against pathogens, and perform several other vital functions.

Think how important your skin is to your well-being and your ability to fully enjoy your journey. Without your skin, you would not be able to regulate your body temperature and would be uncomfortable in any environment. Because the skin is exposed to the external environment, it often needs protection. We paint our houses to protect the outer shell from the elements; likewise, we apply sunscreen when we spend a day at the beach. Although your skin is an important organ, several other accessory components such as nails, hair, and glands are involved, hence the name integumentary *system*.

LEARNING OUTCOMES

At the end of your journey through this chapter, you will be able to:

- Discuss the functions of the integumentary system.
- List and describe the layers of the skin.
- Explain the healing process of skin.
- Explain the two factors used to assess burns.
- Describe the ways in which medication is delivered via the integumentary system.
- Describe the purposes, structure, and growth of nails and hair.
- Explain how the body regulates temperature through the integumentary system.
- Describe common disorders of the integumentary system.

Pronunciation Guide

Correct pronunciation is important in any journey so that you and others are completely understood. Here is a "see and say" Pronunciation Guide for the more difficult terms to pronounce in this chapter. Please note that even though there are standard pronunciations, regional variations of the pronunciations can occur.

apocrine glands (APP oh krin)
avascular (ay VAS cue lair)
carotene (CARE oh teen)
corium (CORE ee um)
eccrine glands (EKK rin)
epidermis (ep ih DER miss)
epithelial cells (ep ih THEE lee al)
integumentary (in teg you MEN tuh ree)
keratin (KAIR eh tin)
keratinization (KAIR eh tin eye ZAY shun)
lesion (LEE zhun)
lunula (LOO nyoo lah)

melanin (MELL an in)
melanocytes (MELL an oh sights)
pustule (PUS tyool)
sebaceous gland (see BAY shus)
sebum (SEE bum)
squamous cells (SKWAY mus)
stratum basale (STRAY tum BAY sell)
stratum corneum (STRAY tum core NEE um)
stratum germinativum
  (STRAY tum JER meh NAY tee vum)
subcutaneous fascia (sub cue TAY nee us FASH ee uh)

SYSTEM OVERVIEW

In this section, we will look at the anatomy, physiology, and related pathology of the **integumentary** system. This system is the protective covering of the body and is the most exposed system. Get ready for this chapter to "get under your skin."

Integumentary System Functions

The integumentary system is comprised of the skin and its accessory components of hair, nails, and associated glands. Your integumentary system performs several vital functions besides protecting you from an invasion of disease-producing microorganisms. This system helps keep the body from drying out, acts as storage for fatty tissue necessary for energy, and, with the aid of some sunshine, produces vitamin D, which is needed to help your body utilize phosphorus and calcium for proper bone and tooth formation and growth. In addition, the skin provides sensory input (pleasant and unpleasant sensations involving pressure and temperature, for example) for your brain and helps regulate your body temperature.

The Skin

Your skin is quite a large organ, easily weighing twice as much as your brain, actually approaching 20 pounds in weight and covering an area of about 20.83 square feet on an average adult-sized body. In fact, the skin is the largest organ. A closer examination of a cross-section of skin reveals three main layers of tissue:

- *Epidermis* (*epi* = upon, *dermis* = true skin)
- *Dermis* (also called *corium*)
- *Subcutaneous fascia* (*sub* = under, *cutane/o* = skin, *fascia* = band; also called the hypodermis layer because it lies *under* the dermis)

As we discuss these three layers, please refer to **FIGURE 8–1** ■ for further clarification.

Epidermis

The **epidermis** is the outer layer of skin that we normally see. It is made up of five even smaller layers of stratified squamous epithelium. The epidermis is interesting for several reasons. First, it's **avascular** (contains no blood vessels, *a* meaning "without" and *vascular* meaning "blood vessels"). Second, the cells on the surface of this layer are constantly shedding and being replaced with new cells that arise from the deeper region of the **stratum basale**, or basal layer, of the epidermis. This region of cell birth is referred to as the **stratum germinativum**. It takes new stratified squamous epithelium cells 2 to 4 weeks to be born and move up to the skin's surface. In fact, the outermost surface of skin is actually a layer of dead cells called the **stratum corneum**, or horny layer. The cells are characteristically flat, scaly, keratinized (hardened) stratified squamous epithelial cells. As they are pushed toward the surface, they die and fill up with the protein keratin. Through everyday activities such as bathing, toweling dry, and moving around, the body sloughs off *500 million* cells a day, equaling about *one and a half pounds* of dead skin a year! This continuous replacement of cells is very

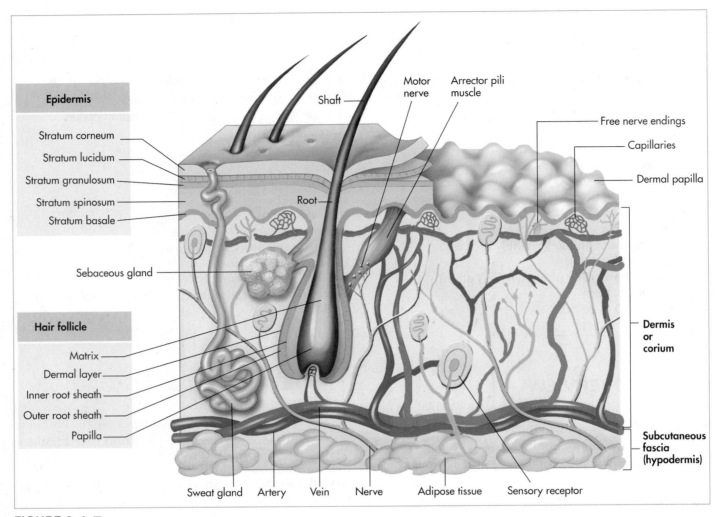

FIGURE 8–1 ■

The three layers of the skin.

important because it allows your skin to quickly repair itself in case of injuries.

Specialized cells called **melanocytes** (melan/o = black, extremely dark hue) are located deep in the epidermis and are responsible for skin color. Melanocytes produce **melanin**, which is the actual substance that helps determine skin color. An interesting note is that all people possess about the same number of melanocytes. The variations of skin color are a result of the amount of melanin that is produced and how it is distributed. Melanin production is obvious when you are exposed to the ultraviolet rays of the sun. To protect your skin, melanocytes produce more melanin, and voila!, you've got a tan. You will also note that in time you will develop a tan line demonstrating that the production of melanin occurs only as needed, in the areas where needed. Regardless of an individual's skin tone or color, all skin types respond to sun exposure. For some of us, the melanin congregates in patches on the skin, forming *freckles*. **Carotene**, which is

another form of skin pigment, gives a yellowish hue to skin. Individuals with a pinkish hue derive that color from the hemoglobin in their blood.

People with the skin condition called *albinism* have very little pigment in their skin, eyes, and hair. This is because they have inherited genes that do not allow their body cells to produce the usual amounts of melanin. Individuals with albinism may have vision problems due to the lack of pigment in their eyes. They may also be at a greater risk for developing skin cancers.

There are times when skin color can indicate an underlying disease. Although carotene gives a yellowish hue to skin, that is normal. In a situation where certain liver diseases exist, the body can't excrete a substance called *bilirubin*. As bilirubin builds up in the body, *jaundice* occurs, giving the skin a deeper yellow color. The changes in color are not as apparent on individuals with darker skin, but the yellowish color is easily seen in the whites of the eyes. Although bronze skin is associated with healthy outdoor living, individuals with a malfunctioning adrenal gland may have the same color due to excessive melanin deposits in the skin. Excessive bruising (black and blue marks called *ecchymosis*) could indicate skin, blood, or circulatory problems as well as possible physical abuse.

Dermis

The layer immediately below, or deep within, the epidermis layer is the thicker **dermis** layer, which is also called the **corium**. This layer of dense, irregular, connective tissue is considered the "true skin" and contains the following structures:

- Capillaries (tiny blood vessels)
- Collagenous and elastic fibers
- Involuntary muscles
- Nerve endings/sensory receptors
- Lymph vessels
- Hair follicles
- Sudoriferous (sweat) glands
- Sebaceous (oil) glands

Small dermal papillae ("fingers" of tissue) project from the surface of the dermis and anchor this layer to the epidermal layer. Fingerprints, toe prints, and other unique skin patterns also arise from this layer. The ridges that form finger and toe prints help improve our ability to grip and hold objects. Due to their individual uniqueness, finger and toe prints can also be used to identify individuals. Nerve fibers are located in this layer so the body can sense what is happening in the environment. Because this layer also possesses blood vessels, this is where your blush comes from when you get embarrassed.

The collagenous and elastic fibers of this layer help your skin flex with the movements that you make. Without that ability, your skin would eventually tear from all the movement your body makes in daily living. In addition to flexing, these fibers allow your skin to return to its normal shape when at rest. In older people and people regularly exposed to high levels of sunlight, the skin's firmness and ability to recoil decrease. To better understand this process, try this experiment. With one of your hands resting palm down, take the thumb and index finger of your other hand and gently pinch and pull up the skin on the back of your resting hand. Let go and observe how quickly the skin recoils. This ability of skin to return back to normal after being deformed is called **turgor**. Try this experiment with an older person and observe how much slower the skin returns to normal. Remember to ask them first! Another example of the skin's resilience due to the collagenous and elastic fibers is when your skin eventually returns to normal after an injury that caused swelling.

Sweat and Sebaceous Glands The sweat (sudoriferous) and sebaceous glands are part of the dermis. Sweat glands are distributed over the entire skin surface, with large numbers under the arms, in the palms, on the soles of the feet, and on the forehead. The perspiration they generate is excreted through pores. The two main types of sudoriferous (or sweat) glands are apocrine and eccrine glands (see **FIGURE 8–2** ■). **Apocrine glands** secrete sweat at the hair follicles in the groin and anal region as well as the armpits. These glands become active around puberty and are believed to secrete a sexual attractant. Located all over your skin, **eccrine glands** are important in the regulation of body temperature. Eccrine glands are found in greater numbers on your palms, feet, forehead, and upper lip. Your body has approximately 3,000,000 sweat glands. You can sweat on average about 500 mL (about 16 ounces) per day. It is interesting to note that sweat is around 99 percent water and by itself does not have a strong odor. However, if it is left on the skin, bacteria degrades substances in the sweat into chemicals that give off strong smells, commonly called *body odor*. Ingestion of certain foods, such as garlic, can also affect the odor of sweat.

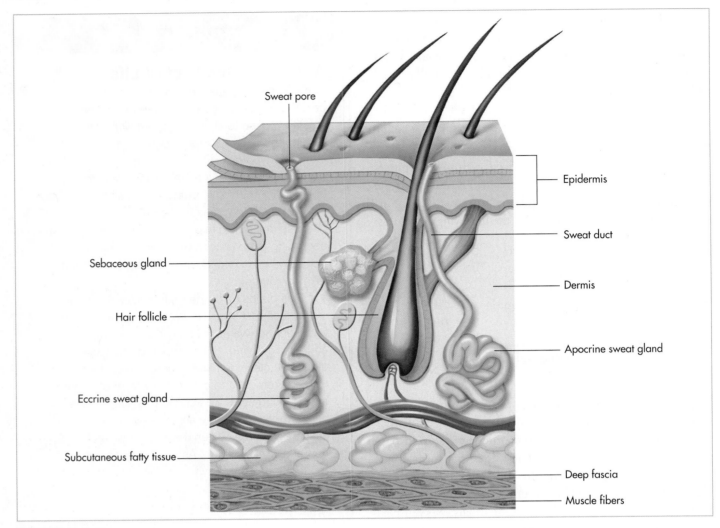

FIGURE 8–2 ■
Sweat and sebaceous glands.

Sebaceous glands play an important role by secreting oil, or **sebum**, that keeps the skin from drying out. Because sebum is somewhat acidic in nature, it also helps destroy some pathogens on the skin's surface. Sebaceous glands are usually found in hair-covered areas, where they are connected to hair follicles. The glands deposit sebum on the hairs that bring it to the skin surface along the hair shaft. Sebaceous glands are also found in areas that do not have hair follicles, such as eyelids, penis, labia minora, and nipples. In these areas, the sebum travels through ducts that terminate in sweat pores on the surface of the skin. A specialized form of sebaceous gland located at the rims of the eyelids called

meibomian glands secrete sebum into the tears that coat the eye, thus slowing their evaporation.

Subcutaneous Fascia

Finally, the deepest layer of skin is the **subcutaneous fascia**, or **hypodermis** (*hypo* = under), which is composed of elastic and fibrous connective tissue and fatty, or adipose, tissue. Within this layer, **lipocytes**, or fat cells, produce the fat needed to provide padding to protect the deeper tissues of the body and act as insulation for temperature regulation. Fat is also an efficient energy storage tissue. The hypodermis is also the layer of skin that is attached to the muscles of your body.

TEST YOUR KNOWLEDGE 8-1

Complete the following:

1. List the three main layers of skin.

   a. _____

   b. _____

   c. _____

2. List four functions of your integumentary system.

   a. _____

   b. _____

   c. _____

   d. _____

Choose the best answer:

3. Which cells are responsible for your normal skin color?

   a. manocytes

   b. jandicytes

   c. eyecytes

   d. melanocytes

4. The two main types of sudoriferous glands are

   a. apocrine and pelicine.

   b. appeltine and eccrine.

   c. eccrine and apocrine.

   d. sudacrine and melocrine.

5. Epidermal cells are created in the

   _____.

   a. horny layer

   b. dermis

   c. basal layer

   d. hypodermis

6. The ability of skin to return to normal after being pulled is called _____.

   a. compliance

   b. turgor

   c. melatonin

   d. rigidity

HOW SKIN HEALS

Just as storms can damage homes by high winds tearing off shingles or siding, lightning burning portions of the exterior, or damage caused by ice, the skin is at risk for injury, too. As a result, the body has developed ways to repair itself when injury threatens its first line of defense—the skin. Refer to **FIGURE 8–3** ■ while you read this section to better understand how wounds heal.

If skin is punctured and the wound damages blood vessels in the skin, the wound fills with blood (see Step 1). Blood contains substances that cause it to clot. The top part of the clot that is exposed to air hardens to form a scab (see Step 2).

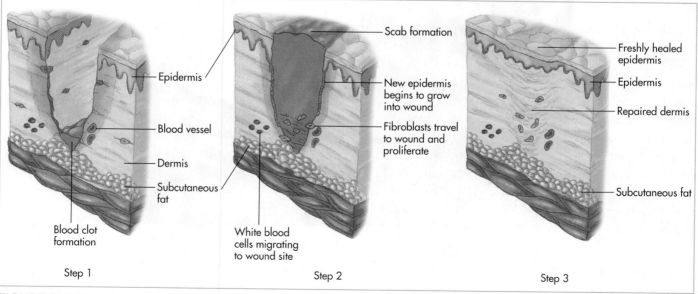

FIGURE 8–3 ■

The steps of wound repair.

This is nature's bandage, forming a barrier between the wound and the outer environment to prevent pathogens from entering. So don't pick your scabs.

Next, the inflammatory response occurs, with the migration of white blood cells to the damaged area to destroy any pathogens that may have entered when the wound occurred. At about the same time, cells called **fibroblasts** (cells that can develop into connective tissue) come in and begin pulling the edges of the wound together. The basal layer of the epidermis begins to hyperproduce new cells for the repair of the wound (see Step 3). If the wound is severe enough, a tough scar composed of collagen fibers may form. Scars usually don't contain any accessory organs of the skin or any sense of feeling. Scar production can be greatly minimized if a specialized glue, stitches, or adhesive strips are used to draw the margins of the wound together before the healing process begins. Sometimes a scar will develop that is excessively large compared to the initial wound, as you will learn in the next Amazing Facts feature. Ideally, the wound starts to heal from the inside before healing toward the outside. This aids in preventing pathogens from becoming trapped between a healed surface and the deeper layers of skin, where they could develop into a major pocket of infection. Diabetic patients often have difficulty with wound healing due to a decrease in both blood flow and white blood cell (WBC) activity to the damaged area.

Amazing Facts

Keloids

A **keloid** can be considered a "scar gone wild." It is a mass of scar tissue that has a raised, firm, irregular shape (see **FIGURE 8–4** ■). A keloid often occurs as a result of trauma or surgical incision, and can even form following an ear piercing. The formation of this mass is a result of an overproduction of connective tissue at the affected site. The formation of keloids appears to be more prominent in the black population. Surgical removal would not make sense (because more keloids would form), so treatment usually consists of steroid injection at the lesion site and cryotherapy (freezing).

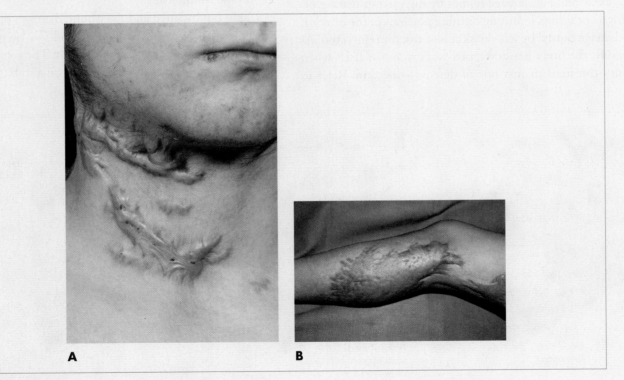

A   **B**

FIGURE 8–4 ■

Examples of keloids.

Burns to the Skin

Burns to the skin present special problems in healing. We naturally think that burns are caused by heat, and that is true. However, burns can also be caused by chemicals, electricity, and radiation. When assessing the damage caused by burns, there are two factors to consider: the *depth* of the burn and the *size of the area damaged* by the burn.

Traditionally, the depth of a burn is classified by the layer or layers of skin affected by the burn. A **first-degree burn** has damaged only the outer layer of skin, the epidermis, and this is considered a **partial thickness burn**. It does not affect the entire depth of the skin. In this case, the skin will be red and painful, but will not blister. The pain usually subsides in about 2 to 3 days with no scarring. The damaged layer of skin usually sloughs off in about a week or so. A sunburn is a classic example of a first-degree burn.

Second-degree burns involve the entire depth of the epidermis and a portion of the dermis, but are still considered *partial thickness* burns. Such burns cause pain, redness, and blistering. The extent of blistering is directly proportional to the depth of the burn. Blisters continue to enlarge even after the initial burn. Excluding any additional complications such as infection, these blisters usually heal within 10 to 14 days, but burns reaching deeper into the dermis require anywhere from 4 to 14 weeks to heal. Scarring in second-degree burn cases is common.

Third-degree burns affect all three of the skin layers and are therefore called **full thickness burns**. Here, the surface of the skin has a leathery feel to it and varies in color: black, brown, tan, red, or white. The victim will feel no pain in the affected area(s) because pain receptors are destroyed by third-degree burns. Also destroyed are the sweat and sebaceous glands, hair follicles, and blood vessels. Third-degree burns are potentially life threatening, but improvements in burn care have decreased the mortality rate.

Fourth-degree burns, also *full thickness burns*, are burns that penetrate to the bone or other underlying structures such as muscles and tendons (see **FIGURE 8–5** ■). These patients also feel no pain at the affected site(s). There are cases that may require full or partial amputation of limbs affected by fourth-degree burns.

A clinician can estimate the extent of the area covered by the burn by using the "rule of nines." As you can see in Figure 8–5, the adult body is divided into regions and given a percentage of body surface area value: head and neck, 9 percent; *each* upper limb, 9 percent; *each* lower limb, 18 percent; *front* of trunk, 18 percent; *back* of trunk and buttocks,

18 percent; and perineum (including the anal and urogenital region), 1 percent. These regions can also be further divided for children and infants, as Figure 8–5 shows.

The clinical concerns for burn patients center on the loss of the skin functions already discussed. Complications can include

- Bacterial infection
- Fluid loss
- Heat loss

Severe burns require healing at an intensity level that the body can't normally achieve on its own. Damaged skin must be removed as soon as possible to allow the process of skin grafting to begin. In this process, healthy skin is placed over damaged areas so it may begin to grow. Ideally, it is best to use the patient's own skin, known as *autografting*, because it generally eliminates the chances of tissue rejection. However, the destruction may be severe enough to require tissue from a donor (*heterografting*). Grafting usually requires repeat surgeries because large areas cannot be done all at once, and often the grafts don't "take." Newer, promising options may include growing sheets of skin in a laboratory from the patient's cells or stem cells or using synthetic materials that act as skin.

FOCUS ON PROFESSIONS

Emergency medical technicians (EMTs) and **paramedics** often deal with burn victims as a result of structural or automobile fires. Learn more about this specialty by visiting the websites of national associations such as the National Association of Emergency Medical Technicians (NAEMT), the National Emergency Medical Services Association (NEMSA), and the International Association of Flight and Critical Care Paramedics (IAFCCP).

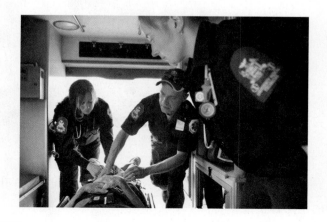

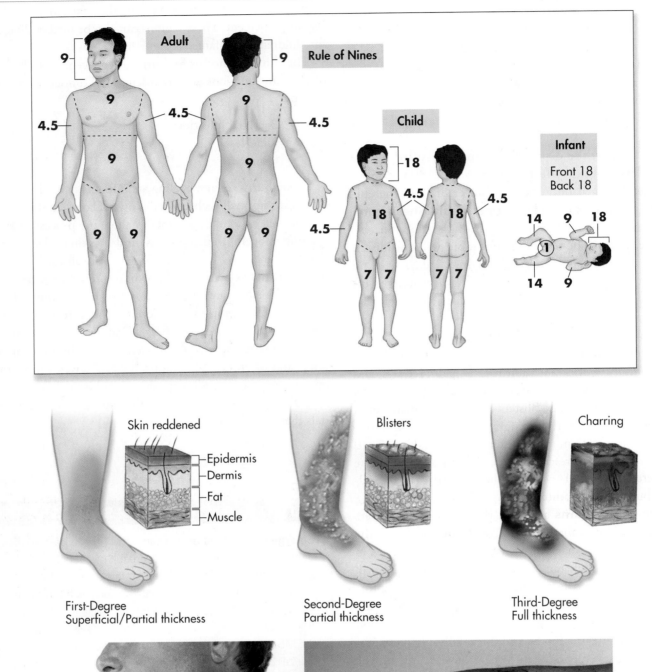

First-Degree
Superficial/Partial thickness

Second-Degree
Partial thickness

Third-Degree
Full thickness

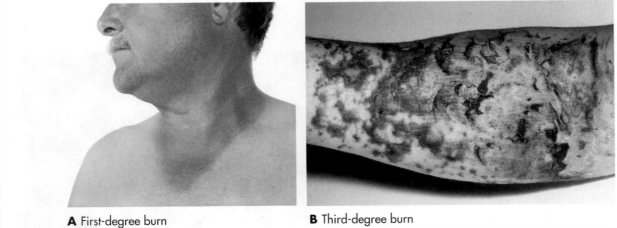

A First-degree burn

B Third-degree burn

FIGURE 8–5 ■

Assessing the degree of the burn. Bottom photos show (A) first-degree burn (sunburn) and (B) third-degree burn.

Clinical Application

MEDICINE DELIVERY VIA THE INTEGUMENTARY SYSTEM

A variety of medicines can be delivered via the integumentary system. Medicines can be applied to adhesive patches that are placed on the skin where it is slowly absorbed into the bloodstream. These are called **transdermal patches**. Nicotine (for smoking cessation), nitroglycerin (for vasodilation in the heart), birth control compounds, and pain medication, for example, can be delivered in this manner. If a more rapid response is required, the cardiac drug nitroglycerin can be placed under the tongue (*sublingually*), where it is rapidly absorbed into the bloodstream because of the high vascularization of the mucosa in that area. Localized skin conditions such as pimples, poison ivy, and wounds can be treated with topical lotions or ointments applied directly to the affected area.

Of course, the other method of drug delivery, injection, is a little more painful but very effective. This method is used when a drug can't be taken by mouth or the digestive system may alter the desired effects of the drug. Medication can be injected utilizing a syringe and needle to deliver the medication either *subcutaneously* (under the skin) or *intradermally* (into the skin). Other routes of injection also include intramuscular, intraspinal, and intravenous (IV) routes.

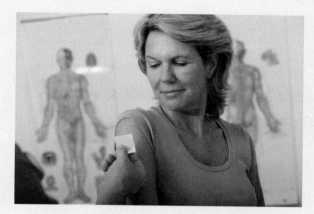

Applying a transdermal nicotine patch for smoking cessation therapy.

NAILS

Specialized **epithelial cells** originating from the *nail root* form your nails (see **FIGURE 8–6** ■). As these cells grow out and over the *nail bed* (actually a part of the epidermis), they go through the process of **keratinization** (*kerat/o* = horny or hard), forming a substance similar to the horns on a bull that is the same protein that fills the cells of the stratum corneum. This process occurs as cells dry and shrink, push to the surface, and become filled with a hard protein called **keratin**. The **cuticle** is a fold of tissue that covers the nail root. The portion that we see is called the *nail body*. The sterile (nail) matrix is a layer of cells that helps the nail body adhere to the nail bed.

Nails normally grow about 1 millimeter every week. Fingernails usually grow faster than toenails. Nail growth can be

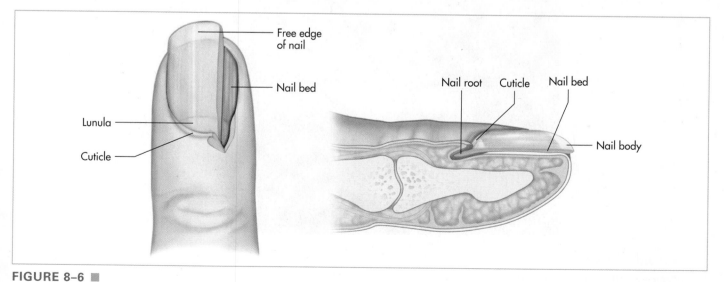

FIGURE 8–6 ■

Structures of the fingernail.

affected by a variety of things. The nails of males generally grow at a faster rate than that of females. The exception is a pregnant female, who will have faster growing nails due to hormonal changes. Nails of your dominant hand will grow faster than the nails of your nondominant hand. Certain chronic illnesses and aging can slow nail growth. Nails usually grow faster in the summer than in the winter. The pink color of your nails comes from the vascularization of the tissue under the nails, whereas the white half-moon shaped area, or **lunula** (*luna* = moon), is a result of the thicker layer of cells at the base.

HAIR

Body hair is normal and served important purposes in our evolutionary past as well as today. Hair helps to regulate body temperature, as you will see in the next section, and it functions as a sensor to help detect things on your skin, such as bugs or cobwebs. Eyelashes help protect our eyes from foreign objects, and hair in the nose helps to filter out gross particulate matter.

Hair is composed of a fibrous protein called **keratin**—just like your fingernails and toenails. The hair that you see is

Clinical Application

ASSESSING PERIPHERAL PERFUSION

The pink color of the nail bed is clinically significant in that it can aid in the assessment of perfusion (blood flow) to the extremities and can be a determinant of oxygenation. If you pinch one of your fingernails straight down with the thumb and index finger of your other hand for 5 seconds and release that pinch, you will note that the nail bed went from a blanched white color back to pink in a matter of seconds. This shows good perfusion as a result of the blood rushing back into the nail bed. In cases of poor perfusion, it takes longer for the nail bed to "pink up." Normally, it takes less than 3 seconds for the nail to return to pink from the blanched white state. If that time is greater than 3 seconds, perfusion to the extremities is considered

sluggish. If the refill time is greater than 5 seconds, there is clearly an abnormal situation occurring. This test is called *capillary refill time* (see **FIGURE 8–7** ■).

One of the complications of diabetes is reduced blood flow to the extremities, known as **peripheral vascular disease (PVD)**. This disease can cause an increase in the time required to reperfuse the nail bed. Blood clots or vascular spasms can decrease blood flow and thereby extend refill time, as can hypothermia, which naturally constricts blood vessels in the periphery to conserve heat. In addition, nail beds can change colors under certain conditions. For example, as the level of oxygen decreases in the tissue, the nail beds become bluish in tint.

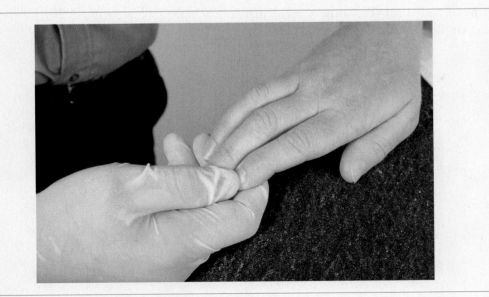

FIGURE 8–7 ■
Clinician performing capillary refill assessment.

called the shaft. The shaft is covered by a protective layer of flat cells called the **cuticle**. The **cortex** layer lies beneath the cuticle. The cortex is made of twisted proteins and the melanin pigments that give hair its color. Coarse hair has another layer of cells beneath the cortex, called the *medulla*. Each hair has a root that extends down into the dermis to the **follicle** (see FIGURE 8–8 ■). The follicle is formed by epithelial cells, which have a rich source of blood provided by the dermal blood vessels. As a result, cells divide and grow in the base of the follicle. As new cells continually form, the older cells are crowded out and pushed upward toward the skin's surface. As these old cells are pushed away from the blood source (which provides their nourishment), they die, becoming keratinized in the process.

So, basically, the hair you see on the person next to you is a bunch of dead cells. This isn't so bad, considering that if your hairs were alive, your haircuts would be extremely painful with a good chance of your bleeding to death if you got more than a light trim! The old, popular belief that shaving or frequent cutting of hair makes it grow quicker or thicker is wrong. Neither shaving nor cutting does anything to affect the rate of cell growth at the base of those hair follicles. On average, each hair on your head grows approximately one-half inch per month. The life span of hair follicles is dependent on their location. Eyelashes last around three to four months, whereas the hair on the scalp lasts for about three to four years. Teachers with difficult classes might pull their own hair out a lot sooner!

If you look at Figure 8–8, you will note that a **sebaceous gland** is associated with the hair follicle. As discussed previously, the sebaceous gland secretes **sebum** (*sebo* = tallow, a term for animal fat), an oily substance that coats the follicle and works its way to the skin's surface. Sebum is somewhat antibacterial, so it aids in decreasing infections on your skin and waterproofs and lubricates the skin and hair. Because its production decreases with age, older individuals have drier skin and more brittle hair.

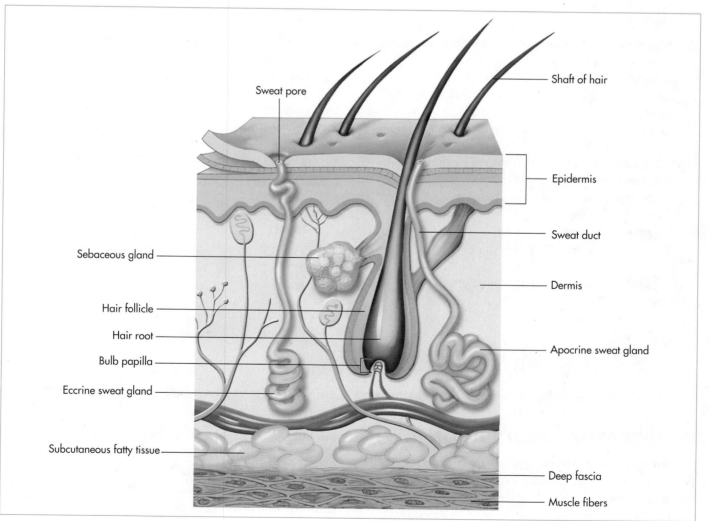

FIGURE 8–8 ■

Diagram of a hair follicle.

APPLIED SCIENCE

Forensics and Hair

An interesting sidelight concerning hair is that its composition can reveal to a pathologist if an individual ingested certain drugs or other substances, such as lead or arsenic. Trace amounts of ingested substances can become part of the hair's general makeup. As a result, analysis of a hair sample can reveal what was ingested and how long ago. The longer the hair, the longer will be the record of what was consumed by that individual.

Like skin color, your hair color is dependent on the amount and type of melanin you produce. Generally, the more melanin, the darker the hair. White hair occurs in the absence of melanin. Red hair is a result of an altered melanin that has iron in it. Did you ever wonder why people get gray hair as they age? European scientists may have finally unraveled the mystery. Apparently our hair follicles produce a small amount of hydrogen peroxide. Hydrogen peroxide historically has been used to lighten or bleach hair. The enzyme *catalase*, which is found in the hair follicle, neutralizes the hydrogen peroxide so our hair color stays the same. As we age, the amount of this enzyme is reduced, and the hydrogen peroxide can now bleach out or gray the hair.

You may be extremely envious of someone with a head full of curly hair or of someone with absolutely straight hair. Don't be envious of the person—just envy his or her hair shafts! Flat hair shafts produce curly hair, whereas round hair shafts produce straight hair.

TEST YOUR KNOWLEDGE 8–2

Choose the best answer:

1. The blood clot that forms in a wound that is exposed to air becomes a
   a. scar.
   b. scab.
   c. hematoma.
   d. keloid.

2. When assessing the skin damage caused by a burn, the two main factors to assess are
   a. temperature and depth.
   b. depth and color.
   c. area of damage and depth.
   d. area of damage and temperature.

3. The white, half-moon–shaped area of your fingernail is called the
   a. cuticle.
   b. lunula.
   c. keratin.
   d. lingual.

4. What layer of the skin has capillaries, nerve endings, and lymph vessels?
   a. hair
   b. hypodermis
   c. epidermis
   d. dermis

5. Hair is composed primarily of the fibrous protein called
   a. carotene.
   b. albumin.
   c. keratin.
   d. collagen.

TEMPERATURE REGULATION

The integumentary system plays a major role in the regulation of the body's temperature. It is amazing how we can stay in a relatively "tight" range of body temperature while we do numerous things in a variety of environments. Of course, clothes do help tremendously, but still it is critical to have a properly functioning temperature regulator like our integumentary system. Temperature regulation is accomplished through a complex series of activities.

Part of temperature regulation is accomplished by changes in the diameter of the blood vessels in your skin. As your temperature rises, your body signals the blood vessels in your skin to get larger in diameter. The correct term is **vasodilation**. This is the body's attempt to get as much "hot" blood as possible exposed to a cooler surrounding environment so the heat radiates away from the body. In addition, sweat glands excrete water (as well as some substances such as nitrogenous wastes and sodium chloride) onto the skin's surface. As the water evaporates, cooling occurs. As long as you stay hydrated so you can produce sweat, this system works pretty well. Hydration is especially important before and during activities to avoid the dangerous effects of dehydration. Thirst indicates the body is already dehydrating. It's pretty easy to dehydrate, especially when you take into consideration that you can have up to 3,000 sweat glands on a square inch of skin on your hands and feet. You can potentially excrete up to 12 liters of sweat in a 24-hour period, not to mention the water vapor you lose with every breath you exhale! The risk of dehydration is very real.

Conversely, if you were in a cold environment and needed to warm up, your peripheral blood vessels would become smaller in diameter, or **vasoconstrict**. This action forces blood away from the skin and back toward the warm core of the body. The perfect visual example of vasoconstriction is a skinny little kid running around a pool on a chilly summer day, shivering, with blue lips. His lips are blue because of vasoconstriction. That your rings have a tendency to slide off your fingers in cold weather more readily than in hot weather is another example of the effects of vasoconstriction.

Body temperature regulation is also aided by the hairs on your skin. Muscles in your skin called *arrector pili*, or erector muscles, are attached to your hairs, and when those muscles contract, they make your hairs stand erect. The contraction of those muscles shows up as goose flesh, or goose pimples, when you are chilled. When the hair stands up, pockets of still air are formed right above the skin, creating a dead air space that insulates the skin from the cooler surrounding environment. This mechanism was much more effective in prehistoric times when humans had much more body hair than we do now. This is also how goose down (feathers) clothing works in protecting against winter's cold. Interestingly, before the now common and effective practice of placing insulation in the walls and ceilings, older homes were actually insulated through the creation of dead air (nonmoving) spaces between the outer and inner walls. **FIGURE 8–9** ■ illustrates how your integumentary system regulates body temperature with the aid of your nervous system.

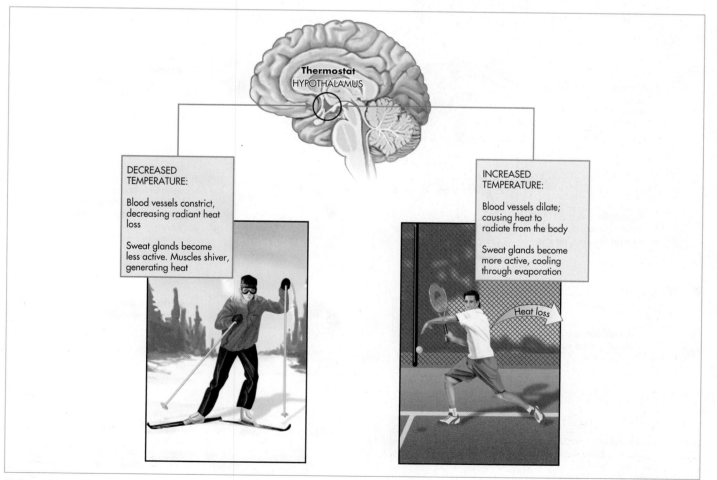

FIGURE 8–9 ■

Integumentary regulation of body temperature.

COMMON DISORDERS OF THE INTEGUMENTARY SYSTEM

Whole sections of medical libraries are dedicated to diseases of the skin. This section will provide you with some basic terms and diseases related to the integumentary system.

Melanoma (*oma* = tumor or growth), a skin cancer, has had a rapid increase in the number of cases in the past several decades. Melanoma is significant for two main reasons. First, it has a very high mortality rate; in fact, it is the cancer with the most rapidly increasing mortality rate. It accounts for approximately 75 percent of all skin cancer deaths. It is the most common form of cancer in people aged 25 to 29. In 1935, one of every 1,500 individuals was diagnosed with melanoma. Now it is about one person in every 75. Second, melanoma is one of the more preventable cancers. The culprit? Excessive sun exposure and tanning. Although the classic patient has fair skin, blue eyes, and blonde or red hair, more darkly pigmented individuals are also at risk, but at a somewhat lower rate. The effects of blistering sunburns have an additive effect. This means that each childhood sunburn you had increases your chance of developing melanoma in adulthood. Protection from excessive sun and early detection are keys to survival.

A **lesion** is a general term for a pathologically altered area of tissue that can include a wound, cancer, injury, or single infected patch of skin. The color of a lesion is usually different from that of normal skin. FIGURE 8–10 ■ shows a variety of lesion types.

In addition to several types of skin lesions, there are many common skin conditions of the integumentary system. TABLE 8–1 ■ describes some of these conditions. See FIGURE 8–11 ■ to view various photos on types of integumentary conditions.

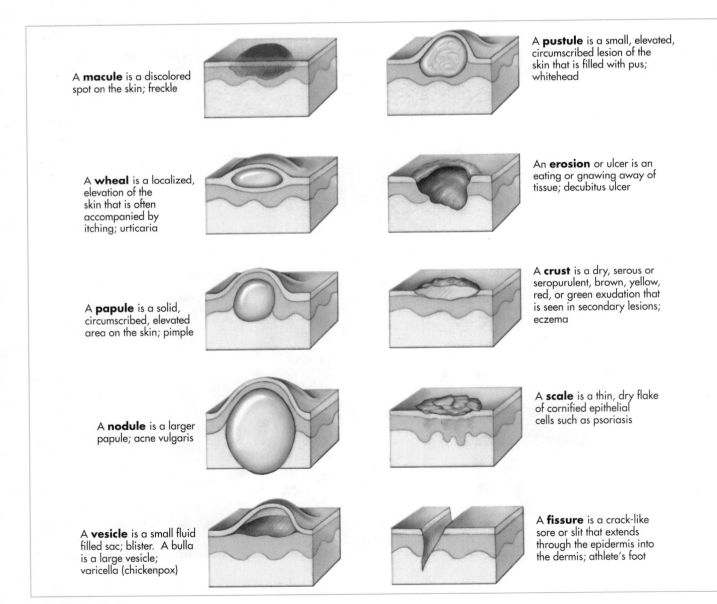

A **macule** is a discolored spot on the skin; freckle

A **wheal** is a localized, elevation of the skin that is often accompanied by itching; urticaria

A **papule** is a solid, circumscribed, elevated area on the skin; pimple

A **nodule** is a larger papule; acne vulgaris

A **vesicle** is a small fluid filled sac; blister. A bulla is a large vesicle; varicella (chickenpox)

A **pustule** is a small, elevated, circumscribed lesion of the skin that is filled with pus; whitehead

An **erosion** or ulcer is an eating or gnawing away of tissue; decubitus ulcer

A **crust** is a dry, serous or seropurulent, brown, yellow, red, or green exudation that is seen in secondary lesions; eczema

A **scale** is a thin, dry flake of cornified epithelial cells such as psoriasis

A **fissure** is a crack-like sore or slit that extends through the epidermis into the dermis; athlete's foot

FIGURE 8–10 ■

Various types of skin lesions.

TABLE 8–1 COMMON PATHOLOGICAL CONDITIONS OF THE INTEGUMENTARY SYSTEM

NAME OF CONDITION	DESCRIPTION
Abrasion	A condition that results from mechanically scraping away a portion of the skin's layer(s). This may be a result of injury or a deliberate clinical procedure.
Acne	Sebaceous glands oversecrete sebum, which, along with the dead keratinized cells, clog the hair follicle. If the blocked follicle becomes infected with bacteria, pimples develop.
Athlete's foot	This is a common fungal infection that occurs in areas of continuous moisture, such as between the toes or on palms or fingers. Jock itch is a fungal infection of the groin area.
Bedsores (decubitus or pressure ulcers)	These sores are a result of a lack of blood flow to skin that has had pressure applied to a bony prominence. This often occurs in bedridden patients who aren't turned often enough. Often called *decubitus* (dee KYOO bih tus) *ulcers*.
Boil (furuncle)	Also known as a furuncle (FOO rung kul), this is an acute inflammatory* process involving the subcutaneous layer of skin, a hair follicle, or a gland.
Cold sore	Often called a fever blister, these watery vesicles are caused by the *Herpes simplex virus*.
Contusion	A traumatic skin injury in which the skin is not broken but an injury still occurs. A contusion can present with pain, discoloration due to breakage of small blood vessels (capillaries), and swelling.
Dermatitis	An inflammatory process that can be caused by a variety of irritants such as plants or chemicals. Patients with dermatitis can exhibit erythema (redness), papules, vesicles, and crusty scabbing. Touching poison ivy or poison oak can lead to the condition called *contact dermatitis*.
Eczema	A superficial form of dermatitis that exhibits redness, papules, vesicles, and crusting.
Hives (urticaria)	This disorder is a result of an allergic reaction and produces reddened patches (wheals) and itching (pruritus) that can be severe.
Psoriasis	From the Greek word meaning "to itch," psoriasis is a chronic, inflammatory skin condition that is characterized by red, dry, crusty papules, which form circular borders over the affected areas.
Scabies	An infectious and contagious disease caused by egg-laying mites, usually seen in children; causes severe itching.
Shingles	This is a very painful inflammatory skin condition that also involves the nervous system. Shingles presents in the form of patches of vesicles mainly on the trunk of the body, but can be found on other body regions. This condition is caused by the virus *Herpes zoster*. *Zoster* is from the Greek word meaning "belt" and relates to the distribution of those patches around the trunk. The pain often remains for some time after the vesicles have healed.
Skin cancer	There are a variety of skin cancers. Basal cell carcinoma and squamous cell carcinoma are the two most common. *Basal cell carcinoma* usually spreads locally and therefore can usually be successfully treated. *Squamous cell carcinoma* may develop deeper into tissue, but it usually doesn't spread. The most serious and least successfully treated skin cancer is *malignant melanoma*. This is a cancer that initially affects the melanocytes, which produce skin pigments. This cancer can spread throughout the body to various organs.

*Inflammation literally means to "flame within." The inflammatory response is tissue's reaction to injury where there is pain, heat, redness, and swelling.

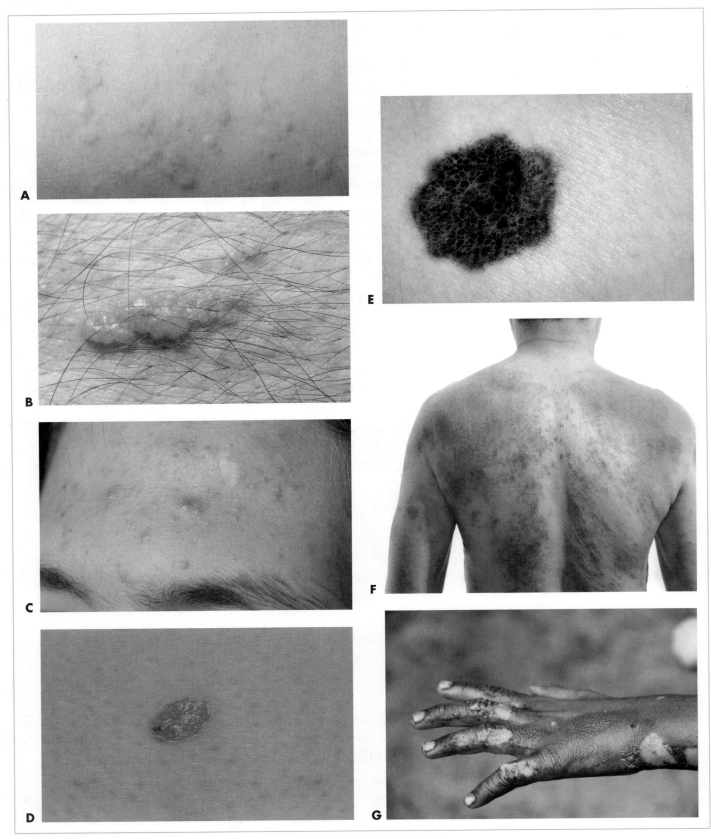

FIGURE 8–11 ■

Various types of integumentary conditions. (A) Urticaria (hives). (B) Herpes simplex. (C) Acne. (D) Psoriasis. (E) Melanoma. (F) Dermatitis. (G) Burn, second degree.

- Your skin is your largest organ.
- Your skin is an amazing organ that has many different functions:

  a. Acts as a barrier to infection both as a physical shield and through secretion of an antibacterial substance

  b. Acts as a physical barrier to injury

  c. Helps keep the body from dehydrating

  d. Stores fat (Yes, you do need some fat!)

  e. Synthesizes and secretes vitamin D with the help of sunshine

  f. Regulates body temperature

  g. By sweating, it provides a minor excretory function in the elimination of water, salts, and urea

  h. Provides sensory input

- The skin is composed of three layers: epidermis, dermis, and subcutaneous fascia.
- The skin has several accessory structures, including various glands, hair, and nails.
- The severity of burns to the skin is evaluated by the depth of the burn and the area that the burn covers.
- Nails are protective structures composed of dead material.
- Hair (also dead material) aids in controlling body temperature.

CASE STUDY

A 27-year-old female presents to her doctor's office with complaints of red, itching, and oozing skin for the past two days. Physical examination and history reveal the following: a well-nourished white female who is in otherwise good health, no known allergies, normal vital signs, pupils normal and reactive, reflexes good, breath sounds normal, liquid-filled vesicles and scabbing on both legs from the top of her sock lines to the bottom of her shorts, new vesicles have formed around her eyes. The patient stated that she returned from a primitive camping and hiking vacation in Virginia two days ago.

a. Based on this information, what do you think is the diagnosis?

_____

_____

b. What caused the vesicles to begin to form around her eyes?

_____

_____

REVIEW QUESTIONS

Multiple Choice

1. The substance that is mainly responsible for skin color is
   a. melanin.
   b. pigmentin.
   c. carrots.
   d. luna.

2. Whether you have naturally curly or straight hair is dependent on the shape of your
   a. hair follicles.
   b. hair shafts.
   c. sebum.
   d. melanin.

3. The fibrous protein that makes up your hair and nails and fills your epidermal cells is called
   a. carotene.
   b. myelin.
   c. keratin.
   d. dermasene.

4. In a cold environment, to maintain a core body temperature, peripheral blood vessels
   a. vasodilate.
   b. venospasm.
   c. shiver.
   d. vasoconstrict.

5. Excess blood loss may cause this sign in the integumentary system.
   a. decreased hair growth
   b. decreased capillary refill
   c. increased wound healing
   d. brittle nails

6. The pinching and release of the nail bed could be used to assess
   a. skin pain.
   b. peripheral perfusion.
   c. body temperature.
   d. skin turgor.

Fill in the Blank

1. The three main layers of skin are the
   _____, _____, and
   _____.

2. The type of sweat gland involved mainly in temperature regulation is _____, and the _____ glands are involved mainly in nervous sweating.

3. Sebaceous glands secrete an oily substance called
   _____.

4. For some individuals, melanin locates in small patches called _____.

5. Jaundice, a condition associated with liver disease, occurs as a result of the buildup of
   _____.

6. The normal life span of a hair follicle located on the scalp is approximately _____.

Short Answer

1. Discuss three functions of the integumentary system.

   _____

   _____

   _____

   _____

2. Explain the organization of the epidermis. What happens to epidermal cells as they rise toward the surface of the skin?

   _____

   _____

   _____

   _____

3. Why is there an increased production of melanin when there is an increased sun exposure?

   _____

   _____

   _____

   _____

4. Explain the classification of burn severity.

   _____

   _____

   _____

   _____

5. List and briefly describe the major accessory structures of skin.

   _____

   _____

   _____

   _____

Visit our new **MyHealthProfessions Lab** to accompany *Anatomy & Physiology for Health Professions*. Here you'll find a rich collection of quizzes, case studies, and animations for deeper understanding and application.

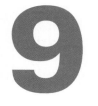

9

The Nervous System (Part I)

THE INFORMATION SUPER HIGHWAY

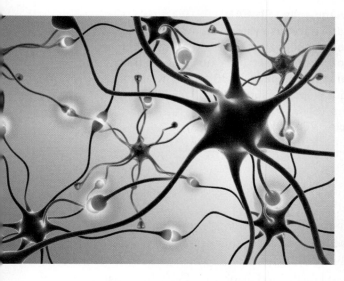

It's often a good idea to take an interesting novel along when traveling. The nervous system, due to its complexity and importance, is our novel for this journey. Don't be dismayed by the length of this novel because the related control system Chapters 11 and 12 ("The Senses" and "The Endocrine System") will be the "short stories" by comparison. So far on our journey, we have seen infrastructure, the building blocks and support systems of the city. Soon we will visit transportation, protection, and energy delivery systems. Like any good city, the body must have control systems—systems that will monitor conditions, take corrective action when necessary, and keep everything running smoothly. Imagine what would happen if a traffic light network in a city were to suddenly fail. The control systems of the body are the nervous and endocrine systems, which receive help from your special senses. Like any control system, they have a large, complex job that is sometimes difficult to understand. They must keep track of everything that is happening in the body. Therefore, the nervous and endocrine systems are perhaps the most complex and vital systems we will visit. To make the trip more manageable, we have subdivided the nervous system into two separate chapters. In this chapter (Part I), we start at the bottom of the control hierarchy, the cells and the spinal cord. In Chapter 10, Part II, we focus on the higher-level control of the brain.

LEARNING OUTCOMES

At the end of your journey through this chapter, you will be able to:

- List and describe the components and basic operation of the nervous system.
- Contrast the central and peripheral nervous systems.
- Define the anatomy and function of neuroglia and neurons.
- Discuss the function of neurons as well as excitable cells, action potentials, graded potentials, and nerve impulse conduction.
- Explain the difference between chemical and electrical synapses.
- Discuss the external and internal anatomy and physiology of the spinal cord.
- Explain how reflexes work.
- List and describe common disorders of the nerves and spinal cord.

Pronunciation Guide Pro·nun·ci·a·tion

Definitions/Parts

Correct pronunciation is important in any journey so that you and others are completely understood. Here is a "see and say" Pronunciation Guide for the more difficult terms to pronounce in this chapter. Please note that even though there are standard pronunciations, regional variations of the pronunciations can occur.

arachnoid mater (ah RACK noyd MAY ter)
astrocytes (ASS troh SITES)
axon (AK sahn)
cerebrospinal fluid (SER eh broh SPY nal)
chemical synapse (SIN aps)
commissures (KAHM ih shoorz)
corticobulbar tract (KOR ti coe BUL bar)
corticospinal tract (KOR ti coe SPY nal)
dendrites (DEN drites)
dorsal root ganglion (GANG lee on)
dura mater (DOO rah MAY ter)
ependymal cells (eh PEN deh mall)
epidural space (epp ih DOO rall)
ganglia (GANG lee ah)
glial cells (GLEE all)
gyri (JIE rie)

meninges (men IN jeez)
microglia (mie crow GLEE ah)
myelin (MY eh lin)
neuroglia (glial cells) (noo ROG lee uh)
nodes of Ranvier (ron vee AYE)
oligodendrocytes (AH li go DEN droe sites)
pia mater (PEE ah MAY ter)
plexus (PLECK sus)
Schwann cells (SHWAN)
somatic nervous system (so MAT ick)
spinocerebellar tract (SPY no ser eh BELL ar)
spinothalamic tract (SPY no THAL uh mic)
subarachnoid space (SUB ah RACK noyd)
subdural space (sub DOO ral)
sulcus (SULL cus)
vesicle (VES ih kuhl)

ORGANIZATION

We begin this journey with an overview of the entire system to show how all the components are connected. Let's start with the basic operations.

The Parts and Basic Operation of the Nervous System

The organization of the nervous system can be compared to a computer. Information is entered into the computer by various means ("senses"): keyboard, mouse, touch screen, voice recognition, Internet connection, and so on. This is similar to our sensory input into the brain.

The main components of the computer's "brain" are the hard drive (long-term memory), random access memory (short-term memory), and central processing unit (thinking and decision making). The computer's output (motor)—its interaction with the world—exits via ports and cables to printers, screen displays, speakers, and other devices.

Typically, we refer to the brain and spinal cord as the **central nervous system (CNS)** and everything outside the brain and spinal cord, which represent the input and output pathways, as the **peripheral nervous system (PNS)**. FIGURE 9–1 ■ is a schematic of the organization of the nervous system.

The peripheral nervous system's "input devices" comprise the **sensory system**. Your senses sample the environment and bring the information to the central nervous system, as explored further in Chapter 11. Everything that can possibly be measured about your body and the world around you is measured by your sensory system. The sensory information goes into the central nervous system, where it is interpreted by the brain and the spinal cord. The brain and the spinal cord compare the sensory input to information from past experiences, and make decisions about how to respond to the information. When the brain and the spinal cord decide what response is required to deal with the new information, the output side is activated. The output side carries out the orders from the brain and the spinal cord.

The output side, called the **motor system**, carries orders to all three types of muscles (skeletal, cardiac, and smooth) and to the body's glands, and tells them how to respond to the new information. The motor system is divided into two different branches: the **somatic nervous system**, which controls skeletal muscle and voluntary movements, and the **autonomic nervous system**, which controls smooth and cardiac muscle in your organs and also several glands. Autonomic output is involuntary and not under conscious control. The autonomic nervous system is further divided into two branches: the

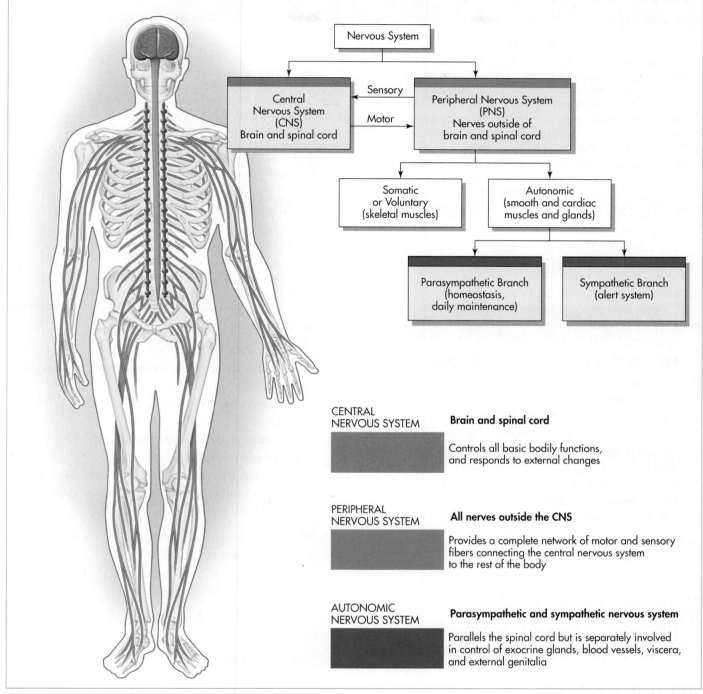

FIGURE 9–1 ■

Organization of the nervous system.

parasympathetic nervous system and the **sympathetic nervous system**. The parasympathetic branch, often called "resting and digesting," controls normal body functioning, whereas the sympathetic branch is the body's alert system, commonly known as the "fight-or-flight" response system. Again, please refer to Figure 9–1.

Each part of the nervous system has separate but unmistakably connected roles to play in assessing a situation and responding to it. The nervous system is active 24 hours a day, seven days a week, for your entire life. Some situations—such as an unfriendly dog, or a sudden drop in blood pressure, or a terrible car accident—may be life threatening. Others—for

APPLIED SCIENCE

The Nervous System in Action

The organization of the nervous system is easier to understand if we look at a real-life event. You drive to your friend's house. As you step onto her walkway, a large dog bounds down the front steps barking and snarling at you. Your sensory system (PNS) gathers the following information about the new stimulus: a large unfriendly dog; you are far from the protection of the car; nobody is coming to help. The information goes into your spinal cord and brain, and several decisions are made (CNS). You are in danger; something must be done. Your brain and spinal cord send directions via your autonomic nervous system (PNS) to your organs

to gear up for action. Your heart rate, blood pressure, and respiration rate rise. You begin to sweat. More blood is delivered to your skeletal muscles and heart to get you fully ready to respond. This is all involuntary, meaning you cannot consciously control it. Your nervous system readies your skeletal muscles to get you out of there. (This fight-or-flight response is discussed later in further depth.) If you can control your fear, you back slowly away from the situation. If you are scared witless, you run from the yard as fast as you can. Either way, you can hopefully escape the danger with your skin and your pride intact.

Amazing Facts

Faster than a Speeding Bullet

Well, not literally! Your nervous system must respond very quickly to stimuli. Think about how fast you pull your hand away from a hot stove or step on the brake when something runs in front of your car. Nerve impulses can move very quickly. Some neurons have speeds as fast as 100 meters per second. That's in the neighborhood of 200 miles per hour. Bullets, on the other hand, can travel 2,000 miles per hour.

example, an ant crawling across your foot or a pencil rolling under the desk just out of reach—are simply annoying. Everything that happens in your world is monitored and responded to by your nervous system. It's a truly Herculean task.

NERVOUS TISSUE

Like all organs, the components of the nervous system are made up of tissue. But unlike tissue in other systems, the nervous system contains no epithelium, connective tissue, or muscle tissue. Nervous tissue is made up of two different types of cells: neuroglia and neurons.

Neuroglia

The **neuroglia**, or **glial cells**, are specialized cells in nervous tissue that allow it to perform nervous system functions. They are like the "glue" that holds the nervous system

together. In fact, *glial* means "glue." In the central nervous system there are four types of glial cells:

- **Astrocytes** are metabolic and structural support cells that are often connected to capillaries and form part of the blood-brain barrier.
- **Microglial cells** can attack microbes and remove debris.
- **Ependymal cells** do the job of epithelial cells, covering surfaces and lining cavities.
- **Oligodendrocytes** hold nerve fibers together and make a lipid insulation called *myelin*, described in more detail a bit later.

In the peripheral nervous system there are only two types of glial cells: **Schwann cells**, which make myelin for the PNS, and **satellite cells**, which are support cells. FIGURE 9–2 ■ shows the CNS and PNS neuroglia.

Neurons

The glial cells do all the support activities for the nervous system, such as lining and covering cavities and supporting and protecting structures. None of the glial cells, however, are capable of measuring the environment, making decisions, or sending orders. All the control functions of the nervous system must be carried out by a second group of cells called **neurons**. Neurons are rather bizarre-looking cells, often with many branches (see FIGURE 9–3 ■). Each part of a neuron has a specific function. The main function of the **neuron body** is that of cell metabolism. Its **dendrites** receive information from the environment or from other cells. The cell body generates and sends signals to other cells. Those signals leave the cell body and travel down the **axon** until it reaches the **axon terminal**, which then connects to a receiving cell.

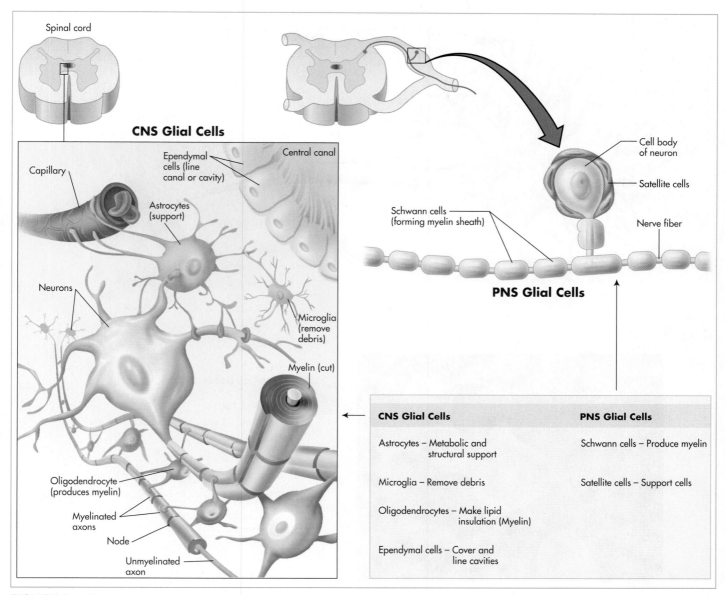

FIGURE 9–2 ■

Glial cells and their functions.

This combination of axon terminal and receiving cell is called a **synapse**. If the receiving cell is a skeletal muscle cell, as in the illustration in Figure 9–3, then this particular synapse is called the *neuromuscular synapse* or *junction*.

Neurons can be classified by how they look (structure) or what they do (function). From a structural point of view, neurons can have one axon and one dendrite (bipolar), one

axon and many dendrites (multipolar), or one process that splits into a central and a peripheral projection (unipolar). Classified by function, input neurons are known as **sensory neurons**, and output neurons are known as **motor neurons**. Neurons that carry information between neurons are called **interneurons** (*inter* means "between") or **association neurons** as you can see in the illustration in Figure 9–3B.

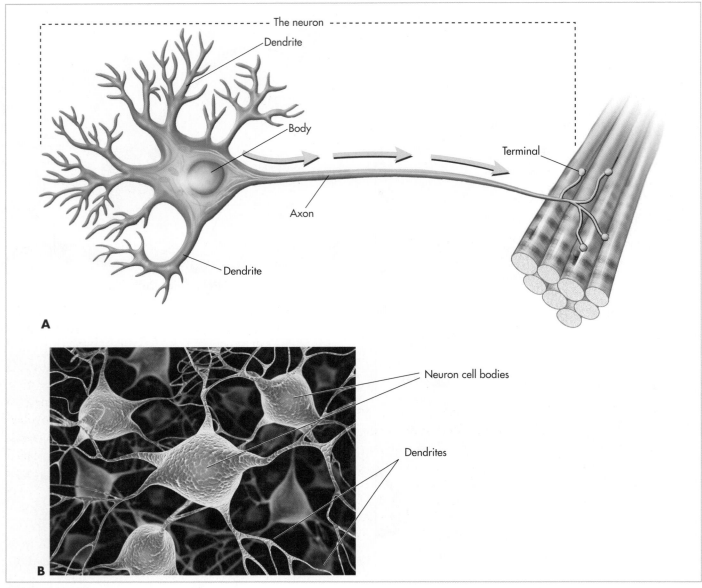

The neuron

Dendrite

Body

Terminal

Axon

Dendrite

Neuron cell bodies

Dendrites

A

B

FIGURE 9–3 ■

(A) A neuron connecting to a skeletal muscle. (B) Interneurons or association neurons.

TEST YOUR KNOWLEDGE 9-1

Choose the best answer:

1. Which cells are the support cells in the nervous system?
   a. neurons
   b. neuroglia
   c. epithelium
   d. all of the above

2. The output side of your nervous system is called
   a. sensory.
   b. motor.
   c. central.
   d. exit.

3. The part of the nervous system that integrates and processes information is known as the
   a. PNS.
   b. PBS.
   c. CNS.
   d. CIA.

4. The lipid insulation of nervous tissue is called
   a. glia.
   b. myelin.
   c. Schwann cells.
   d. astrocytes.

5. The fight-or-flight response is controlled by the
   a. spinal cord.
   b. autonomic nervous system.
   c. brain.
   d. hormones.

HOW NEURONS WORK

Now that we know the basic structure of neurons, let's look more closely at how they function.

Excitable Cells

A neuron is a kind of cell called an **excitable cell**. An excitable cell carries a small electrical charge when stimulated. Each time charged particles flow across a cell membrane, a tiny electrical current is generated. Electricity is just the flow of charges from one place to the other. All three types of muscle cells are excitable cells, as are many gland cells. Because neurons are excitable cells, it makes sense that the way neurons send and receive signals is via tiny electrical currents. This is also one of the reasons electrocution can cause nervous system damage and even death. It literally shorts out the electrical pathways in the neurons.

How, you might ask, can cells carry electricity? It seems hard to believe, but cells are like miniature batteries, able to generate tiny currents simply by changing the permeability of their membranes. Perhaps the plot of the *Matrix* movies in which humans are used by machines as batteries is not so far-fetched.

Action Potentials

Action potentials in neurons are known as *nerve impulses* and allow for signals to travel for cell-to-cell communication. In other cells, action potentials can activate intracellular processes such as skeletal and cardiac muscle contractions or even the release of insulin. Since the concept of action potential is sometimes difficult to grasp, you may want to refer to **FIGURE 9–4** ■ as you read through this section.

A cell that is not stimulated or excited is called a **resting cell** and is said to be **polarized**. This means it has a difference in charge across its membrane such that it is more negative on the inside than on the outside. The difference in charge is called the *membrane potential*. When that cell is stimulated (excited), gates in the cell membrane spring open. When these gates, called *sodium gates*, open, they allow sodium ions (Na^+) to travel across the cell membrane into the cell. These sodium ions are positively charged, so when they go into the cell, the cell becomes more positive than it was at rest. A cell that is more positive than at rest is called **depolarized**. As more sodium ions enter, it makes it easier for even more sodium ions to enter. This causes the cell to become even more depolarized. This act of allowing more and more ions to enter is known as a *positive feedback loop*. In less than a millisecond, the gates on the sodium channels shut, just like the automatic doors at the supermarket shut by themselves. This shuts off the positive feedback loop. At around the same time, gates on potassium channels in the cell membrane open. Potassium (K^+), which is also positive, leaves the cell, taking its positive charges with it. The inside of the cell becomes more negative again, eventually returning to rest. This is **repolarization**, an example of negative feedback (see Figure 9–4). This movement of Na^+ into and K^+ out of the cell creates a flow of ions that generate an electrical charge.

Sometimes a cell overshoots and becomes more negative than when it is at rest. Then the cell is **hyperpolarized**. (This hyperpolarization is often called an *after potential*.) Eventually, the cell will return to resting. It should be noted that the cell is unable to accept another stimulus until it repolarizes (returns to its resting state). This time period during which it cannot accept another stimulus is called the **refractory period**. This whole series of permeability changes within the cell and the resultant changes of the internal and external charges is called the *action potential*.

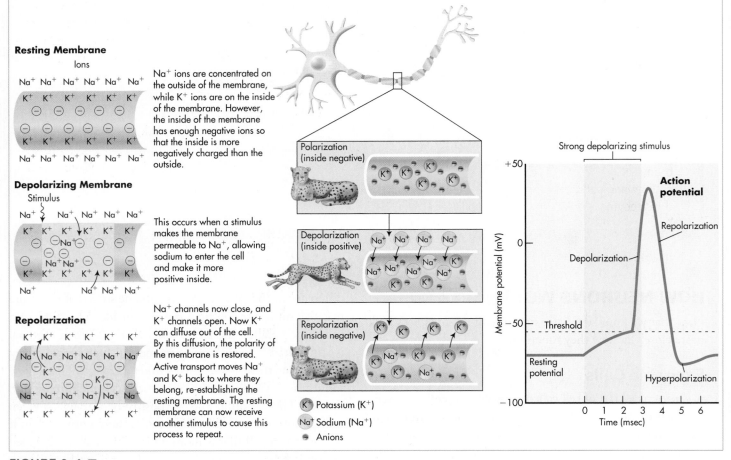

Resting Membrane

Ions

Na$^+$ Na$^+$ Na$^+$ Na$^+$ Na$^+$ Na$^+$

K$^+$ K$^+$ K$^+$ K$^+$ K$^+$ K$^+$
⊖ ⊖ ⊖ ⊖ ⊖
⊖ ⊖ ⊖ ⊖ ⊖
K$^+$ K$^+$ K$^+$ K$^+$ K$^+$ K$^+$

Na$^+$ Na$^+$ Na$^+$ Na$^+$ Na$^+$ Na$^+$

Na$^+$ ions are concentrated on the outside of the membrane, while K$^+$ ions are on the inside of the membrane. However, the inside of the membrane has enough negative ions so that the inside is more negatively charged than the outside.

Depolarizing Membrane

Stimulus

Na$^+$ Na$^+$ Na$^+$ Na$^+$ Na$^+$

K$^+$ K$^+$ K$^+$ K$^+$ K$^+$
⊖ ⊖Na$^+$⊖ ⊖ ⊖
⊖ Na$^+$Na$^+$ ⊖ ⊖
K$^+$ K$^+$ K$^+$ K$^+$ K$^+$

Na$^+$ Na$^+$ Na$^+$ Na$^+$

This occurs when a stimulus makes the membrane permeable to Na$^+$, allowing sodium to enter the cell and make it more positive inside.

Repolarization

K$^+$ K$^+$ K$^+$ K$^+$ K$^+$ K$^+$

Na$^+$Na$^+$Na$^+$Na$^+$Na$^+$Na$^+$
⊖ K$^+$ ⊖
⊖ ⊖ ⊖ K$^+$ ⊖ ⊖
Na$^+$Na$^+$Na$^+$Na$^+$Na$^+$Na$^+$

K$^+$ K$^+$ K$^+$ K$^+$ K$^+$ K$^+$

Na$^+$ channels now close, and K$^+$ channels open. Now K$^+$ can diffuse out of the cell. By this diffusion, the polarity of the membrane is restored. Active transport moves Na$^+$ and K$^+$ back to where they belong, re-establishing the resting membrane. The resting membrane can now receive another stimulus to cause this process to repeat.

Polarization
(inside negative)

Depolarization
(inside positive)

Repolarization
(inside negative)

K$^+$ Potassium (K$^+$)
Na$^+$ Sodium (Na$^+$)
⊖ Anions

Strong depolarizing stimulus

Action potential

Repolarization

Depolarization

Threshold

Resting potential

Hyperpolarization

Membrane potential (mV)

+50

0

−50

−100

Time (msec)
0 1 2 3 4 5 6

FIGURE 9–4 ■

The action potential.

Graded Potentials

Neurons can use their ability to generate electricity to send, receive, and interpret signals. Let's look at an example of how this works. You are hammering a picture hanger into the wall of your newly painted bedroom, and you hit your thumb. The blow from the hammer stimulates the dendrites in your thumb and they become depolarized. If you hit your thumb softly, the cell is stimulated only a little and the cell does not depolarize very much. (The pain isn't too bad, either.) If you hit your thumb really hard, the cell depolarizes much more. (It hurts a lot more, too.) This phenomenon is known as a *graded potential*. In a graded potential, the size of the stimulus determines the excitement of the cell. A big stimulus causes a bigger depolarization than a small stimulus. Many sensory cells work via graded potentials. That's often how your CNS tells the size of the environmental change.

The dendrites carry the depolarization to the sensory neuron cell body. The cell body takes that information and generates an action potential, if the stimulus is big enough. One difference between action potentials and graded potentials

is that action potentials are "all or none," which means that the action potential, once it starts, will always finish and will always be the same size. You either have one or you don't. There are no small action potentials or big ones, unlike graded potentials.

APPLIED SCIENCE

Fugu

The puffer fish, fugu, is considered a delicacy in Japan because if you eat it, you could die. Fugu can be served only by specially certified chefs trained to prepare the fish so it is safe to eat. Puffer fish contain a poison, tetrodotoxin (TTX), in their tissues that blocks sodium channels, preventing sodium from entering cells. Cells exposed to TTX cannot depolarize. Thus, neurons cannot fire action potentials. People who consume improperly prepared fugu become paralyzed. Symptoms develop as paralysis within 15 minutes to 20 hours after ingestion. If untreated, death can result in 4 to 6 hours after the onset of symptoms.

Impulse Conduction

Once an action potential is formed, it travels down the axon from the cell body to the terminal. This movement is called **impulse conduction**. The speed of impulse conduction along an axon is determined by two characteristics: the presence of myelin and the diameter of the axon.

Myelin

Myelin is a lipid insulation or sheath formed by the oligodendrocytes in the CNS and the Schwann cells in the PNS. In preserved brains, the myelinated axons look white. Unmyelinated parts of the CNS, like cell bodies, look gray. Therefore, what we call "white matter" is typically made of myelinated axons, and what we call "gray matter" is made of cell bodies. The cell membranes of oligodendrocytes or Schwann cells are wrapped around an axon like a bandage. Between adjacent glial cells are tiny bare spots called **nodes of Ranvier** (see **FIGURE 9–5** ■).

When an axon is wrapped in myelin, it is called a *myelinated axon*. Myelin is essential for the speedy flow of action potentials down axons. In an *unmyelinated axon*, the action potential can only flow down the axon by depolarizing each and every millimeter of the axon. Every single sodium channel must open, and every single potassium channel must open. It is a relatively slow process. In a myelinated axon, only the channels at the nodes must open for the action potential to flow down the axon. Myelin prevents ions from passing through channels, because ions are water soluble, and myelin is a lipid. (Remember, charged particles cannot get through lipids.) The action potential therefore "hops" down the axon from node to node (nodal transmission) rather than creeping along the entire length of the axon. This type of conduction is called *saltatory conduction*. It works the same way as if you try to walk across the floor heel to toe, never missing a spot and then skip across the floor in large leaps. Which is faster?

Axon Diameter

The diameter of the axon also affects the speed of action potential flow. Think about moving through two different pipes, say on a playground or obstacle course. One pipe is one-half meter in diameter (less than 2 feet). To move through the pipe, you must crawl. The other pipe is 2 meters in diameter (more than 6 feet). Most of you can stand in this pipe with room to spare. Which trip would be faster? Obviously, it's the one through the larger diameter pipe. You don't have to crawl, you don't get hung up on the side. Heck, you could even run through the big pipe. For ions, the axon is essentially a pipe. The wider the axon, the faster the ions flow. The combination of myelination and large diameter makes a huge difference in speed.

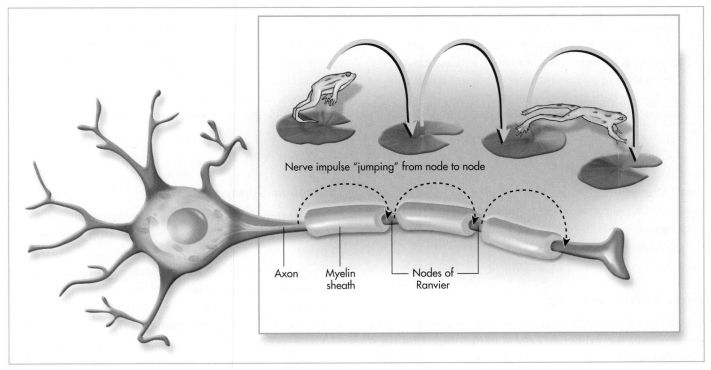

Nerve impulse "jumping" from node to node

Axon   Myelin   Nodes of
        sheath   Ranvier

FIGURE 9–5 ■
Impulse conduction via a myelinated axon.

TEST YOUR KNOWLEDGE 9–2

Choose the best answer:

1. Which ions move *into* neurons during the action potential?
   a. potassium
   b. calcium
   c. sodium
   d. acetylcholine

2. Which of the following is all or none?
   a. graded potential
   b. action potential
   c. chemical synapse
   d. impulse conduction

3. Membrane potential is
   a. current flow across a membrane.
   b. separation of charge across a membrane.
   c. the energy needed to flow across a membrane.
   d. the ability to become a membrane.

4. An excitable cell is one that can
   a. change its membrane potential.
   b. separate its charge.
   c. use active transport.
   d. have different moods.

5. During hyperpolarization a cell becomes
   a. more positive than resting.
   b. more negative than resting.
   c. colder than resting.
   d. none of the above

Clinical Application

MULTIPLE SCLEROSIS

Multiple sclerosis (MS) is a disorder of the myelin sheath in the CNS. Patients with multiple sclerosis have many areas in which the myelin has been destroyed. In areas without myelin, impulse conduction is slow or impossible. Imagine an electrical wire with many bare spots or with no insulation. These bare or exposed parts can "short out" and prevent the current from passing further down the wire. Symptoms of multiple sclerosis differ from patient to patient, depending on where the myelin damage occurs. Patients may have disturbances in vision, balance, speech, or movement. This disorder is more common in women than in men and is diagnosed most often in people under the age of 50.

Small, unmyelinated axons have speeds as low as 0.5 meter per second, whereas large-diameter, myelinated axons may be as fast as 100 meters per second. That's 200 times faster.

How Synapses Work

For neurons to communicate, there must be some way for a message to be sent from one neuron to the other. This communication occurs at the synapse after an action potential is generated and flows toward the axon terminal. There are two types of synapses: chemical and electrical.

Chemical Synapses

When an impulse arrives at the axon terminal, the *terminal* depolarizes, and this causes calcium gates to open. Calcium flows into the cell. When calcium flows in, it triggers a change in the terminal. There are tiny sacs in the terminal called **vesicles**, which release their contents from the cell via exocytosis when calcium flows in. These vesicles are filled with molecules called **neurotransmitters**.

These neurotransmitters are used to send the signal from the neuron across the synapse to the next cell in line. The neurotransmitter binds to the cell receiving the signal and causes gates to open or close. Some neurotransmitters excite the receiving cell, and some calm it down. In the case of the hammered thumb, the neurotransmitter would be released in your spinal cord and would excite a pain neuron. The receiving neuron would be stimulated and take the information about your thumb to your brain, where your brain would register the pain.

Since chemicals are used to send the signals, the final phase is a chemical cleanup. The neurotransmitter must be taken away from the synapse or it will continually bind to the receiving cell. This cleanup is accomplished through an inactivator. For example, if the neurotransmitter chemical is *acetylcholine (ACh)*, it will be inactivated by *acetylcholinesterase (AChE)*, an enzyme that breaks down ACh. Note that the ending "ase" means enzymes that break down the substance, in this case acetylcholine. This type of information flow, using neurotransmitters, is called a **chemical synapse** because chemicals (neurotransmitters) are used to carry the information from one cell to another. See **FIGURE 9–6** ■ for the steps in chemical synaptic transmission.

The Neuromuscular Junction One chemical synapse, the **neuromuscular junction**, is particularly important to the function of your motor system, as we mentioned briefly in Chapter 7, "The Muscular System." The neuromuscular junction is a specialized synapse between somatic (voluntary) motor neurons and the skeletal muscles they innervate. The surface of the muscle is studded with sodium channels that are *ligand-gated*. A ligand-gated channel opens or closes when a molecule binds to a receptor that is part of the channel, like a key fitting into a lock. In the case of skeletal muscles, the ligand, or key, is the neurotransmitter acetylcholine. Acetylcholine is released from the terminal of a motor neuron and binds to the surface of skeletal muscle, opening sodium channels and causing the skeletal muscle to be depolarized. This depolarization leads to the changes described in Chapter 7, and the muscle contracts. Like all chemical synapses, the neuromuscular junction must be cleaned up at the end of transmission. The enzyme responsible for cleaning up the synapse is called *acetylcholinesterase*.

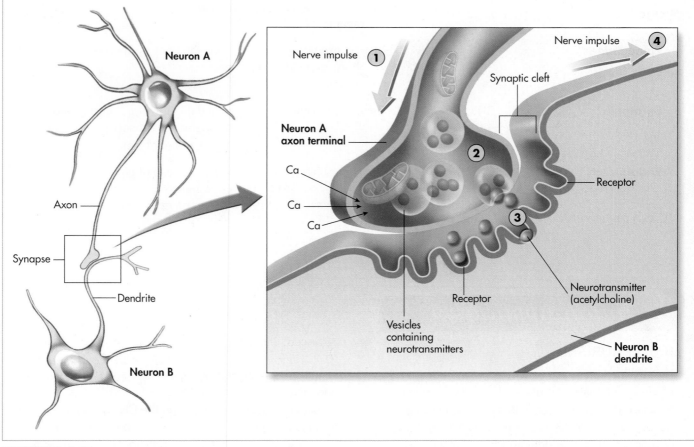

FIGURE 9–6 ■

The chemical synapse. Step 1: The impulse travels down the axon. Step 2: Vesicles are stimulated to release neurotransmitter (exocytosis). Step 3: The neurotransmitter travels across the synapse and binds with the receptor site of the postsynaptic cell. Step 4: The impulse continues down the dendrite.

MANIPULATING CHEMICAL SYNAPSES IN MEDICINE

Our understanding of chemical synapses has led to several breakthroughs for treating mental illness. Many medications on the market today are designed to modify synapses. Selective serotonin reuptake inhibitors (SSRIs) are good examples. These medications prevent the cleanup of the neurotransmitter serotonin from synapses, thereby increasing the effects of serotonin on the receiving cell. Serotonin is thought to be involved in controlling mood. Having more serotonin in the synaptic cleft is associated with feelings of well-being and happiness. Many antidepressants, obsessive compulsive disorder medications, and anti-anxiety medications are SSRIs. TABLE 9–1 ■ contains other examples of clinically important neurotransmitters.

TABLE 9–1 SELECTED COMMON NEUROTRANSMITTERS

NEUROTRANSMITTER	SYSTEM	EXCITATORY OR INHIBITORY	LOCATION/ ACTION
Acetylcholine	CNS* and PNS*	Generally excitatory, but is inhibitory to some visceral effectors	Stimulates skeletal muscles, excites smooth muscle, and inhibits cardiac muscle
Norepinephrine	CNS and PNS	May be excitatory or inhibitory, depending on the receptors	Stimulation of sympathetic pathways
Epinephrine	CNS and PNS	May be excitatory or inhibitory, depending on the receptors	Stimulation of sympathetic pathways
Serotonin	CNS	Generally inhibitory	Found in pathways that regulate temperature, sensory perception, mood, onset of sleep
Endorphins	CNS	Generally inhibitory	Inhibit release of pain neurotransmitters

*CNS = central nervous system; PNS = peripheral nervous system

BIOTERRORISM

If acetylcholinesterase activity is prevented, acetylcholine continually stimulates the muscle, eventually paralyzing it. Some insecticides and the nerve gas Sarin, which killed 12 people and injured hundreds of others during a terrorist attack in a Tokyo subway tunnel in 1995, are acetylcholinesterase inhibitors. Victims of Sarin or overexposure to organophosphate insecticides may die from respiratory arrest. Organophosphates have effects that could interfere with respiration, including effects on the CNS, on the neuromuscular junction, and directly on the lungs, causing increased secretions and bronchoconstriction. Not all acetylcholinesterase inhibitors are poisons. Some are used as medications.

Electrical Synapses

Some cells do not need chemicals to transmit information from one cell to another. These synapses are called **electrical synapses**. The cells in an electrical synapse can transfer information freely because they have special connections called **gap junctions**. Such connections can exist between many types of excitable cells. They are found, for example, in the intercalated discs between cardiac muscle fibers.

TEST YOUR KNOWLEDGE 9–3

Choose the best answer:

1. The molecules used to send signals across synapses are called
   a. hormones.
   b. ions.
   c. neurotransmitters.
   d. messengers.

2. Which axons are fastest?
   a. small, myelinated
   b. small, unmyelinated
   c. large, unmyelinated
   d. large, myelinated

3. What is another name for myelinated axons?
   a. gray matter
   b. dura mater
   c. white matter
   d. duzitmater

4. After a neurotransmitter is released from the presynaptic neuron, what happens next?
   a. nothing
   b. the postsynaptic cell engulfs the neurotransmitter
   c. the neurotransmitter binds to the postsynaptic cell
   d. the neurotransmitter is cleaned up

5. If an illness could be treated by increasing the activity of chemical synapses, which treatment would work?
   a. decreasing the amount of neurotransmitter
   b. inhibiting the "cleanup" enzyme
   c. blocking the receptors on the receiving cell
   d. blocking action potentials

SPINAL CORD AND SPINAL NERVES

So far we've discussed the nervous system at the cellular and tissue level. In addition, we've described how impulses are transmitted in the nervous system. Now let's focus on the main neural highway that these impulses travel.

External Anatomy

The **spinal cord** is located in a hollow tube (vertebral cavity) running inside the vertebral column from the *foramen magnum* to the second lumbar (L2) vertebra. You can think of your spinal cord as a very sophisticated neural information superhighway connecting the central and peripheral nervous systems. It is divided into 31 segments, each with a pair of **spinal nerves**. The spinal cord segments and the spinal nerves are named for their corresponding vertebrae. The spinal cord ends at L2 in a pointed structure called the *conus medullaris*. Hanging from the conus medullaris is the **cauda equina** (literally "horse's tail"). The cauda equina consists of spinal nerves L2 through the coccygeal (Co) nerve dangling loosely in a bath of **cerebrospinal fluid (CSF)**, which acts as a shock absorber for both the brain and the spinal cord. The spinal cord has two widened areas, the cervical and lumbar enlargements, which contain the neurons for the limbs. See **FIGURE 9–7** ■.

Meninges

The CNS, both brain and spinal cord, are surrounded by a series of protective membranes called the **meninges**. The purpose of the meninges is to cover the delicate structures of the brain and the spinal cord. In essence, they help to set up layers that act as cushioning and shock absorbers for the brain as well as the spinal cord (see **FIGURE 9–8** ■). The meninges form three distinct layers. The outer layer of thick, fibrous tissue is called the **dura mater**. The middle layer, a wispy, delicate layer resembling spider webs, is the **arachnoid mater**. The third, innermost layer, which is fused to the neural tissue of the CNS, is the **pia mater**. This layer contains blood vessels that serve the brain and the spinal cord.

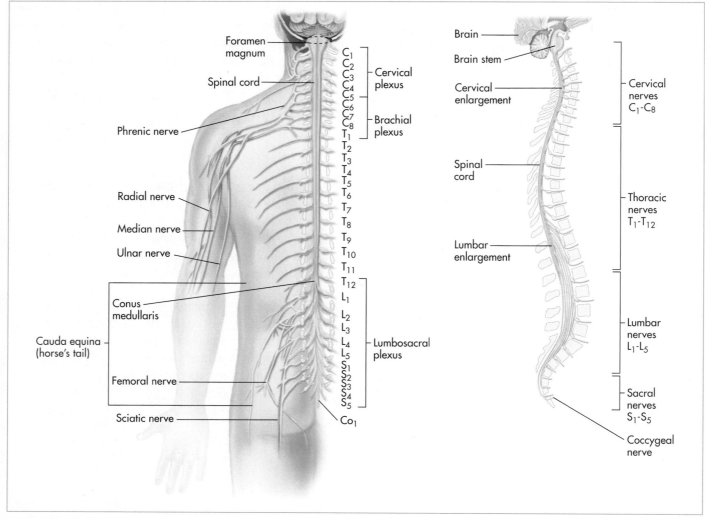

FIGURE 9–7 ■

The spinal cord. Although there are only seven cervical vertebrae, there are eight cervical spinal cord segments. One set of spinal nerves comes off the spinal cord superior to the first cervical vertebra, so the numbers in the cervical spinal cord do not match the cervical vertebrae exactly.

A series of spaces are associated with the meninges. Between the dura and the vertebral column is a space filled with fat and blood vessels called the **epidural space**. Between the dura mater and the arachnoid mater is the **subdural space**, which is filled with a tiny bit of fluid. Between the arachnoid mater and the pia mater is the large **subarachnoid space**, which is filled with cerebrospinal fluid and acts as a fluid cushion for the CNS. In addition, cerebrospinal fluid can also transport dissolved gases and nutrients as well as chemical messengers and waste products. These three membranes and their fluid-filled spaces, together with the bones of the skull and the vertebral column, form a strong protection system against CNS injury.

Clinical Application

EPIDURAL ANESTHESIA

Often, during labor or in preparation for a Cesarean section, a woman receives an *epidural*. An epidural is an injection of local anesthetic into the epidural space. The anesthetic is usually delivered via a catheter (a small tube). Ideally, epidural anesthesia allows a woman to continue to participate actively in the birth without severe labor pains. Epidural injections of steroids are sometimes prescribed for patients with chronic lower back injuries to relieve pain and inflammation.

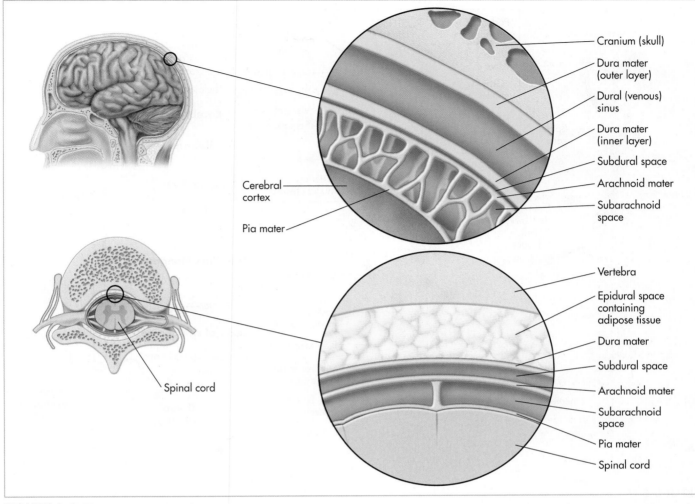

Cranium (skull)
Dura mater (outer layer)
Dural (venous) sinus
Dura mater (inner layer)
Subdural space
Arachnoid mater
Subarachnoid space

Cerebral cortex
Pia mater

Vertebra
Epidural space containing adipose tissue
Dura mater
Subdural space
Arachnoid mater
Subarachnoid space
Pia mater
Spinal cord

Spinal cord

FIGURE 9–8 ■

The meninges of the brain and spinal cord.

LEARNING HINT

Directional Terms

In the spinal cord, directional terms—anterior, posterior, dorsal, and ventral—are very important because function is linked to location. It is easy to get confused by the use of anterior and posterior for some structures and dorsal and ventral for others. Just keep in mind that in humans, anterior is ventral and posterior is dorsal. The names are interchangeable for all the structures except the spinal roots. The spinal roots are *always* called dorsal and ventral.

Internal Anatomy of the Spinal Cord

The spinal cord is divided in half by a *ventral median fissure* and a *dorsal median sulcus*. Please see **FIGURE 9–9A** ■. A **fissure** is a deep groove on the CNS surface, whereas a **sulcus** is a shallow groove on the CNS surface. The interior of the spinal cord is then divided into a series of sections of white matter **columns** and gray matter **horns**. There are three types of horns. The posterior or dorsal horn is involved in *sensory* functions, the anterior or ventral horn in *motor* functions, and the lateral horn in *autonomic* functions. The horns are the regions in which the neurons have their cell bodies.

There are also dorsal, lateral, and ventral columns, the white matter of the spinal cord. These columns act as nerve tracts, pathways, or axons, running up and down the spinal cord to and from the brain. Whether the tracts are ascending or descending, it helps to think of the columns as communication wires, part of a vast network of wires, transporting information to the appropriate parts of the system. This is the neural information superhighway.

Three ascending pathways—the dorsal column tract, the spinothalamic tract, and the spinocerebellar tract—carry information from your sense of touch to the spinal cord and then to your brain from all parts of the skin, joints, and tendons. (Figure 9–9B shows the dorsal column tract and the

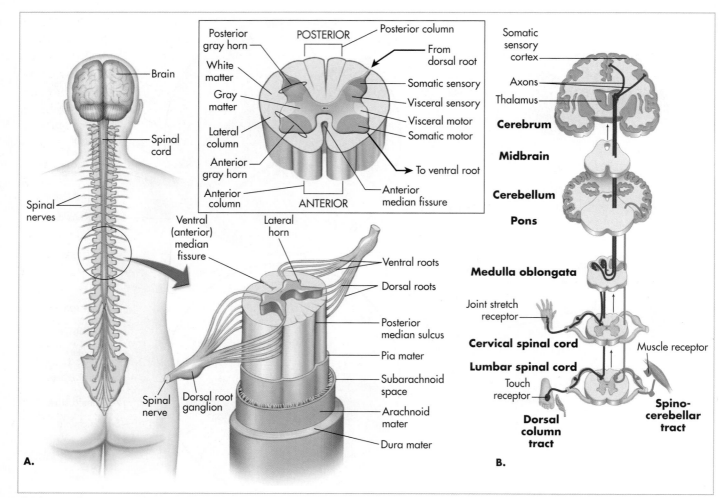

FIGURE 9–9 ■

(A) Internal anatomy of the spinal cord. (B) Ascending spinal tracts.

spinocerebellar tract.) These ascending pathways carry the following information:

- The **dorsal column tract** carries fine-touch and vibration information to the cerebral cortex.
- The **spinothalamic tract** carries temperature, pain, and crude touch information to the cerebral cortex.
- The **spinocerebellar tract** carries information about posture and position to the cerebellum.

Several descending pathways carry motor information (orders for voluntary movements) from the brain to the spinal cord, including the corticospinal tract, corticobulbar tract, reticulospinal tract, and rubrospinal tract. The axons from all pathways synapse on motor neurons in the ventral horn of the spinal cord. These descending pathways carry the following information:

- The **corticospinal tract** carries orders from the cerebral cortex to the motor neurons in the ventral horn of the spinal cord.

- The **corticobulbar tract** carries orders from the cerebral cortex to motor neurons in the brain stem.
- The **reticulospinal tract** and the **rubrospinal tract** (along with several other tracts) carry information from the various regions of the brain to the brain stem and ventral horn, which helps to coordinate movements.

Although this may all seem very complicated, keep in mind that the ascending pathways or tracts carry sensory information to the brain to process. The descending tracts transmit motor output in response to the sensory information.

In addition to the horns and columns, the spinal cord has several other features. The **commissures**, gray and white, connect left and right halves of the cord so the two sides of the CNS can communicate. (So the right hand does usually know what the left hand is doing, even if it doesn't always seem like it.) The central canal is a cavity in the center of the spinal cord that is filled with cerebrospinal fluid. The **spinal roots**, projecting from both sides of the spinal cord in pairs, fuse to form spinal nerves. The roots are the on-ramps and off-ramps of the neural superhighway. The dorsal root, with the embedded **dorsal root ganglion**, a collection of sensory neurons, carries sensory information, whereas the **ventral root** carries motor information. Refer to Figure 9–9A.

Spinal Nerves

Nerves are the connection between the CNS (brain and spinal cord) and the world outside the CNS. Nerves are therefore part of the PNS. Isn't it amazing that the brain, which is totally encased in darkness, can receive and interpret the nerve messages from the PNS to allow us to see the wonderful world around us? All nerves consist of bundles of axons, blood vessels, and connective tissue. Nerves run between the CNS and organs or tissues, carrying information into and out of the CNS. The nerves connected to the spinal cord are called **spinal nerves**. There are 31 pairs of spinal nerves, each named for the spinal cord segment to which they are attached. Because each spinal nerve is a fusion of dorsal and ventral roots, spinal nerves carry both sensory and motor information. A nerve that carries both types of information is called a **mixed nerve**. All spinal nerves are mixed. When spinal nerves leave the vertebral column, they can go through a number of different pathways to reach the peripheral tissues. Spinal nerves from the thoracic spinal cord project directly to the thoracic body wall without branching. Spinal nerves from the cervical, lumbar, and sacral regions of the spinal cord go through complex branching patterns, recombining with nerves from other spinal cord segments before projecting to peripheral structures. These complex branching patterns are called **plexuses**. See **FIGURE 9–10** ■. The sensory information carried on each spinal nerve can be mapped on the body into dermatomes. Dermatomes will be discussed in more detail in Chapter 10.

LEARNING HINT

Degrees of Touch

Crude touch does not provide very much detailed information, only that something is touching the skin. Fine touch, on the other hand, provides details, including texture. For example, if you just had crude touch and were holding a peach, you would only know you were holding something round and firm in your hand. Fine touch allows you to distinguish between a peach and a nectarine because of the "fuzz" on the peach.

Clinical Application

A MATTER OF CENTIMETERS

Did you know that the difference between being able to breathe on your own after a spinal cord injury and being dependent on a ventilator is literally a matter of centimeters? It's true. One of the nerves that projects from the cervical plexus is called the *phrenic nerve*. This nerve is the motor nerve for your diaphragm, your main breathing muscle. If the spinal cord is damaged below the cervical plexus, say in the high thoracic region, the phrenic nerve can receive signals from the brain and send them to the diaphragm, and the injured person is able to breathe. However, if the damage to the spinal cord is between the brain and the cervical plexus, the path from the brain to the phrenic nerve is blocked, and the signals can't get to the diaphragm from the brain. The diaphragm is paralyzed, and the person cannot breathe on his or her own. The difference is a matter of only a few centimeters.

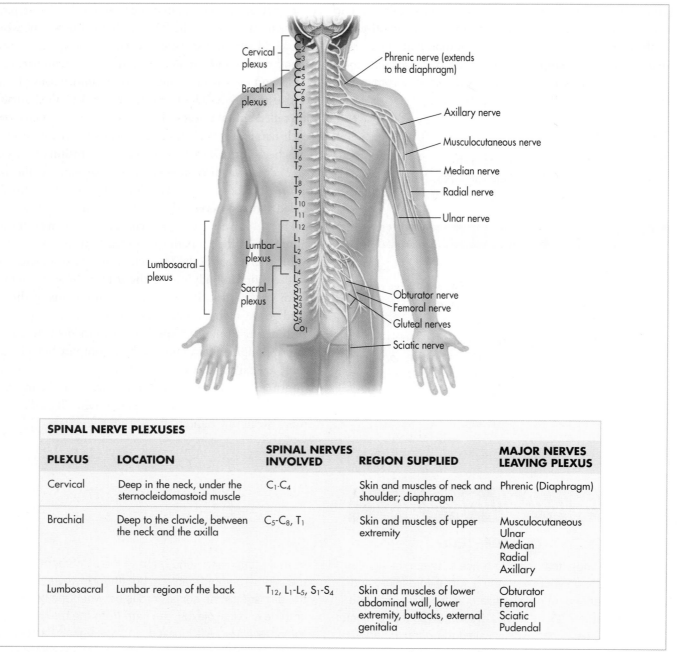

SPINAL NERVE PLEXUSES				
PLEXUS	**LOCATION**	**SPINAL NERVES INVOLVED**	**REGION SUPPLIED**	**MAJOR NERVES LEAVING PLEXUS**
Cervical	Deep in the neck, under the sternocleidomastoid muscle	C_1-C_4	Skin and muscles of neck and shoulder; diaphragm	Phrenic (Diaphragm)
Brachial	Deep to the clavicle, between the neck and the axilla	C_5-C_8, T_1	Skin and muscles of upper extremity	Musculocutaneous Ulnar Median Radial Axillary
Lumbosacral	Lumbar region of the back	T_{12}, L_1-L_5, S_1-S_4	Skin and muscles of lower abdominal wall, lower extremity, buttocks, external genitalia	Obturator Femoral Sciatic Pudendal

FIGURE 9–10 ■

Spinal cord plexuses. *Note:* Although there are seven cervical vertebrae, the first spinal nerve begins above the first vertebrae, leading to eight cervical spinal nerves.

Reflexes

Reflexes are the simplest form of motor output. Reflexes are generally protective, keeping you from harm. They are involuntary, and usually the response is proportionate to the stimulus. Some familiar reflexes are the *withdrawal reflex*, activated, for example, when you pound your thumb with a hammer or touch a hot stove; the *vestibular reflex*, which keeps you vertical; and the *startle reflex*, which causes you to jump at loud sounds. The amazing thing about reflexes is that they can often occur without your brain being involved. For many reflexes, only the spinal cord is necessary and no impulse needs to travel to the brain.

The most common example of a reflex is the *patellar tendon (knee-jerk) reflex*. You may have experienced this reflex at the doctor's office. The doctor taps your knee with a hammerlike instrument, and your leg kicks, seemingly against your will. What exactly is going on? When the doctor taps your knee, the hammer gently tugs on a tendon that is connected to your quadriceps muscles. The quads are gently tugged. This causes them to lengthen slightly. This length change is perceived by a sensory neuron and transmitted back to the spinal cord. The sensory neuron synapses with a motor neuron in the ventral horn. The motor neuron sends a signal to the quadriceps to stop the stretch. How do the quads stop the stretch? They shorten (contract). When a muscle shortens, it causes a movement. The shortening of

the quadriceps muscles extends your knee, causing your leg to kick. All of this is occurs by a simple tapping of the knee! By testing this reflex, a physician can test the basic workings of the nervous system. If the reflex is somehow abnormal, that may indicate muscle, nerve, or spinal cord problems. This action is totally reflexive (no pun intended). You can't stop yourself from kicking, even if you try. You do not have to think about kicking. The action happens without your brain. Only the spinal cord is necessary. **FIGURE 9–11** ■ illustrates this process in detail.

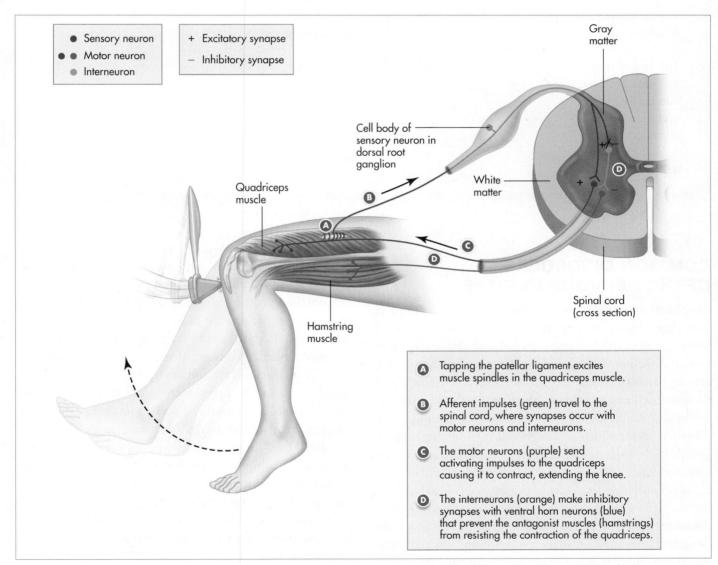

FIGURE 9–11 ■

The patellar reflex. (A) Striking the patellar ligament excites the quadriceps muscle spindles. (B) Sensory input travels to spinal cord and synapses with motor neurons and interneurons. (C) Motor neurons send impulses to contract the quadriceps, thus extending the lower leg. (D) Interneurons make inhibitory connections in the ventral horn of the spinal column to prevent hamstrings (antagonist muscles) from contracting so they do not resist the movement.

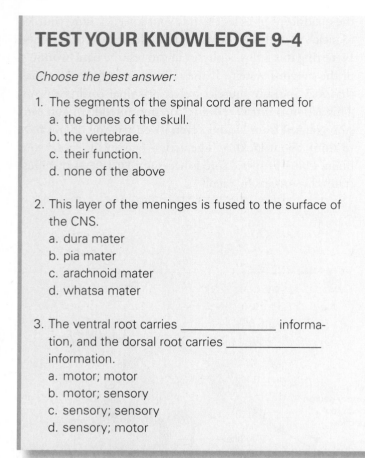

TEST YOUR KNOWLEDGE 9–4

Choose the best answer:

1. The segments of the spinal cord are named for
   a. the bones of the skull.
   b. the vertebrae.
   c. their function.
   d. none of the above

2. This layer of the meninges is fused to the surface of the CNS.
   a. dura mater
   b. pia mater
   c. arachnoid mater
   d. whatsa mater

3. The ventral root carries _____ information, and the dorsal root carries _____ information.
   a. motor; motor
   b. motor; sensory
   c. sensory; sensory
   d. sensory; motor

4. What is the term for the axon pathways carrying information up and down the spinal cord?
   a. horns
   b. roots
   c. columns
   d. ganglia

5. The ascending spinal cord tracts are
   a. sensory.
   b. motor.
   c. mixed.
   d. autonomic.

COMMON DISORDERS OF THE NERVOUS SYSTEM

Peripheral neuropathy encompasses a number of disorders involving damage to peripheral nerves. Because peripheral nerves are involved in sensory, motor, and autonomic function, the symptoms of peripheral neuropathy vary greatly among patients. Symptoms include muscle weakness and decreased reflexes, numbness, tingling, paralysis, pain, difficulty controlling blood pressure, abnormal sweating, and digestive abnormalities. Nongenetic neuropathy can be grouped into three broad categories: trauma, systemic disease, and infection or autoimmune disorders. *Trauma*, such as falls or automobile accidents, causes mechanical injury to nerves. Nerves may be severed, crushed, or bruised. *Systemic disorders* that cause peripheral neuropathy include kidney disorders, hormonal imbalance, alcoholism, vascular damage, repetitive stress (like carpal tunnel), chronic inflammation, diabetes, toxins, and tumors. *Infections* such as shingles, Epstein-Barr virus, herpes, HIV, Lyme disease, and polio cause peripheral neuropathy. Guillain-Barré syndrome is an acute form of peripheral neuropathy. Some forms of neuropathy are inherited.

Even though the spinal cord is well protected by the bones and meninges, trauma can cause damage to the delicate neural tissue. The spinal cord may be partially or completely severed, crushed, or bruised. Bruises to the spinal cord may resolve with time and rehabilitation, but a severed or crushed spinal cord is usually a permanent injury. **Spinal cord injury** usually results in paralysis and sensory loss below the injury, and the extent of the paralysis is related to the location of the spinal cord injury. Patients with injuries to the cervical region are quadriplegics, paralyzed in all four limbs. Some quadriplegics, with damage very high in the cervical region, have paralyzed diaphragms and cannot breathe on their own. Patients with injuries in the thoracic region and lower have paraplegia. They can move their arms, but their legs are paralyzed.

Guillain-Barré syndrome (GBS) is a paralysis caused by inflammation of peripheral nerves. Patients develop, over variable periods of time, weakness and ascending paralysis of the limbs, face, and diaphragm. Some patients may have a mild form of Guillain-Barré syndrome, but those with severe disease must be kept on a ventilator until the paralysis resolves. The cause of the disease is not known, although some patients develop Guillain-Barré syndrome after a viral infection. Other evidence suggests that an autoimmune attack of peripheral myelin may be to blame. There is no effective treatment except supportive care. Fortunately, the disorder is usually temporary. Many patients need rehabilitation after their PNS recovers.

Myasthenia gravis is an autoimmune disorder in which the immune system attacks and destroys acetylcholine receptors at the neuromuscular junction. Motor neurons continue to release acetylcholine, but the receptor number is reduced, so motor neurons cannot communicate with skeletal muscles. Eye muscles are typically the first muscles affected, but some patients initially experience difficulty chewing, swallowing, or talking. The disorder, like most autoimmune disorders, is progressive, though the course of the disease varies widely among patients. Treatment for myasthenia gravis includes acetylcholinesterase inhibitors, corticosteroids, immunosuppressant drugs, and plasma exchange. In a few patients, the disease disappears spontaneously.

Botulism is a form of paralysis caused by toxins produced by the bacterium *Clostridium botulinum*. Botulism can be caused by ingesting the toxin in food and can also result from wound infections. The bacteria grow most commonly in improperly prepared canned food, especially home-canned food. The toxin keeps neurotransmitters from being released at the neuromuscular junction, causing paralysis. Initial symptoms include vision disturbances, slurred speech, dry mouth, and muscle weakness. If left untreated, paralysis will spread to limbs and respiratory muscles. Botulism can be treated by administration of antitoxin and supportive care. Botulism is a rare disorder. According to the CDC, the United States averages 145 cases per year.

Meningitis is an infection, usually from viruses or bacteria, of the meninges, the lining of the brain and the spinal cord. Bacterial meningitis is a potentially fatal infection. The bacteria first infect the upper respiratory tract and then travel to the meninges. High-risk groups include older adults, people with suppressed immune systems, very young children, and college students who live in dorms. Patients who survive bacterial meningitis often have severe neurological impairment, including deafness and severe brain damage. Viral meningitis is a much milder disease caused by viruses that enter the mouth and travel to the meninges.

The relationship between the muscular system and nervous system can be seen in the condition of **carpal tunnel syndrome (CTS)**, which occurs with an inflammation and swelling of the tendon sheaths surrounding the flexor tendon of the palm. Although the classic etiology of this condition can be the result of a repetitive motion such as typing on a keyboard, CTS can also be caused by certain prescription drugs, high cholesterol levels, and even diabetes. As a result of this inflammation and swelling, the median nerve is compressed, producing a tingling sensation or numbness of the palm and first three fingers.

LEARNING HINT

Scenic Overview

Often when you are on a journey, you cannot see or appreciate the big picture. For example, if you are in a portion of the Grand Canyon, it can be quite impressive, but when you stand on top at the rim of the Grand Canyon, the "whole picture" becomes clear and spectacular. This chapter on the nervous system has given you a picture of the nervous tissue and how nerve transmission occurs. In addition, this chapter has begun to develop the role of the spinal cord. The next chapter focuses on the brain and then pulls everything together so you can see the big picture.

- The nervous system is the body's control system. It has a sensory (input) system, an integration center, the CNS, and a motor (output) system. The input and output nerves are in the PNS, and the brain and spinal cord are the CNS.

- The tissue of the nervous system is made up of two types of cells: neurons, which send, receive, and process information, and neuroglia, which support the neurons.

- Neurons are excitable cells. They do their jobs by carrying tiny electrical currents caused by changes in cell permeability to certain ions. These tiny electrical currents can be all-or-none responses (action potentials), can change depending on the size of the stimulus (graded potentials), can travel down axons (impulse conduction), or can be used to transmit information from one cell to another (synaptic transmission).

- Your CNS is surrounded by a three-layered membrane system: dura mater, arachnoid mater, and pia mater,

collectively known as the meninges. Cerebrospinal fluid is also contained in the space between the arachnoid and pia maters.

- The spinal cord has 31 segments, each with a pair of spinal nerves. The spinal nerves are a part of the peripheral nervous system.

- The spinal nerves are made of a pair of spinal roots. The ventral root is integral to motor function, and the dorsal root is integral to sensory function. Spinal nerves are mixed; they carry both sensory and motor information.

- A series of tracts run up and down the spinal cord to and from the brain. The tracts going toward the brain carry sensory information to the brain. The tracts coming from the brain toward the spinal cord carry motor information from the brain.

CASE STEUDY

During the biggest game of his high school football career, Dylan, the best wide receiver in the league, leaps high into the air in the end zone to score the game-winning touchdown. A player for the other teams hits him hard, knocking him into the goalpost. Dylan crumples to the ground,

unmoving. When the EMTs get to him, Dylan is paralyzed on both sides of his body and in respiratory arrest.

Given your knowledge of the nervous system, can you pinpoint the location of Dylan's injury? Explain how you arrived at your conclusion.

REVIEW QUESTIONS

Multiple Choice

1. The input side of your nervous system is known as
   a. motor.
   b. sensory.
   c. association.
   d. all of the above

2. The ascending spinal tracts carry _____ information to the brain.
   a. hormonal
   b. motor
   c. sensory
   d. sensory and motor

3. During depolarization, _____ ions move _____ a neuron.
   a. K^+, out of
   b. K^+, into
   c. Na^+, out of
   d. Na^+, into

4. The ventral root of the spinal cord is
   a. sensory.
   b. motor.
   c. association.
   d. none of the above

5. Spinal nerves carry what kind of information?
   a. sensory
   b. motor
   c. mixed
   d. vertebral

6. A spinal cord injury at T3 would cause
   a. paralysis in all four limbs.
   b. paralysis from the chest down.
   c. paralysis in all four limbs and respiratory arrest.
   d. paralysis of the arms.

7. Sodium channel blockers, which prevent sodium channels from working, would block which part of the action potential?
   a. hyperpolarization
   b. depolarization
   c. repolarization
   d. afterpotential

8. Multiple sclerosis is often associated with a decrease in these neuroglia.
   a. astrocytes
   b. Schwann cells
   c. oligodendrocytes
   d. microglia

Fill in the Blank

1. The speed of impulse conduction is determined by _____ and _____.

2. _____ potentials are all or none.

3. The spinal cord has white matter _____ and gray matter _____.

4. _____ fluid is contained in the _____ space between the arachnoid mater and pia mater.

5. A(n) _____ is an involuntary, protective movement that is sometimes generated without the brain.

6. The virus polio causes loss of motor function but not of sensory function, because it infects neurons. These neurons are located in the _____ horn of the spinal cord.

Short Answer

1. Explain the changes in a neuron during an action potential.

   _____

   _____

   _____

   _____

2. List the steps in chemical synaptic transmission.

   _____

   _____

   _____

   _____

3. List the layers of protection around the CNS.

   _____

   _____

   _____

   _____

4. List the types of neuroglia and their functions.

   _____

   _____

   _____

   _____

5. Explain the results of spinal cord injuries in the following locations: C_2, T_3, and L_2.

   _____

   _____

   _____

   _____

Visit our new **MyHealthProfessions Lab** to accompany *Anatomy & Physiology for Health Professions.* Here you'll find a rich collection of quizzes, case studies, and animations for deeper understanding and application.

10

The Nervous System (Part II)

THE TRAFFIC CONTROL CENTER

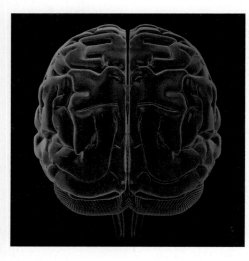

Welcome to the final leg of your trip through the nervous system. In this chapter, we focus on the main controller of the nervous system—the brain—and then pull everything together to see how all the pieces of the puzzle form the big picture. Staying with our journey analogy, the previous chapter focusing on the spinal cord and nerves presented the roadways we travel. There are all kinds of roads that lead to all kinds of places. However, the flow of traffic must be precisely controlled, or chaos and wrecks would occur. The control system of the roadways includes such things as traffic signs and lights, tollbooths, and drawbridges. The brain is the control system of the nervous system superhighway, attempting to keep everything running smoothly. Let's hope this journey is not as "nerve wracking" as some of the highways you may have been on.

LEARNING OUTCOMES

At the end of your journey through this chapter, you will be able to:

- Locate and define the internal and external structures of the brain and their corresponding functions.
- List and describe the cranial nerves and their functions and discuss how they differ from spinal nerves.
- Discuss the integration of the brain, spinal cord, and peripheral nervous system.
- Describe the somatic sensory system.
- Describe the motor system functions of the brain with related structures.
- Contrast the parasympathetic and sympathetic branches of the autonomic nervous system.
- Discuss the limbic system and reticular formation.
- Discuss some representative diseases of the nervous system.

Pronunciation Guide

Correct pronunciation is important in any journey so that you and others are completely understood. Here is a "see and say" Pronunciation Guide for the more difficult terms to pronounce in this chapter. Please note that even though there are standard pronunciations, regional variations of the pronunciations can occur.

anterior commissure (KAHM ih shur)
basal nuclei (BAY zal NOO klee eye)
cerebellum (ser eh BELL um)
cerebrum (ser EE brum)
corpus callosum (KOR pus kah LOH sum)
diencephalon (DYE in SEFF ah lon)
fornix (FOR niks)
gyri (JIE rie)
hypothalamus (high poh THAL ah mus)

limbic system (LIM bick)
medulla oblongata (meh DULL ah OB long GA ta)
occipital lobe (awk SIP eh tal)
parietal lobe (pah RYE eh tal)
pineal body (PIN ee al)
subarachnoid space (sub ah RACK noyd)
sulcus (SULL cus)
thalamus (THAL ah mus)

THE BRAIN AND THE CRANIAL NERVES

The brain and the cranial nerves represent the major control system of the nervous system. The brain acts as the main processor and director of the entire system. The cranial nerves leave the brain and go to specific body areas, where they receive information and send it back to the brain (sensory), and the brain then sends back instructions for the appropriate response (motor). Let's again begin with an overview and then get more specific.

At the top of the spinal cord, beginning at the level of the foramen magnum of the skull and filling the cranial cavity, is the brain. Just like a grocery store needs to be organized into sections such as produce, meats, and deli, the brain can be divided into several anatomical and functional sections. We will talk about each section separately and then describe the interactions between the brain parts and the spinal cord.

The Brain's External Anatomy

Let's start our journey looking at the outside of the brain, and then we will zoom in on the internal structures. From the outside, you can see that the brain consists of a cerebrum, cerebellum, and brain stem. See **FIGURE 10-1** ■.

Cerebrum

The **cerebrum**, which is the largest part of the brain, is divided into two **hemispheres**, a right and left, by the **longitudinal fissure** and divided from the cerebellum ("little brain") by the **transverse fissure**. The surface of the cerebrum is not smooth; rather, it is broken by ridges, or **gyri**, and grooves, or **sulci** (plural of sulcus), collectively known as *convolutions*. These convolutions serve a very important

purpose by increasing the surface area of the brain, yet allowing it to be "folded" into a smaller space. Most of the sulci are extremely variable in their locations among humans, but a few are in basically the same place in every human brain. These less variable sulci are used to divide the brain into four large sections called **lobes**, much like the major departments in a grocery store are separated by aisles.

Amazing Facts

Why Not a Smooth Brain?
The surface of the brain is folded and rippled into a series of convolutions. These convolutions allow lots of brain surface area to fit into a very small space. If you could lay the convolutions flat, they would be the size of a pillow case. Talk about your big heads! Another fact to keep in "mind" is that the brain can die if deprived of oxygen in as little as 4 to 8 minutes.

Just some food for thought as you travel through this chapter. The scarecrow on *The Wizard of Oz* "thought" he needed a brain. As you work through this chapter, can you "think" of several reasons why you knew all along he had a brain?

The lobes (see **TABLE 10-1** ■) are named for the skull bones that cover them, and they occur in pairs, one in each hemisphere. The most anterior lobes, separated from the rest of the brain by the central sulci, are the frontal lobes. The **frontal lobes** are responsible for motor activities, conscious thought, and speech. A major portion of the frontal lobes control personality, planning, and impulsiveness. Posterior

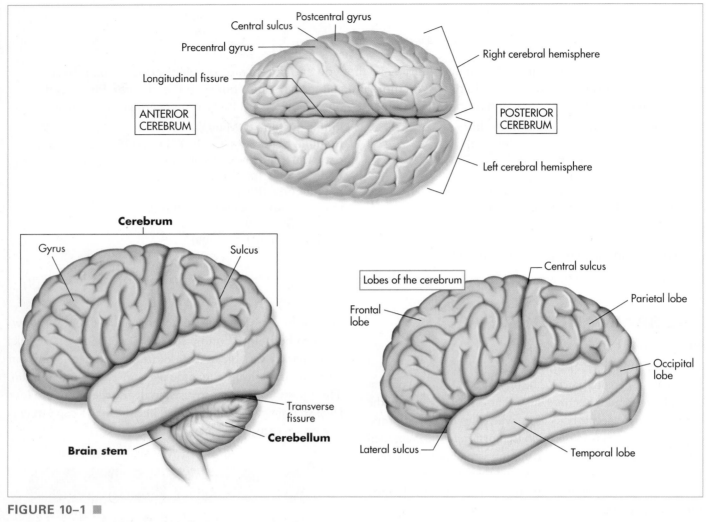

FIGURE 10–1 ■
External brain anatomy and lobes.

to the frontal lobe are the parietal lobes. The **parietal lobes** are involved with body sense, perception, and understanding language. Posterior to the parietal lobes are the **occipital lobes**, which are responsible for vision. There is no obvious external dividing line between the parietal and occipital lobes, the most posterior lobes at the back of the skull. The most inferior lobes, separated by the lateral fissures, are the **temporal lobes**, which are involved in hearing and the integration of sensory information and memory. Again, refer to Figure 10–1, which shows the lobes of the brain and the sulci that separate them. The **insula** is a section of the brain located deep inside the temporal lobes that is often listed as a fifth lobe, but it is not visible on the surface of the cerebrum. The insula helps coordinate autonomic (visceral) functions. In addition, there is evidence that the insula is involved in many other functions.

Much of the information coming into your cerebrum is *contralateral*. That is, the left side of the body is controlled by the right side of your brain, and the right side of the body is controlled by your left brain.

Here, we should point out some specific regions within each lobe. On either side of the central sulcus are two gyri named for their locations: the **precentral gyrus**, in the frontal lobes, anterior to the central sulcus, and the **postcentral gyrus**, in the parietal lobes, posterior to the central sulcus. The importance of these gyri will become obvious when we discuss brain function later in the chapter. The frontal lobe also contains **Broca's area**, which controls motor output for speech. In the parietal and temporal lobes is **Wernicke's area**, which was long thought to control sensory aspects of language, including understanding. However, new evidence in the field of neuroscience supports that this area is actually part of a larger general interpretive area for many types of sensory information and may integrate much of the sensory information coming to the cerebral cortex. In most people, Broca's and Wernicke's areas are in the left hemisphere.

TABLE 10–1 CEREBRAL LOBES AND CEREBELLUM

STRUCTURE	MAJOR FUNCTIONS
Cerebral Lobes	
Frontal lobe	Motor function, behavior and emotions, memory storage, thinking, smell
Parietal lobe	Body sense, perception, and understanding language
Occipital lobe	Vision
Temporal lobe	Hearing, integration of sensory information, memory
Insula	Autonomic (visceral) functions, many others (e.g., taste)
Cerebellum	The "little brain"; sensory and motor coordination and balance, cognitive functions, social behavior

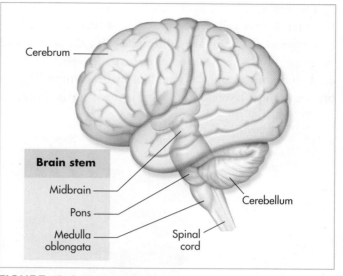

FIGURE 10–2 ■
The brain stem.

Cerebellum

The **cerebellum** is posterior to the brain stem and plays an important role in sensory and motor coordination, balance, and cognitive functions. Its surface is also convoluted like that of the cerebrum and it is divided into lobes. From its external appearance, it is easy to see why anatomists named the cerebellum the "little brain." Again, please see Figure 10–1 and Table 10–1.

The Brain Stem

The **brain stem** (see **FIGURE 10–2** ■) is a stalklike structure inferior to and partially covered by the cerebrum. It is divided into three sections. The **medulla oblongata** is continuous with the spinal cord. It is responsible for impulses that control heartbeat, breathing, and the muscle tone in blood vessels, which controls blood pressure. The **pons** is just superior to the medulla oblongata and connects the medulla oblongata and the cerebellum with the upper portions of the brain. The pons also plays a role in breathing. The **midbrain**, which is the most superior portion of the brain stem, acts as a two-way conduction pathway to relay visual and auditory impulses and other information to the cerebrum (see **TABLE 10–2** ■). The brain stem receives sensory information and contains control systems for vital functions such as blood pressure, heart rate, and breathing. The brain stem controls the vital functions of life.

TABLE 10–2 THE BRAIN STEM

STRUCTURE	FUNCTION
Midbrain	Relays sensory and motor information
Pons	Relays sensory and motor information; role in breathing
Medulla oblongata	Regulates vital functions of heart rate, blood pressure, breathing, and reflex center for coughing, sneezing, swallowing, and vomiting

Clinical Application

SURVIVING BRAIN INJURIES

Patients with severe brain injuries but with an intact brain stem can continue in a coma or a vegetative state as long as they are nutritionally supported. They may have sleep–wake cycles and even respond to some stimuli but they cannot interact in a meaningful way with their environment.

The brain, like the spinal cord, is covered with protective membranes called *meninges*. See **FIGURE 10–3** ■. The meninges of the brain are continuous with the spinal cord meninges but there are some differences between the spinal cord and brain meninges. The dura mater surrounding the brain is double layered. One layer is fused to the inside of the skull (there is no epidural space). Between that layer and the second layer are several blood-filled spaces called *dural sinuses*. A potentially fatal condition is an infection of the meninges called **meningitis**, which can rapidly spread and affect the brain and spinal cord through this common covering (see Chapter 9).

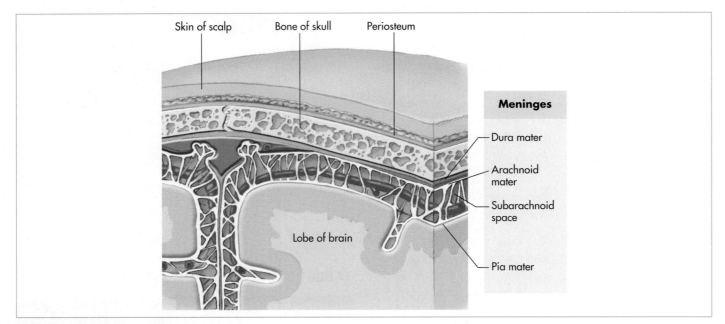

FIGURE 10–3 ■

The meninges.

TEST YOUR KNOWLEDGE 10–1

Choose the best answer:

1. Which of the following is *not* part of the brain stem?
   a. pons
   b. medulla oblongata
   c. midbrain
   d. diencephalon

2. This lobe contains the primary visual cortex.
   a. frontal
   b. temporal
   c. occipital
   d. parietal

3. The cerebrum is divided into right and left hemispheres by the
   a. central sulcus.
   b. transverse fissure.
   c. corpus callosum.
   d. none of the above

4. The raised areas on the surface of the cerebrum are called
   a. sulci.
   b. convolutions.
   c. gyri.
   d. lobes.

5. The role of Broca's area is
   a. sensory control of speech.
   b. integration of sensory inputs.
   c. motor control of speech.
   d. personality.

6. After hitting the left side of her head, Kim has difficulty speaking and cannot move the right side of her body. Where is her injury?
   a. occipital lobe
   b. frontal lobe
   c. parietal lobe
   d. temporal lobe

The Brain's Internal Anatomy

Like the spinal cord, the inside of the brain has white matter, gray matter, and hollow cavities containing cerebrospinal fluid. (See! We really do have holes in our heads.) Unlike the spinal cord, however, the white matter is surrounded by the gray matter in the cerebrum and cerebellum. (Remember, in the spinal cord, the white matter surrounds the gray matter.) The layer of gray matter surrounding the white matter in the brain is called the **cortex** (see **FIGURE 10–4** ■). In the cerebrum it is called the *cerebral cortex*, and in the cerebellum it is called the *cerebellar cortex*. Throughout the brain there are deep "islands" of gray matter surrounded by white matter. These islands are called **nuclei**.

The fluid-filled cavities in the brain are called **ventricles**, and they are continuous with the central canal of the spinal cord and the **subarachnoid space** of both the brain and the spinal cord. These ventricles allow for the circulation of cerebrospinal fluid throughout the brain. The lateral ventricles (ventricles 1 and 2) are in the cerebrum; the third ventricle is in the diencephalon, a region between the cerebrum and brain stem; and the fourth ventricle is in the inferior part of the brain between the medulla oblongata and the cerebellum.

The Cerebrum

The inside of the cerebrum reflects its external anatomy (see **FIGURE 10–5** ■). The right and left hemispheres are connected by a collection of white matter surrounding the lateral ventricles, called the **corpus callosum**. This connection allows for cross-communication between the right and left sides of the cerebrum. Many of our day-to-day activities, like walking or driving, require both sides of the body, and therefore both sides of the brain, to be well coordinated. Imagine walking if your legs were acting independently. Several prominent cerebral nuclei are also involved in motor coordination, sensation, and motor control.

The Diencephalon

Inferior to the cerebrum is a section of the brain that is not visible from the exterior, called the **diencephalon**. The diencephalon consists of several parts: the **thalamus**, **hypothalamus**, **pineal body**, and **pituitary gland** (see **TABLE 10–3** ■). The thalamus relays and processes information going to the cerebrum. The hypothalamus, pineal body, and pituitary gland represent an interface with the endocrine system (the other control system), covered in Chapter 12. The diencephalon contains the third ventricle and a number of nuclei. Specific nuclei of the diencephalon are responsible for controlling hormone levels, hunger and thirst, body temperature, and sleep–wake cycles, and for coordinating the flow of information around the brain.

TABLE 10–3 DIENCEPHALON

STRUCTURE	FUNCTION
Thalamus	Relays and processes information going to the cerebrum
Hypothalamus	Regulates hormone levels, temperature, water balance, thirst, appetite, sleep–wake cycles, and some emotions (pleasure and fear); regulates the pituitary gland and controls the endocrine system
Pineal body	Responsible for secretion of melatonin (body clock)
Pituitary gland	Secretes hormones for various functions (explained in Chapter 12)

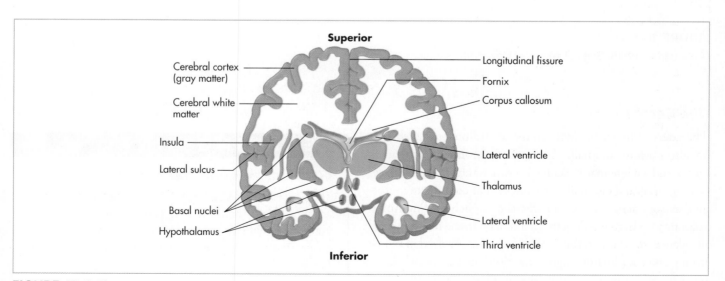

FIGURE 10–4 ■

Frontal sectional view of the brain.

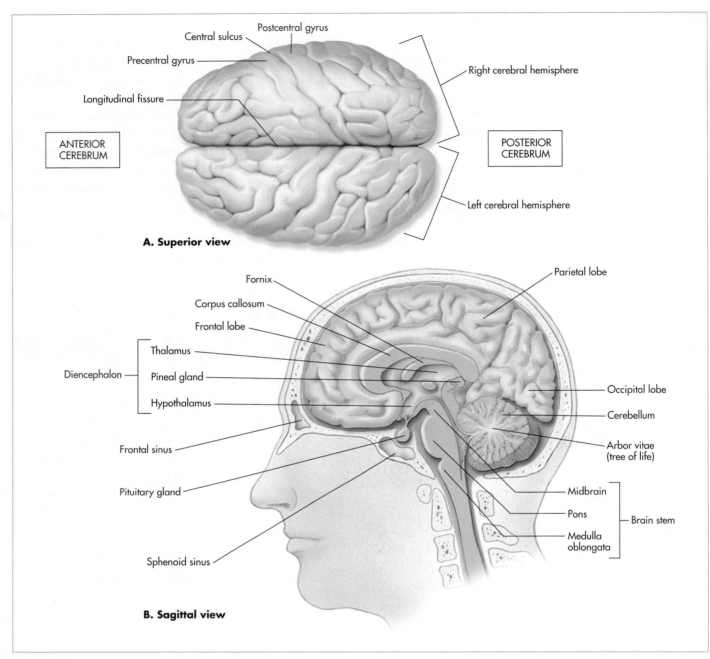

FIGURE 10–5 ■

(A) Superior and (B) Sagittal sectional views of the brain.

The Cerebellum

The external similarities between the cerebellum and cerebrum are also obvious internally. The cerebellum has a gray matter cortex and a white matter center, known as the *arbor vitae* (tree of life). The cerebellum also has nuclei that coordinate motor and sensory activities. Essentially, the cerebellum fine-tunes voluntary skeletal muscle activity and helps in the maintenance of balance. In addition, the cerebellum is also involved in monitoring and coordinating higher functions such as social behavior, attention, and memory. Again, please see Figure 10–5.

LEARNING HINT

Gray versus White Matter

The gray matter is composed of the cell bodies of the neurons. White matter is composed of axons, which are surrounded with myelin. Remember from the previous chapter that myelin allows messages to be transmitted faster.

Clinical Application

CEREBROSPINAL FLUID CIRCULATION AND HYDROCEPHALUS

The ventricles of the brain, the central canal of the spinal cord, and the subarachnoid space, surrounding both parts of the CNS, are all filled with cerebrospinal fluid (CSF). The CSF is secreted by tissue in the ventricles called *choroid plexus*. Produced at the rate of 750 milliliters daily, CSF made in the lateral ventricles flows through the interventricular foramen into the third ventricle and then through the cerebral aqueduct into the fourth ventricle. From the fourth ventricle, CSF flows into the central canal of the spinal cord and the subarachnoid space. Cerebrospinal fluid is returned to the blood via special "ports" (the arachnoid villi) between subarachnoid space and blood spaces in the dura mater (the dural sinuses). See **FIGURE 10–6** ■.

The balance of CSF made and CSF reabsorbed by the blood is very important. The brain is a very delicate organ captured between the liquid CSF and the bones of the skull. If there is too much CSF, pressure inside the skull rises, eventually crushing brain tissue. This condition, in which there is too much CSF, is called **hydrocephalus** (literally, "water in the head"). Hydrocephalus can be caused by blockage of the narrow passages between the ventricles due to trauma, by birth defects or tumors, or by decreased reabsorption of CSF due to subarachnoid bleeding. Hydrocephalus may be treated by medication, but the most common treatment is insertion of a shunt, a tube that drains the extra CSF into the patient's heart or abdominal cavity.

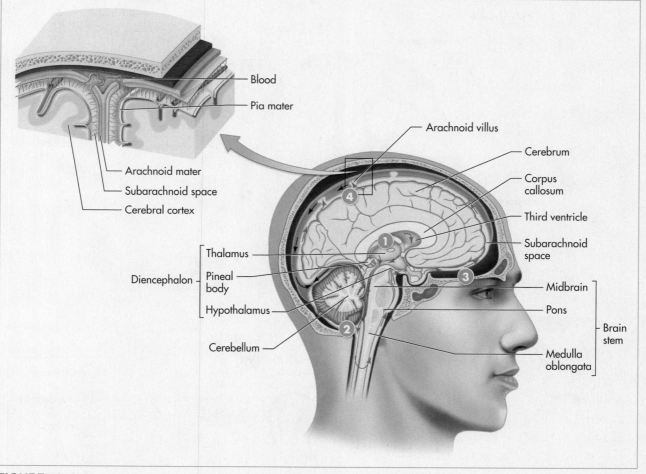

FIGURE 10–6 ■

Cerebral spinal fluid (CSF) circulation and internal anatomy of the brain. CSF flow: (1) CSF is produced by the choroid plexus in each of the four ventricles. (2) CSF flows from the ventricles to the central canal of the spinal cord. (3) CSF also flows from the ventricles into the subarachnoid space surrounding the brain. (4) CSF is absorbed into the dural venous sinuses via the arachnoid villi.

CRANIAL NERVES

For the central nervous system to function, it must be connected to the outside world via nerves of the peripheral nervous system. We have already seen that the spinal cord is connected to the outside via spinal nerves. The brain also has nerves to connect it to the outside, aptly named **cranial nerves** (see FIGURE 10–7 ■). Cranial nerves are like spinal nerves in that they are the input and output pathways for the brain, just as the spinal nerves are the pathways for the spinal cord. However, there are some important differences. You should remember that there are 31 pairs of spinal nerves and that *all* of them are *mixed nerves*: They carry both sensory and motor information because they are formed by a combination of dorsal and ventral roots. There are far fewer cranial nerves—only 12 pairs. All but the first two pairs arise from the brain stem. Cranial nerves are not *all* mixed as are spinal nerves. Some cranial nerves are mainly sensory nerves, providing input; some are mainly motor nerves, directing activity; and some are mixed. Cranial nerves are much more specialized than spinal nerves and are named based on their specialty. Some cranial nerves carry sensory and motor information for the head, face, and neck, whereas others carry visual, auditory, smell, or taste sensation. TABLE 10–4 ■ lists cranial nerves and their functions.

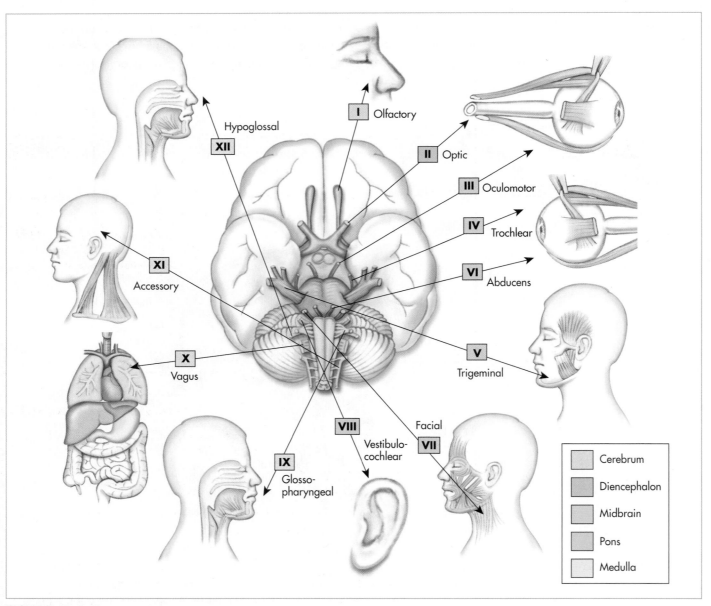

FIGURE 10–7 ■

Cranial nerves.

TABLE 10–4 CRANIAL NERVES AND FUNCTIONS

NERVE	FUNCTION
Olfactory (I)	Sensory (smell)
Optic (II)	Sensory (vision)
Oculomotor (III)	Mixed, chiefly motor for eye movements
Trochlear (IV)	Mixed, chiefly motor for eye movements
Trigeminal (V)	Mixed, sensory for face, motor for chewing
Abducens (VI)	Mixed, chiefly motor for eye movements
Facial (VII)	Mixed; motor for face; sensory for taste
Vestibulocochlear (VIII)	Sensory, hearing, and balance
Glossopharyngeal (IX)	Mixed, motor for tongue and throat muscles; sensory for taste and physiology
Vagus (X)	Mixed, motor for autonomic heart, lungs, viscera; sensory for viscera, taste buds
Accessory (XI)	Motor for larynx, soft palate, trapezius, and sternocleidomastoid muscles
Hypoglossal (XII)	Motor for tongue muscles

LEARNING HINT

Mnemonic Devices

A mnemonic device is a tool used to help you memorize long lists. It can be very useful in anatomy. To make a mnemonic device, take the first letter of each part of the list you are trying to memorize and make it into a sentence. For example, the five great lakes in order from west to east are Superior, Michigan, Huron, Erie, and Ontario. The mnemonic device used to remember the right order is **S**am **M**ade **H**arry **E**at **O**nions, much easier to remember than the lakes themselves. An example for the cranial nerves is this one: **O**n **O**ld **O**lympus **T**owering **T**ops **A** **F**inn **V**ith **G**erman **V**alked **A**nd **H**opped. It's goofy but it works for us. You may want to find your own sentence that works better for you.

TEST YOUR KNOWLEDGE 10–2

Choose the best answer:

1. Deep islands of gray matter are known as
   a. hemispheres.
   b. gyri.
   c. nuclei.
   d. nerves.

2. Which of the following is *not* found in the diencephalon?
   a. thalamus
   b. pineal body
   c. postcentral gyrus
   d. hypothalamus

3. The right and left hemispheres are connected by the
   a. ventricles.
   b. corpus callosum.
   c. cerebellum.
   d. cranial nerves.

4. Which of the following is true of cranial nerves?
   a. They are all mixed.
   b. They all project from the cerebrum.
   c. They may carry motor, sensory, or both kinds of information.
   d. They carry information for the body below the neck.

(continued)

THE BIG PICTURE: INTEGRATION OF BRAIN, SPINAL CORD, AND PNS

So how does the brain work with the spinal cord and peripheral nervous system? Let's begin to put the pieces together by revisiting the overall organizational chart of the nervous system, to serve as our guide or GPS to keep our location clear. See **FIGURE 10–8** ▇ to show our current location.

The Somatic Sensory System

We have already mentioned the parts of your brain that are dedicated to your special senses: vision (occipital lobe), hearing (temporal), taste (insula), and smell (frontal lobe). The **somatic sensory system** provides sensory input for your nervous system. The term *somatic* relates to sensations that are perceived as originating from superficial (skin) or muscular structures of the body. We have not yet talked about the sense of touch, called **somatic sensation**. Somatic sensation allows you to feel the world around you. Somatic sensation includes not just fine touch, which allows you to tell the difference between a peach and a nectarine or a golf ball and a ping-pong ball, but also crude touch, vibration, pain, temperature, and body position. Although your special senses are all carried on cranial nerves, information for somatic sensation comes into *both* the brain and the spinal cord. Ultimately, for you to attach meaning to touch sensation, the sensory information must get to your brain via the peripheral nervous system.

Let's start with the spinal cord. When we talked about reflexes, we saw somatic sensory information come into the

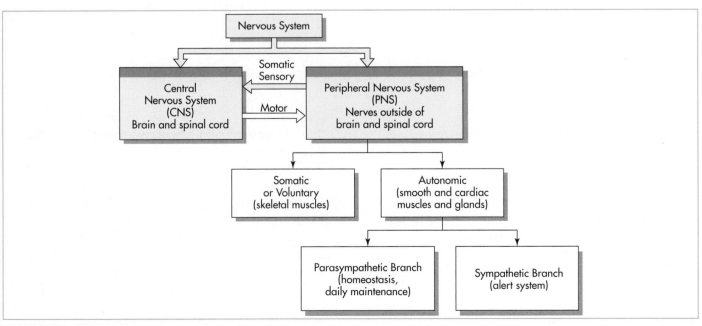

FIGURE 10–8 ▇

Nervous system flowchart highlighting our current location.

TABLE 10–5 SPINAL CORD PATHWAYS FOR SENSORY INFORMATION

PATHWAY	INFORMATION	FROM	TO
1. Spinothalamic		Skin	Somatic sensory cortex
a. lateral	Pain; temperature		
b. anterior	Itch; pressure; tickle		
2. Dorsal column	Fine touch; limb position	Skin; joints	Somatic sensory cortex; cerebellum
3. Spinocerebellar	Posture	Joints; tendons	Cerebellum

spinal cord via the dorsal root and synapse with a motor neuron in the ventral horn. Let's say you place your hand on a hot iron. The sensory neuron carries pain information to your spinal cord. The motor neuron then activates the muscle, allowing you to respond to the stimulus *immediately* and pull your hand away to minimize injury. The same pain neurons that carried the pain signal to your spinal cord join the spinothalamic tract in your spinal cord and simultaneously send a pain signal to your brain.

Because there are so many variations of "touch" information that must come in from all parts of the body, different neural highways are needed to more effectively take that information to the brain. See **TABLE 10–5** ■ for a description

of spinal cord pathways. (Reminder: These pathways were already discussed in Chapter 9.)

The sensory information coming into the brain must reach a specific area for processing. As you can see from Table 10–5, the dorsal column and spinothalamic tracts both transport sensory information from your skin and joints to the **primary somatic sensory cortex**, in the postcentral gyrus of the parietal lobe, described earlier in the chapter.

The axons transport information to specific parts of the somatic sensory cortex that correspond to parts of the body. This route can be mapped out, as in **FIGURE 10–9** ■, to provide the primary somatic sensory area showing the relationship between the body part and the sensory input provided for that part.

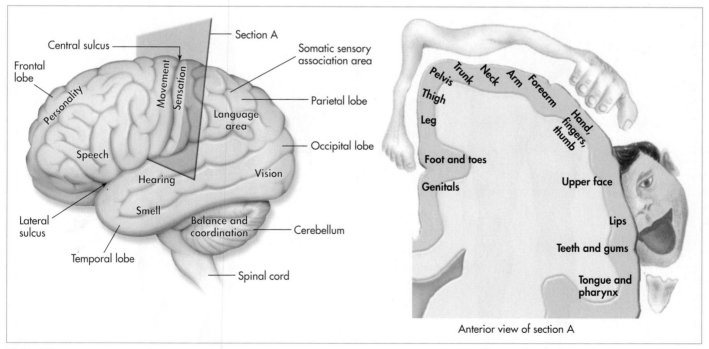

FIGURE 10–9 ■

Primary somatic sensory area. Notice the size of the body parts are proportional to the amount of the sensory input provided. For example, the hands provide much more sensory input due to touch than your neck would, and as a result, the area devoted to the neck is much smaller. Remember that the map is contralateral.

The neurons in the somatic sensory cortex are the neurons that allow conscious sensation. You feel an insect crawling on your arm because the "arm" neurons in your somatic sensory cortex are stimulated by the insect. The map is also evident on your body surface. The map of the body surfaces innervated by each spinal nerve consists of a band or region of skin supplied by a single spinal nerve. Each band is called a dermatome (see **FIGURE 10–10** ■).

Somatic Sensory Association Area: How Do We Interpret Touch?

Another area of the cerebral cortex allows *understanding* and *interpretation* of somatic sensory information. It is located in the parietal lobe just posterior to somatic sensory cortex and is known as the **somatic sensory association area**.

The somatic sensory system works on a kind of hierarchy, with the sensory neurons in the spinal cord and brain stem (brain stem neurons transport information in the same fashion as the spinal sensory neurons, but without going to the spinal cord first) collecting information and passing it to areas in the thalamus, cerebellum, and cerebrum for processing. The *actual* understanding of complex sensory input happens only *after* the information is passed to the somatic sensory cortex and somatic sensory association area.

Let's go back to hitting your thumb with a hammer. The pain neurons, with bodies in the dorsal root ganglion, are depolarized and send signals to the spinal cord via the spinal nerve and dorsal root. The neurons synapse with motor neurons, causing you to pull your hand away from the stimulus. These same pain neurons join the spinothalamic tract in your spinal cord and simultaneously send a pain signal to your brain. The signal goes first to the thalamus and other parts of the diencephalon, causing physiological symptoms, like sweating and increased heart rate. The pain then continues

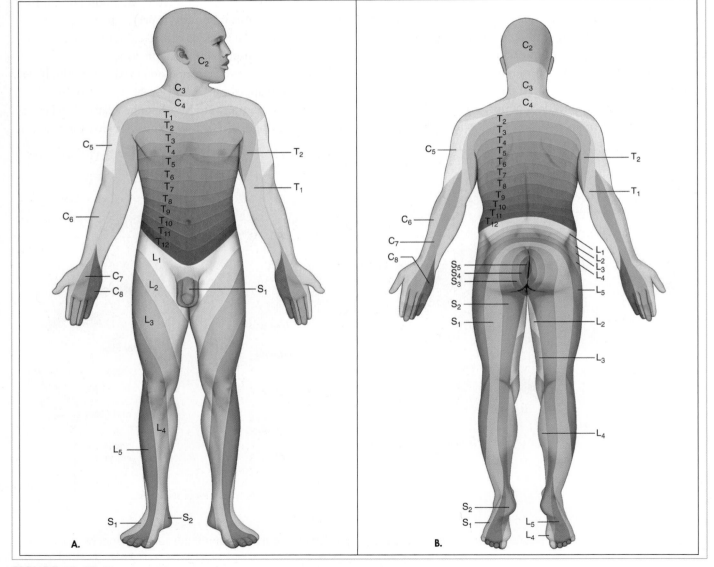

FIGURE 10–10 ■

Dermatomes: Body map showing the band or region innervated by each spinal nerve. For example an injury to L3 (lumbar vertebra 3) would cause a pain sensation in the corresponding colored region.

along the pathway to your somatic sensory cortex. There, the exact location of the pain becomes apparent to you. Now you know *where* the pain is, but still may not recognize it as pain. The *understanding* occurs when the information is integrated with sensation in the *somatic sensory association area.* Now you know that you have hurt yourself. All this receiving of information and processing and associated actions happen almost instantaneously.

TEST YOUR KNOWLEDGE 10–3

Choose the best answer:

1. This form of sensation includes fine and crude touch.
   a. somatic sensation
   b. palpatory sensation
   c. motor sensation
   d. all of the above

2. The role of the somatic sensory association area is
   a. understanding and interpreting touch information.
   b. comparing planned movement to actual movement.
   c. feeling textures.
   d. finding the position of objects in space.

3. Which of the following spinal cord pathways carries pain and temperature information?
   a. dorsal column
   b. spinothalamic
   c. corticospinal
   d. thermostatic

4. Where are the sensory neurons located that receive pain information from your body and send it to the brain?
   a. thalamus
   b. primary somatic sensory cortex
   c. dorsal root ganglion
   d. ventral horn of spinal cord

5. How does somatic sensory information from your face get to your brain?
   a. neurons in dorsal root ganglion
   b. via cranial nerves to brain stem nuclei
   c. up the spinal cord
   d. from the thalamus

The Motor System

The motor system is also a hierarchy, working in parallel with the somatic sensory system. However, now information is moving in the opposite direction, from brain to spinal cord to body instead of from body to spinal cord to brain. Refer to **FIGURE 10–11** ■ to see our current position on the nervous system organizational chart.

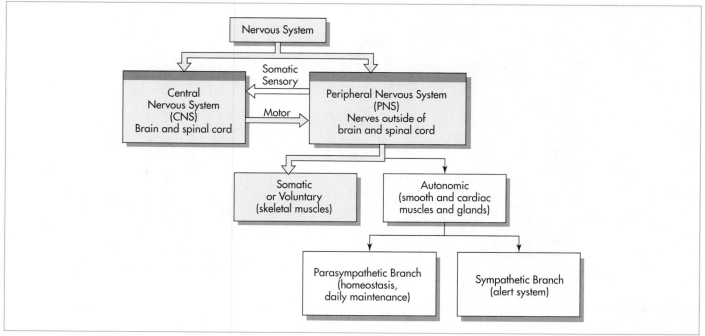

FIGURE 10–11 ■

Our current position on the nervous system flowchart.

The **somatic motor system** controls voluntary movements under orders from the cerebral cortex. In the frontal lobe is the premotor area, which *plans* movements. The plan from this area is then sent to the primary motor cortex. The primary motor cortex is located in the precentral gyrus, in the frontal lobe, anterior to the somatic sensory cortex just discussed. The primary motor cortex should seem familiar. Just like the somatic sensory cortex, the motor cortex has a map of the body. The size of the map in the motor cortex is proportional to the amount of movement control. Therefore, the hands and the tongue, both of which require finer movements, have larger maps than the trunk or forearms. Like the somatic sensory cortex, the primary motor cortex is contralateral. See **FIGURE 10–12** ■.

Amazing Facts

Size Matters

Check out the size of the primary motor cortex dedicated to each body part in Figure 10–12. Does the size of the map make sense given the size of the body parts? Not really: The hands, lips, and head have very large maps, whereas the legs and arms have very small maps compared to each body part's size.

What determines map size? What do the hand and lips have in common that makes them different from the arms and legs? They are required to perform more finely coordinated movements, such as speaking and handwriting (or typing), and therefore have more motor output. If you aren't convinced, think about how much harder it would be to type with your feet than with your hands. This map can be drawn as a homunculus (little man) with huge hands, lips, and head (see Figure 10–12).

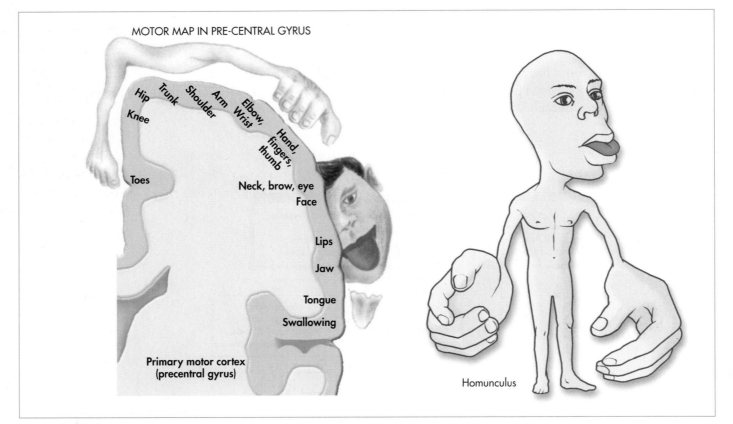

FIGURE 10–12 ■

Motor areas of the brain, with homunculus. (See an explanation of homunculus in the Amazing Facts box.)

Subcortical Structures

Deep in the cerebrum are nuclei. The nuclei in the cerebrum can be part of the **basal nuclei** (sometimes called basal ganglia, but technically because they are in the brain they are nuclei), which is a motor coordination system, or part of the **limbic system**, which controls emotion and mood. We are concerned with motor neurons now, so the basal nuclei are our focus.

The plan for movement leaves the motor cortex and connects with neurons in the thalamus, which is located in the diencephalon. The thalamus, basal nuclei, and cerebellum are part of a complicated *motor coordination loop*. Here, the movement must be fine-tuned, posture and limb positions are taken into account, other movements are turned off, and movement and senses are integrated. This loop is fundamental. Without the coordination loop among the subcortical structures (subcortical = "under the cortex"), movements would be at best jerky and inaccurate. Some movements would be impossible.

> ### *Clinical Application*
>
> #### PARKINSON'S DISEASE
>
> Patients with Parkinson's disease have a disorder of one of the basal nuclei and are unable to start new movements or turn off other movements. Patients have difficulty walking and swallowing and usually have an uncontrollable tremor when trying to sit still.

Spinal Cord Pathways

After the movement information is processed by the thalamus, basal nuclei, and cerebellum, it moves to the spinal cord and brain stem via the **corticospinal tract** and the **corticobulbar tract** as well as several other tracts. (See the discussion in Chapter 9.) The corticospinal and corticobulbar tracts from your motor cortex are direct pathways, whereas others coming from subcortical structures are considered indirect pathways (there are many of these). The axons from all pathways synapse on motor neurons in the ventral horn of the spinal cord or in brain stem nuclei. These motor neurons connect to skeletal muscles via the cranial nerves (in the brain stem) or the ventral roots and spinal nerves (spinal cord), sending orders to the skeletal muscles to carry out the planned movement or coordinate ongoing movements. (Remember, these neurons communicate with the muscles via the neuromuscular junction and therefore release the neurotransmitter acetylcholine across the synapse.) A second function of the motor tracts is the fine-tuning of reflexes. These tracts inhibit reflexes, making them softer than they would be if they had no influence from the brain. For a list of motor pathways, see TABLE 10–6 ■.

Let's go back again to hitting your thumb with the hammer. After you hit your thumb, the first motor activity is a withdrawal reflex. You pull your thumb away from the painful stimulus. As we mentioned before, this is not a voluntary movement. It isn't planned. Only your spinal cord motor neurons are necessary for withdrawal. However, after the initial withdrawal, some jumping up and down, and perhaps some cursing, you stop and think. What do you do next? You look at your thumb. That is a planned movement. It requires coordination between your motor system, to uncover your thumb and move it into you visual field, and your visual system to look at your thumb. You walk to the kitchen, open the freezer, get out the ice, and make an ice pack. Then you grab a cold drink from the fridge and walk back into the living room, nursing your wounds. All this activity requires motor planning and coordination. You must reach for the freezer door and open it accurately. You must stay upright with respect to gravity. You must open a plastic bag and put ice in it. None of this happens without careful motor planning and coordination.

TABLE 10–6 SPINAL CORD PATHWAYS FOR MOTOR INFORMATION

PATHWAY	INFORMATION	FROM	TO
Direct	Voluntary movement		
Corticospinal	Body below neck	Motor cortex	Ventral horn
Corticobulbar	Face/head	Motor cortex	Brain stem nuclei
Indirect	Unconscious movements	Subcortical structures	
Reticulospinal	Posture adjustment	Reticular formation	Ventral horn/brain stem
Rubrospinal	Movement coordination	Basal nuclei	Ventral horn/brain stem

The Role of the Cerebellum

We have really glossed over the important function of the cerebellum in the motor system. The cerebellum has both motor and sensory inputs and outputs from the cerebral cortex, the thalamus, the basal nuclei, and the spinal cord. The cerebellum gets information about the *planned* movement and the *actual* movement and *compares* the plan to the actual. If the plan and the actual do not match, the cerebellum can adjust the actual movement to fit the plan. The function of the cerebellum is subtle and still a bit of a mystery, but without the cerebellum, movements would be inaccurate at best.

TEST YOUR KNOWLEDGE 10–4

Choose the best answer:

1. The size of the map for a particular body part in the precentral gyrus is determined by
   a. the amount of fine motor control.
   b. the size of the body part.
   c. the importance of the body part.
   d. all of the above

2. The cerebellum compares
   a. shapes of objects.
   b. planned movement to actual movement.
   c. textures.
   d. the position of objects in space.

3. The motor plan is made in this part of the brain.
   a. cerebellum
   b. frontal lobe
   c. medulla oblongata
   d. thalamus

4. Parkinson's disease results from damage to this brain structure.
   a. cerebellum
   b. basal nucleus
   c. brain stem
   d. limbic system

5. The somatic nervous system controls
   a. emotions.
   b. involuntary movements.
   c. temperature.
   d. voluntary movements.

THE AUTONOMIC NERVOUS SYSTEM

The peripheral nervous system is divided into two systems: the **somatic** or voluntary system, which controls skeletal muscles, and the **autonomic system**, which controls involuntary muscles. Involuntary muscles are the smooth muscles found in structures such as the blood vessels and airways and the cardiac muscle found in the heart. Glands are also controlled by this system. The autonomic system, then, controls physiological characteristics such as blood pressure, heart rate, respiration rate, digestion, and sweating.

The neurons for the autonomic system, like the somatic motor neurons, are located in the spinal cord and brain stem and also release neurotransmitters. This is where the similarity ends. All the autonomic motor neurons are located in the lateral horns rather than the ventral horns, and, unlike the somatic motor neurons, autonomic neurons do not connect directly to muscles. Instead, these neurons, the *preganglionic neurons*, make synapses in ganglia outside the CNS. A **ganglion** is group of nerve cell bodies outside the CNS. You can think of this as a junction box where the signal can be passed on to the next part of the circuit. A second motor neuron, called a *postganglionic neuron*, connects from the ganglion to the smooth muscle or gland.

The Sympathetic Branch

The autonomic nervous system is divided into two subdivisions: the sympathetic and the parasympathetic divisions. Please see **FIGURE 10–13** ■. The **sympathetic** division controls the fight-or-flight response. It is charged with getting your body ready to expend energy. Sympathetic effects include increased heart rate, increased blood pressure,

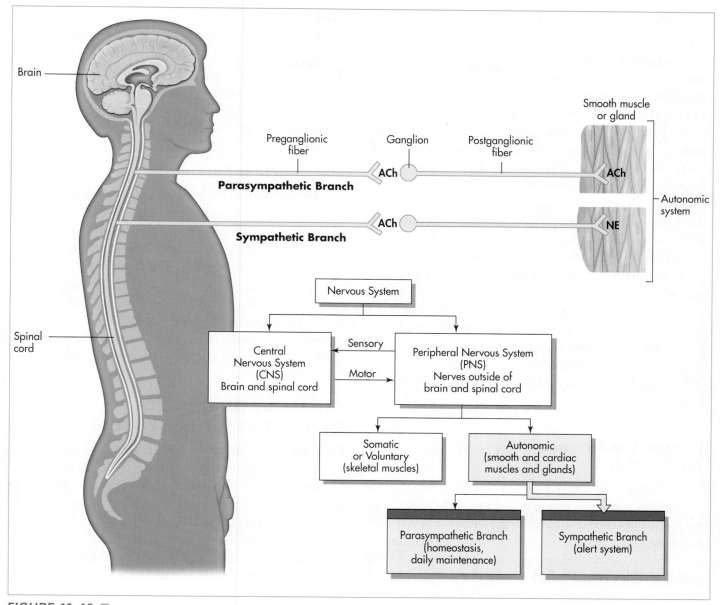

FIGURE 10–13 ■

General representation of autonomic nervous system (ACh = acetylcholine; NE = norepinephrine).

sweating, and dry mouth, all the symptoms of an adrenaline rush. This part of the autonomic system was responsible for your racing heart, rapid breathing, and intense sweating when confronted with the snarling dog. Your heart pumped more blood to your muscles, and your lungs took in more oxygen, both of which got you "up" to either fight or, more likely, flee. Another sympathetic response is dilation of your pupils to help you see the situation at hand much better. Sympathetic output is pretty strong when you hit your thumb with the hammer, too.

The *preganglionic neurons f*or the sympathetic system are located in the thoracic and first two lumbar segments of

the spinal cord and they are referred to as *thoracolumbar*. The preganglionic neurons, which secrete acetylcholine, synapse with the postganglionic neurons in the sympathetic ganglia. The ganglia for the sympathetic division form a pair of chainlike structures that run parallel to the spinal cord. These are called *paravertebral ganglia*. The postganglionic neurons release the *neurotransmitter* **norepinephrine**. One of the most important effects of the sympathetic system is its stimulation of the adrenal gland to release the *hormone* **epinephrine** (adrenaline), the chemical that causes that familiar adrenaline rush by circulating in the bloodstream.

The Parasympathetic Branch

If you have a gas pedal, you also need a brake. The **parasympathetic** division of the autonomic nervous system is often called "resting and digesting" because it has the opposite effect of the sympathetic division. The parasympathetic division is responsible for maintenance of everyday activities. It also helps bring you back down to normal from a sympathetic response. Parasympathetic effects include decreased heart rate, respiration, and blood pressure and increased digestive activity, including salivation and even stomach rumbling. The parasympathetic system allows you to calm down after you get the ice pack on your thumb or the dog is safely locked inside its cage.

The *preganglionic neurons* of the parasympathetic system are in the brain stem and the sacral spinal cord and thus are called *craniosacral*. They, too, release acetylcholine. The preganglionic neurons synapse with postganglionic neurons in the parasympathetic ganglia. Parasympathetic ganglia are located near the organs. Postganglionic neurons release the neurotransmitter **acetylcholine**. (Acetylcholine excites skeletal muscle but inhibits cardiac and some smooth muscle activity.)

Putting the Autonomic System All Together

Let's revisit the snarling dog. When you encounter it, your sympathetic nervous system is stimulated, and the impulses are sent from the thoracolumbar region of the spinal cord to preganglionic fibers, which release the neurotransmitter acetylcholine. Acetylcholine combines with receptors on the postganglionic neurons, which generate an action potential and carry the impulse to the target area, where norepinephrine is released. When this occurs at the heart (cardiac muscle), the rate and force of contraction will supply more blood for the fight-or-flight response.

When the emergency is over, the sympathetic pathway will not be as active, and the norepinephrine will be metabolized so you don't remain in that stimulated state. The parasympathetic system now takes over to slow your system down to normal. This is another example of homeostasis in which normal heart rate is regulated by a balance between these two systems. **FIGURE 10–14** ▪ shows a comparison of the sympathetic and parasympathetic systems.

OTHER SYSTEMS

Two other systems that do not have a single, specific location but are found throughout the brain are the limbic system and the reticular formation.

The Limbic System

The **limbic system** is a series of nuclei in the cerebrum and the diencephalon. These nuclei are involved in mood, emotion, and memory. One nucleus helps attach emotion or intensity to movement. Another coordinates emotion and your sense of smell. Still another is responsible for storing and retrieving memories.

The Reticular Formation

The **reticular formation** is a diffuse network of nuclei in the brain stem. Some of these nuclei are responsible for "waking up" your cerebral cortex, as part of the reticular activating system. This activity is vital for the maintenance of conscious awareness of your surroundings. When your alarm clock wakes you in the morning, your reticular system is responsible for nudging your cortex out of slumber. General anesthesia inhibits the reticular system, rendering surgery patients unconscious. Injury due to ischemia, mechanical damage, or drugs can damage the reticular system and lead to persistent unconsciousness.

COMMON DISORDERS OF THE NERVOUS SYSTEM

Paralysis, which is the inability to control voluntary movements, can be spastic or flaccid. *Spastic paralysis* is characterized by muscle rigidity or increased muscle tone (*hypertonia*) and overactive reflexes (*hyperreflexia*). In spastic paralysis, the muscles are rigid and the reflexes are overactive because of decreased communication from the brain to the ventral horn motor neurons in the spinal cord. Muscles contract randomly, and the reflexes do not have any control signals from the brain. Stroke, head injuries, and spinal cord injuries can cause spastic paralysis.

Flaccid paralysis is characterized by floppy muscles (decreased muscle tone, or *hypotonia*) and decreased reflexes (*hyporeflexia*). In flaccid paralysis, the damage is to the spinal nerves. Impulses cannot get to the muscles from the motor neurons. Therefore, the muscles are floppy and the reflexes are absent. Flaccid paralysis can be caused by peripheral injury or disorders such as polio and Guillain-Barré syndrome.

Cerebral palsy (CP) is a collection of movement disorders that initially occur in young children and are not progressive. Patients with cerebral palsy exhibit signs of classic spastic paralysis. The disorder is caused by improper development of or damage to the motor system of the brain. Symptoms of cerebral palsy can range from minor motor loss to significant motor deficits, including the inability to walk or speak. Patients with cerebral palsy may have significant developmental delays or may have average or above-average intelligence.

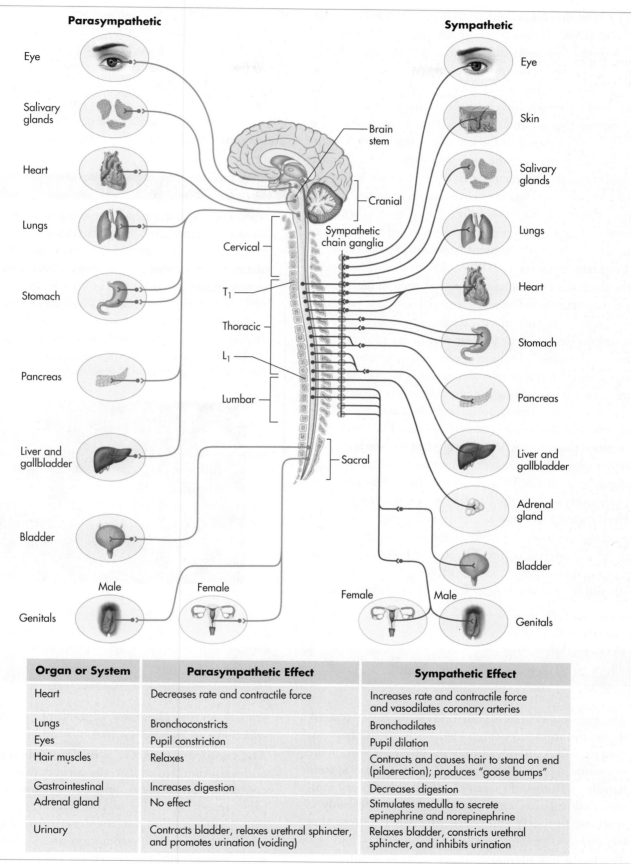

Organ or System	Parasympathetic Effect	Sympathetic Effect
Heart	Decreases rate and contractile force	Increases rate and contractile force and vasodilates coronary arteries
Lungs	Bronchoconstricts	Bronchodilates
Eyes	Pupil constriction	Pupil dilation
Hair muscles	Relaxes	Contracts and causes hair to stand on end (piloerection); produces "goose bumps"
Gastrointestinal	Increases digestion	Decreases digestion
Adrenal gland	No effect	Stimulates medulla to secrete epinephrine and norepinephrine
Urinary	Contracts bladder, relaxes urethral sphincter, and promotes urination (voiding)	Relaxes bladder, constricts urethral sphincter, and inhibits urination

FIGURE 10–14 ◼

A comparison of the parasympathetic and sympathetic nervous systems.

The condition known as a **stroke**, or a **cerebral vascular accident (CVA)**, is caused by the disruption of blood flow to a portion of the brain due to either hemorrhage or blood clot. If the oxygen is disrupted for long enough, brain tissue will die. The symptoms of stroke vary, depending on the location of the stroke. Muscle weakness, paralysis, or the lack of sensation due to stroke is contralateral (remember, the right hemisphere controls the left side of the body). Strokes can also rob patients of the ability to speak and can cause blindness and destroy memory. Symptoms of stroke appear suddenly. Some patients may have a series of minor strokes (almost like tiny earthquakes before the big one) with minor, temporary symptoms before they have a major stroke. These ministrokes are called **transient ischemic attacks (TIAs)**.

Traumatic brain injury (TBI) occurs when force is applied to the skull and causes brain damage. A mild brain injury is called a **concussion**. For many years concussions were dismissed as unimportant injuries. Recently the effects of repeat concussions have become so clear that major sports organizations such as the NFL have implemented rigorous testing before allowing a player with a concussion to play again. In more serious cases, swelling and bleeding may occur at the site of the injury. These may cause increases in pressure inside the skull, which may cause permanent damage. This increase in intracranial pressure not only damages brain tissue but it also puts pressure on the brain stem, sometimes pushing it through the foramen magnum. This can decrease blood flow and damage respiratory centers, thus causing even more damage.

Huntington's disease is a progressive genetic disorder causing deterioration of neurons in the basal nuclei and eventually of the cerebral cortex. The disease begins with mood swings and memory disturbances, writhing movements of the hands and face, or clumsiness. Eventually, the disease causes difficulty swallowing, speaking, and walking, as well as memory loss, psychosis, and loss of cognitive function. There is no cure for Huntington's disease, and most patients die from accidental injuries, infections, or other complications. A genetic test can determine whether a person carries the gene for the disease. Offspring of parents who have the disease have a 50 percent chance of inheriting the gene for Huntington's disease. A carrier of the gene will eventually develop the disease.

FOCUS ON PROFESSIONS

Many drugs are used to treat nervous system disorders. There are various career opportunities and levels within the pharmaceutical profession—including **pharmacist**, **pharmacy technician**, and **pharmaceutical sales representative**, just to name a few. Learn more about this exciting field by visiting the websites of national organizations, such as the National Community Pharmacists Association (NCPA), the American Pharmacists Association (APhA), the National Pharmacy Technician Association (NPTA), and the American Association of Pharmacy Technicians (AAPT).

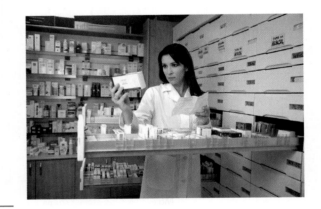

SUMMARY: Points of Interest

- The nervous system is your body's computer system, its information superhighway. Without the nervous system, you could not sample the environment, make decisions, or respond to stimuli. The nervous system handles millions of pieces of information every minute, making sure that every system in the body is working properly and correcting any problem that occurs.

- The brain is a hierarchical organ. It is divided into compartments (lobes), each with very specific functions. The brain also has nerves attached to it, called cranial nerves. There are 12 pairs of cranial nerves, and they can be sensory, motor, or mixed.

- The cerebrum controls your conscious movement and sensation. Inferior to the cerebrum are the diencephalon, brain stem, and cerebellum. Each part plays important roles in coordinating sensory and motor information for the cerebrum. Other parts of the brain, called association areas, allow you to make connections between different types of sensory information and to compare current experience to memories.

- There are motor and sensory maps of the body in the cerebral cortex. Orders for voluntary movements originate in the primary motor cortex in the precentral gyrus of the frontal lobe and travel down the spinal cord via direct spinal cord tracts. Subcortical structures coordinate this information via indirect tracts. The somatic sensory cortex is in the postcentral gyrus of the parietal lobe. Sensory information from the spinal cord tracts eventually ends up in this part of the cortex. When the information arrives there, you become aware of your sense of touch.

- The nervous system also controls smooth muscle, cardiac muscle, and endocrine glands via a part of the system known as the autonomic nervous system. The autonomic nervous system has two branches. The sympathetic division controls the fight-or-flight response, and the parasympathetic division controls day-to-day activities.

CASE STUDY

A young woman finds her elderly father lying in bed well past his usual rising time. He is still in his pajamas and is semiconscious. He is paralyzed on his right side, but he seems to be able to feel that side of his body. At the hospital, he is diagnosed with a stroke.

What part of his brain is damaged? How can you tell?

What would you expect to happen to his ability to speak and understand language?

_____

_____

REVIEW QUESTIONS

Multiple Choice

1. One of the following brain parts is a cortical structure. Which one?
   a. hypothalamus
   b. medulla oblongata
   c. precentral gyrus
   d. pineal body

2. This cranial nerve controls the abdominal viscera.
   a. olfactory (I)
   b. trigeminal (V)
   c. vestibulocochlear (VII)
   d. vagus (X)

3. The size of the map of each body part in the postcentral gyrus is determined by the
   a. sensitivity of the body part.
   b. size of the body part.
   c. importance of the body part.
   d. fine-motor control of the body part.

4. The sympathetic nervous system
   a. causes decreased heart rate.
   b. has ganglia near the organs.
   c. has ganglia near the spinal cord.
   d. all of the above

5. This part of the brain contains the body's set points and controls most of its physiology, including blood pressure and hunger level.
   a. thalamus
   b. hypothalamus
   c. amygdala
   d. hippocampus

6. After a severe blow to the head, Jill has uncontrollable hunger and thirst, her body temperature varies wildly, and she keeps passing out because her blood pressure is not well controlled. Neurological tests discover a hemorrhage. Where is the bleed located?
   a. frontal lobe
   b. hypothalamus
   c. basal nuclei
   d. spinal cord

7. After having meningitis, Charlie loses his sight. What part of his nervous system may be damaged?
   a. frontal lobe
   b. occipital lobe
   c. spinal cord
   d. Broca's area

8. During a party, Ramón begins to feel just awful. His heart is racing, he can't catch his breath, and he is sweating and beginning to panic. He suspects somebody has spiked his drink. What part of his nervous system is stimulated?
   a. hypothalamus
   b. parasympathetic
   c. frontal lobe
   d. none of the above

Fill in the Blank

1. The _____ are nuclei that coordinate motor output.

2. The occipital lobe is responsible for this sensation: _____.

3. The white matter of the spinal cord contains _____ tracts, which are motor, and _____ tracts, which are sensory.

4. Emotion, mood, and memory are controlled by this collection of nuclei: _____.

5. This portion of the brain stem has vital nuclei for respiration and the cardiovascular system: _____.

6. Bea has become very uncoordinated lately, her movements slow and stilted. She can move, but not easily. A neurologist determines that she has had a small stroke that has damaged this part of the motor system: _____.

Short Answer

1. List the differences between cranial and spinal nerves.

   _____

   _____

   _____

   _____

2. List the differences between the sympathetic and parasympathetic nervous systems.

   _____

   _____

   _____

   _____

3. Explain how the cerebral cortex and subcortical structures interact to produce motor output.

   _____

   _____

   _____

   _____

4. Explain how somatic sensory information travels from skin sensation to understanding.

   _____

   _____

   _____

   _____

5. Explain the overall hierarchy of the nervous system that exists between cerebral cortex, subcortical structures, and the spinal cord.

   _____

   _____

   _____

   _____

Visit our new **MyHealthProfessions Lab** to accompany *Anatomy & Physiology for Health Professions.* Here you'll find a rich collection of quizzes, case studies, and animations for deeper understanding and application.

11

The Senses

THE SIGHTS AND SOUNDS

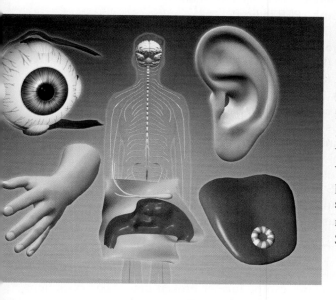

As we stroll through the city on our journey, we take in many sights, sounds, and smells. As you look around, you will likely see many different buildings and types of people. The city is also noisy, full of car horns honking, brakes squealing, and people talking. You will smell delicious food wafting out restaurant windows or the stench of garbage in overflowing dumpsters. Our special senses receive all this input and send it to the brain for interpretation so we can understand and appreciate what is happening around us. These special senses are highly integrated with the nervous system, enabling us to respond quickly and thereby protecting us from harm. For example, we need to *see* that oncoming speeding car as we step away from the curb and *hear* the blaring horn to respond by quickly stepping back to the safe confines of the sidewalk. See how sensory input can determine motor response?

LEARNING OUTCOMES

At the end of your journey through this chapter, you will be able to:

- Distinguish between general and special senses.
- Describe the process of seeing.
- Describe the external and internal anatomy and functions of the eye.
- Describe the external and internal anatomy and functions of the ear.
- Explain the process of hearing.
- Discuss the processes involved with the senses of taste, smell, and touch.
- Contrast the types of pain and the pain response.
- Explain several common disorders of the eye and ear.

Pronunciation Guide Pro·nun·ci·a·tion

Correct pronunciation is important in any journey so that you and others are completely understood. Here is a "see and say" Pronunciation Guide for the more difficult terms to pronounce in this chapter. Please note that even though there are standard pronunciations, regional variations of the pronunciations can occur.

amblyopia (AM blee OH pee ah)
anesthesia (an ess THEE zee ah)
aqueous humor (AY kwee us)
auricle (AW rih kul)
cataract (KAT ah rakt)
cerumen (seh ROO men)
ceruminous glands (seh ROO men us)
choroid (KOH royd)
ciliary muscles (SILL ee AIR ee)
cochlea (KOCK lee ah)
conjunctiva (KON junk TIH vah)
conjunctivitis (kon JUNK tih VYE tis)
cornea (KOR nee ah)
endolymph (EN doh limf)
eustachian tubes (yoo STAY she an)
external auditory meatus
   (AW dih TOH ree mee AYE tus)
glaucoma (glaw KOH mah)
gustatory sense (GUS ta TOH ree)
hyperopia (HIGH per OH pee ah)
incus (ING kus)

labyrinth (LAB ih rinth)
lacrimal apparatus (LAK rim al app ah RAT us)
malleus (MALL ee us)
Ménière's disease (MAIN ee airz)
myopia (my OH pee ah)
ossicle (AHS ih kull)
otitis media (oh TYE tis MEH dee ah)
perilymph (PER ih limf)
pinna (PIN ah)
presbyopia (PREZ bee OH pee ah)
retina (RET eh nah)
sclera (SKLAIR ah)
stapes (STAY peez)
tactile corpuscles (TACK tile KOR pus el)
tinnitus (tin EYE tus)
tympanic membrane (tim PAN ik)
umami (you MA me)
vestibulocochlear nerve
   (VESS tih byool oh KOHK lee are)
vestibule chamber (VES tih byool)
vitreous humor (VIT ree us)

TYPES OF SENSES

Our body senses allow us to experience all aspects of our journey. They are truly remarkable sensors through which we see, hear, smell, taste, and feel the world around us. These amazing senses monitor and detect changes in the environment and send this information from a receptor to the brain via sensory (afferent) neurons. The brain interprets the information and in many circumstances makes the appropriate motor (efferent) response.

Traditionally, we are taught that we possess five senses: vision, hearing, smell, taste, and touch. However, there are other types of sensory input into the brain. What about pain and pressure sensations? How do we "feel" hot and cold? How does our body sense position and balance (equilibrium)? What about feelings of hunger and thirst? These, too, are senses that are very important to our survival.

The senses of sight (eyes), sound and equilibrium (ears), taste (tongue), and smell (nose) are referred to as our *special senses*. These senses are found in a well-defined region of the body. However, other senses, called *general senses*, are scattered throughout various regions of the body. These include the sensations of heat, cold, pain, nausea, hunger, thirst, and pressure or touch.

The senses can be further broken down. For example, the receptors of the skin are called the *cutaneous senses* and include touch, heat, cold, and pain. The *visceral senses* include nausea, hunger, thirst, and the need to urinate and defecate.

Before finishing this discussion of the various senses, we should also mention a final, more controversial sense. By "reading your mind," we see you already identified it as extrasensory perception, or ESP. *Extrasensory* means senses outside the normal sensory perceptions. Although there is still debate over whether this phenomenon exists, we just "know" this chapter will be an "eye-opening" experience for you. We hope the puns aren't stimulating your visceral senses and making you nauseous.

SENSE OF SIGHT

While on our journey, we see many amazing sights. To record these sights for later viewing, most of us will take along a smart phone; others will bring a camera and film. The eye has many similarities to an older-type film camera. The light rays from the images photographed with a camera pass through the small opening (comparable to the pupil) and through the transparent lens (lens of the eye), where the rays are then focused on a photoreceptive film (retina). The shutter of a camera opens and closes at various speeds to adjust the amount of light exposure on the film. The shutter (iris) must allow just the right amount of light to enter and focus properly on the film for a clear image. A camera may be packed away in a suitcase or thrown in a car and therefore needs protection from being dropped or exposed to a harsh environment. You will soon see how the external structures of the eye help protect it from injury, much like a camera case protects a camera. In addition, the camera lens must be kept clean to ensure a clear picture. The lacrimal glands that secrete tears help perform this function. Now that you have this analogy to give you the "big picture," let's explore the specific structures and functions of the eye.

The External Structures of the Eye

The **orbit** (orbital cavity) is a cone-shaped opening formed by the skull that houses and protects the *eyeball*, a one-inch sphere. This cavity is padded with fatty tissue that cushions and protects the eye from injury and has several openings through which nerves and blood vessels can pass. The eyeball is connected to the orbital cavity with six short muscles that provide support and allow rotary movement so you can see in all directions. Also protecting the eye is a pair of movable folds of skin, commonly called *eyelids*, which contain eyelashes to help prevent gross particles from entering. The *eyelashes* act as sensors to cause rapid closure as a foreign object approaches the eyeball. The eyelids close over the eye much like the lens cover of a camera to protect it from intense light, foreign particles, or impact injuries. The eyelids also contain sebaceous glands that secrete the oily substance *sebum* onto the eyelids to keep them soft, pliable, and a little sticky to trap particles.

A protective membrane called the **conjunctiva** covers the exposed surface of the eyeball and acts as a protective covering. Each eye has a **lacrimal apparatus** that produces and stores tears. The lacrimal apparatus includes the **lacrimal gland** and its corresponding ducts or passageways that transport the tears. The lacrimal glands (which are exocrine glands because their secretion of tears goes outside the body) produce the tears needed for constant cleansing and lubrication, which are spread over the eye surfaces by blinking. Our eyes are constantly tearing, but they do not overflow because excess tears drain into the nose via two small openings or ducts in the inner corner of the eye. However, when we cry, the excess runs down our cheeks, and drains into our nose, causing it to run. The tears also act as an **antiseptic** to help reduce eye infections. See FIGURE 11–1 ■ for the structures involved with tearing.

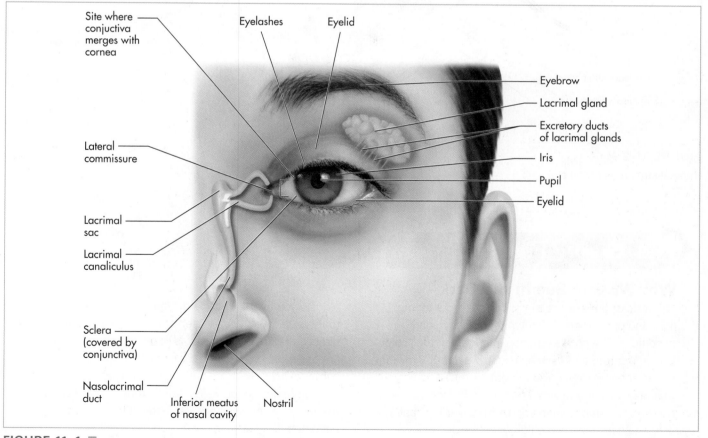

FIGURE 11–1 ■

Lacrimal structures of the eye.

The Internal Structures of the Eye

The globe-shaped eyeball is the organ of vision and is separated into two chambers of fluid that help protect the eye. These "fluids of the eye" are called *humors*. The **aqueous humor** ("watery" humor) bathes the iris, pupil, and lens, and fills the anterior and posterior chambers of the eye. The second humor is called the **vitreous humor** and is a clear, jelly-like fluid that occupies the entire eye cavity behind the lens.

The eyeball has three layers: the *sclera, choroid,* and *retina.* **FIGURE 11-2** ■ shows these layers and the internal structures of the eye. The **sclera** is the outermost layer and is a tough, fibrous tissue that serves as the protective shield we commonly call the "whites of the eyes." The sclera contains a specialized portion called the **cornea,** which is transparent to allow light rays to pass into the eye. The cornea has a curved surface that allows it to bend the entering light

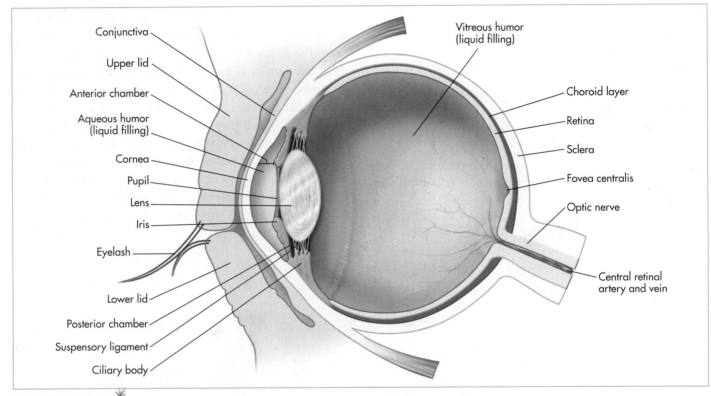

FIGURE 11-2 ■ ✳
Internal structures of the eye.

Amazing Facts

Why We Can See in the Dark

The rods of the eye are the photoreceptors for dim light and provide black-and-white images in dark conditions. The cones function in bright light for color vision. The retina of each eye contains about 3 million cones and 100 million rods. Together they enable you to see in a variety of light conditions. In fact, your eyes can distinguish between approximately 500 shades of gray and can spot candle light over a mile away!

Do you ever wonder why you have to look off to the side if you want to see stars at night that are directly in front of you? That is because rods and cones are not evenly distributed throughout the eye. The center of your eye is densely populated with cones, and the perimeter contains mostly rods. This means that when you look directly at a star, it disappears or becomes dim because cones cannot "see" it.

waves to focus them on the surface of the retina. It was previously believed that the cornea was composed of five layers: the corneal epithelium as the front layer, Bowman's layer, the corneal stroma, Descemet's membrane, and the corneal endothelium as the back layer. Recently, a sixth layer, dubbed the Dua layer (after Harminder Dua, professor of ophthamology and visual sciences at the University of Nottingham), was discovered between the corneal stroma and Descemet's membrane.

The middle layer, or **choroid**, is a highly vascularized (rich blood supply) and pigmented region that provides nourishment to the eye. This layer also contains the *iris* and the *pupil*. The **iris** is the colored portion of the eye that controls the size of the opening (pupil) where light passes into the eye. The iris is a sphincter, which means it can relax or contract, thereby making the center opening, or **pupil**, larger or smaller, depending on light conditions. In low light, the iris relaxes, causing the pupil to dilate and thereby allowing more light into the eye for a better image.

Located behind the pupil is the **lens**, which is surrounded by **ciliary muscles**. These muscles can alter the shape of the lens, making it thinner or thicker to allow the incoming light rays to focus on the retinal area. This process is called *accommodation*, which basically combines changes in the size of the pupil and the lens curvature to make sure the image converges in the same place on the retina and therefore is properly focused.

The third and innermost layer is the **retina**. This area contains the nerve endings that receive and help interpret the rays of light as images. The retina is a delicate membrane that continues posteriorly and joins the *optic nerve*. It contains two types of light-sensing receptors called *rods* and *cones*. The **rods** are active in dim light and do not perceive color,

whereas the **cones** are active in bright light and do perceive color. These receptors contain **photopigments** that cause a chemical change when light hits them. This chemical change causes an impulse to be sent to the optic nerve and then to the brain, where the impulse is interpreted, and we "see" the object. This interpretation occurs in the visual part of the cerebral cortex located in the occipital lobe.

In summation, light rays enter the eye and pass through the cornea, aqueous humor, pupil, lens, and vitreous humor, and are focused on the retina. Here, the photoreceptors in the retina cause an impulse to be sent to the optic nerve (Cranial Nerve II), which carries it to the visual area of the cerebral cortex located in the occipital lobe of the brain for the interpretation we call vision. Refer to TABLE 11–1 ■, which summarizes the major structures and their corresponding functions of the eye.

Amazing Facts

Eye Dominance
Most people have a dominant eye. To find yours, look at a small, distant object with both eyes open. Extend both arms with both palms facing that object. Slowly bring your hands together so there is a small opening or window formed in the space between the thumbs and the index figure. Now locate your distant object in that opening with both eyes open. Now alternately close each eye to determine which eye still sees that object. This is your dominant eye. Generally speaking, right-handed people have right-dominant eyes.

TABLE 11–1 STRUCTURES AND FUNCTIONS OF THE EYE

ORGAN OR STRUCTURE	PRIMARY FUNCTION
Orbit	Cone-shaped cavity that contains the eyeball; padded with fatty tissues, the orbit has several openings for nerves and blood vessels to pass through
Eye muscles	Six short muscles that provide support and rotary movement
Eyelid	Movable fold of skin containing eyelashes to protect eye from intense light, foreign particles, and impact injuries
Conjunctiva	Protective membrane that lines the exposed surface of eyeball
Lacrimal apparatus	Includes the lacrimal gland that produces tears that lubricate and cleanse the eye and the corresponding ducts or passageways to transport the tears

(continued)

TABLE 11–1 STRUCTURES AND FUNCTIONS OF THE EYE *(continued)*

ORGAN OR STRUCTURE	PRIMARY FUNCTION
Eyeball	Globe-shaped organ of vision
Sclera	Outermost layer known as the "white of the eye"; contains the transparent curved cornea, which bends outside light rays to focus them on the surface of the retina
Choroid	The middle layer that has rich blood vessels and pigmentation to prevent internal reflection of light rays; also contains the iris and pupil
Iris	Colored portion of eye that controls the size of the opening (pupil) where light passes into the eye
Pupil	The opening through which light passes into the eye
Retina	Innermost layer that contains the nerve endings that receive and interpret the rays of light for vision
Lens	Located behind the pupil, the lens is controlled by ciliary muscles that shape the lens by thinning or thickening the lens to allow light to focus on the retinal surface; this process, called accommodation, combines changes in pupil size and the lens curvature to ensure the light rays focus properly on the retina

TEST YOUR KNOWLEDGE 11–1

Choose the best answer:

1. Which of the following is *not* a layer of the eye?
   a. photo optic
   b. sclera
   c. choroid
   d. retina

2. Which layer of the eye contains the iris and the pupil?
   a. cornea
   b. sclera
   c. choroid
   d. retina

3. The _____ is the colored portion of the eye that controls the opening, or _____, where light passes through.
   a. retina; pupil
   b. pupil; iris
   c. sclera; pupil
   d. iris; pupil

4. This layer contains the actual sensory cells that respond to light.
   a. choroid
   b. retina
   c. conjunctiva
   d. sclera

5. These cells allow vision in low light.
   a. cones
   b. rods
   c. iris cells
   d. corneal cells

6. The eye can differentiate _____ shades of gray.
   a. 50
   b. 5
   c. 500
   d. 2

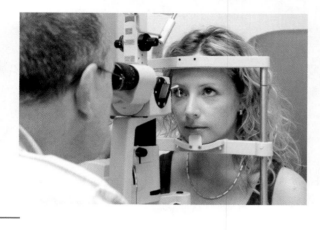

THE SENSE OF HEARING

On our journey, we hear many interesting sounds. Without our ears, we would miss all the pleasant noises—as well as the not-so-pleasant ones—that add to the appreciation of the journey. Our brain processes sounds much faster than it processes images; it is even aware of sounds as we sleep. Sounds can have positive effects, such as promoting relaxation, or negative effects, such as disturbing our concentration and impacting our health. Along with potentially damaging your hearing, constant exposure to loud noises can actually raise your blood pressure. Your ears are able to detect the direction of the source of a sound quite well but have less accuracy in determining the distance of that source.

Also on our journey, we might walk over some rough and uneven terrain. Our ears are responsible for our sense of balance so we don't fall and get hurt. We can "hear" your heart pounding with anticipation, so let's explore the specific structures and functions of the ear.

Structures of the Ear

The ear is responsible for the senses of hearing and *equilibrium*, or balance. We hear by receiving vibrations usually via the air (unless we are under water) and translating them into an interpretable sound via the eighth cranial nerve. The ear can be separated into three divisions: the *external ear*; the *middle ear*, or the *tympanic cavity*; and the *inner ear* (also called the *labyrinth*). See **FIGURE 11–3** ■ for the structures of the ear.

The External Ear

The **external ear** is the outer group of structures, the part we can see. It comes in all shapes and sizes (see Dumbo the Elephant). It also includes the canal (where we put cotton swabs, despite the warning label) leading into the middle ear. The projecting part is called the **pinna**, or **auricle**, which collects and directs sound waves into the **auditory canal**, or **external auditory meatus**. The canal contains earwax, called **cerumen**, which is secreted by the **ceruminous glands** to lubricate and protect the ear. At the end of the canal is the **eardrum**, or **tympanic membrane** (*tympanon* = Greek word for drum), where the external ear ends and the middle ear begins. Don't you wish there was just *one* term everyone agreed on for these structures!

The Middle Ear

The **middle ear**, or **tympanic cavity**, is basically a space that contains the three smallest bones of your body. The three bones, or **ossicles**, are joined so they can amplify the sound waves received by the tympanic membrane from the external ear (sound travels best through a solid). Once amplified, the sound waves are transmitted to the *fluid* contained in the internal ear. Again, this is another example of sound waves being transmitted more efficiently though a liquid medium than in air.

The bones of the middle ear are named according to their shapes. The first ossicle attached to the tympanic membrane is the *hammer*, or **malleus**. The *anvil*, or **incus**, is attached to the hammer. Finally, the *stirrup*, or **stapes**, connects to a membrane called the **oval window**. The oval window begins the internal ear and transmits the amplified vibrations from the tympanic ossicles. During transmission, the sound or vibrations can be amplified as much as 22 times their original level.

Also contained within the middle ear are the **eustachian tubes**. These tubes allow for air pressure on either side of the eardrum to be equalized. The tubes connect the nasal cavity and pharynx to the middle ear. Therefore, they transmit both the outside atmospheric pressure through the nose and throat opening and the middle ear pressure, where they are located, to allow for an equalization of pressure between the atmosphere and the middle ear. This equalizing of pressure between the middle ear and external atmosphere allows the eardrum to freely vibrate with incoming sound waves. Sudden pressure changes, such as one caused by flying in an airplane, can affect this area. This is why, when flying, you are instructed to chew gum or swallow so the inner ear can better sense and adjust to the rapidly changing outside atmosphere via the eustachian tubes.

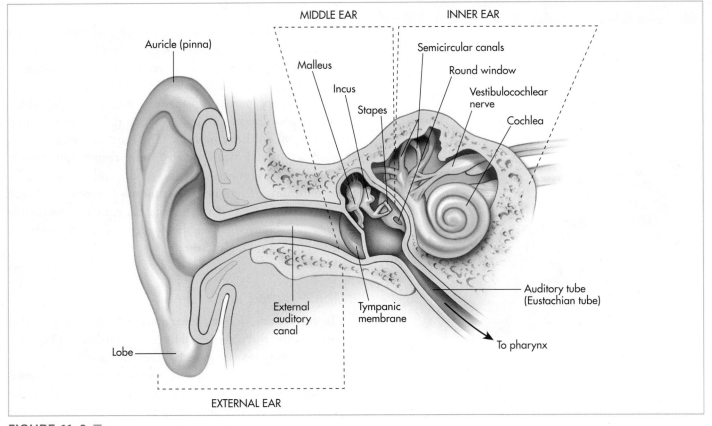

FIGURE 11–3 ■

Structures of the ear.

The Inner Ear

The oval window membrane is the portal into the **inner ear**, or **labyrinth**. This area contains three separate, hollow bony spaces that form a complex maze of winding and twisting channels. Because another name for a maze is labyrinth, this area can also be called the *bony labyrinth*. The three areas are the **vestibule chamber**, which houses the internal ear, the **cochlea** (Latin word for "snail shell"), and the **semicircular canals**.

The cochlea is the bony spiral or snail shell–shaped entrance to the inner ear connected to the oval window

membrane (see **FIGURE 11–4** ■). The cochlea contains fluid called **perilymph**, which helps transmit the sound through this area. The sound is then transmitted to the back of the maze, which contains another fluid called **endolymph**. Here, the sound is carried to tiny hairlike receptors that are stimulated and conduct the signal to the brain via the acoustic nerve, or **vestibulocochlear nerve** (**cranial nerve VIII**). **TABLE 11–2** ■ lists the major structures and functions of the ear.

Hearing Summarized

In summary (and you may want to view **FIGURE 11–5** ■ as you read this), sound waves enter the external canal and vibrate the eardrum, or tympanic membrane, in a process called *sound conduction*. The middle ear then amplifies the sound through the respective ossicles. This process is called *bone conduction* of sound. The last ossicle (stapes) vibrates and causes a gentle pumping against the oval window membrane. This causes cochlear fluid to vibrate small hairlike neurons found in an area called the *organ of Corti*. As a result of the vibration, sensory cells send a nerve impulse to the temporal lobe of the brain, where it is interpreted as sound, a process called *sensorineural conduction*.

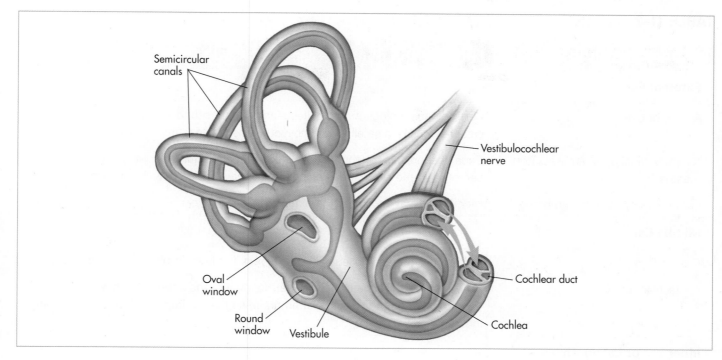

FIGURE 11–4 ■

The structures of the inner ear.

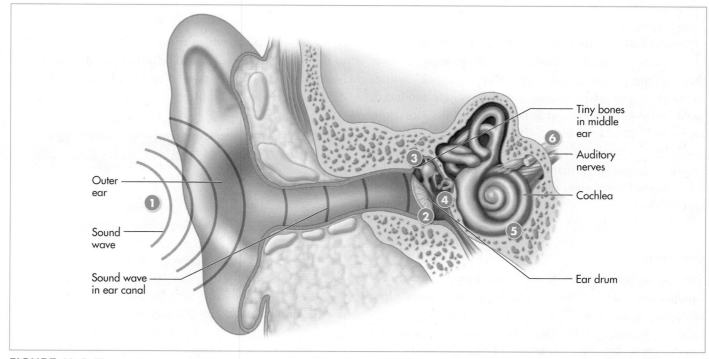

FIGURE 11–5 ■

The steps in the hearing process. (1) Sound waves enter the outer ear and travel through the ear canal. (2) Sound waves vibrate the ear drum. (3) The vibrations now vibrate the auditory ossicles in the middle ear. (4) Pressure waves created by stapes transfer to the oval window, causing cochlea fluid to vibrate hairlike nerve cells. (5) Vibrations travel through the cochlear duct. (6) Signals travel to the brain's auditory center via the auditory nerves.

TABLE 11–2 STRUCTURES AND FUNCTIONS OF THE EAR

ORGAN OR STRUCTURE	FUNCTION
External Ear	
Auricle or pinna	Cartilaginous projection that collects and directs sound waves into the auditory canal, much like a satellite dish collects transmissions from space
Auditory canal or external auditory meatus	Canal responsible for conduction of sound that contains earwax, or cerumen, secreted by the ceruminous glands to lubricate the canal and trap foreign particles
Eardrum or tympanic membrane	Membrane that separates the external and middle ear
Middle Ear	
Ossicles	Three small bones (malleus, incus, stapes) that help amplify and transmit sound
Eustachian tubes	Allows for equalization of external (atmospheric) and internal (within the middle ear) pressure on the tympanic membrane so the eardrum can freely vibrate with incoming sound
Inner Ear or Labyrinth	
Cochlea	Bony, snail-shaped entrance to the internal ear containing perilymph fluid, which helps to transmit sound
Semicircular canals	Three canals containing endolymph fluid, which transmits positional changes to tiny, hairlike receptors that are stimulated and conduct the signal to the brain via the vestibulocochlear nerve (eighth cranial nerve) to help maintain balance

Low-intensity sound waves, similar to a clock ticking, send vibrations that cause the sensory cells to move in waves that are interpreted by the brain as at "tick-tock" sound. In extreme cases when intense sound waves are produced, such as from a gun blast, it is believed that the vibrations are so great that they may knock over the hairlike cells, much like an earthquake knocks over tall trees. Repeated assaults can lead to permanent hearing damage. Therefore, it is a "sound" investment to wear proper hearing protection around loud noises.

Balance

The ear is also responsible for your sense of balance, or equilibrium. The semicircular canals process sensory input related to equilibrium. They contain nerve endings or receptors in the form of hair cells. The semicircular canals are three loops within the inner ear that help maintain balance. Like the cochlea, they are filled with endolymph fluid, and each canal contains a sensory receptor. This fluid moves when you change body position. The movement is picked up by sensory receptors, which trigger a nerve impulse to travel to the brain stem and the cerebellum. Here, the impulse is interpreted as body position to help maintain muscle coordination and body equilibrium.

Amazing Facts

Vertigo

The term **vertigo** is often used incorrectly when trying to describe the symptom of dizziness or light-headedness. Vertigo is actually the sensation of moving around in space or the illusion of objects moving around the person. This condition may be caused by a variety of disorders such as middle-ear disease or toxic conditions as the result of the ingestion of high levels of alcohol, streptomycin, salicylates, or food poisoning. Vertigo can also be caused by sunstroke, infectious diseases, and postural hypotension.

TEST YOUR KNOWLEDGE 11–2

Complete the following:

1. The structure that marks the end of the external ear and the beginning of the middle ear is called the
   a. pinna.
   b. hammer.
   c. tympanic membrane.
   d. labyrinth.

2. The structures of the ear that are important for balance are the
   a. ceruminous glands.
   b. incus, malleus, and stapes.
   c. semicircular canals.
   d. eustachian tubes.

Provide the synonymous terms for each of the following:

3. auricle _____

4. earwax _____

5. malleus _____

6. anvil _____

7. stirrups _____

8. A sense of your body moving through space or objects swirling around you is termed _____.

OTHER SENSES

Other senses also help us to interpret the world around us. These include the senses of taste, smell, and touch.

Taste

The sense of taste is referred to as the **gustatory** sense. During our hunting and gathering days, this sense kept us from eating harmful foods. Due to this role, your sense of taste is extremely fast in detecting bad food. A taste can be detected in as little as .0015 second! As you develop taste experiences, your brain attaches emotions to certain tastes. For example, you will be repulsed by the taste of spoiled milk and yet may have pleasurable feelings about chocolate-covered strawberries (unless you are allergic to either one!).

The tongue is covered by tiny bumps called *papillae*, as seen in **FIGURE 11–6** ■, each of which contains several taste receptors. These receptors, called *taste buds*, can also be found in other parts of the mouth, including the lips, palate, and inner cheeks. Taste buds die off and are replaced on a regular basis. As we age, the replacement process slows down, making our ability to taste less acute. This is why many geriatric patients tend to prefer foods that are more highly seasoned.

Taste buds send signals to the brain via three distinct cranial nerves. One nerve detects the anterior two-thirds of the tongue, a second detects the posterior portion of the tongue, and the third detects the throat area. Taste buds detect five tastes: *sweet, sour, salty, bitter,* and *umami.* **Umami** has been included with the traditional four because it is the distinct taste of glutamates, which cannot be duplicated by the combination of any of the other four tastes. Newer research indicates that the old taste map of the tongue that identified specific locations for taste buds that registered bitter, sweet, and so forth was incorrect. The taste buds for each taste are actually spread out over the whole surface of the tongue. Quite often, taste preferences change with the body's need, which is why, for example, pregnant women may crave a variety of foods throughout their pregnancy. The refinement of food taste is primarily dependent on the sense of smell and the number of functioning taste buds.

Smell

The sense of smell arises from the receptors located in the olfactory region, or the upper part of the nasal cavity. We "sniff" to bring smells up to this area, where they can be interpreted. Remember that taste and smell are closely related, which is why we can't taste foods very well when we have a severe head cold. Pleasant food odors also initiate digestive enzymes, so when you smell that cinnamon apple pie baking, your mouth really may water in anticipation.

Smell is also closely linked to memory. Have you ever smelled cookies and automatically thought about a holiday or special family celebration? Smell has been known to trigger memories. It is believed that this occurs due to the fact that the temporal lobe of the brain processes smells as well as memories and emotions. This may be useful some day

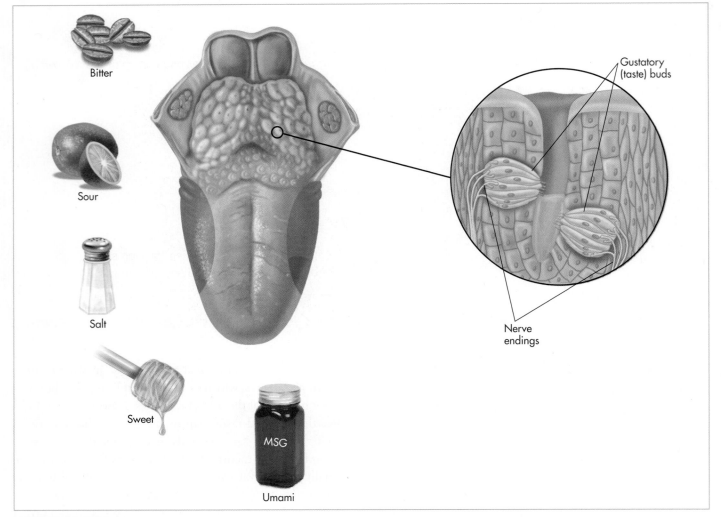

FIGURE 11–6 ■

The sense of taste. Note: taste buds are located on the anterior and posterior portions of the tongue, as well as in the throat.

for the treatment of dementia in which smells are used to try to retrieve past memories (see **FIGURE 11–7** ■).

Touch

Touch receptors are small, rounded bodies called **tactile corpuscles** located in skin and especially concentrated in the fingertips (see **FIGURE 11–8** ■). There are about 4 million of these sensory receptors in your skin! It is interesting to note that even when a patient is locally anesthetized (and awake), there are no pain sensations, but the patient is still conscious of pressure through deep touch sensors. Traction and pressure are similar; pressure is a downward force, whereas traction is more like a squeeze or pinch. Tickle is a peculiar sensation-caused touch that elicits reflex muscular movements and laughter or some other form of emotional expression.

Temperature

Temperature sensors are also found in the skin. Thermoreceptors stop being stimulated once the surface temperature of your skin drops to below 40 degrees Fahrenheit (this is when your skin starts to become numb) and over 113 degrees Fahrenheit, at which point pain receptors then take over to help avoid getting burned. These thermoreceptors may cause an interesting phenomenon called **adaptation** to occur. Continued sensory stimulation causes the sensors to desensitize, or adapt. For example, if you are continually exposed to the cold, the receptors adjust, and you don't feel so cold. That is why an outside temperature of 50 degrees seems warm after a long cold winter, but that same temperature seems cold after a long hot summer. Another example is when you first enter a hot bath, it may feel extremely hot. After a few seconds, it doesn't feel so hot, yet the actual temperature of the water has not yet changed appreciably.

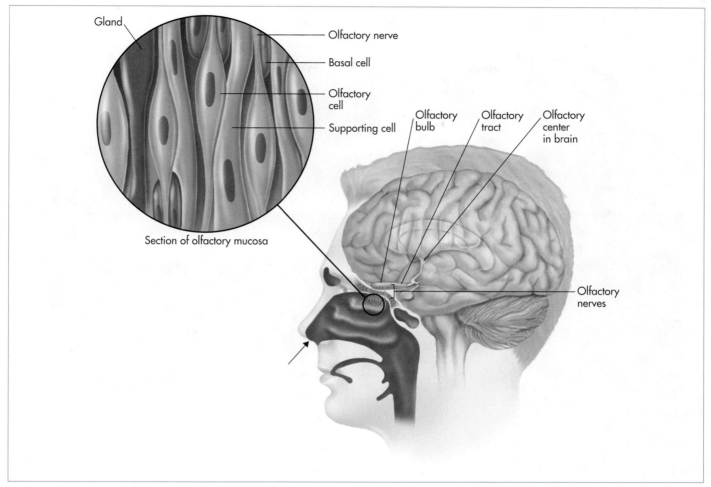

Gland
Olfactory nerve
Basal cell
Olfactory cell
Supporting cell
Olfactory bulb
Olfactory tract
Olfactory center in brain
Olfactory nerves
Section of olfactory mucosa

FIGURE 11–7 ■

The sense of smell.

Pain

Pain is a very important protective sense. It is the body's way of drawing attention to a particular danger, such as the "hitting your finger with a hammer" example used earlier in the book. Pain is the most widely distributed sense, and these receptors are in greater numbers than the receptors for any other sensation. Pain receptors are merely branches of nerve fibers called *nociceptors* (free nerve endings). They are found in skin, muscles, joints, and internal organs, which makes sense since this sensation is crucial for one's survival.

There are even different types of pain. *Referred pain* originates in an internal organ, yet is felt in another region of the skin. For example, liver and gallbladder diseases often cause pain in the right shoulder. See **FIGURE 11–9** ■ for various sites of referred pain. *Phantom pain* can result from an amputated limb—an individual can feel pain or sensations in an arm or leg he or she no longer has.

Pain receptors do not adapt as heat and cold receptors do. Pain is felt for as long as the stimulus is there that is causing it or unless a person is under **anesthesia**. An interesting debate is whether or not some people have higher or lower thresholds of pain.

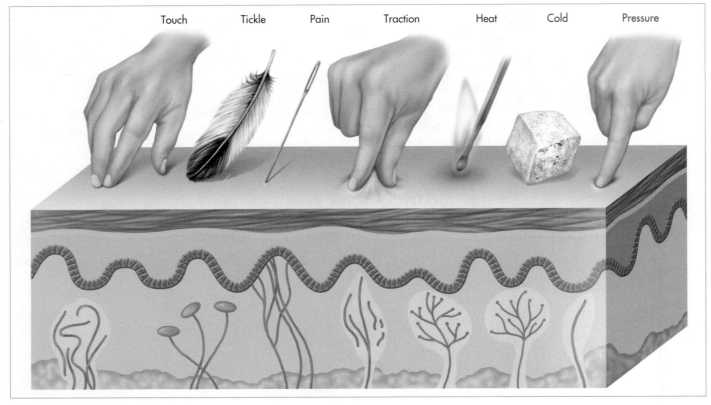

Touch   Tickle   Pain   Traction   Heat   Cold   Pressure

FIGURE 11–8 ■

The sense of touch.

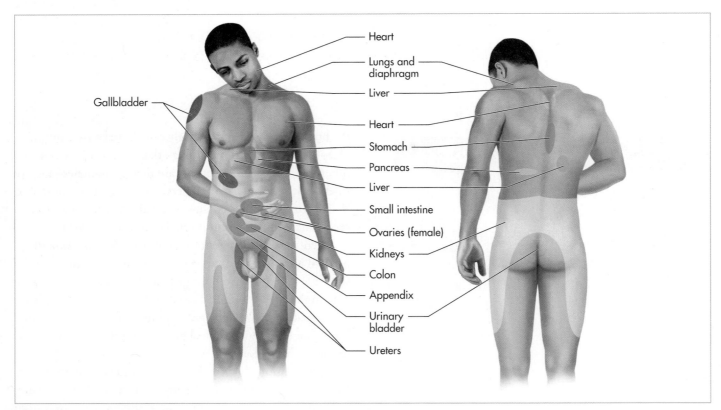

FIGURE 11–9 ■

Various sites of referred pain.

COMMON DISORDERS OF THE EYE AND EAR

Conjunctivitis is an inflammation of the membrane that lines the eye (conjunctiva). This condition can either be acute or chronic and is caused by a variety of irritants and pathogens. The acute phase is commonly called *pinkeye* and is a highly contagious form caused by bacteria.

A **cataract** is a condition in which the lens loses its flexibility and transparency, and light cannot easily pass through the clouded lens. Most cataracts are age-related, but it has been shown that increased exposure to sunlight may speed up the development of cataracts. When untreated, this condition can lead to blindness. It is interesting to note that cataract surgery was one of the earliest recorded surgical procedures, dating back to ancient Greece.

Glaucoma, known as the "silent thief of sight" because it can often go undetected, can lead to blindness. It is caused by increased pressure in the fluid of the eye, which interferes with optic nerve functioning. Glaucoma occurs in 20 percent of adults over age 40 and accounts for 15 percent of the cases of blindness in America. This is a tragic loss because glaucoma can be readily diagnosed and treated.

The eye can have several defects that impair vision. The eyes may have difficulty focusing on near or far objects because the light rays are not focusing properly on the retina. **Hyperopia** (farsightedness) occurs when the eye cannot focus properly on nearby objects. This condition results from the flattening of the globe of the eye or a refraction problem where light rays focus behind the retina. **Presbyopia** (*presby* = old, *opia* = refers to vision) is farsightedness that occurs with age, usually between ages 40 and 45. The lens becomes stiff and yellowish. Such age-related changes make it difficult for older adults to focus as well as make them more sensitive to glare, which can impair their nighttime driving abilities. **Myopia** (nearsightedness) causes objects at a distance to appear blurred.

Amblyopia, or lazy eye, usually occurs in childhood. Here, poor vision in one eye is caused by the abnormal dominance of the other eye, which does most of the work. In addition, the eyes can be used to help diagnose a variety of nonvisual diseases. For example, a yellow tint to the conjunctiva (jaundice) may indicate a liver disease. A neurological assessment called PERRLA, which stands for *Pupils Equal, Round, Reactive to Light and Accommodation*, can be used to assess brain injury. The **rapid eye movement (REM)** stage of sleep is measured during sleep studies and helps diagnose sleep disorders.

Otitis media (*oto* = ear, *it is* = inflammation, *media* = middle) is an infection of the middle ear, usually caused by a bacteria or virus, and is frequently found in infants and young children. It is commonly associated with an **upper respiratory infection (URI)**, such as a cold. By examining the structure of the ear, can you see how a sinus infection can spread to the ear and vice versa?

Labyrinthitis is an inflammation of the inner ear and usually is caused by high fevers. Labyrinthitis can cause **vertigo**, which is a feeling of dizziness or whirling in space. If you are not sure what vertigo is, watch the Alfred Hitchcock classic movie of the same name. Not only does it clearly demonstrate vertigo, but it is a great mystery movie. **Ménière's disease** is a chronic condition that affects the labyrinth and leads to progressive hearing loss and vertigo.

Deafness can be either partial or complete and is caused by a variety of conditions, ranging from inflammation and scarring of the tympanic membrane to auditory nerve and brain damage. Finally, **tinnitus** is a ringing sound in the ears, which according to superstition, means someone is talking about you. Clinically, it can occur as a result of chronic exposure to loud noises, Ménière's disease, some medications, wax buildup, or various disturbances to the auditory nerve. **FIGURE 11–10** ■ shows some common eye disorders.

FOCUS ON PROFESSIONS

Audiologists are health care professionals who evaluate, diagnose, treat, and manage hearing loss, tinnitus, and balance disorders in children and adults. Learn more about the exciting profession of audiology by visiting the websites of national organizations, such as the American Academy of Audiology (AAA), the American Speech Language Hearing Association (ASHA), and the Audiology Resource Association (ARA).

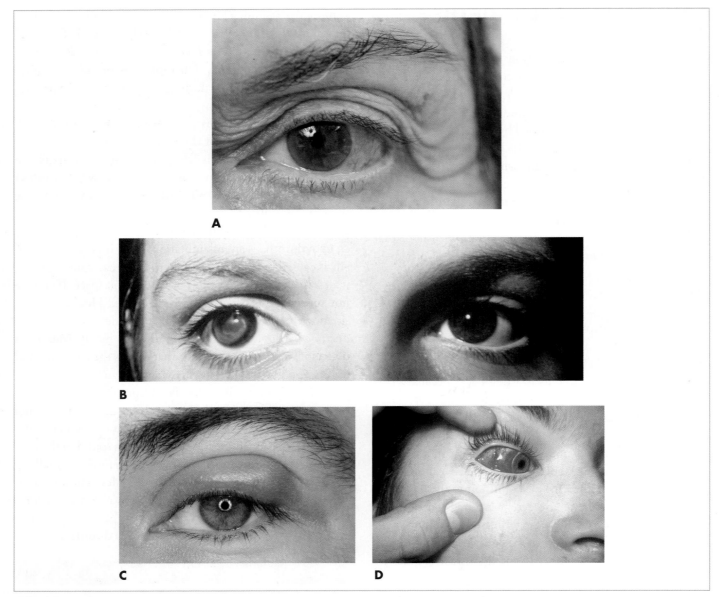

FIGURE 11–10 ■

Some common eye disorders. (A) Conjunctivitis ("pinkeye"). (B) Cataract of right eye. (C) Stye. (D) Conjunctival hemorrhage of the right eye of this patient with infectious mononucleosis.

SUMMARY: Points of Interest

- The senses of sight (eyes), sound and equilibrium (ears), taste (tongue), and smell (nose) are called special senses. The body feels other sensations, such as touch, heat, cold, and pain, which are called general senses.

- The eye is very similar to a camera, with lens cover (eyelids), opening (pupils), shutter (iris), lens (eye lens), and photoreceptive film (retina). Light rays enter the eye and pass through the cornea, aqueous humor, pupil, lens, and vitreous humor and are focused on the retina. The photoreceptors in the retina cause an impulse to be sent to the optic nerve, which carries it to the brain for the interpretation we call vision.

- The ear has three major divisions: the external, middle, and inner ear. The ear is the organ for hearing and maintaining our sense of balance. Sound waves enter the external canal and vibrate the eardrum, or tympanic membrane. The middle ear then amplifies the sound through the respective tiny bones, or ossicles. The last ossicle (stapes) vibrates and causes a gentle pumping against the oval window membrane. This causes cochlear fluid to move and vibrate tiny, hairlike neurons, which transmit an impulse to the hearing centers in the brain, where the sound is interpreted.

- The semicircular canals are responsible for maintaining body balance.

- Our sense of taste, or gustatory sense, has traditionally been thought to consist of sweet, sour, salty, and bitter, but a fifth taste, umami, has recently been distinguished as its own category. The sense of taste originates on taste buds on the tongue and is closely associated with the sense of smell.

- The sense of smell arises from the olfactory region of the nose.

- The sense of touch allows perceptions of pain, temperature, pressure, traction, and the sensation of being "tickled."

CASE STUDY

A 40-year-old male patient presents with complaints of tinnitus and vertigo. He complains that his hearing is getting progressively worse over the last three years, and he is having dizzy spells and nausea.

1. Describe the patient's complaints in your own words.

   _____

   _____

2. What possible disease is present?

   _____

   _____

3. What part of the ear is affected and why?

   _____

   _____

REVIEW QUESTIONS

Multiple Choice

1. The part of the eye that allows for varying amounts of light onto the retina is the
   a. lens.
   b. humor.
   c. iris.
   d. optic nerve.

2. The photopigment structures responsible for the ability to see colors are the
   a. cones.
   b. rods.
   c. iris.
   d. pupil.

3. The incus is found in the
   a. inner ear.
   b. middle ear.
   c. external ear.
   d. region of South America.

4. What is the correct descending order for the media through which sound travels, with the most efficient conductor of sound listed first?
   a. liquid, air, solid
   b. solid, liquid, air
   c. air, liquid, solid
   d. they are all equal

5. Another word for the sense of taste is
   a. olfactory.
   b. vertigo.
   c. mastication.
   d. gustatory.

6. Damage to the tympanic membrane can cause this kind of deafness.
   a. nerve
   b. conduction
   c. membranous
   d. all of the above

7. Which part of the body has the highest density of touch receptors?
   a. fingers
   b. forearm
   c. back
   d. buttocks

Fill in the Blank

1. The two functions of the auditory system are _____ and _____.

2. The three ossicles of the ear are the _____, _____, and _____.

3. A man with red/green color blindness is missing one type of _____, a retinal cell.

4. A woman presents with pain in her upper right abdomen and back. What organ may be inflamed? _____

5. People who spend a lot of time in the sun are more likely to develop this eye disorder. _____

Short Answer

1. Differentiate between special and general senses.

   _____
   _____
   _____
   _____

2. What are the five basic tastes? How are taste and smell related?

   _____
   _____
   _____
   _____

3. Define *adaptation* in relation to temperature sensors.

   _____
   _____
   _____
   _____

4. Trace the path of light rays from the world to the brain. Explain how the rays are focused.

   _____
   _____
   _____
   _____

5. Explain the journey of sound waves from the environment to the brain.

   _____
   _____
   _____
   _____

6. Which condition is known as the "silent thief of sight" and why?

   _____
   _____
   _____

12

The Endocrine System

THE BODY'S OTHER CONTROL SYSTEM

ENDOCRINE SYSTEM

Adrenal gland

Pituitary gland

Pineal gland

Testicle

Thymus

Thyroid

Pancreas

Ovary

Here we are again, talking about control. We have already visited one of the control systems: the complex structure of cells and connections known as the nervous system. Now we visit yet another control system, the endocrine system. They seem like separate systems, but they are totally integrated and always monitor each other's activities. The nervous system collects information and sends orders with a speed that is truly mind boggling. Although the endocrine system also collects information and sends orders, it's a slower, more subtle control system. The endocrine system's orders to the body also last much longer than those made by the nervous system. You might think of the endocrine system as sending "standing orders," which are orders meant to be obeyed indefinitely unless changed by another set of orders. The orders change subtly on a regular basis, but their purpose is to maintain consistency. The nervous system, on the other hand, issues orders that are to be obeyed instantaneously but are used for short-term situations. The endocrine system demands organs to "carry on," whereas the nervous system expects them to respond immediately.

On our journey, suppose we stop at an amusement park to ride a roller coaster. Afterward, en route to our next destination, we are forced off the road because of a near miss with a truck. In both cases—when the roller coaster ride is over and the truck is long gone—your legs still shake, your heart continues to race, and your blood pressure remains elevated, even though you are no longer in danger. We call such lingering effects the "adrenaline rush." These lingering effects are not due to continued activity of the nervous system, but rather to endocrine activity deliberately triggered by the autonomic nervous system.

LEARNING OUTCOMES

At the completion of your journey through this chapter, you will be able to:

- Describe the purpose and effects of hormones within the body.
- Explain the difference between a hormone and a neurotransmitter.
- Explain how hormones work.
- Describe the control of endocrine activity within the body, including homeostasis, negative feedback, and the three mechanisms of control of hormone levels.
- Discuss the location and function of major endocrine organs and glands to include the hypothalamus, pituitary gland, thyroid gland, thymus gland, pineal gland, pancreas, adrenal glands, and gonads.
- Discuss common disorders of the endocrine system

ORGANIZATION OF THE ENDOCRINE SYSTEM

The endocrine system has many organs that secrete a variety of chemical substances. Let's begin by looking at the basic organization of the system.

Endocrine Organs and Glands

The **endocrine system** (*endo* = into; *crine* = to secrete) is a series of organs and glands in your body that secretes chemical messengers (called *hormones*) *into* your bloodstream (see **FIGURE 12–1** ■). There are also glands that secrete *outside* the body, such as sweat glands (*exocrine* glands), but they are not part of the *endo*crine system because their secretions leave the body. Sometimes there is confusion in differentiating between glands and organs. A *gland* is an organized cluster of cells or tissues whose sole function is to manufacture a substance that is either secreted from or used within the body. *Organs* are collections of more than one type of specialized tissues that may be able to secrete substances but also have additional functions. The kidneys, for example, produce and release the hormone erythropoietin and also function to filter blood and maintain electrolyte and fluid balance.

We have already discussed some of the endocrine glands, such as the hypothalamus, pituitary gland, and pineal gland, because they are part of the nervous system and provide a link *between* the two control systems. We visit some of the other endocrine organs and glands in later chapters when we journey through the urinary, reproductive, and digestive systems. It may seem like an overwhelming task to learn all the endocrine glands and their associated hormones; therefore, we will begin our discussion with a concise overview

to lay a foundation on which to build. As we travel through this chapter, these concepts are reinforced and expanded. For now, see **TABLE 12–1** ■, which lists the wide variety of functions of endocrine organs and glands.

Amazing Facts

Lesser-Known Endocrine Organs

Did you know that many organs, such as the heart, kidney, small intestine, stomach, and placenta, can also secrete hormones? These and many other organs are not listed as endocrine organs because their primary jobs are focused on other tasks, such as pumping blood, storing and digesting food, or nourishing an embryo. But the hormones secreted by other organs are still an important part of the body's control systems. We will learn more about them when we discuss the body's other systems in those respective chapters.

Hormones

The chemical messengers released by endocrine glands are called **hormones**. Neurotransmitters are one type of chemical messenger; they are released by neurons at chemical synapses. They diffuse across the synapse, a very tiny space, to a cell on the other side and bind to that cell. Neurotransmitters are cleaned up quickly, so their effects are localized and short lived. Hormones, on the other hand, are released into the bloodstream and travel all over your body. Some hormones can affect millions of cells simultaneously.

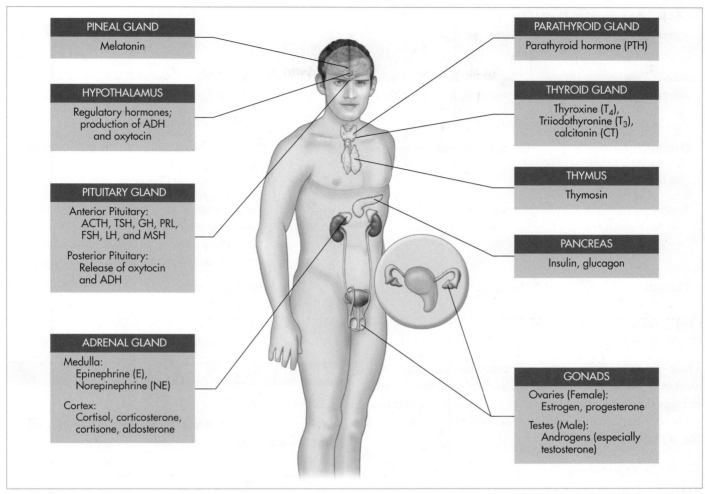

FIGURE 12–1 ■

The endocrine glands and their hormones.

TABLE 12–1 ENDOCRINE GLANDS/ORGAN FUNCTIONS

ENDOCRINE GLANDS/ORGANS	HORMONE RELEASED	EFFECT
Hypothalamus	Numerous hormones that will be discussed in dedicated upcoming section (Table 12–3)	Controls pituitary hormone levels
Pineal	Melatonin	Believed to regulate sleep
Pituitary	Numerous hormones that will be discussed in dedicated upcoming section (Table 12–3)	Controls other endocrine organs
Thyroid	Thyroxine, triiodothyronine	Controls cellular metabolism
	Calcitonin	Decreases blood calcium
Parathyroid glands	Parathyroid hormone	Increases blood calcium
Pancreas	Insulin	Lowers blood sugar
	Glucagon	Raises blood sugar

(continued)

TABLE 12–1 ENDOCRINE GLANDS/ORGAN FUNCTIONS (continued)

ENDOCRINE GLANDS/ORGANS	HORMONE RELEASED	EFFECT
Adrenal glands	Epinephrine, norepinephrine	Flight-or-fight response
	Adrenocorticosteroids	Many different effects
Ovaries	Estrogen, progesterone	Controls sexual reproduction and secondary sexual characteristics, such as pubic and axillary hair, and breast development
Testes	Testosterone	Controls secondary sexual characteristics such as growth of beard or other hair, deepening of voice, increase in musculature, and production of sperm
Thymus	Thymosin	Immune system, causes maturation of white blood cells

Their effects last for minutes or even hours or days. Many hormones are secreted constantly, and the amount secreted changes as needed. To help clarify the similarities and differences between a neurotransmitter and a hormone, please see TABLE 12–2 ■.

TABLE 12–2 COMPARISON OF NEUROTRANSMITTERS AND HORMONES

NEUROTRANSMITTERS	HORMONES
Chemical messengers	Chemical messengers
Bind to receiving cell	Bind to receiving cell
Control cell excitation	Control cell activities
Released by neurons	Released by neurons, glands, or organs
Released at chemical synapse	Released into bloodstream
Intended target very close	Travel to distant target
Effects happen quickly (less than a second)	Effects take time (seconds or minutes)
Effects wear off quickly (few seconds)	Effects long lasting (minutes or hours)
Affect single cell	Can affect many cells, whole systems

LEARNING HINT

Hormone Names

Most hormones are named according to where they are secreted or what they do. If you learn the meanings of their names, you can usually tell something about the hormone. For example, growth hormone stimulates cells to grow. **Prolactin** increases milk production. Even a complicated hormone name such as adrenocorticotropic hormone can be picked apart fairly easily. *Adreno* refers to the adrenal gland, *cortico* refers to the cortex, and *tropic* means "influences the activity of." Therefore, adrenocorticotropic hormone is a hormone that binds to (in this case increases the activity of) the adrenal cortex. Also keep in mind that most hormones are known by their abbreviations, for obvious reasons. Adrenocorticotropic hormone, for example, is abbreviated ACTH, which is much easier to say and write.

How Hormones Work

Like neurotransmitters, hormones work by binding to extracellular receptors on target cells. But hormones may bind not only to sites on the outside of the cell, like neurotransmitters, but also to sites inside the cell. If hormones bind to extracellular receptors, they send the target cell a message that changes cellular activity. Thus, the target cell changes what it has been doing, usually by making a new protein, turning off a protein it has been making, or changing the amount it is making. These hormones are generally modified amino acids or polypeptides.

Two types of hormones—**steroids** and **thyroid hormones**—are particularly powerful because they can bind to sites *inside* cells (intracellular sites). These hormones, which can pass through the cell membrane, can interact directly with the cell's DNA, the genetic material, to change cell activity. These hormones are carefully regulated by the body because of their ability, even in very small amounts, to control target cells. See the section titled "The Adrenal Glands" for further discussion of steroid hormones and the dangers of taking steroids. Thyroid hormones will be discussed later in this chapter in "The Thyroid Gland."

Amazing Facts

Prostaglandins: Short-Range Hormones

There are other ways to send signals from cell to cell. There are two types of cell signaling that should be mentioned here: **autocrine** and **paracrine**. Autocrine signaling occurs when a cell sends out a signal that affects the cell itself. We will discuss autocrine signaling in Chapter 15, "The Lymphatic and Immune Systems." Paracrine signaling occurs when a cell sends out a signal that affects nearby cells that are different from the cell sending out the signal. **Prostaglandins** are an example of paracrine signaling. Prostaglandins are molecules that are short-range hormones that are formed rapidly and act in the immediate area. Many different body tissues produce prostaglandins. These molecules have a variety of functions depending on where they were produced. Some prostaglandins help to constrict or dilate smooth muscle, in blood vessels, the digestive tract, or the bronchial tubes of the lungs. Others are involved in tissue inflammation. Each one acts in a small area of the body. Prostaglandins have a short but powerful effect on these local tissues. Nonsteroidal anti-inflammatory drugs (NSAIDs) such as ibuprofen work by inhibiting the prostaglandin release associated with inflammation.

TEST YOUR KNOWLEDGE 12–1

Choose the best answer:

1. What chemical, when secreted into the bloodstream, controls the metabolic processes of target cells?
   a. neurotransmitter
   b. secretion
   c. hormone
   d. ligand

2. Steroid hormones are very powerful because they
   a. are hormones.
   b. are medicine.
   c. interact directly with DNA.
   d. are secreted outside the body.

3. Which of the following is true of hormones?
   a. They last a short time.
   b. They are fast acting.
   c. They affect distant targets.
   d. They leave the body.

4. Which of the following organs is not a primary endocrine organ though it secretes hormones?
   a. thyroid
   b. pituitary
   c. kidney
   d. adrenal gland

5. Why can steroids pass into the cell when other hormones cannot?
   a. There are special steroid channels.
   b. Lipids can pass through cell membranes.
   c. Inhibitors block nonsteroid hormones.
   d. Steroids are tiny molecules.

6. Short-range hormones that are formed rapidly and act only in the immediate area are:
   a. steroids
   b. prostaglandins
   c. amino acids
   d. mucoids

CONTROL OF ENDOCRINE ACTIVITY

Many endocrine glands are active all the time. The amount of hormone they secrete changes as the situation demands, but unlike neurons, the cells in the endocrine glands often secrete hormones continuously. How is the activity controlled? How do the glands know how much hormone to secrete?

Homeostasis and Negative Feedback

To understand how the endocrine system is controlled, we first have to revisit the concept of **homeostasis** discussed at the beginning of our journey in Chapter 1 (see FIGURE 12–2 ■). Recall that many of the chemical and physical characteristics of the body have a standard level, or **set point**, that is the ideal level for that particular value. Blood pressure, blood oxygen, heart rate, and blood sugar, for example, all have "normal" ranges. Your nervous and endocrine control systems work to keep the levels at or near ideal. There is a way for your body to measure the variable, a place where the "ideal" level is stored, and a way for the body to correct levels that are not near ideal. For example, neurons measure your body temperature. The hypothalamus stores the set point. If your temperature falls below the set point temperature, the hypothalamus causes shivering to produce additional heat. If body temperature rises above the set point, the hypothalamus causes sweating.

If any of the body's dozens of homeostatic values become seriously disrupted, the control systems work to bring them back to set point. This process is called **negative feedback** (see FIGURE 12–3 ■). Most of you are familiar with negative feedback in real life. When you pump gas, a sensor in the nozzle turns *off* the flow of gas when the tank is full. That is negative feedback. The gas is flowing, the tank is filling, and when the goal is reached, the gas stops flowing. A "time-out" for a toddler who has misbehaved is also negative feedback. The time-out is designed to turn *off* the naughty behavior. In the body, negative feedback counteracts a change. As blood pressure rises, for example, your body works to bring it down to "normal," the set point. If blood pressure falls, your body works to raise it back to set point. Hormones work the same way. If hormone levels rise, negative feedback turns off the endocrine organ that is secreting the hormone.

The body is also capable of **positive feedback**, which increases the magnitude of a change. The flow of sodium into a neuron during depolarization is a real-life example we have already visited. The more depolarized a neuron becomes, the more sodium flows in, so it becomes more depolarized, so more flows in, and so on. Such a process is also known as a *vicious cycle*. Therefore, positive feedback is not a way to regulate your body because it increases a change away from set point. What if instead of shivering when you got cold, to raise your body temperature, you got colder and colder and colder?

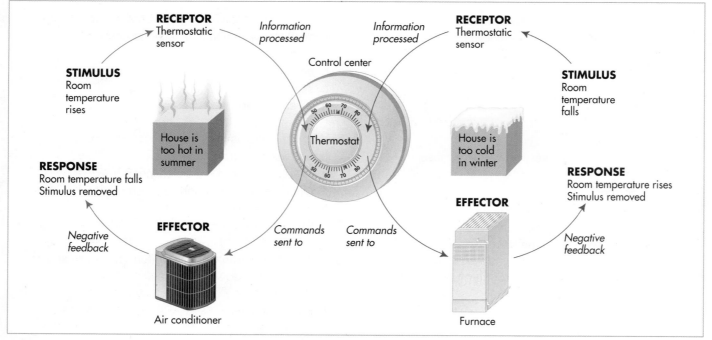

FIGURE 12–2 ■

Homeostasis is analogous to regulation of temperature via a thermostat.

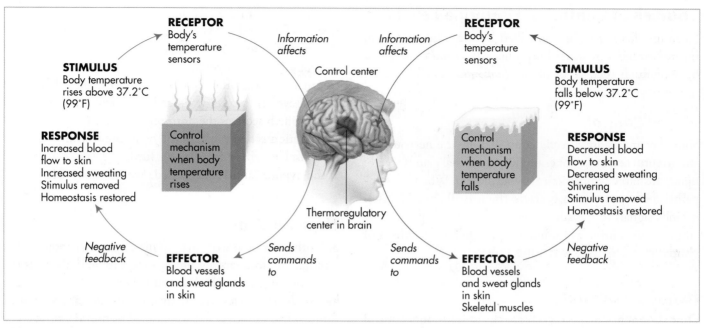

FIGURE 12–3 ■

Homeostasis and negative feedback as related to control of body temperature.

Amazing Facts

Fever

When you get an infection, sometimes your body temperature rises above normal (set point). Lay terminology may refer to this as "running a fever." The medical term for a patient with a fever is *febrile*. A fever is the deliberate raising of your body temperature set point by your hypothalamus. Initially, the new set point is higher than your normal temperature.

Your body thinks you are cold and takes steps to raise your body temperature to the new set point. Now you have a fever. Your head aches as blood vessels expand; your heart rate and blood pressure rise. You feel miserable, and you have your hypothalamus to blame! Sometimes the creation of fever is attributed to invading bacteria releasing toxins that can stimulate a fever.

Clinical Application

CHILDBIRTH AND POSITIVE FEEDBACK

Often, positive feedback is harmful if the vicious cycle cannot be broken, but sometimes positive feedback is necessary for a process to run to completion. A good example of necessary positive feedback is the continued contraction of the uterus during childbirth. When a baby is ready to be born, a signal, not well understood at this time, tells the hypothalamus to release the hormone **oxytocin** from the posterior pituitary. Oxytocin increases the intensity of uterine contractions. As the uterus contracts, the pressure inside the uterus caused by the baby moving down the birth canal increases the signal to the hypothalamus: More oxytocin is released, and the uterus contracts harder. As pressure gets higher inside the uterus, the hypothalamus is signaled to release more oxytocin, and the uterus contracts even harder. This cycle of ever-increasing uterine contractions due to an ever-increasing release of oxytocin from the hypothalamus continues until the pressure inside the uterus decreases—that is, when the baby is delivered. This is one of the relatively rare examples of positive feedback control of hormone levels.

Sources of Control of Hormone Levels

Hormone levels can be controlled by the nervous system (*neural control*), by other hormones (*hormonal control*), or by body fluids such as the blood (*humoral control*).

Neural Control

Some hormones are directly controlled by the nervous system (**neural control**). For example, the adrenal glands receive signals from the sympathetic nervous system. When the sympathetic nervous system is active (fight-or-flight response), it sends signals to the adrenal glands to release epinephrine and norepinephrine as hormones, prolonging the effects of sympathetic activity (see **FIGURE 12–4** ■).

Hormonal Control

Other hormones are part of a hierarchy of **hormonal control** in which one gland is controlled by the release of hormones from another gland higher in the chain, which is controlled by another gland's release of hormones yet higher in the chain. Orders are sent from one organ to another. This is very similar to a relay race at a track meet, where the baton is smoothly handed from one runner to the next to send the baton to the finish line. Negative feedback controls the flow of orders via hormones from one part of the "chain of command" to the other. For example, the hypothalamus has control over the pituitary, which has control over the adrenal gland, which secretes the hormone cortisol. Increased cortisol secretion is one way that the body copes with stress, and as cortisol levels rise in the blood, further release of hormones at the hypothalamus is depressed. See **FIGURE 12–5** ■.

Humoral Control

Still other endocrine organs can directly monitor the body's internal environment by monitoring the body fluids, such as the blood, and respond accordingly via negative feedback loops. *Humoral* pertains to body fluids or substances; control through body fluids is therefore called **humoral control**. For example, the pancreas secretes insulin in response to rising blood sugar, as shown in **FIGURE 12–6** ■, and insulin in turn increases glucose uptake by tissues, which reduces total blood glucose levels.

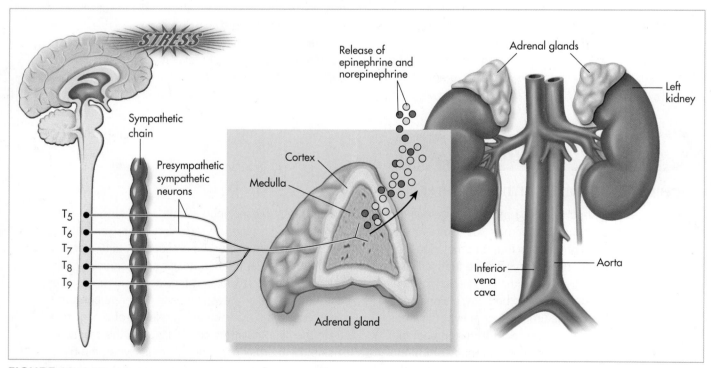

FIGURE 12–4 ■

Sympathetic control of adrenal gland.

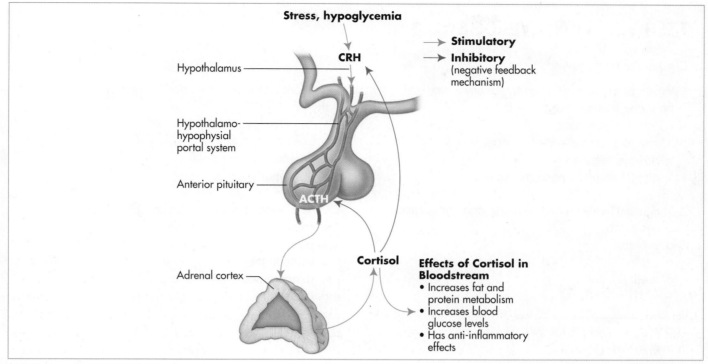

FIGURE 12–5 ■

Hormonal control of adrenal gland. CRH = corticotropin releasing hormone; ACTH = adrenocorticotropic hormone.

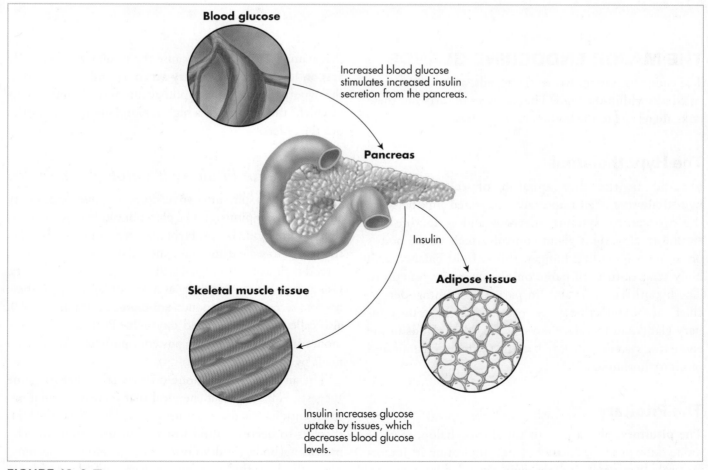

FIGURE 12–6 ■

Humoral control of blood sugar levels.

TEST YOUR KNOWLEDGE 12–2

Choose the best answer:

1. Which of the following is *not* typically a way that hormone levels are regulated?
   a. negative feedback
   b. control by other endocrine organ
   c. positive feedback
   d. direct control by nervous system

2. The "ideal" value for a body characteristic is called the
   a. set point.
   b. average.
   c. goal.
   d. feedback point.

3. _____ feedback enhances a change in body chemistry.
   a. Negative
   b. Positive
   c. Regular
   d. Cyclic

4. If a hormone is under humoral control, what controls the hormone?
   a. negative feedback
   b. positive feedback
   c. another endocrine gland
   d. the hypothalamus

5. What hormone is involved in childbirth that is an example of positive feedback?
   a. oxytocin
   b. epinephrine
   c. testosterone
   d. glucagon

THE MAJOR ENDOCRINE GLANDS

The endocrine system has several glands, and each has specific tasks within the body. The messages to carry out these tasks are related to the hormones they release.

The Hypothalamus

Located in the diencephalon of the brain, the **hypothalamus** is an important integrated link between the two control systems—nervous and endocrine (see **FIGURE 12–7** ■). This gland controls much of the body's physiology, including hunger, thirst, fluid balance, and body temperature, to name only a few of its functions. The hypothalamus is also, in part, the "commander-in-chief" of the endocrine system because it controls the pituitary gland and therefore most of the other glands in the endocrine system. **TABLE 12–3** ■ lists the hypothalamic and pituitary hormones.

The Pituitary

The **pituitary**, also a part of the diencephalon, is commonly known as the "master gland," indicating its important role in control of other endocrine glands. However, that name is misleading because the pituitary gland rarely acts on its own. The pituitary acts only under orders from the hypothalamus. If the hypothalamus is the "commander-in-chief," the pituitary is a high-ranking soldier who carries out the orders.

The Posterior Pituitary (Neurohypophysis)

The pituitary is split into two sections: the *posterior* pituitary and the *anterior* pituitary. The posterior pituitary is an extension of the hypothalamus. Hypothalamic neurons, which are specialized to secrete hormones instead of neurotransmitters, extend their axons through a stalk to the posterior pituitary. Using the posterior pituitary as a sort of launch pad, these neurons secrete two hormones: **antidiuretic hormone (ADH)**, also called vasopressin, and **oxytocin**. Both of these hormones are secreted from the posterior pituitary, but they are made by the hypothalamus.

The antidiuretic hormone does exactly what its name suggests. A *diuretic* is a chemical that increases urination, so an antidiuretic decreases urination. The effect of ADH, then, is to decrease fluid lost due to urination, thereby increasing body fluid volume. The hormone is secreted when the hypothalamus senses decreased blood volume

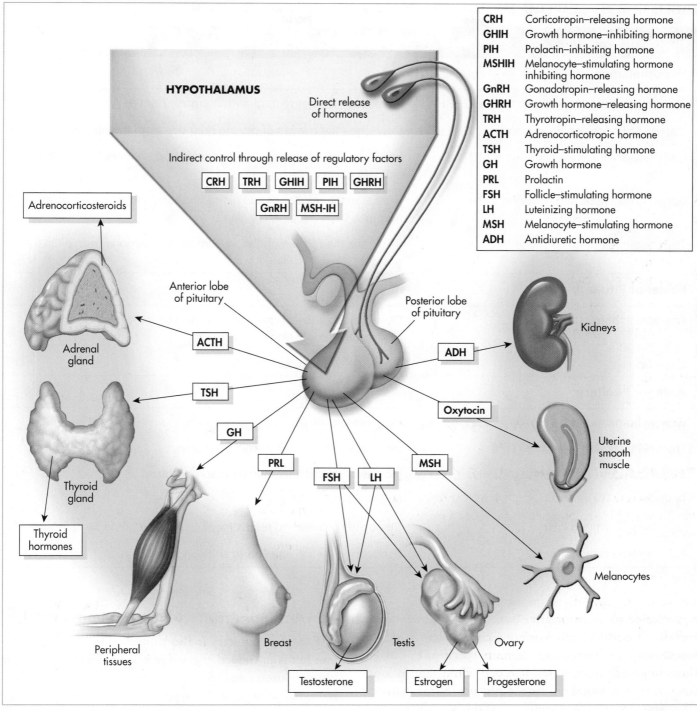

CRH	Corticotropin–releasing hormone
GHIH	Growth hormone–inhibiting hormone
PIH	Prolactin–inhibiting hormone
MSHIH	Melanocyte–stimulating hormone inhibiting hormone
GnRH	Gonadotropin–releasing hormone
GHRH	Growth hormone–releasing hormone
TRH	Thyrotropin–releasing hormone
ACTH	Adrenocorticotropic hormone
TSH	Thyroid–stimulating hormone
GH	Growth hormone
PRL	Prolactin
FSH	Follicle–stimulating hormone
LH	Luteinizing hormone
MSH	Melanocyte–stimulating hormone
ADH	Antidiuretic hormone

FIGURE 12–7 ◾

The hypothalamus, anterior and posterior pituitary glands, and their targets and associated hormones.

TABLE 12–3 SELECTED HYPOTHALAMIC AND PITUITARY HORMONES

HORMONE	FUNCTION
Hypothalamus	
Growth hormone–releasing hormone (GHRH)	Increases the release of growth hormone from the pituitary gland
Growth hormone–inhibiting hormone (GHIH)	Decreases the release of growth hormone from the pituitary gland
Corticotropin-releasing hormone (CRH)	Increases the release of adrenocorticotropic hormone from the pituitary gland
Gonadotropin-releasing hormone (GRH)	Increases the release of luteinizing hormone and follicle-stimulating hormone from the pituitary gland
Thyrotropin-releasing hormone (TRH)	Increases the release of thyroid-stimulating hormone from pituitary gland
Posterior Pituitary	
Antidiuretic hormone (ADH)	Dilutes blood and increases fluid volume by increasing water reabsorption in the kidney
Oxytocin	Increases uterine contractions
Anterior Pituitary	
Growth hormone (GH)	Increases tissue growth
Thyroid-stimulating hormone (TSH)	Increases secretion of thyroid hormones
Adrenocorticotropic hormone (ACTH)	Increases steroid secretion from adrenal gland
Prolactin	Increases milk production
Luteinizing hormone (LH)	Stimulates ovaries and testes for ovulation and hormone secretion
Follicle-stimulating hormone (FSH)	Estrogen secretion and sperm and egg production

or increased blood osmolarity (more solutes suspended in blood). The antidiuretic hormone circulates through the bloodstream and targets the kidneys specifically, causing them to absorb more water. It is very important in long-term control of blood pressure, especially during dehydration. (For more information on ADH, see Chapter 13, "The Cardiovascular System," and Chapter 17, "The Urinary System").

The second hypothalamic hormone released from the posterior pituitary is oxytocin. This hormone is important in maintaining uterine contractions during labor in women and is involved in milk ejection in nursing mothers. Oxytocin's function in males is under investigation. Pitocin, which is given to women to increase contractions, is a synthetic form of oxytocin.

The Anterior Pituitary (Adenohypophysis)

The anterior pituitary is also controlled by the hypothalamus but is an endocrine gland in its own right. The anterior pituitary makes and secretes a number of hormones, under hormonal control of the hypothalamus, that control other endocrine glands. (Growth hormone and prolactin are exceptions to this rule.) Refer to Table 12–3 and Figure 12–7 for a list of hypothalamic and pituitary hormones. We discussed this relationship previously when we talked about hormonal control. The hypothalamus secretes a hormone that controls hormone secretion by the anterior pituitary, which usually controls the secretion of hormones by another endocrine gland. The hormone levels are controlled by negative feedback to both the pituitary and the hypothalamus.

Amazing Facts

ADH and Alcohol

Drinking too much alcohol can lead to several unpleasant consequences, not the least of which is the development of a hangover. The symptoms of a hangover are due to many side effects from alcohol consumption, but the most important may be that alcohol turns off ADH. The more alcohol you drink, the less ADH you secrete, and the more dehydrated you become. That makes you thirsty, so you drink some more beer, and you secrete even less ADH and become even more dehydrated. (This is another example of a vicious cycle.) The more beer you drink, the more you urinate and the more dehydrated you are. This is part of the reason why consuming too much alcohol on Friday night can make you miserable on Saturday morning.

Clinical Application

STATURE DISORDERS

Stature disorders are those disorders that result in well-below-average height (called *dwarfism*) or well-above-average height (called *giantism* or *gigantism*). Some of these disorders are caused by abnormalities in skeletal development or nutritional deficiencies. However, growth hormone (GH) problems are often implicated. If GH secretion is insufficient during childhood, children do not grow to "standard" height. This type of dwarfism results in stunted adult height. However, if GH deficiency is diagnosed before closure of the growth zones of the long bones, it can be treated with GH injections. Children treated with GH injection attain full height. On the other end of the spectrum are those who secrete too much GH. If the oversecretion occurs during childhood, people grow extremely tall. The tallest man to ever live, according to *Guinness Book of World Records*, was more than 8 feet tall. Gigantism causes many health problems. The body can become so big that it cannot support itself. Surgery and medication are the only treatments. If GH oversecretion begins after a person has stopped growing (bone closure), he or she does not get any taller, but the tissues of the hands, feet, face, and many internal organs continue to grow out of control, causing pain and organ dysfunction. Most oversecretion of growth hormone is caused by noncancerous pituitary tumors. The use of GH to enhance performance is banned by the major sports associations.

TEST YOUR KNOWLEDGE 12–3

Choose the best answer:

1. Oxytocin
   a. is secreted from the anterior pituitary.
   b. decreases uterine contractions.
   c. is released from the posterior pituitary.
   d. is a way to get more oxygen to your toes.

2. The _____ is controlled by hormones from the hypothalamus, and the _____ actually secretes hypothalamic hormones.
   a. posterior pituitary; posterior pituitary
   b. anterior pituitary; anterior pituitary
   c. anterior pituitary; posterior pituitary
   d. posterior pituitary; anterior pituitary

(continued)

The Thyroid Gland

The **thyroid gland**, located in the anterior portion of your neck, is a butterfly-shaped organ. It is responsible for secreting the hormones thyroxine (T_4) and triiodothyronine (T_3), under orders from the pituitary gland (see **FIGURE 12–8** ■). These two hormones, T_4 and T_3, contain iodine and control cell metabolism and growth. The thyroid gland also secretes a third hormone, calcitonin, which decreases blood calcium by stimulating bone-building cells. Thyroxine and triiodothyronine are generally referred to as "thyroid hormones" and are of great clinical importance. Overproduction (hyperthyroidism) or underproduction (hypothyroidism) can cause a variety of clinical symptoms because the level of these hormones is essential in controlling growth and metabolism of body tissues, particularly in the nervous system. These hormones are so important that table salt contains added iodine to ensure that people get enough iodine in their diets to make thyroid hormones.

The thyroid gland has two small pairs of glands embedded in its posterior surface. These glands are called the **parathyroid glands**, and they produce **parathyroid hormone (PTH)**, which regulates the levels of calcium in the bloodstream. If calcium levels get too low, the parathyroid glands are stimulated to release PTH, which stimulates bone-dissolving cells and thereby releases needed calcium in the bloodstream. Again, see Figure 12–8.

The Thymus Gland

The **thymus gland** is located in the upper thorax and plays an important function in the immune system. It produces a hormone called **thymosin**, which helps with the maturation

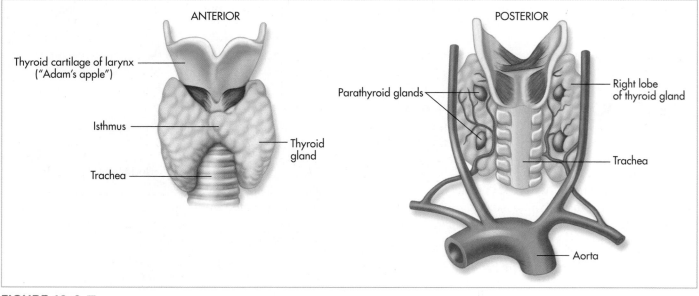

ANTERIOR

Thyroid cartilage of larynx ("Adam's apple")

Isthmus

Trachea

Thyroid gland

POSTERIOR

Parathyroid glands

Right lobe of thyroid gland

Trachea

Aorta

FIGURE 12–8 ■

The thyroid and parathyroid glands.

of white blood cells during childhood to fight infections. This gland is further discussed in Chapter 15, "The Lymphatic and Immune System."

The Pineal Gland

The tiny **pineal gland** is found in the diencephalon, and its full function still remains unknown. However, it has been shown to produce the hormone **melatonin**, which rises and falls during the waking and sleeping hours. It is believed this hormone is what triggers our sleep by peaking at night and causing drowsiness.

The Pancreas

The **pancreas** is largely responsible for maintaining blood sugar (glucose) levels at or near set point. The normal clinical range for a fasting (not eating for 12 hours) blood glucose level is 70 to 105 mg/dL (milligrams per deciliter). The pancreas can measure blood sugar, and if the blood glucose is high or low, the pancreas releases a hormone to correct the level. To understand the importance of the pancreas, let's go back in your journey to the chapter on cells. Why does it matter how much glucose is in your blood? Why devote an organ, and a pretty big one at that, to controlling blood sugar? There are two reasons why blood glucose is important. Too much glucose floating around in your blood causes many problems with the fluid balance of your cells. Recall that if the concentration of the fluid outside a cell is high in solutes, the cell will lose water to the surroundings. If the solutes are low outside the cell, the cell will fill with water and eventually can even burst. Obviously, that's a serious problem. It does not matter if the solutes are salts or glucose, the result is the same. Blood glucose must therefore be maintained at a certain level for cells to neither gain nor lose water. Why else is glucose important? Glucose is vital for cellular respiration. Cellular respiration is needed to make energy, by making adenosine triphosphate (ATP), so cells need to have enough glucose that they can make sufficient ATP to carry out their daily activities.

The pancreas makes two hormones that control blood glucose: *insulin*, which should sound familiar, and *glucagon*, both produced in the pancreatic islets. Insulin, the hormone that is missing or ineffective in diabetes, removes glucose from the blood by directing the liver to store excess glucose as the polysaccharide glycogen and by helping glucose to get inside the cells so it can be used to make ATP. Glucose, a carbohydrate, is pretty big and hydrophilic, so it cannot get into cells by itself. When would insulin be secreted by the pancreas: When blood glucose is high or when blood glucose is low? Because insulin removes glucose from the blood, it lowers blood sugar, so it is released when blood sugar is high (hyperglycemia), like right after a meal.

Clinical Application

DIABETES MELLITUS

Diabetes mellitus is a condition characterized by abnormally high blood glucose (hyperglycemia). Type 1 diabetes (formerly called insulin-dependent diabetes mellitus (IDDM) or juvenile onset diabetes) is caused by the destruction of the insulin-producing cells of the pancreas. Patients with type I diabetes do not produce enough insulin. They are always dependent on daily insulin injections. Type 2 (formerly called noninsulin-dependent diabetes mellitus (NIDDM) or late onset diabetes) is caused by insensitivity of the body's tissues to insulin. Patients with type 2 diabetes can often be treated with a carefully controlled diet and weight-loss regimen. In both types of diabetes, abnormally high blood glucose must be resolved. If blood glucose remains high, the kidneys work overtime to secrete the excess sugar. Increased urination and dehydration are the most obvious symptoms. But the stress of trying to get rid of the excess blood sugar eventually causes kidney damage. In addition, if insulin is not effective, glucose cannot get into cells. Cells must have glucose to make ATP. If cells can't get glucose and can't make ATP, they will look for other sources of energy, breaking down lipids and proteins.

Untreated diabetics often lose weight as their body searches for other energy sources. Often, their blood becomes increasingly acidic as waste products from abnormal cell metabolism accumulate in the bloodstream. The changes in blood chemistry lead to tissue and organ damage. Left untreated, diabetes mellitus may lead to coma and death. See **TABLE 12–4** ■ that compares type 1 and type 2 diabetes.

(continued)

Clinical Application (continued)

TABLE 12–4 COMPARISON OF TYPE 1 AND TYPE 2 DIABETES

	TYPE 1 DIABETES	TYPE 2 DIABETES
Cause	Autoimmune destruction of pancreas; not enough insulin is produced	Insulin resistance, obesity and sedentary lifestyle; insulin produced by pancreas does not work effectively
Age at onset	Typically before the age of 40	Typically later in life, though some obese and/or sedentary children are being diagnosed
Treatment	Insulin injections, insulin pump, pancreas transplant	Diet and exercise, medications, insulin in later stages
Symptoms	Usually sudden and severe, excess urination, extreme thirst, weight loss	Often more subtle than type 1 symptoms, excess urination, thirst

The hormone glucagon produced by the pancreas, does the opposite of insulin. Glucagon puts glucose into the bloodstream mainly by directing the liver to release stored glucose in the form of glycogen. Glucagon is released typically several hours after a meal to prevent blood glucose from dropping too low (hypoglycemia). These two hormones (insulin and glucagon) control blood glucose very tightly in healthy humans (see **FIGURE 12–9** ■). Other hormones, like the adrenal hormone cortisol, also aid in the control of blood sugar.

The Adrenal Glands

The **adrenal** glands are a pair of small glands that sit on top of your kidneys, similar to baseball hats. The adrenal glands are split into two regions: the *adrenal cortex*, an outer layer, and the *adrenal medulla*, the middle of the gland. (Note that it is best to be specific when talking about the adrenal cortex because your cerebrum has a cortex, too.)

The Adrenal Medulla

The **adrenal medulla** releases two hormones: **epinephrine** (also known as adrenaline) and **norepinephrine**. These hormones increase the duration of the effects of your sympathetic nervous system. (Remember your friend's snarling dog.) Cells of the adrenal medulla receive the neurotransmitter norepinephrine (it is both a hormone and a neurotransmitter, depending on where it is released) from the sympathetic nervous system.

FOCUS ON PROFESSIONS

It is critically important to monitor blood glucose levels and maintain an appropriate diet for patients with diabetes. **Phlebotomists** are specially trained health professionals who draw and test blood samples. Learn more about this important profession by visiting the websites of national organizations, including the American Society of Phlebotomy Technicians (ASPT), the National Association of Phlebotomists (NAP), and the National Phlebotomy Association.

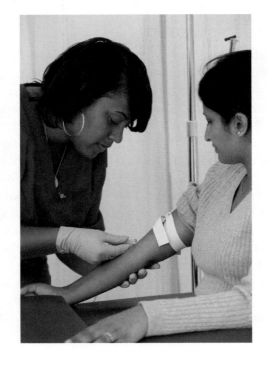

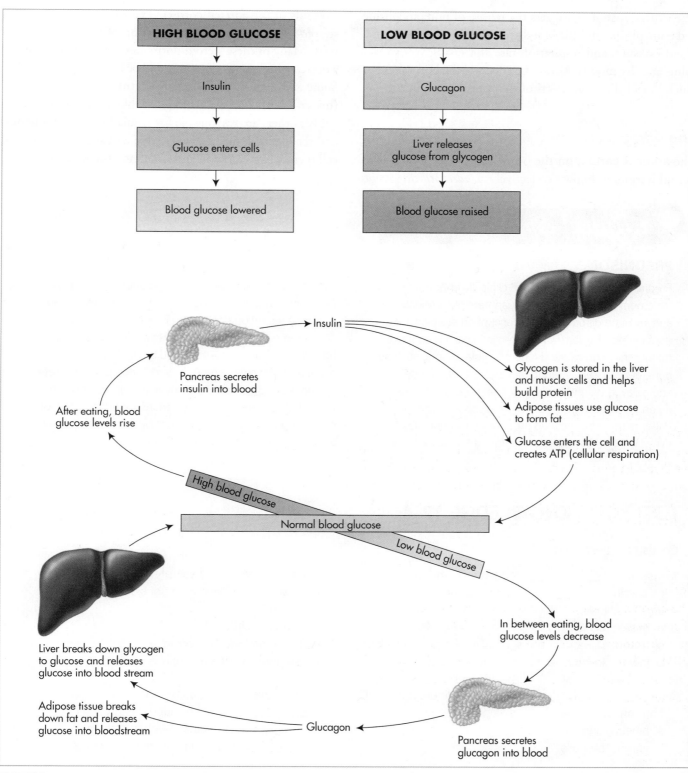

FIGURE 12–9 ■

Control of blood glucose by pancreatic hormones.

The neurotransmitter triggers the release of norepinephrine and epinephrine into the bloodstream, increasing heart rate, blood pressure, and respiration rate and giving you sweaty palms and dry mouth. Again, the effects of the hormones last much longer than the effects of the neurotransmitter.

The Adrenal Cortex

The **adrenal cortex**, on the other hand, makes dozens of steroid hormones known collectively as *adrenocorticosteroids* (steroids in the adrenal cortex). The adrenal cortex releases steroid hormones under the direction of the anterior pituitary. Many of these steroid hormones are so important that a decrease in their production could be fatal relatively quickly. Some of these hormones regulate electrolyte and fluid balance (mineralocorticoids); others regulate blood sugar (glucocorticoids); others are responsible for regulation of reproduction and secondary sexual characteristics; and still others control cell metabolism, growth, and immune system function.

Clinical Application

PREDNISONE

Prednisone (hydrocortisone) is clinically important in the treatment of inflammation, organ transplant rejection, and immune disorders, but prescription steroids are a double-edged sword. These medications are so powerful that they can cause dangerous side effects, such as bone density loss, weight gain, hair growth, fat deposits, and delayed wound healing. These drugs, even when taken for a short time, cannot be discontinued suddenly. Patients must be weaned off their medication slowly. Why? When a patient takes a steroid medication, the adrenal gland decreases steroid production in response. Remember negative feedback: As hormone levels rise, hormone secretion decreases. Therefore, if the medication is removed suddenly, patients are left with a severe hormone deficiency, which could be fatal. Their adrenal gland must be given some time to "gear up" to secrete hormones at the appropriate level. It is no surprise, then, that taking steroid medications for the purpose of increasing athletic performance is prohibited by amateur and professional sports organizations.

TEST YOUR KNOWLEDGE 12–4

Choose the best answer:

1. Insulin _____ blood sugar, whereas glucagon _____ blood sugar.
   a. raises; lowers
   b. raises; raises
   c. lowers; raises
   d. lowers; lowers

2. The _____ secretes many different steroid hormones.
   a. pineal gland
   b. adrenal medulla
   c. thyroid
   d. none of the above

3. Excess secretion of hormones from this gland can cause rapid heart beat, high blood pressure, and anxiety.
   a. adrenal cortex
   b. anterior pituitary
   c. thyroid gland
   d. pancreas

4. These two hormones secreted by the thyroid and parathyroid glands control blood calcium.
   a. T_4 and T_3
   b. T_3 and calcitonin
   c. T_3 and parathyroid hormone
   d. calcitonin and parathyroid hormone

5. Classify the following as type 1 or type 2 diabetes.
   _____ autoimmune destruction of pancreas
   _____ usually develops later in life
   _____ insulin may not be required

The Gonads

The chief function of the gonads—the **testes** in males and the **ovaries** in females—is to produce and store gametes, eggs, and sperm. However, the gonads also produce a number of sex hormones that control reproduction in both males and females, including testosterone in males and estrogen and progesterone in females. For more details on the hormones produced by the gonads, see Chapter 18.

COMMON DISORDERS OF THE ENDOCRINE SYSTEM

Anabolic steroids are a class of steroid molecules that cause large increases in muscle mass when compared to working out without steroids. Remember that anabolism is the building of molecules by cells? *Anabolic* means to build up. Some athletes use anabolic steroids to enhance performance or to develop big muscles much faster than they would without steroids. Because steroid hormone levels are so tightly controlled by the body, anabolic steroids have a number of side effects.

Think back to the discussion of prednisone at therapeutic levels; abuse levels are much higher. Men abusing steroids may experience changes in sperm production, enlarged breasts, and shrinking of their testicles. Women may experience deepening of the voice, decreased breast size, and excessive body hair growth. Steroid abuse may lead to cardiovascular diseases and increased cholesterol levels. Many steroids suppress immune function, and because steroid use is illegal without a prescription, many abusers expose themselves to hepatitis B and HIV when sharing needles. Steroid abuse has also been linked to increased aggressive behavior. All major professional and amateur athletic organizations ban the use of steroids.

Syndrome of inappropriate antidiuretic hormone secretion (SIADH) is a condition characterized by severe hyponatremia (low blood sodium), usually due to overproduction of ADH. It leads to fluid retention and very dilute plasma. The dilution of plasma leads to dangerously low sodium levels in the blood. Causes of SIADH include pulmonary disease, cancer, some medications, and central nervous system disorders. One of the most common causes of SIADH is traumatic brain injury (TBI). Symptoms of SIADH include confusion, altered consciousness, fatigue, nausea, muscle cramps, and loss of appetite. Untreated hyponatremia can lead to brain herniation and coma and can be fatal. Given that the symptoms of SIADH overlap with those of TBI, it is often difficult to diagnose SIADH. Also, since this is a disorder caused by too much water retention, giving

IV fluids may exacerbate the problem. Current research is aimed at finding better ways to diagnose SIADH.

Hashimoto's disease (also called *Hasimoto's thyroiditis*) is a form of hypothyroidism caused by an autoimmune attack on your thyroid gland. For unknown reasons, the immune system begins to attack the cells in the thyroid, causing inflammation and damage to the gland. This damage eventually leads to decreased production of thyroid hormones—hypothyroidism. In addition, the thyroid may swell, causing pain and difficulty swallowing. Symptoms of hypothyroidism include fatigue, feeling cold, thinning hair, weight gain, muscle pain and dry, itchy skin. Hashimoto's disease, like many autoimmune disorders, is most common in women between 30 and 50 years old. It can be treated by taking thyroid hormones daily.

Congenital hypothyroidism, in which babies do not produce enough thyroid hormone, can cause developmental disabilities. It can be easily treated with hormone injections. The disorder is relatively common. In the United States, babies are tested for the disorder at birth so they can be treated.

Graves' disease is also an immune disorder that affects the thyroid, but in this case the immune system stimulates the thyroid, resulting in hyperthyroidism. Symptoms include arrhythmia, irritability, and weight loss. Graves' disease can result in a potentially fatal condition called a *thyroid storm*. Treatment for Graves' disease involves decreasing the activity of the thyroid with medication. If medication does not work, the thyroid may be removed, and the patient must then take thyroid hormones. A goiter is an enlargement of the thyroid gland that may be caused by thyroiditis, benign nodules, malignancies, or iodine deficiencies. See **FIGURE 12–10** ■ for a comparison between the signs and symptoms of hypothyroidism and hyperthyroidism.

A **pheochromocytoma** is a tumor of the adrenal gland that causes the gland to secrete excess epinephrine. The symptoms of these tumors are what you might expect: an adrenaline rush. Patients experience severe headaches, excessive sweating, racing heart, anxiety, abdominal pain, heat intolerance, and weight loss. Pheochromocytomas are not generally cancerous, but they must be removed or the effects of excess epinephrine can be fatal.

Addison's disease is caused by insufficient production of the adrenocorticosteroid cortisol. The deficiency causes weight loss, muscle weakness, fatigue, low blood pressure, and excessive skin pigmentation. Aldosterone may also be deficient. Many cases of Addison's disease have an autoimmune etiology. Addison's disease is treated with hormone replacement.

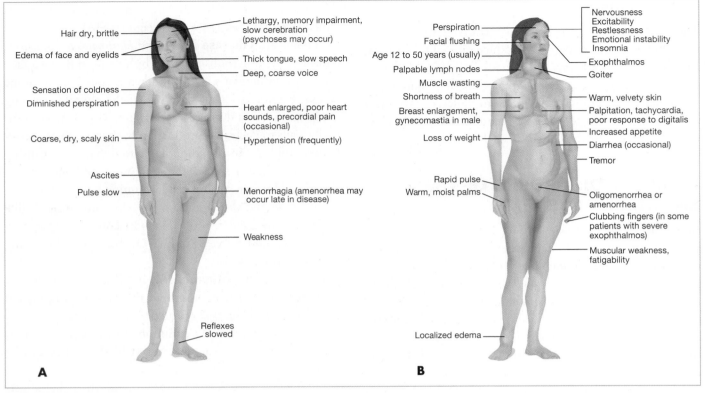

FIGURE 12–10 ■

A comparison of the signs and symptoms of (A) hypothyroidism and (B) hyperthyroidism.

Cushing's syndrome is caused by oversecretion of cortisol. Symptoms include upper body obesity, round face, easy bruising, weakened bones, fatigue, high blood pressure, and high blood sugar. Women may have excess facial hair and irregular periods; men may have decreased fertility and decreased sex drive. Cushing's syndrome may be a side effect of the medical use of steroids, like prednisone, or may be due to pituitary tumors, lung tumors, adrenal tumors, or one of several genetic disorders. Treatment depends on the underlying cause of the disorder. Typically, the cause of the excess production must be removed, and patients generally must take hormone replacement. **FIGURE 12–11** ■ shows examples of some common endocrine disorders.

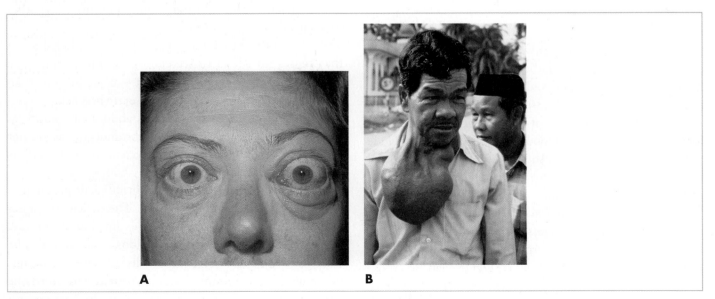

FIGURE 12–11 ■

Examples of endocrine disorders. (A) A patient with exophthalmos, a symptom of hyperthyroidism (Graves' disease). (B) A patient with a goiter.

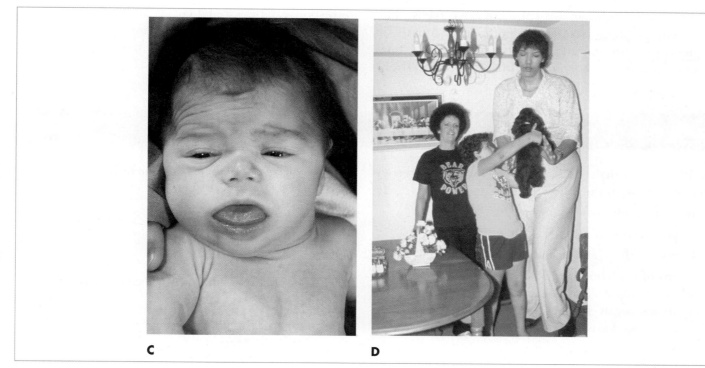

FIGURE 12-11 ■ (*Continued*)
(C) A patient with congenital hypothyroidism. (D) A patient with gigantism.

SUMMARY: Points of Interest

- The endocrine system works together with the nervous system to regulate the activities of all the body systems. The endocrine system is linked to the nervous system but works very differently. The endocrine system secretes hormones that act very slowly on distant targets. Their effects are long lasting. Some organs, such as the pancreas and the thyroid gland, function mainly to release hormones. However, many other organs, such as the heart and stomach, can also release hormones. They aren't considered primary endocrine glands because hormone release isn't their primary role.

- Most hormones act on cells by binding to external receptors, causing changes in enzyme activity inside the target cell. Steroids and thyroid hormones, however, can enter cells and interact with DNA, which makes steroids very powerful.

- Hormone levels are controlled largely by negative feedback. When hormone levels rise, signals are transmitted to the endocrine organ releasing the hormone, telling the organ to decrease the amount of hormone released. Hormone levels will then decrease.

- Hormone levels can be regulated via three mechanisms: changes in the body's internal environment (humoral), control by hormones released by another endocrine gland (hormonal), and direct control by the nervous system (neural).

- The hypothalamus, a part of the diencephalon, controls much of the endocrine system by controlling the pituitary gland. The pituitary gland has two parts: the posterior pituitary, which is part of the hypothalamus and actually secretes hypothalamic hormones (ADH and oxytocin), and the anterior pituitary, which secretes several different hormones under the influence of hormones from the hypothalamus. The hormones secreted by the anterior pituitary typically control other endocrine glands (growth hormone is an exception).

- Several other endocrine glands have important control functions. The thyroid gland secretes the iodine-containing hormones triiodothyronine (T_3) and thyroxine (T_4), which control growth and cellular metabolism. The pancreas secretes two hormones: insulin, which lowers blood sugar, and glucagon, which raises blood sugar. Diabetes is caused by a decrease in insulin secretion or decreased sensitivity to insulin. Very high blood sugar is the result.

- The adrenal glands are split into two parts. The adrenal medulla is an extension of the sympathetic nervous system, releasing epinephrine and norepinephrine as hormones during fight-or-flight response. The adrenal cortex releases many different adrenocorticosteroid hormones, which control reproduction, inflammation, tissue growth, and immunity.

CASE STUDY

A 50-year-old male patient arrives in the emergency department with the following symptoms:

- Recent weight loss
- Generalized weakness
- Excessive thirst and urination

Portions of his laboratory values show a blood glucose level of 280 mg/dL and acidic urine and blood. He has a family history of diabetes, but this is the first time he has experienced these symptoms.

1. What type of diabetes does he have?

_____

2. What organs will be affected if he is not properly diagnosed and treated?

_____

3. What treatment and lifestyle changes would you suggest?

_____

REVIEW QUESTIONS

Matching

1. Match the hormone or neurotransmitter on the left with the description on the right.

_____ ADH	A. decreases blood sugar
_____ insulin	B. increases thyroid hormone secretion
_____ glucagon	C. regulates cell metabolism
_____ oxytocin	D. increases steroid release
_____ epinephrine	E. increases uterine contractions
_____ thyroxine	F. decreases urination
_____ prolactin	G. prolongs sympathetic response
_____ ACTH	H. stimulates tissue growth
_____ TSH	I. increases blood sugar
_____ growth hormone	J. increases milk production in females

Multiple Choice

1. ADH stands for
   a. antidiuretic hormone.
   b. androdoginin hormone.
   c. American Department of health.
   d. all-diglyceride hormone.

2. The "master gland" is the
   a. adrenal.
   b. pituitary.
   c. pineal.
   d. pancreas.

3. The thymus gland's main function is for
   a. reproduction.
   b. growth.
   c. immunity.
   d. RBC levels.

4. The pineal gland is located in/on the
   a. kidneys.
   b. brain.
   c. thorax.
   d. abdomen.

5. Glucagon performs the opposite action of
   a. glucose.
   b. insulin.
   c. ATP.
   d. WBCs.

6. Some of these disorders are associated with weight gain: (I) type II diabetes; (II) hyperthyroidism; (III) Cushing's syndrome; (IV) Addison's disease. Which ones?
   a. I, II
   b. I, II, III
   c. I, II, IV
   d. I, III

7. If an adult patient is treated for gigantism by removal of her or his pituitary gland, which hormone would have to be replaced with drug therapy?
   a. thymosin
   b. melatonin
   c. thyroid-stimulating hormone
   d. insulin

Fill in the Blank

1. Glucagon _____ blood sugar.

2. Thyroxine _____ cell metabolism.

3. _____ increases uterine contractions.

4. Sympathetic response is enhanced by epinephrine secreted by the _____.

5. Increased secretion of aldosterone, a corticosteroid could be caused by a tumor on the _____ or _____ glands.

6. Damage to the _____ in the brain could cause widespread endocrine abnormalities.

7. This hormone is less important in adults than in children. _____

Short Answer

1. Compare and contrast neurotransmitters and hormones.

   _____
   _____
   _____
   _____

2. Explain negative feedback and its role in controlling hormone levels.

   _____
   _____
   _____
   _____

3. Discuss why the use of anabolic steroids should be outlawed for performance enhancement.

   _____
   _____
   _____
   _____

4. What is the difference between neural control and humoral control of endocrine glands?

   _____
   _____
   _____
   _____

The Cardiovascular System

TRANSPORT AND SUPPLY

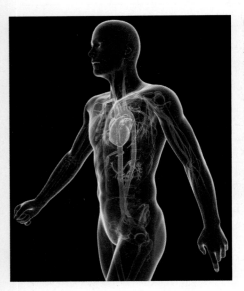

On our cross-country journey, we will see a series of rivers and streams and perhaps some canals. Historically, these waterways have been used as a way of transporting food and supplies to people. These very same waterways also had by-products of industry dumped back into them. This is very similar to the cardiovascular system, where nutrients and oxygen are transported to the cells in the body, and carbon dioxide and other waste products of cells' metabolism are filtered and removed. The cardiovascular system is also a lot like a hot water heating system in your house or hotel where you are staying. The furnace has a pump (heart) to circulate the hot water (blood) through the piping system (vessels) to deliver the much needed heat to every room throughout the building. So let's get right to the "heart" of the matter.

LEARNING OUTCOMES

Upon completion of your journey through this chapter, you will be able to:

- Identify structures and functions of the cardiovascular system.
- Explain the cardiac cycle and trace the blood flow through the vessels and chambers of the heart.
- Explain coronary circulation.
- Describe the conduction system of the heart.
- List the major components of blood and their functions.
- Discuss the importance of blood typing.
- Explain the process of blood clotting.
- Differentiate between arteries, veins, and capillaries.
- Explain regulation of blood pressure.
- Explain the relationship of the lymphatic system to the cardiovascular system.
- Describe various cardiovascular diseases.

Pronunciation Guide

Correct pronunciation is important in any journey so that you and others are completely understood. Here is a "see and say" Pronunciation Guide for the more difficult terms to pronounce in this chapter. Please note that even though there are standard pronunciations, regional variations of the pronunciations can occur.

agglutinate (ah GLUE tin ate)
albumin (al BYOO men)
anastomoses (ah NASS toh MOE sis)
anemia (ah NEE mee ah)
aneurysm (AN yoo riz em)
arterioles (are TEE ree ohlz)
arteriosclerosis (are TEE ree oh skleh ROH sis)
atherosclerosis (ATH er oh skleh ROH sis)
atrioventricular node
  (AY tree oh vehn TRIK yoo lahr)
atrium; atria (AY tree um; AY tree ah)
autorhythmicity (AW toe rith MIH sih tee)
basophils (BAY soh filz)
bundle of His (HISS)
capillaries (KAP ih lair eez)
cor pulmonale (KOR pull moh NAH lee)
diastole (dye ASS toe lee)
embolus (EM boh lus)
endocardium (EHN doh KAR dee um)
eosinophils (EE oh SIN oh filz)
erythrocytes (eh RITH roh sights)
fibrinogen (fye BRINN oh jenn)
hemophilia (HEE moh FILL ee ah)

hemopoiesis (HEE moh poy EE sus)
hemostasis (HEE moh STAY sis)
infarct (in FARKT)
inotropism (EYE no TROPE iz em)
ischemia (iss KEE mee ah)
leukocytes (LOO koh sights)
lysosomes (LIE so soamz)
phagocytosis (fag oh sigh TOH sis)
plaque (plack)
polycythemia (PALL ee sigh THEE mee ah)
prothrombin (pro THROM bin)
septum wall (SEHP tum)
sinoatrial (SIGN oh AYE tree al)
systole (SIS toh lee)
thrombin (THROM bin)
thrombocytes (THROM boh sights)
thrombocytopenia
  (THROM boh SIGH toh PEE nee ah)
tunica externa (TOO nik ah ex TERN ah)
tunica interna (TOO nik ah in TERN ah)
tunica media (TOO nik ah mee DEE ah)
venules (VEHN yulz)

SYSTEM OVERVIEW

The cardiovascular system includes the heart, blood, and blood vessels. The circulatory system can include the cardiovascular system, which will be discussed directly, and the lymphatic system, which will be further covered in the immune system chapter. The cardiovascular system has four main functions. First, it is designed specifically to transport blood to various parts of the body. Second, it pumps a variety of substances along with the blood throughout the body. Third, this movement of materials facilitates the delivery of vital materials, such as oxygen and nutrients, to the cells and picks up cellular waste for removal. Finally, the circulatory system returns excess tissue fluid, often in the form of lymph, to general circulation and possible elimination as needed.

The major components of the **cardiovascular system** include the *heart*, which is the organ that pumps blood through the system; *blood*, which is a form of connective tissue comprised of a fluid component (**plasma**) and a variety of cells and substances; and *blood vessels*, a network of passageways to transport the blood to and from the body's cells.

Circulation is the movement of blood to and from the heart. Circulation can be split into two systems: *pulmonary circulation*, from the heart to the lungs and back to the heart, and *systemic circulation*, from the heart to the body tissues and back to the heart. Regardless of whether you are considering systemic or pulmonary circulation, the vessels that carry blood *away* from the heart are called **arteries**. These main vessels branch out into ever smaller vessels called **arterioles**, which eventually divide and become even smaller **capillaries**. Capillaries are where the exchange of nutrients, gases, and waste products occurs at the cellular level. Capillaries deliver oxygenated blood to the body's tissues and take away carbon dioxide to be exhaled by the lungs. At the lungs, the opposite occurs. The capillaries drop off carbon dioxide to be exhaled and leave with freshly oxygenated blood to then be carried to the tissues. Capillaries are also the transition vessels where blood begins its trip back to the heart through ever-merging vessels, the tiniest of which are called **venules**, that merge to form the larger **veins**. To view this transitional region along with the cardiovascular system, see **FIGURE 13–1** ■.

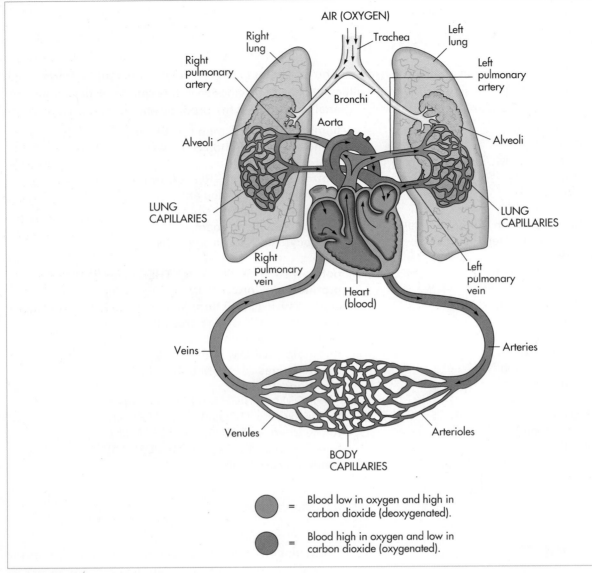

AIR (OXYGEN)

Right lung
Trachea
Left lung

Right pulmonary artery
Left pulmonary artery

Bronchi

Aorta

Alveoli
Alveoli

LUNG CAPILLARIES
LUNG CAPILLARIES

Right pulmonary vein
Left pulmonary vein

Heart (blood)

Veins
Arteries

Venules
Arterioles

BODY CAPILLARIES

= Blood low in oxygen and high in carbon dioxide (deoxygenated).

= Blood high in oxygen and low in carbon dioxide (oxygenated).

FIGURE 13–1 ■

Overview of the cardiovascular system.

LEARNING HINT

Arteries or Veins?

Remembering what arteries and veins do can be confusing. One easy way to remember is that arteries take blood *away* from the heart. Both words start with *a*. Obviously, then, veins have to bring blood back to the heart.

In general, veins differ from arteries not only because veins bring blood *back* to the heart but also because the blood is now deoxygenated (contains less than a normal arterial amount of oxygen) and has a higher level of carbon dioxide and other waste products of cellular metabolism. Veins also have thinner walls than arteries, have one-way valves on their

APPLIED SCIENCE

Color-Coded Blood

Notice in Figure 13–1 that blood is depicted as being blue or red, depending on the area in which it is located. When the blood contains high amounts of oxygen (oxygenated), it causes a chemical change within the red blood cells. This occurs in the blood of most arteries. As a result of that change, the arterial blood turns a bright red color. As the oxygen is being delivered to the tissues in the body, the blood begins to turn darker red. This occurs mostly in the veins that have lower levels of oxygen (deoxygenated) due to their delivery or dumping of oxygen to the tissues. You can see the darker veins within your wrist or arms as they appear to have a bluish tint through the skin. However, when you cut a vein, the blood is no longer darker red because it immediately mixes with the oxygen in the atmosphere and becomes bright red.

inner surface to prevent a backflow of blood, are more numerous, and have a larger capacity to hold blood. The movement of blood back to the heart is enhanced by the *skeletal muscle pump*. Working in conjunction with the one-way valves in the veins, repeated contraction of skeletal muscles squeeze the veins, thus increasing blood pressure in that area. The one-way valves closer to the heart open, allowing blood to move forward toward the heart while the valves farther away from the heart close, thus preventing a backflow. This increase in pressure forces the blood to move toward the heart.

INCREDIBLE PUMPS: THE HEART

Let's begin our journey with the main organ of the cardiovascular system: the heart. Although it is often described as the "pump" of the cardiovascular system, you will soon see that it is actually *two* pumps working together.

General Structure and Function

The heart is a specially shaped muscle about the size of your fist and is located slightly left of the center of your chest and above your diaphragm. The heart is surrounded by a tough membrane, the **fibrous pericardium**. Inside the fibrous pericardium is the **serous pericardium**. The parietal layer of the serous pericardium lines the fibrous pericardium. The visceral layer is fused to the heart surface, and there is a very fine space between the layers called the **pericardial cavity**. The outer layer of the heart wall, the same layer as the visceral pericardium, is also known as the **epicardium**. The middle layer of the heart wall, the **myocardium**, is made of cardiac muscle. The heart is lined by epithelium, called the **endocardium**. See **FIGURE 13–2** ■.

As strange as it may initially appear, the **base** of the heart is proximal to your head, whereas the **apex** of the heart is distal. Although the heart is a single organ, it is easier to

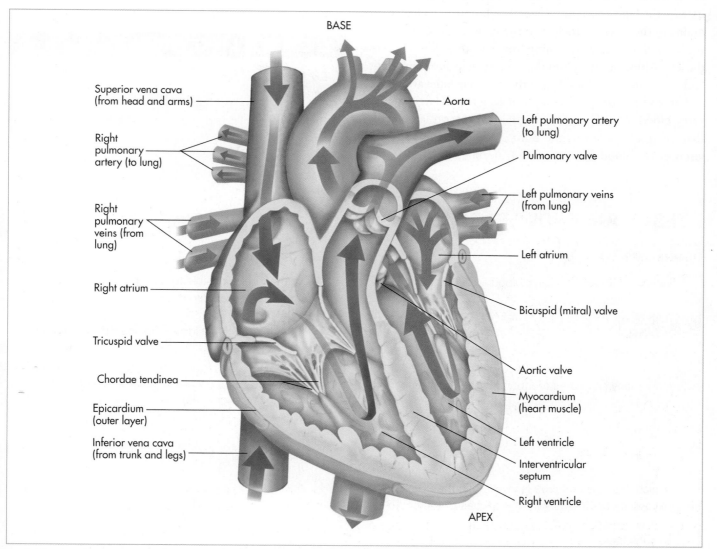

BASE

Superior vena cava (from head and arms)

Right pulmonary artery (to lung)

Right pulmonary veins (from lung)

Right atrium

Tricuspid valve

Chordae tendinea

Epicardium (outer layer)

Inferior vena cava (from trunk and legs)

Aorta

Left pulmonary artery (to lung)

Pulmonary valve

Left pulmonary veins (from lung)

Left atrium

Bicuspid (mitral) valve

Aortic valve

Myocardium (heart muscle)

Left ventricle

Interventricular septum

Right ventricle

APEX

FIGURE 13–2 ■

Anatomy of the heart. Remember: It is labeled right and left based on the patient's perspective.

understand its function if you think of it as *two separate pumps working together*. The right side of the heart is responsible for collecting blood from the body and sending it to the lungs to pick up oxygen and get rid of carbon dioxide. The left side of the heart collects blood from the lungs and pumps it through the body.

Opening the heart reveals four chambers (see Figure 13–2). The small upper chambers are the **atria**; the large lower chambers are the **ventricles**. The chambers of the right side of the heart are separated from the chambers of the left side of the heart, so there is no mixing of blood from one side to the other. The wall that separates the two atria is called the *interatrial* **septum**, and the wall between the ventricles is called the *interventricular* **septum**. When looking at Figure 13–2, notice the small chamber in the upper left quadrant of the picture. That is the *right* atrium (remember, locations are based on the *patient's* perspective). This is a collecting chamber where blood is returned to the heart via large veins after its trip through the body. Once the blood is collected, it drains to the *right* ventricle. On the upper right quadrant is the left atrium. Blood returning from the lungs flows into to the left atrium and then into the left ventricle. From the right and left ventricles, blood leaves the heart via large arteries.

Large veins bring blood to the atria, whereas large arteries carry blood away from the ventricles. The two large veins that bring the blood to the right atrium are the **superior vena cava** (blood from the head, neck, chest, and upper extremities) and **inferior vena cava** (blood from the trunk, organs, abdomen, pelvic region, and lower extremities). The large veins that bring blood back to the left atrium are the **pulmonary veins**. Large arteries carry blood away from the ventricles. The **pulmonary trunk** (which splits into smaller pulmonary arteries) carries blood from the right ventricle to the lungs. The **aorta** carries blood from the left ventricle to the body (again, see Figure 13–2).

To keep blood flowing in the correct direction through the heart, there are two sets of valves. The valves between each atrium and the ventricle on the same side are called **atrioventricular (AV) valves**. On the right side is the **tricuspid** valve because the valve is formed with three cusps, or folds. The valve on the left is the **bicuspid**, or **mitral**, valve. Between the ventricles and the large arteries that carry blood away from the heart are the **semilunar** valves. The *pulmonary semilunar* valve is on the right, and the *aortic semilunar* valve is on the left.

LEARNING HINT

Getting It Right

Tri = Right

Remember the Tricuspid valve is on the Right side of the heart.

TEST YOUR KNOWLEDGE 13–1

Answer the following:

1. Which blood vessels carry blood away from the heart?
   a. capillaries
   b. venules
   c. veins
   d. arteries

2. How many chambers are found in the human heart?
   a. one
   b. two
   c. three
   d. four

3. Which blood vessel type is involved in the exchange of oxygen and nutrients with the tissues of the body?
   a. arterioles
   b. sphincters
   c. arteries
   d. capillaries

4. The chamber responsible for pumping blood to the body's various organs is the _____.

5. The _____ side of the heart pumps blood to the lungs.

6. The _____ valve is located between the right atrium and right ventricle.

Cardiac Cycle

The movements of the heart, called the cardiac cycle, can be divided into two phases called systole and diastole. **Systole** is contraction of a chamber, whereas **diastole** is relaxation. During systole, a contraction is pumping blood out of the chamber. During diastole, the chamber is filling with blood. Both atria and ventricles undergo systole and diastole, but usually when discussing heart movement, we refer to *ventricular activity*.

When the right ventricle is full of blood, the ventricle contracts. Because the tricuspid valve is a one-way valve, as the right ventricular pressure increases, the valve shuts so that blood doesn't squirt back into the right atrium. As the pressure increases, the blood has to go somewhere. Now the only way for the blood to travel is through the *pulmonary semilunar valve* to the pulmonary trunk, which divides into the left and right **pulmonary arteries.**

Each pulmonary artery goes to its respective lung and branches down into ever smaller vessels to the point where they become capillaries that form a network around each air sac in the lungs. This is where the blood gives up one of the waste products of metabolism by cells (carbon dioxide) and picks up a fresh supply of oxygen from the lungs. These capillaries containing freshly oxygenated blood converge into increasingly larger vessels until they form the left and right pulmonary veins. **FIGURE 13–3** ■ illustrates the blood flow through the heart.

The pulmonary veins meet and pour their contents into the *left* atrium. When the left atrium is filled, blood flows through the left AV valve and into the *left* ventricle. When the left ventricle is full, the ventricle contracts (squeezes) again. The ventricular pressure increases, forcing the left AV valve shut and ejecting the blood out of the left ventricle through the aortic semilunar valve to the ascending aorta, sending it on its way throughout the body. Now the ventricles and atria can rest (**diastole**) as the atria fill with blood before they squeeze another load of blood into the ventricles. Remember, the chambers of the heart fill during diastole, or the relaxation phase, and eject blood during systole, or the contraction phase.

Amazing Facts

Pulmonary Arteries and Veins

True to what we have told you, the pulmonary arteries take blood away from the heart to the lungs. What is amazing is that they are the *only* arteries in the body that normally carry deoxygenated blood. The pulmonary veins collect this oxygenated blood and return it to the left side of the heart, and therefore it is the only vein to normally carry oxygenated blood.

Here are some points to remember:

- Both atria fill at the same time.
- Both ventricles fill at the same time.
- Both ventricles eject blood at the same time when the heart contracts.

Do you ever get yelled at or get mad at the *other* person for squeezing the toothpaste tube in the middle? What's the big deal? When you eat a freeze pop, do you squeeze it in the middle or from the bottom and work the contents up to your mouth? These two examples are important to visualize because the heart has to contract in a certain way to make sure that all the blood is squeezed out during each contraction. To do this, the contraction begins at the apex and travels upward. As you trace the flow of blood in Figure 13–3, you will see how efficient this is.

If you further examine the heart illustration, you will notice that the walls of the atria are thinner than the ventricular walls. This is because higher pressures are generated in the ventricles to move blood. You should also note that the walls of the left ventricle are thicker than the walls of the right ventricle. When you think about it, this makes total sense. The right ventricle has to pump blood only a short distance through the vasculature of the lungs and back to the heart. The left ventricle, on the other hand, has to pump all the blood throughout the body and back to the right atrium. The resistance of all those blood vessels in the body is six times greater than the resistance of the lung **vasculature** (network of blood vessels).

Coronary Circulation

It is obvious that the heart muscles need to have a blood-rich environment. In **FIGURE 13–4** ■, you can see that a portion of the newly oxygen-enriched blood is diverted from the aorta by the right and left **coronary arteries.** These arteries continuously divide into smaller branches, forming a web of interconnections known as **anastomoses**, which enable the heart muscle to constantly and fairly consistently receive a rich supply of blood. It is interesting to note that regular aerobic exercise can increase the density of these blood vessels that supply the heart. The number of anastomoses also increases, as does their number of locations. This is important for people with blockage of a small coronary artery. They have an increased survival rate because blood now has alternate routes to travel, which helps prevent heart muscle damage.

The right coronary artery provides blood for the right ventricle, posterior portion of the interventricular septum, and inferior parts of the heart. The left coronary artery provides blood to the left lateral and anterior walls of the left ventricle and to portions of the right ventricle and interventricular septum.

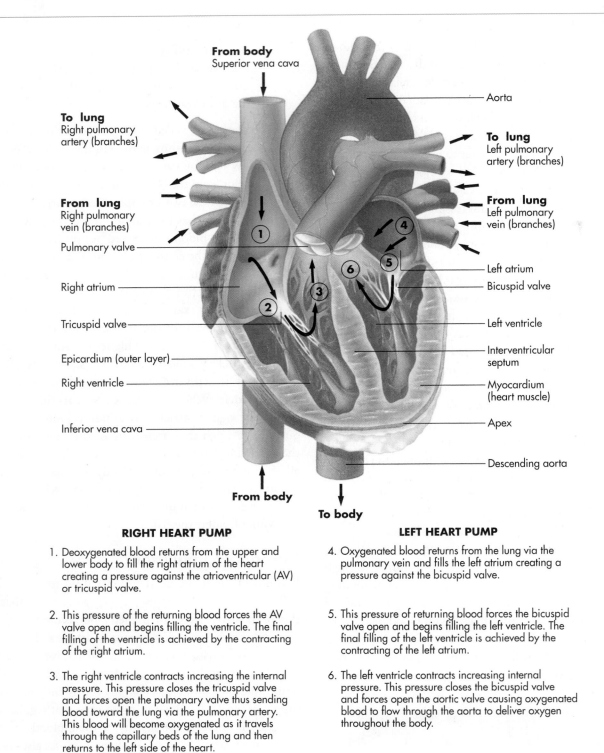

RIGHT HEART PUMP

1. Deoxygenated blood returns from the upper and lower body to fill the right atrium of the heart creating a pressure against the atrioventricular (AV) or tricuspid valve.

2. This pressure of the returning blood forces the AV valve open and begins filling the ventricle. The final filling of the ventricle is achieved by the contracting of the right atrium.

3. The right ventricle contracts increasing the internal pressure. This pressure closes the tricuspid valve and forces open the pulmonary valve thus sending blood toward the lung via the pulmonary artery. This blood will become oxygenated as it travels through the capillary beds of the lung and then returns to the left side of the heart.

LEFT HEART PUMP

4. Oxygenated blood returns from the lung via the pulmonary vein and fills the left atrium creating a pressure against the bicuspid valve.

5. This pressure of returning blood forces the bicuspid valve open and begins filling the left ventricle. The final filling of the left ventricle is achieved by the contracting of the left atrium.

6. The left ventricle contracts increasing internal pressure. This pressure closes the bicuspid valve and forces open the aortic valve causing oxygenated blood to flow through the aorta to deliver oxygen throughout the body.

FIGURE 13–3 ■

Functioning of the heart valves and blood flow.

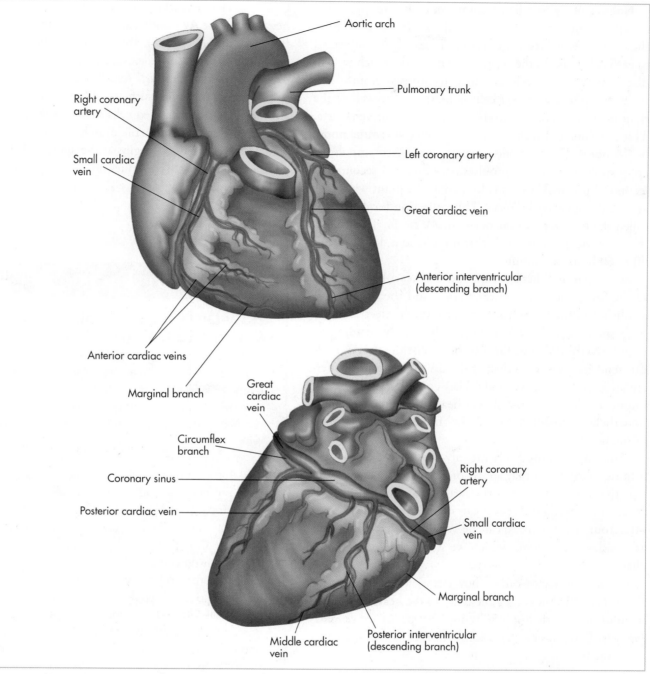

FIGURE 13–4 ■

Coronary circulation.

The Conduction System: The Electric Pathway

Unlike skeletal muscles (remember the neuromuscular junction?), cardiac muscles don't need nerve impulses or hormones to contract. In fact, they can contract on their own. This unique ability is known as **autorhythmicity**. The problem with this ability is that uncontrolled *individual* contractions would prohibit the heart from contracting effectively. This potential problem is solved through the use of specialized cardiac cells that create and distribute an electrical current that causes a *controlled* and *directed* heart contraction. Think of this as the electric company that supplies electricity to your home and the fine educational institution you are attending.

Nodal cells (also called **pacemaker cells**) are specialized cells that not only create an electrical impulse but also create these impulses at a regular interval. These cells are connected to each other and to the conducting network, which we will discuss soon. Nodal cells are divided into two groups. The main group of pacemaker cells is found in the wall of the right atrium, near the entrance of the superior vena cava. This collection of pacemaker cells forms the **sinoatrial node**, or **SA node**. The SA node generates an electric impulse at approximately 70 to 80 impulses per minute. A second collection of pacemaker cells is located at the point where the atria and the ventricles meet. This collection forms what is called the **atrioventricular node**, or **AV node**. The cells in the AV node generate an electric impulse at a slower rate of 40 to 60 beats per minute.

So, which one dictates how fast the heart beats? Think of the SA node as the power station and the AV node as a substation that supplies electricity via an electrical grid for a small city. The SA node sets the rate by sending its impulse to the AV node for distribution before the AV node can send its own. However, *if* the SA node cannot generate an impulse, the AV node takes control and sends out impulses that result in a slower heartbeat, but a heartbeat nonetheless. FIGURE 13–5 ■ shows the conduction system of the heart.

"So, why isn't my heart rate always 70 to 80 beats per minute, like when I play sports or get scared?" you ask. It's true that the SA node sets the heart rate when the body is at rest, but several influences can increase or decrease heart rate. Your heart activity can be regulated by the nervous and endocrine systems, which we will discuss later in the chapter.

On our journey we can see how electricity is moved in the form of electric lines along the road. In the heart, the movement of the electric impulses is done by specialized *conducting* cells. This power grid of electric distribution has to be set up so the following actions can occur:

1. First, the right and left atria contract together and *before* the right and left ventricles.
2. Next, the two ventricles must contract together.
3. Finally, the direction of the wave of ventricular contraction has to be from the *apex* to the *base* of the heart. This ensures that all the blood is squeezed out of the ventricles (remember the tube of toothpaste?).

So let's retrace the electrical "wiring," as illustrated in Figure 13–5. When an electric impulse is generated at the SA node, several pathways composed of conducting cells transmit that impulse to the AV node. A slight signal delay allows for the atria to fill with blood before contraction occurs.

Once this charge reaches the AV node, it continues its journey through the **AV bundle**, also known as the **bundle of His** (which sounds like "hiss"). Traveling down the interventricular septum, the AV bundle eventually divides into the *right bundle branch* and the *left bundle branch*. These branches spread across the inner surfaces of both ventricles. Finally, another type of specialized cells called *Purkinje fibers* carry the impulse to the contractile muscle cells of the ventricles. And so the contraction begins at the apex, and the wave of contraction smoothly continues up the ventricles, squeezing out all the blood.

Amazing Facts

How Does It Keep Going and Going and Going?

One of the amazing things about your heart is that it continues to beat day after day without you even thinking about it. Each day, your heart works to move blood 12,000 miles, which is FOUR times the distance between the U.S. east coast and west coast!

Here is a neat experiment. Previously, we said that your heart is about the size of your fist. Let's pretend that your fist is your heart. To mimic the pumping action of your heart, open your fist with your fingers fully extended. Now make a tight fist. Continue this action of fully opening and tightly closing your hand for the next *60 seconds*. Chances are good that your hand will feel like it's ready to fall off your arm! If this is how your hand feels after 60 seconds, how does your heart constantly beat approximately 100,000 times and move approximately 1,800 gallons of blood each day for decades and decades? Think back to Chapter 7 on muscles. Cardiac muscle cells have specialized connections called **intercalated discs**. These connections, along with associated pores, provide an efficient connection with adjacent muscle cells so electrical impulses, ions, and various small molecules can readily travel throughout the heart, allowing a smooth contraction from one area of the heart to another. The vasculature of the heart takes approximately 5 percent of oxygenated blood from each heartbeat to ensure there is a blood-rich environment with plenty of oxygen and nutrients available.

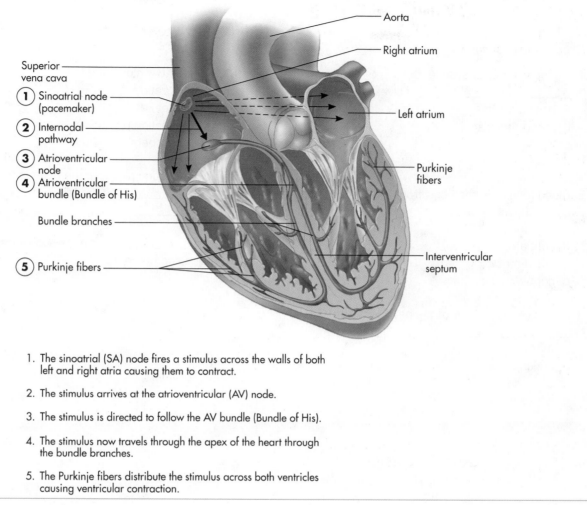

1. The sinoatrial (SA) node fires a stimulus across the walls of both left and right atria causing them to contract.

2. The stimulus arrives at the atrioventricular (AV) node.

3. The stimulus is directed to follow the AV bundle (Bundle of His).

4. The stimulus now travels through the apex of the heart through the bundle branches.

5. The Purkinje fibers distribute the stimulus across both ventricles causing ventricular contraction.

FIGURE 13–5 ■

Conduction system of the heart.

FOCUS ON PROFESSIONS

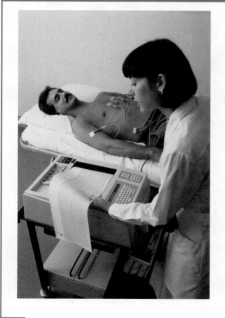

Cardiovascular technicians perform EKGs and other cardiovascular tests, such as Holter monitors, cardiac computerized tomography (CT) scans, cardiac catheterization, and cardiac magnetic resonance imaging (MRI). Learn more about this exciting profession by visiting the websites of national organizations, such as the Joint Review Committee on Education in Cardiovascular Technology (JRC-CVT), the American Registry of Radiologic Technologists (ARRT), and the Commission on Accreditation of Allied Health Education Programs (CAAHEP).

TEST YOUR KNOWLEDGE 13–2

Choose the best answer:

1. During ventricular systole, the
   _____ valves are closed.
   a. semilunar
   b. atrioventricular
   c. all
   d. none

2. Blood returns to the heart from the body via the vena cavae and into the
   a. left atrium.
   b. right atrium.
   c. left ventricle.
   d. right ventricle.

3. The main pacemaker of the heart is the
   _____.
   a. AV node
   b. Purkinje fibers
   c. SA node
   d. left ventricle

4. Cardiac valves close due to
   a. depolarization.
   b. pressure.
   c. cardiac action potentials.
   d. Purkinje fibers.

5. The contraction phase of the heart is termed
   _____, and the relaxation phase is termed
   _____.

6. The _____ arteries supply the heart with oxygen and nutrients.

Clinical Application

EKGs

Because the myocardial contraction is initiated and continues due to an electrical impulse, that charge can actually be detected on the surface of the body. This surface detection of the electric impulse traveling through the heart can be recorded by using an *electrocardiograph*, which records an *electrocardiogram* (*ECG* or, more commonly, the German form *EKG*). See **FIGURE 13–6** ■.

The normal EKG has three distinct waves that represent specific heart activities. The *P wave* is the first wave on the EKG and represents the impulse generated by the SA node and depolarization of the atria right before they contract. The next wave is called the *QRS complex* (a combination of *Q, R,* and *S waves*). It represents the depolarization of the ventricles that occurs right before the ventricles

contract. The ventricles begin contracting right after the peak of the *R wave*. Due to the greater muscle mass of the ventricles compared to the atria, this wave is greater in size than the *P wave*. The final wave is the *T wave*, which represents the repolarization of the ventricles where they are at rest before the next contraction. "Aha," you say, "where is the repolarization of the atria?" It occurs during the QRS complex but is usually overshadowed by the ventricles' activity. In the recording of a healthy heart, there are set ranges for the height, depth, and length of time for each of the waves and wave complexes. Changes in those parameters, or the addition of other abnormal types of waves, known as cardiac **arrhythmias** or **dysrhythmias**, can indicate health problems that involve the heart.

Clinical Application (continued)

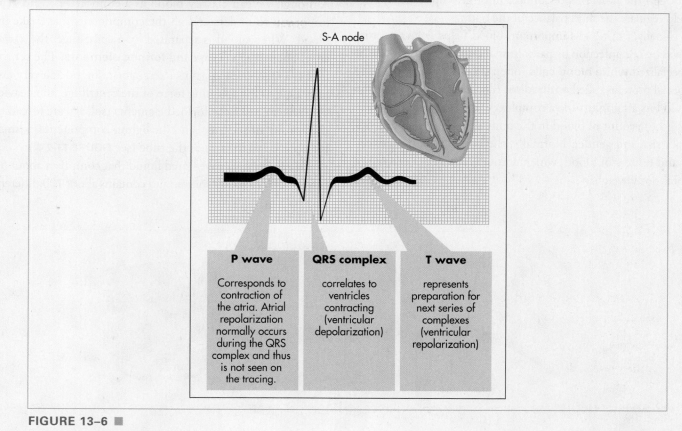

S-A node

P wave

Corresponds to contraction of the atria. Atrial repolarization normally occurs during the QRS complex and thus is not seen on the tracing.

QRS complex

correlates to ventricles contracting (ventricular depolarization)

T wave

represents preparation for next series of complexes (ventricular repolarization)

FIGURE 13–6 ■

Typical EKG tracing.

BLOOD

Now that we understand the pump, let's talk about what exactly is pumped. Blood is a fluid form of connective tissue that is responsible for three very important functions: transport, regulation, and protection.

Blood *transports* oxygen from the lungs, nutrients from the digestive system, and hormones from endocrine glands to the approximately *75 trillion* cells in the body. On the return trip from those cells, blood transports carbon dioxide and other waste products that were formed from metabolic activities of the cells to the kidneys, lungs, and other organs for removal from the body.

Blood helps in *regulating* a variety of levels in the body to maintain homeostasis. For example, the blood ensures that **pH** (levels of acidity or alkalinity) and **electrolyte** (ion) values are within normal parameters for proper cell functioning. Blood also helps regulate body temperature by absorbing heat generated by skeletal muscles, spreading it throughout the rest of the body.

Amazing Facts

What's in a Drop of Blood?

In *one drop* of blood, you will find *5 million* red blood cells, *250,000* to *500,000* platelets, and *7,500* white blood cells. Don't forget that there are a lot of other substances, such as plasma proteins, nutrients, oxygen, carbon dioxide, hormones, and electrolytes, in there too. These substances help to make blood *5 times thicker* than water. With a life expectancy of approximately 120 days, new red blood cells are created to replace old ones at the rate of *2 million each second*. Even more amazing is that the total surface area of all the red blood cells in your body is greater than the surface area of a football field.

Conversely, blood can radiate excess heat out of the body through the skin. Blood can take in or give up more fluid to help regulate the fluid balance of the body.

Finally, but no less important, blood helps *protect* us from invasion and infection by pathogens and toxins. This is done by specialized **white blood cells** (often shortened to **WBCs**) and special proteins called **antibodies**. Blood also protects us from fluid loss after injury via a complex process of blood clotting.

The amount of blood in the body depends on an individual's size and gender. Normally, the body contains between 4 and 6 liters of blood, which accounts for 7 to 9 percent of total body weight.

Blood Composition

Although we can classify blood as a connective tissue, it is important to understand all the components that make up blood. When blood is separated by a centrifuge, the *major* components are **plasma** and **formed elements**. The centrifuge is a machine that spins a test tube of blood at a very fast rate. Due to the spinning force of the centrifuge, the heavier components, like the formed elements (solids), are forced to the bottom of the tube, and the lighter component (plasma) is displaced to the top of the tube (see **FIGURE 13–7** ■).

Plasma is the straw-colored liquid that comprises about 55 percent of the blood's volume and contains about 100 different

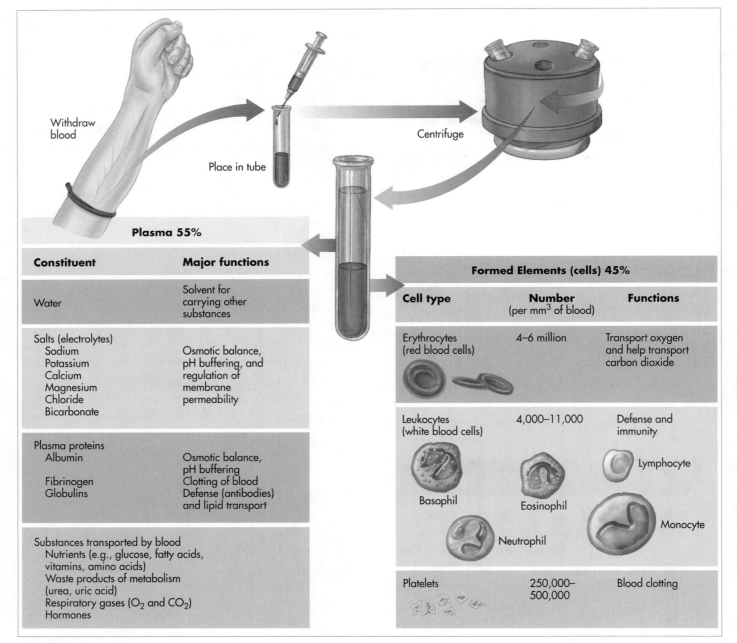

FIGURE 13–7 ■

Composition of blood.

dissolved substances. So, if your total blood volume is 5 liters, you have about 2.6 liters of plasma. Plasma is about 90 percent water; nutrients, salts, CO_2, and a small amount of oxygen is also dissolved into the plasma for transport to the body's cells. Hormones and other cell activity–regulating substances are also found in plasma. **Plasma proteins** are an important group of dissolved substances that includes **albumin**, which aids in controlling fluid balance; **fibrinogen**, which is a substance needed for blood clotting; and **globulins**, which form antibodies that protect us from infection.

Formed or solid elements include the following:

1. **Red blood cells (RBCs)**, or **erythrocytes**, which carry oxygen
2. **White blood cells (WBCs)**, or **leukocytes**, which protect us from infection
3. **Thrombocytes** (also known as **platelets**), which aid in clotting

Red Blood Cells

Lacking a nucleus, and therefore unable to divide to form new cells, red blood cells are created by the red bone marrow through a process called **hemopoiesis** (*poiesis, poietic* = making

or producing) and are similar in shape to a donut. On average, RBCs have a life span of 120 days and are filtered out of circulation by the liver and spleen once they are no longer useful. Reusable substances such as iron are saved while the remaining substances are eliminated by the body. Red blood cells perform two crucial functions. With the aid of an iron-containing red pigment called **hemoglobin**, red blood cells transport oxygen from the lungs to the cells in the body. Every healthy red blood cell contains between 200 to 300 *million* molecules of hemoglobin and each of those molecules has four potential sites on which to attach an oxygen molecule! In addition, the molecules help transport carbon dioxide, a by-product of cellular respiration (see Chapters 3 and 4), from the cells to the lungs for removal from the body through the simple act of breathing.

White Blood Cells

There are several types of white blood cells. Polymorphonuclear granulocytes originate from red bone marrow. Also originating from bone marrow, but maturing in lymphoid and myeloid tissues, are mononuclear agranulocytes. White blood cells are our guardians from invasion and infection (see **FIGURE 13–8** ■).

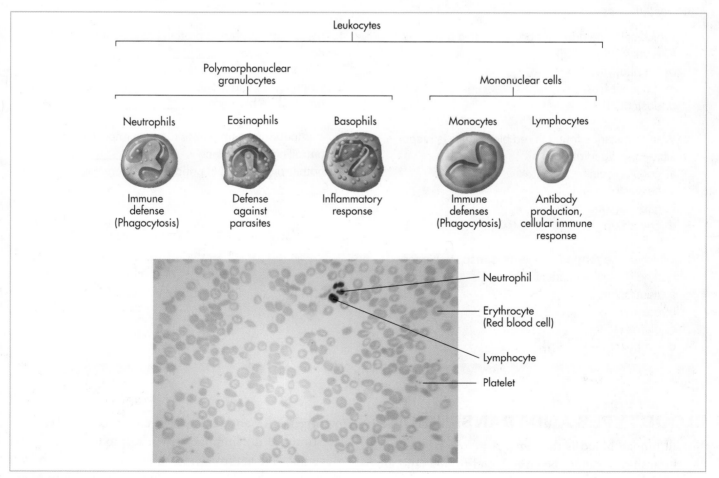

FIGURE 13–8 ■

Functions of white blood cells.

The types of white blood cells that compose the polymorphonuclear granulocyte group are neutrophils, eosinophils, and basophils. **Neutrophils** are the most aggressive white blood cells in cases where bacteria attempt to destroy tissue. **Phagocytosis** is the process in which neutrophils surround and ingest the invader and attempt to destroy it by utilizing organelles called **lysosomes** that release powerful enzymes. As an infection occurs, the body produces a higher-than-normal number of neutrophils. **Eosinophils** are utilized to combat parasitic invasion and a variety of body irritants that lead to allergies. **Basophils** are involved with allergic reactions by enhancing the body's response to irritants that cause allergies. In addition, basophils are important because they secrete the chemical **heparin**, which helps keep blood from clotting as it courses through blood vessels.

The types of white blood cells that comprise the mononuclear agranulocytes are monocytes and lymphocytes.

Monocytes are found in higher-than-normal amounts when a chronic (long-term) infection occurs in the body. Like neutrophils, monocytes destroy invaders through phagocytosis. Even though it takes longer for monocytes to arrive on the scene of infection, their numbers are greater than neutrophils, and therefore they destroy more bacteria. **Lymphocytes** are unique cells that protect us from infection. Instead of utilizing phagocytosis, they are involved in a process that produces antibodies that inhibit or directly attack invaders. The details are discussed in Chapter 15.

Thrombocytes

Thrombocytes, also known as platelets, are the smallest of the formed elements and are responsible for the blood's ability to **clot**. In addition, thrombocytes can release a substance called *serotonin*, which can cause smooth muscle constriction and decreased blood flow.

TEST YOUR KNOWLEDGE 13–3

Choose the best answer:

1. Which cell type does not belong in this group?
   a. erythrocyte
   b. lymphocyte
   c. monocyte
   d. eosinophil

2. What substance found in red blood cells is responsible for oxygen transport?
   a. gobuloglobin
   b. hemoglobin
   c. gammaglobulin
   d. cytoplasm

3. Which of the formed elements is responsible for defending against parasites?
   a. neutrophils
   b. eosinophils
   c. platelets
   d. lymphocytes

4. This important plasma protein helps maintain fluid balance of your blood: _____.

5. Lymphocytes and monocytes belong to this classification of white blood cells _____.

6. An important plasma protein that is important for controlling fluid balance is _____, while another protein that is needed for blood clotting is _____.

BLOOD TYPES AND TRANSFUSIONS

Not all human blood is the same. A person in need of a blood transfusion cannot be given blood from a randomly selected donor. Incompatibility of blood types is due in part to antigens. An **antigen** is a protein on cell surfaces that can stimulate the immune system to produce antibodies, which fight foreign invaders. Antigens are typically foreign proteins introduced into the body through wounds, blood transfusions, and so on. Because they are not "native" to the body, they are called "nonself" antigens. They differ from our own "self-antigens" that exist on the cell membrane of every cell in the body. The chain of events that occurs between antigens and antibodies is called the *antigen–antibody reaction*, which is the basis for immune response, as you will see in Chapter 15. Antibodies often react with the antigens that caused them to form, and this reaction causes the antigens to stick together, or **agglutinate**, in little clumps. Although at least 50 different antigen types are found on the surface of a red blood cell, our main focus is on the A, B, and Rh antigens. The A and B antigens and their antibodies are found in a group of blood types called the A, B, O blood group.

Everybody has only *one* of the following blood types:

- Type A
- Type B
- Type AB
- Type O

Type A blood is very common. Approximately 41 percent of the U.S. population has this type of blood. *A* represents a specific type of self-antigen that is found on the cell membrane of each red blood cell in the body of a person with type A blood. Because that person was born with type A blood, no antibodies were created to fight it, so there are no anti–A antibodies in that person's plasma. Interestingly, type A blood *does* contain anti–B antibodies.

Type B red blood cells possess type B self-antigens, and the plasma contains anti–A antibodies. Type AB contains *both* of the A and B self-antigens with neither A nor B antibodies in the plasma. Type O red blood cells contain *no* A or B antigens, but its plasma contains *both* A and B antibodies. (*Hint*: Think O = zero antigens.) This information is important to know if there is a need to transfuse blood. If the donor's antigens and the antibodies in the blood recipient's plasma agglutinate, serious harm and even death can occur.

If a *donor* gives blood that contains no A or B antigens, agglutination by anti–A and/or anti–B antibodies in the *recipient's* blood is prevented. Because type O doesn't have A or B antigens, it can be given to anyone, so a donor with type O blood is a **universal donor**. Because type AB doesn't contain plasma anti–A antibodies or anti–B antibodies, it can't clump with any donated blood that contains A or B antigens. Because of this, a type AB person is labeled a **universal recipient**. See **FIGURE 13–9** ■, which shows blood types with matching antigens and antibodies

and which recipient blood would safely match the donor's blood.

Are you with us so far? Good. Now there is one more thing we need to add: the **Rh factor**. Based on a discovery of a special blood antigen first found in the blood of rhesus monkeys, it was discovered that approximately 85 percent of the white and 88 percent of the African American population of the United States possess the Rh antigen in their blood. Individuals with this antigen in their blood are said to be **Rh-positive**. Conversely, those without this antigen are referred to as **Rh-negative**. When typing an individual's blood, the term *Rh* is eliminated, so an individual would be O-positive or AB-negative, for example. A problem arises when there is an Rh-positive father and an Rh-negative mother. If their first baby inherits the father's Rh-positive blood trait, the mother will develop anti–Rh antibodies (remember the foreign invader scenario?). This baby will be okay, but any future baby born to these parents may be attacked by the anti–Rh antibodies of the mother *if* that baby has the Rh-positive trait in its blood.

Amazing Facts

Coconut Juice Transfusions and Artificial Blood

There are reports that in the Pacific Theater during World War II, coconut juice was used on injured soldiers to bring their blood volumes up when there was a lack of real blood. The juice was supposedly sterile when taken directly from the coconut and transfused into their veins.

Currently, there is much research on the development of artificial blood or blood substitutes. The main objective is to develop a blood form that can be universally used for all humans without the need to match specific blood types. Other objectives include making a substitute that is free of blood-borne diseases, has the ability to be rapidly infused, has increased oxygen-carrying capacity, and has an extended shelf life. Some artificial blood is made by chemically altering and refining natural blood components, and some artificial blood is synthetic in nature.

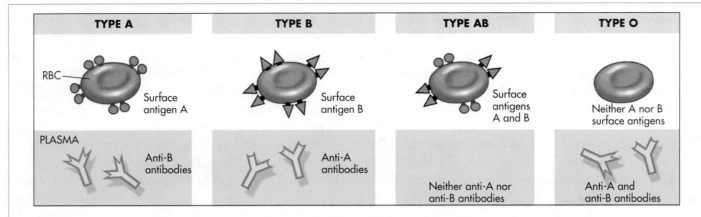

Recipient's blood		Reactions with donor's blood			
RBC antigens	**Plasma antibodies**	**Donor type O**	**Donor type A**	**Donor type B**	**Donor type AB**
None (Type O)	Anti-A Anti-B				
A (Type A)	Anti-B				
B (Type B)	Anti-A				
AB (Type AB)	(None)				

Normal blood   Agglutinated blood

FIGURE 13–9 ■

Blood types and results of donor and recipient combinations.

BLOOD CLOTTING

As we have discussed, the cardiovascular system is a closed and pressurized system. Imagine what could happen if a leak or a break in the system occurred. You have probably seen cars along the road with blown radiator hoses. The steam shoots out, and the car goes nowhere. A similar condition can occur in your body; no steam shoots out of your blood vessels, of course, but if enough blood is lost, you won't go anywhere and could die. Thanks to several substances in your blood, most leaks or breaks that occur can be stopped.

Hemostasis (the stoppage of bleeding) is accomplished through a chain of events shown in **FIGURE 13–10** ■.

Damage to the innermost wall of a vessel exposes the underlying collagen fibers. Platelets that are floating around in the blood begin attaching to the rough, damaged site. The attached platelets release several chemicals that draw more platelets to that site, creating a *platelet plug*. These platelets also release *serotonin*, which causes blood vessels to spasm, thereby decreasing blood flow to that area. Within approximately 15 seconds from the time of the initial injury, the

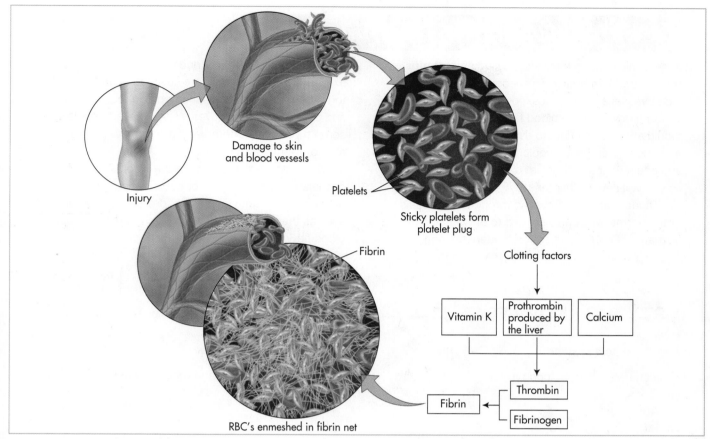

FIGURE 13–10 ■

The clotting process.

actual **coagulation** (clotting) of blood begins. A chain reaction starts with the help of calcium ions and 11 different plasma proteins (clotting factors). One of the clotting proteins, **prothrombin**, which is produced by the liver with the help of vitamin K, converts to **thrombin**. Thrombin transforms **fibrinogen**, which is dissolved in the blood, into its insoluble, hairlike form called **fibrin**. Fibrin forms a netlike patch at the injury site and snags more blood cells and platelets, and within 3 to 6 minutes, a clot is created. Once the clot is formed, it eventually begins to retract and, as a result, pulls the damaged edges of the blood vessel together. This allows the edges to regenerate the necessary epithelial tissue to make a permanent repair over time. Once the clot has outlived its usefulness, it is dissolved. Again, please see Figure 13–10.

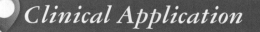

Clinical Application

CLOTTING GONE BAD

The chain reaction that causes a clot must be stopped when it has accomplished its purpose, or else clotting would continue throughout the vascular system. However, there are times when unwanted clotting occurs. A rough surface on an otherwise smooth lumen of a blood vessel may allow platelets to begin "sticking" there, forming a type of clot called a **thrombus**. A thrombus that forms in the vascular system of the heart can partially or totally block blood flow to

a portion of the heart, resulting in a coronary thrombosis, which can cause a heart attack. The degree of blockage along with the heart area affected determines the severity of the attack. If allowed to increase in size as more blood cells attach to it, total blockage of blood flow can happen.

Another scenario is the potential for a portion, or several portions, of the thrombus to break off and flow through the circulatory system like an iceberg

(continued)

Clinical Application (continued)

at sea. This floating thrombus, called an **embolus**, is not a problem until it travels down too narrow a blood vessel and becomes lodged, partially or totally blocking downstream blood flow. A cerebral embolus would affect blood flow to the brain, causing a stroke; a pulmonary embolus would lodge in the lung region and affect your ability to get oxygen into your blood, as you will see in Chapter 14.

Blood that is not traveling through the vessels at the normal rate can also lead to unwanted clot formation. People who are bedridden, on long

plane flights or bus or car rides, or immobile for extended periods of time are susceptible to thrombus formation. It also appears that women who smoke and use oral contraceptives, as well as individuals on some types of chemotherapy, are also at a higher risk for clot formation.

Substances that decrease the blood's ability to coagulate, such as aspirin or heparin, help prevent unwanted clotting. Once a clot forms, "clot busters," such as the drug alteplase, are given to regain proper blood flow.

TEST YOUR KNOWLEDGE 13–4

Choose the best answer:

1. The universal donor blood type is
   a. O.
   b. AB.
   c. Rh.
   d. B.

2. Blood type AB has _____ antigens and _____ antibodies.
   a. A & B; no
   b. O; anti A & Anti B
   c. Anti A & Anti B; O
   d. no; Anti A & Anti B

3. A type of unwanted blood clot is a
   a. bolus.
   b. thrombus.
   c. omnibus.
   d. skoolbus.

4. Blood clotting is dependent on a series of proteins called
   a. albumins.
   b. antibodies.
   c. clotting factors.
   d. thromboids.

5. When antigens stick together or form clumps it is termed _____.

6. The vitamin needed for normal clotting is vitamin _____.

BLOOD VESSELS: THE VASCULAR SYSTEM

So far, we have a pump and some fluid. We now need a way to transport the blood away from and then back to the heart. The arteries and veins we discussed previously now come into play.

Structure and Function

Initially, blood leaves the heart through the aorta, which branches into large vessels called *arteries*. Arteries divide into smaller and smaller ones as they spread out through the body.

The smallest form of arteries is classified **arterioles**. Arterioles feed the capillaries that form the capillary beds in your body's tissues. Here is where fresh oxygen and nutrients are supplied to the cells of your body, and carbon dioxide and other waste products are picked up by the blood for removal.

Blood from the capillary beds begins its return trip to the heart by draining into tiny veins called **venules**. Venules combine into veins, which eventually combine into the great veins (superior and inferior vena cavae) that empty back into your heart.

For most blood vessels, the walls are composed of three layers, often called *coats* or *tunics*. See **FIGURE 13–11** ■.

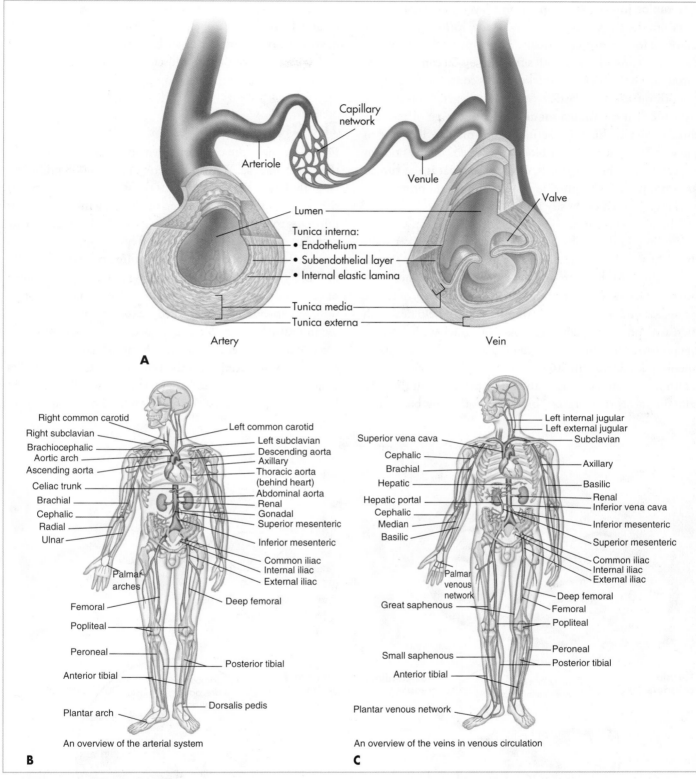

Capillary network

Arteriole

Venule

Lumen

Valve

Tunica interna:
• Endothelium
• Subendothelial layer
• Internal elastic lamina

Tunica media
Tunica externa

Artery

Vein

A

Right common carotid
Right subclavian
Brachiocephalic
Aortic arch
Ascending aorta
Celiac trunk
Brachial
Cephalic
Radial
Ulnar

Left common carotid
Left subclavian
Descending aorta
Axillary
Thoracic aorta (behind heart)
Abdominal aorta
Renal
Gonadal
Superior mesenteric
Inferior mesenteric
Common iliac
Internal iliac
External iliac

Palmar arches

Femoral
Popliteal
Peroneal
Anterior tibial

Deep femoral

Posterior tibial

Plantar arch
Dorsalis pedis

An overview of the arterial system

B

Superior vena cava
Cephalic
Brachial
Hepatic
Hepatic portal
Cephalic
Median
Basilic

Left internal jugular
Left external jugular
Subclavian
Axillary
Basilic
Renal
Inferior vena cava
Inferior mesenteric
Superior mesenteric
Common iliac
Internal iliac
External iliac

Palmar venous network

Great saphenous

Small saphenous
Anterior tibial

Plantar venous network

Deep femoral
Femoral
Popliteal
Peroneal
Posterior tibial

An overview of the veins in venous circulation

C

FIGURE 13–11 ■

(A) Blood vessels and the capillary connection. (B) Locations of major arteries. (C) Locations of the major veins.

The **tunica interna** is the innermost layer and is composed of a thin, tightly packed layer of *squamous epithelial* cells over a layer of loose connective tissue. The compacting of the epithelial cells provides a smooth surface so blood can easily pass through. The next layer is thicker and is composed mainly of smooth muscle and elastic tissue and collagen. This middle layer is called the **tunica media**. By contracting or relaxing those muscles, this layer actually controls the diameter of the vessels to meet certain blood flow needs of the body at a given time. The outermost, or external, coat is the **tunica externa**. Its job is to provide vessel support and protection, so it is composed of mostly fibrous tissue.

The differences in the structure of the blood vessels vary, depending on their job. Arteries possess much thicker walls than veins. As we said earlier, this makes sense because arteries are closer to the heart and have to deal with higher pressures. In fact, larger arteries contain complete sheets of elastic tissue, *elastic laminae*, in their middle walls to help deal with increased pressure. Veins can possess thinner walls because the pressure on them is lower than in arteries, but the inside opening, known as the **lumen**, is larger than in arteries. In addition, the larger veins of the body, especially in the legs, contain valves that prevent blood from flowing backward.

Remember, the venous side is lower in pressure. Another means the body has to help move venous blood toward the heart is through the use of skeletal muscle. The relaxation and contraction of skeletal muscles that surround veins help to "milk" the blood toward the heart.

The Capillaries

Finally, we have the capillaries, which are composed of only the tunica interna. With a diameter of only 0.008 millimeter (slightly larger than the diameter of single red blood cell), this wall is only one cell layer thick, allowing oxygen and nutrients to move easily into the tissues, and carbon dioxide and wastes to move into the blood. This is important because even at rest, metabolizing cells require approximately 250 milliliters of oxygen while producing almost 200 milliliters of carbon dioxide *every minute*. Dozens of capillaries form a web, or network, of vessels called a **capillary bed**. As you can see in **FIGURE 13–12** ■, capillary beds are composed of two types of blood vessels: a **vascular shunt**, which is a main road connecting the arteriole to the venule, and **true capillaries**, which make the actual exchanges with body cells. True capillaries can be considered the on-ramps and off-ramps to and

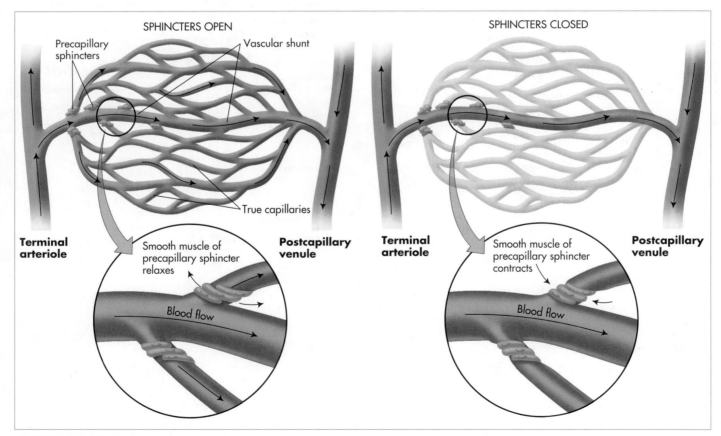

FIGURE 13–12 ■
Capillary beds and sphincters.

from the vascular shunt. In Figure 13–12, you will notice a group of structures called **precapillary sphincters**. These structures are composed of smooth muscle and act as tollbooths either allowing blood to flow through or stopping blood flow when they contract. If the blood flows through, it travels through the true capillaries and to cells of the tissue. If the blood is stopped at the precapillary sphincters, then the blood travels through the vascular shunt.

Regulation of Blood Pressure

Blood pressure (BP), like many of your body's functions is controlled to maintain homeostasis. As BP rises, homeostatic actions will bring it down back to normal, if BP falls, homeostatic actions will bring it back up to set point. Blood pressure can be homeostatically controlled by blood vessel diameter (**peripheral resistance**), the amount of blood pumped by the heart (**cardiac output**), and changes in fluid volume. Cardiac output is a function of heart rate and the amount of blood pumped with each contraction (**stroke volume**). Stroke volume is influenced mainly by blood volume. For example, increased fluid volume, increased heart rate, and increased peripheral resistance would lead to increased blood pressure.

Heart rate and stroke volume are regulated by the *autonomic nervous system*. The autonomic nervous system (both the sympathetic and parasympathetic divisions) has direct connections to the SA and AV nodes, as well as to the myocardium (sympathetic only). The sympathetic division can release neurotransmitters that increase the heart rate and the force of the contraction (**inotropism**). To counteract this, the parasympathetic division, through the **vagus nerve**, releases a neurotransmitter that can decrease the heart rate.

In addition, ions, hormones, and body temperature can influence heart rate. For example, as body temperature increases, so does the rate and force of contractions because of the increased metabolic rate of cardiac muscle cells. Conversely, as the body cools down below normal temperature, the rate and force of cardiac contractions decrease. Electrolytes are important players, especially when there is an imbalance of too many or too few specific ones. Low sodium or potassium can alter heart activity, as can abnormal levels of calcium. Low potassium can lead to a weak heartbeat, whereas high levels of calcium can prolong heart muscle contractions to the point where the heart can stop beating. These are just a few examples of what can happen when electrolyte levels are outside normal range. Age, gender, a history of exercise, or lack thereof—all of these can alter your heart rate. Normally, the resting heart rate for a female is 72 to 80 beats per minute, whereas the average resting heart rate for males is 64 to 72 beats per minute.

Peripheral resistance is controlled by the sympathetic nervous system. When blood pressure drops, sympathetic signals to blood vessels cause **vasoconstriction** (decrease the inner diameter or lumen), increasing peripheral resistance and increasing blood pressure. If BP increases, blood vessels **vasodilate** (increase the inner diameter or lumen) as needed to lower blood pressure.

Fluid volume is controlled by many hormones, including the antidiuretic hormone (ADH), as discussed in the endocrine chapter. All these hormones affect the kidney, causing either increased or decreased urination. Decreased urination increases fluid volume, thereby increasing BP. Thus, if you become dehydrated and your blood pressure falls, ADH will be secreted, decreasing urination and bringing your BP back to normal. For details of the role of kidney function on BP, see Chapter 17, "Urinary System."

Clinical Application

OSMOTIC VERSUS HYDROSTATIC PRESSURE: THE GREAT BALANCING ACT

Knowing that your circulatory system is pressurized and that capillary walls are semipermeable, did you ever wonder why blood doesn't continually leak out of them or how swollen tissue from an injury, such as a contusion, finally "goes down"? These are normally a result of an amazing balancing act between hydrostatic pressure and osmotic pressure. *Hydrostatic pressure* is the force that the liquid portion of blood exerts on the inner wall of blood vessel trying to "push" fluid through the wall and out into surrounding tissue. Normally, a hydrostatic pressure of 10 to 15 mmHg tends to push fluid out of the capillaries and into surrounding tissue. To counteract this "pushing" force, plasma proteins in the blood (albumin and globulin particles), which are too large to pass though the vessel wall, create what is called *colloid osmotic pressure* (also known as *oncotic pressure*). This "pulling" force, which is normally 25 to 30 mmHg, tends to draw fluid from the tissues back into the blood vessels because it is a greater force than the hydrostatic pressure. Whenever hydrostatic pressure is greater than oncotic pressure, fluid "leaks out." Whenever oncotic pressure is greater than hydrostatic pressure, fluid is drawn back into the blood vessels.

Clinical Application

TAKING A BLOOD PRESSURE

An important diagnostic test is the determination of arterial blood pressure (BP). This is done with a stethoscope and a sphygmomanometer. As shown in **FIGURE 13–13** ■, an inflatable cuff is placed around the arm, above the elbow, so when the cuff is inflated, it squeezes the brachial artery shut. Your stethoscope is placed over the brachial artery in the proximity of the inner bend of the patient's elbow. The cuff can then be inflated by repeatedly squeezing the bulb while listening with the stethoscope. As you listen while you inflate the cuff, continue squeezing the bulb until you raise the pressure to about 30 millimeters of mercury (mm Hg) *beyond* the point that the pulse is no longer heard.

When the pressure is 30 mm Hg above the point where the pulse sound is lost, the release valve is opened *slightly* so the cuff slowly deflates as you listen to the brachial artery. As the cuff pressure decreases to slightly below systolic pressure (pressure when the heart contracts), the sound of blood being pushed through the artery by the heart can be heard because the arterial pressure is now greater than cuff pressure. This is the peak systolic pressure, or top number of the BP reading.

As the cuff pressure decreases, the sound intensity of the pulse decreases and then disappears. That point when the sound disappears is where the cuff pressure is equal to the arterial pressure when the

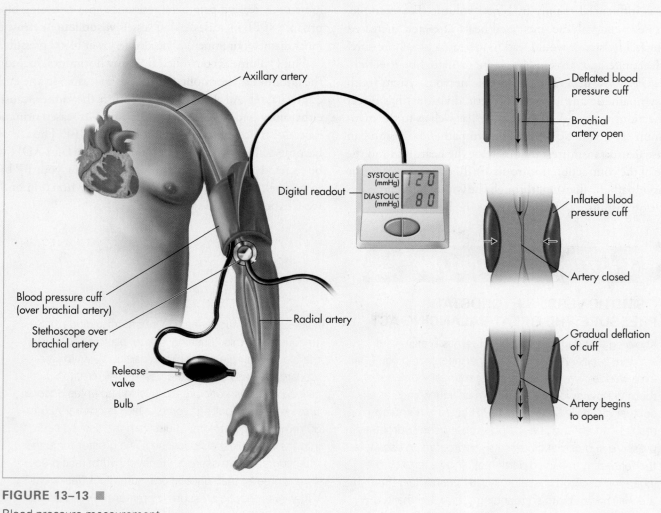

FIGURE 13–13 ■

Blood pressure measurement.

heart is at rest (diastole). This is the bottom number in the BP reading. Traditionally, one-twenty over eighty (120/80) has been accepted as a normal BP for healthy young adults. Recently, lower values are being considered as more in line with a healthy value.

Conversely, there is currently much discussion on what values constitute prehypertension. Time and continued study will tell which will be the accepted values. Please see TABLE 13–1 ■ to see where various values currently fall within low, normal, or high ranges of BP evaluation.

TABLE 13–1 BLOOD PRESSURE CLASSIFICATIONS

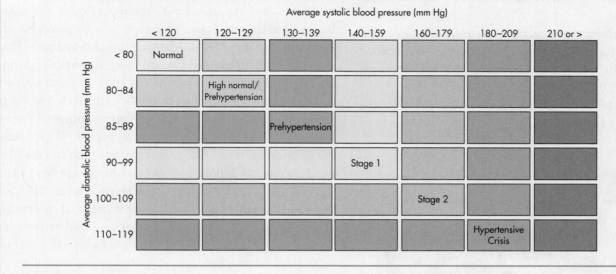

TEST YOUR KNOWLEDGE 13–5

Complete the following:

1. The smallest form of arteries are
   a. arterules.
   b. capillaries.
   c. arterioles.
   d. vesicles.

2. Vasoconstriction controls BP by causing
   a. decreased cardiac output.
   b. decreased peripheral resistance.
   c. increased cardiac output.
   d. increased peripheral resistance.

3. Which of the following is a regulator of BP?
   a. fluid volume
   b. cardiac output
   c. peripheral resistance
   d. all are

4. List the three layers commonly found in a blood vessel:
   a. _____.
   b. _____.
   c. _____.

5. The _____ is the layer of blood vessels that changes the diameter of vessels, controlling peripheral resistance.

6. The term used for the force of a heart contraction is _____.

THE LYMPHATIC CONNECTION

The lymphatic system, the topic of Chapter 15, has an important relationship with the cardiovascular system (see **FIGURE 13–14** ■). The lymphatic system runs parallel to the cardiovascular system and has three major responsibilities:

1. It helps maintain the body's fluid balance by returning interstitial fluid to the venous side of the cardiovascular system.
2. It assists the cardiovascular system in distributing nutrients and hormones that may not easily enter the blood system directly and assists in the removal of waste products from tissues.
3. It helps prevent infection and disease by utilizing lymphocytes.

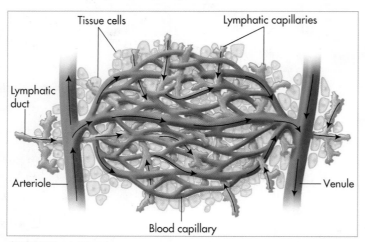

FIGURE 13–14 ■

Relationship of the lymphatic system to the cardiovascular system.

COMMON DISORDERS OF THE CARDIOVASCULAR SYSTEM

The following are several types of cardiovascular conditions. This section discusses heart problems, blood vessel problems, and blood disorders.

Pump Problems

So far, we have discussed how a healthy heart works. However, certain events can affect the efficiency of the heart's pumping action. Remember that this is a *two-pump* system.

What may damage one pump may not always damage the other pump.

Let's look at the right side of the heart first. **Right-side heart failure** (formerly known as **cor pulmonale**) is a potentially serious condition in which the right-side pump can't move blood as efficiently as it should. This is a result of the heart muscles working harder than they normally do. As with any muscle that you exercise, heart muscle also becomes larger.

In this case, the muscles on the right side of the heart become too large and can no longer efficiently pump blood. Remember that the left side is pumping normally, and we are working with a closed system, much like a water pump and cooling system in a car. As the left side pumps blood through your body and back to the right side, the right side cannot take all the returning blood to pump it to the lungs. As a result, the blood begins to back up. The vessels in the body are flexible and can expand a little to take that extra volume of blood, so extended neck veins can be a sign of right-sided heart failure. Certain organs can hold more blood than usual, so an engorged liver and spleen can also be signs. Tissues in the periphery can hold extra fluid, so swollen ankles, feet, and/or hands are also indicators of right-sided heart failure.

Disease conditions such as **polycythemia**, in which the blood is thicker than normal and is harder to pump, or blood vessels in the lungs that constrict more than normal, making it harder to push blood through them, can cause the heart muscles to work harder. Because these two conditions are related to certain lung diseases, it is no surprise that 85 percent of the patients with chronic obstructive pulmonary disease develop right-sided heart failure.

Left-side heart failure is a potentially life-threatening condition. The healthy right pump pushes blood through the vasculature of the lungs on its way to the left-side pump. If the left side can't keep up with the blood being delivered to it, the blood backs up into the lungs, increasing the pressure in those blood vessels. Once that pressure reaches a certain point, fluid leaks out of the vessels and into the lung tissue. Pulmonary edema is the term for fluid that forms in the lungs and causes difficulty breathing. See **FIGURE 13–15** ■.

Sometimes the heart muscle is fine, but there is a problem with one or more of the heart valves that seal off the chambers during contraction. There are two possible types of problems: either the passageway through the valve is too small (**valvular stenosis**) and restricts sufficient blood flow, or the passageway is too large and blood squirts backward into the chamber on contraction

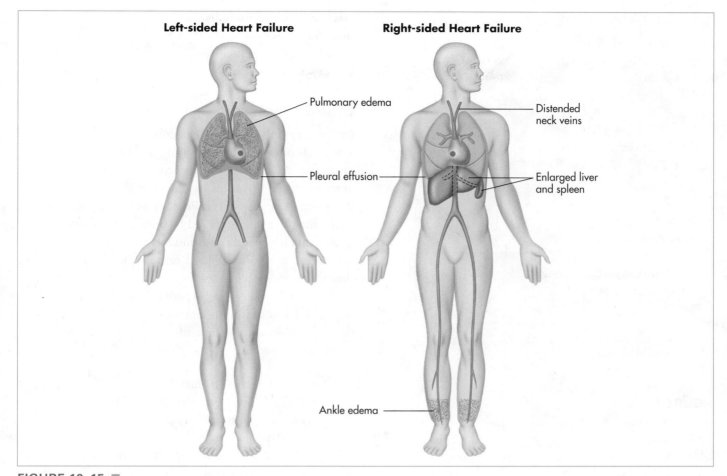

FIGURE 13–15 ■

Left-side and right-side heart failure.

(**valvular insufficiency**). A problem that can occur in either case is the increased tendency to form clots in the damaged valve area. Such clots can detach, flow through the blood vessels, and cause a pulmonary embolus in the lungs or can travel to the brain and cause a stroke. There are also potential problems with the small, specialized muscles called the *papillary muscles* that attach to the undersides of the cusps and contract when the ventricles contract so the cusps don't flap back up into the atria. The failure of the papillary muscles to properly contract will allow blood to flow backward into the atrium instead of flowing forward.

Vessel Problems

A common problem with blood vessels occurs to some degree for all of us as we age. **Arteriosclerosis** (*arteri/o* = artery, *sclerosis* = hardening), also known as *hardening of the arteries*, is a result of the thickening of the interna, which causes the involved vessels to become less flexible or even brittle. Blood vessels in this condition have a tendency to rupture. Because these vessels are less flexible and can't readily accommodate increases in blood volume, the body is more susceptible to high blood pressure.

Normally, blood vessels have a smooth inner lining, which promotes efficient blood flow by decreasing resistance. **Atherosclerosis** (*ather/o* = fatty or porridge-like) is a potentially life-threatening condition in which fatty deposits, called **plaque**, build up on the inner lining of blood vessels. As a result, blood flow can become greatly restricted or totally blocked. The fatty material that makes up plaque is composed mostly of **cholesterol**. Interestingly, all blood vessels are susceptible to atherosclerosis, but the aorta and coronary arteries seem particularly susceptible to developing this condition (see **FIGURE 13–16** ■). Note that cerebral arteries can also be affected.

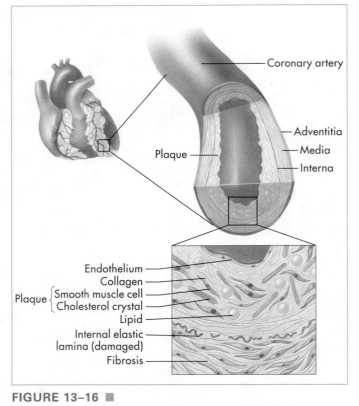

FIGURE 13–16 ■

Atherosclerosis.

If blood flow is restricted through one or more coronary arteries, heart muscle may become oxygen starved and cause tissue death. This would be a **myocardial infarct** (MI), or heart attack. If there is blockage of blood flow to the brain, a **cerebral vascular accident (CVA)**, or stroke, can occur. Reduced blood flow to tissues that leads to tissue *injury* but not tissue *death* is called tissue **ischemia**.

Heredity seems to be one factor for atherosclerosis, and atherosclerosis is also a common complication of diabetes. It is interesting that many medical professionals feel that diabetes should be classified as a cardiovascular disease. Diet and lifestyle also seem to predispose some individuals to atherosclerosis.

Arteries are designed to handle the increased pressures generated by a beating heart. In some individuals, those walls may not always be able to maintain their integrity. An **aneurysm** is a localized weakened area of a blood vessel wall that may have been caused by a congenital defect, disease, or injury. There also appears to be a familial tendency for abdominal aneurysms, which often present no warning symptoms. The danger is when the aneurysm expands to the point that it ruptures, causing hemorrhaging. If a major

artery is involved, an individual can bleed out in a matter of minutes. If the aneurysm is detected on an x-ray or ultrasound, surgical intervention can remedy the situation. Early detection is important.

Blood Problems

Secondary polycythemia is a condition in which chronic low levels of oxygen (due to lung disease or living in high altitudes) cause the body to produce more than normal amounts of erythrocytes to transport more efficiently the decreased oxygen available. **Primary polycythemia** does the same thing but can be caused by bone marrow cancer.

Anemia is a blood condition in which there is a less than normal number of red blood cells or there is abnormal or deficient hemoglobin, resulting in decreased oxygen delivery to tissues. Anemia can be a result of bone marrow dysfunction, low levels of iron or vitamins, or the improper formation of red blood cells. Individuals with anemia share these common symptoms:

- Pale skin tone (pallor)
- Pale mucous membrane and nail beds
- Fatigue and muscle weakness
- Shortness of breath
- Chest pains in some heart patients due to decreased levels of oxygen being supplied to the heart

Sickle cell anemia is an inherited condition in which red blood cells and hemoglobin molecules do not form properly. The resultant red blood cells are crescent- or sickle-shaped and have a tendency to rupture. As they are destroyed, the body is stimulated to produce greater numbers of red blood cells to replace them. Unfortunately, at that high production rate, the blood cells cannot mature fast enough. The ruptured cells also clog up smaller blood vessels. Clogged vessels combined with the increased thickening of the blood from excess red blood cells and cell parts lead to increased clotting and an impaired ability to carry oxygen.

Several blood problems involve white blood cells. **Leukemia**, usually due to bone marrow cancer, is a condition in which a higher-than-normal number of white blood cells are produced. You might think this would be a good thing; however, the problem is that the white blood cells produced are immature and therefore ineffective in protecting the body from infection. **Leukocytosis** also presents as a situation in which there is a higher-than-normal number of white blood cells. In this case, the cause is often an infection

Clinical Application

HEART ATTACKS

A true heart attack occurs when there is an insufficient supply of blood from the coronary artery to the tissues of the heart. This could be a result of plaque buildup in the arteries decreasing flow or a piece of that plaque breaking off and occluding the artery. If the decreased blood flow is sufficient to kill heart tissue, the condition is called *myocardial infarction (MI)*. You may think that the classic heart attack is when the victim clutches his or her chest in extreme pain and falls over. However, most heart attacks start out slowly with little or no pain (often called a *silent MI*) and may progress over a few hours, days, or even weeks, showing only subtle signs.

Symptoms that can be indicative of an MI are centrally located chest pain, chest heaviness, or vague discomfort; pain in the left shoulder or shoulder blade, neck, and jaw (where it mimics a toothache), radiating down the left arm; nausea, heartburn, weakness, or a clammy, sweaty feeling. Shortness of breath and/or dizziness can also be a warning sign. Women often exhibit "nontraditional" signs and symptoms, such as pain in the shoulder blade or jaw, and such symptoms are missed as indicators of a heart attack, often with tragic results.

Another big problem is that the victim often goes into denial, trying to explain away the symptoms as the result of some other problem, such as indigestion from eating too much or food that "doesn't agree with me" or feeling that it's a gallbladder problem or a pulled muscle. This can cost the patient valuable time in the treatment for a heart attack. Indeed, the first hour is when much of the heart damage can occur.

Call 911 *immediately* if you even suspect a heart attack. Research shows that an individual who is experiencing a heart attack should also immediately chew and swallow an aspirin tablet, preferably baby aspirins or a plain, nonenteric-coated adult aspirin. The anticoagulating ability of aspirin helps to keep blood flowing through the coronary vasculature, hopefully decreasing the amount of damage to the heart muscle. Most heart attacks are survivable *if* you act quickly and seek treatment immediately. It is better to be safe than sorry!

---

that is being fought. **Leukopenia** is a condition in which the number of white blood cells is lower than normal. This can be a result of drugs that suppress their production, such as corticosteroids and anticancer agents. Chronic infections can also wear the body down to the point that it cannot produce the necessary numbers of white blood cells.

Sometimes, there is a problem with the ability of blood to clot properly. **Hemophilia** is a general term used to describe inherited blood conditions that prohibit or slow down the blood's ability to clot. **Thrombocytopenia** is a condition in which there are fewer-than-normal circulating platelets. If the platelet count is low enough, even normal movement can lead to bleeding. This condition can be caused by liver dysfunction, vitamin K deficiency, radiation exposure, or bone marrow cancer.

- The cardiovascular system is a closed, pressurized system, much like the engine cooling system of a car, responsible for transportation of oxygen, hormones, and nutrients to the tissues of the body and for removing the by-products of metabolism by the cells. The cardiovascular system also helps maintain proper fluid balance of the body, assists in the control of body temperature, and is a major player in the body's defense from infection.

- The heart is an organ that is actually two pumps working together to move blood. The heart's right pump moves blood collected from the body to the lungs, where oxygen is loaded and carbon dioxide is removed to be exhaled by the lungs, while the heart's left pump takes the freshly oxygenated blood and pushes it through the body so tissue cells can be kept healthy.

- Arteries carry blood away from the heart. Veins carry blood toward the heart.

- Capillaries are blood vessels with walls the thickness of only one cell, which readily allows the transfer of oxygen and nutrients to the tissues in the body. This thinness of capillary walls also allows for waste products of the cells' metabolism to be picked up by the blood for removal.

- The major components of blood are plasma, erythrocytes (red blood cells, the main transporter of oxygen), leukocytes (white blood cells, protectors from infection), and platelets (aid in the clotting of blood).

- Blood pressure is controlled by cardiac output, peripheral resistance, and changes in fluid volume.

CASE STUDY

A 55-year-old male arrives at the emergency room, complaining about vague chest pains for the past several days. A quick patient history revealed the following: a two-packs-a-day smoker since the age of 15; height of 67 inches; weight 240; lives alone and doesn't prepare meals, preferring cookies, snack foods, and diet cola; sedentary lifestyle; uses oxygen daily to relieve shortness of breath; and complains of occasional chest pains.

a. Given these facts, what disease process(es) do you think this individual may be experiencing?

_____

b. Once the patient condition is stable, what discharge education and lifestyle changes would you suggest?

_____

REVIEW QUESTIONS

Multiple Choice

1. The valve between the right atrium and the right ventricle is the
   a. sinoatrial.
   b. bicuspid.
   c. tricuspid.
   d. semilunar.

2. During ventricular systole, these valves are closed.
   a. sinoatrial
   b. atrioventricular
   c. semilunar
   d. retroventricular

3. When cardiac output increases, what happens to BP?
   a. It increases.
   b. It decreases.
   c. It goes up and then back down.
   d. It doesn't change.

4. The _____ wave of the EKG occurs during depolarization of the ventricles.
   a. P
   b. QRS
   c. PDQ
   d. T

5. After the electrical impulse leaves the AV node it travels down the
   a. Purkinje fibers.
   b. left bundle branch.
   c. AV bundle.
   d. SA node.

6. During what part of the ECG are ventricles relaxing?
   a. PR
   b. T
   c. QRS
   d. PT

7. If a heart attack damages the interventricular septum, what part of the conduction system will be damaged?
   a. SA node
   b. Purkinje fibers
   c. AV bundle branches
   d. all of the above

8. An infection would generally cause increased numbers of which formed element?
   a. erythrocytes
   b. leukocytes
   c. thrombocytes
   d. antibodies

Fill in the Blank

1. List the three main functions of blood:
   a. _____
   b. _____
   c. _____

2. Decreased blood flow to cardiac muscle that only *injures* the tissue creates a condition known as _____.

3. The structures composed of smooth muscle that direct the flow through capillary beds are called _____.

4. _____ is an important vitamin that is needed for the proper clotting of blood.

5. _____ is a term used for the dividing wall between the ventricles.

6. Damage to the SA node causes a(n) _____ (increase or decrease) in heart rate.

7. A young woman falls, putting her hand through a window. She is bleeding profusely. To try to maintain her blood pressure, her heart rate will _____ (increase or decrease)?

8. Many endurance athletes live and train at high elevation because high elevation causes an increase in _____, which may give the athletes a competitive advantage.

Short Answer

1. Explain the control of blood pressure.

_____

_____

_____

_____

2. Describe the flow of blood beginning at the right atrium and ending at the aorta.

_____

_____

_____

_____

3. Explain the antigens and antibodies of the A, B, and O blood types.

_____

_____

_____

_____

4. Explain hemostasis.

_____

_____

_____

_____

5. List the types of formed elements and their functions.

_____

_____

_____

_____

6. What is one reason that iron is an important nutrient to include in your diet?

_____

_____

_____

_____

7. Why is the direction of the wave of contraction in the heart so important?

_____

_____

_____

_____

8. Contrast the terms thrombus and embolus.

_____

_____

_____

_____

Visit our new **MyHealthProfessions Lab** to accompany *Anatomy & Physiology for Health Professions.* Here you'll find a rich collection of quizzes, case studies, and animations for deeper understanding and application.

14
The Respiratory System

IT'S A GAS

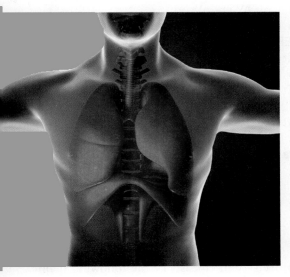

Without fuel, we wouldn't get very far on our trip. Our car won't start without gasoline, our plane would be grounded without jet fuel, and our bodies would die without the fuel necessary for metabolism—glucose. The respiratory system's primary function is to transport the oxygen from the atmosphere into the bloodstream to be used by cells, tissues, and organs for the processes necessary to sustain life. Remember, during cellular respiration, glucose is broken down to make adenosine triphosphate (ATP). Your body needs oxygen to "burn" glucose, just as your car needs oxygen to burn gasoline. This amazing system is often taken for granted. We don't even consciously realize that the respiratory system is moving 12,000 quarts of air a day into and out of our lungs. On our journey, the fuel for our means of transportation also produces a waste by-product, or exhaust. For example, our car produces waste gases that it eliminates through its exhaust system. The body also produces a waste gas, carbon dioxide, during metabolism that needs to be eliminated via the respiratory system so it does not build up to toxic levels. In this chapter, we explore the journey that oxygen molecules must take from our surrounding atmosphere to our cells and tissues. Hopefully, your journey through the respiratory system will be a "breathtaking" experience.

LEARNING OUTCOMES

At the end of the journey through this chapter, you will be able to:

- List the basic functions of the respiratory system.
- Differentiate between respiration and ventilation.
- Name and explain the functions of the structures of the upper and lower respiratory tracts.
- State the purpose and function of the mucociliary escalator.
- Discuss the process of gas exchange at the alveolar level.
- Describe the various skeletal structures related to the respiratory system.
- Explain the actual process and regulation of ventilation.
- Discuss several common respiratory system diseases.

Pronunciation Guide Pro·nun·ci·a·tion

Correct pronunciation is important in any journey so that you and others are completely understood. Here is a "see and say" Pronunciation Guide for the more difficult terms to pronounce in this chapter. Please note that even though there are standard pronunciations, regional variations of the pronunciations can occur.

adenoid (AD eh noid)
alveoli (al VEE oh lye)
atelectasis (AT eh LEK tah sis)
bronchi (BRONG kye)
bronchioles (BRONG kee ohlz)
capillaries (KAP ih lair eez)
carina (kah RINE uh)
cilia (SILL ee ah)
conchae (KONG kay)
diaphragm (DIE ah fram)
emphysema (em fih SEE mah)
empyema (em pye EE mah)
epiglottis (ep ih GLAH tiss)
erythropoiesis (eh RITH roh poy EE sis)
esophagus (eh SOFF ah gus)
eustachian tubes (yoo STAY she ehn)
glottis (GLAH tiss)
hilum (HIGH lim)
larynx (LAIR inks)

lingula (LING gu lah)
mediastinum (MEE dee ah STY num)
medulla oblongata (meh DULL lah OB long GAH tah)
nasopharynx (NAY zoh FAIR inks)
oropharynx (OR oh FAIR inks)
palatine tonsils (PAL ah tine)
parietal pleura (pah RYE eh tal PLOO rah)
pneumocyte (NEW moh site)
respiration (res pir AY shun)
rima glottidis (RIE mah GLAH ti diss)
sternum (STER num)
surfactant (sir FAC tant)
thoracic cage (tho RASS ik)
trachea (TRAY kee ah)
tuberculosis (too BER kew LOH sis)
ventilation (ven tih LAY shun)
vibrissae (vie BRISS ee)
visceral pleura (VISS er al PLOO rah)

SYSTEM OVERVIEW

Along your journey, you will undoubtedly have plenty of exercise walking to see the sights. Have you ever wondered why you feel out of breath or why breathing faster and deeper helps you recover from strenuous exercise? Our body uses energy from the food we eat, but cells can obtain the energy from food only with the help of the vital gas oxygen (O_2), which allows for cellular respiration. Luckily, oxygen is found in relative abundance in the atmosphere and therefore in the air we breathe. However, when the cells use oxygen, they produce the gaseous waste carbon dioxide (CO_2). If allowed to build up in the body, carbon dioxide would become toxic, so the bloodstream carries the carbon dioxide to the lungs to be exhaled and eliminated from the body. The respiratory system's primary role, therefore, is to bring oxygen from the atmosphere into the bloodstream and to remove the gaseous waste by-product carbon dioxide. As you can see from this discussion, the respiratory system works closely with the heart and circulatory system. Because of this relationship, these two systems are often grouped together in medicine to form the **cardiopulmonary system**.

The respiratory system consists of the following major components:

- Two lungs, the vital organs of the respiratory system
- Upper and lower airways that *conduct,* or move, gas into and out of the system
- Terminal air sacs called *alveoli* surrounded by a network of capillaries that provide for *gas exchange*
- A thoracic cage that houses, protects, and facilitates the function of the system
- Muscles of breathing that include the main muscle, the diaphragm, and accessory muscles

Please take a few minutes to look at **FIGURE 14–1** ■. We will explore each of these components as we travel through the respiratory system.

Ventilation versus Respiration

Before beginning our journey, it is important to pave the way with a solid understanding of some commonly confused concepts. The air we breathe is a mixture of several gases, as can be seen from **TABLE 14–1** ■. The predominant gas is nitrogen (N_2), but this is an *inert* gas, which means it does not combine

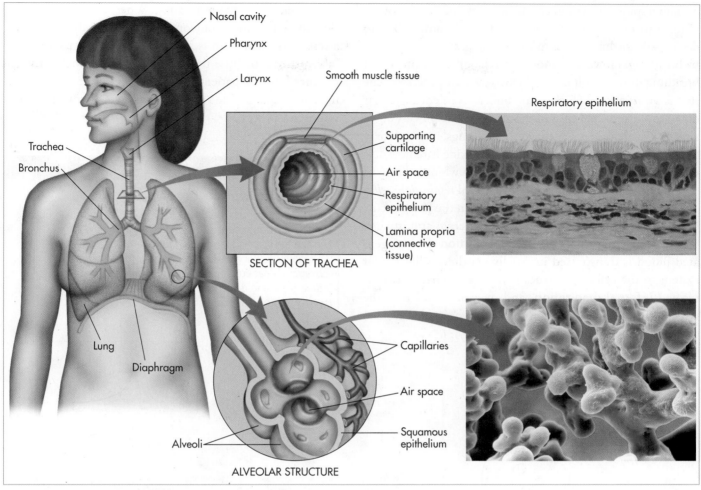

FIGURE 14–1 ■

The components of the respiratory system with micrographs of the respiratory epithelium and alveoli.

or interact with anything in the body. Even though nitrogen travels into the respiratory system and comes out virtually unchanged, it is vitally important as a support gas that keeps the lungs open with its constant volume. The next greatest concentrated gas is oxygen, and it is very physiologically active within our bodies. You'll notice that carbon dioxide is in low concentration in the air we inhale, but it is in much higher concentration in the air we exhale.

TABLE 14–1 GASES IN THE ATMOSPHERE

GAS	% OF ATMOSPHERE
Nitrogen (N_2)	78.08
Oxygen (O_2)	20.95
Carbon dioxide (CO_2)	.03
Argon	.93

Note: The atmosphere also contains trace gases such as neon and krypton.

Amazing Facts

Autocontrol of the Cardiopulmonary System

The cardiovascular and the respiratory, or pulmonary, systems function without any conscious effort on your part. You probably didn't realize it, but as you read the previous paragraph and these last two sentences, your heart beat approximately 70 times and pumped approximately 5 liters of blood around your body. During that same time, you breathed approximately 12 times, moving over 6,000 milliliters of air. Homeostatic control mechanisms, including the autonomic nervous system and the hypothalamus, regulate ventilation rate, cardiac output, and blood pressure.

The respiratory system contains a very intricate network of tubes that moves, or conducts, gas from the atmosphere to deep inside the lungs. This movement of gas is accomplished by breathing. However, a more precise look at the process of breathing shows that it is actually two separate processes. The first is **ventilation**, which is the bulk movement of the air down to the terminal ends of the airways. The process of *gas exchange,* which occurs deep within the lungs, in which oxygen is added to the blood and carbon dioxide is removed, is termed **respiration**. (*Note:* The process by which cells make ATP by breaking down glucose is also called *respiration: cellular respiration.*) Because the gas exchange in the lungs occurs between the blood and the air in the external atmosphere, it is more precisely called **external respiration**. The oxygenated blood is transported internally via the cardiovascular system to the cells and tissues where gas exchange is now termed **internal respiration**, and oxygen moves into the cells as carbon dioxide is removed. Therefore, ventilation is not the same thing as respiration. When you watch a television show in which someone says to place the patient on a respirator, that term is incorrect. The person should say "a ventilator" because the machine is only moving the gas mixture into the patient's lung (ventilating) and not causing gas exchange. See **FIGURE 14–2** ■, which contrasts these important processes.

APPLIED SCIENCE

Gas Exchange in Plants

Fortunately for us, the physiology of gas exchange in plants is exactly opposite that of humans. Plants take in the CO_2 in the atmosphere and use it for energy, then release oxygen into our atmosphere. The earth's largest source of oxygen released is the Amazon rainforest, which is unfortunately being destroyed at a high rate. We truly need a green earth to survive, so thank the next plant you see.

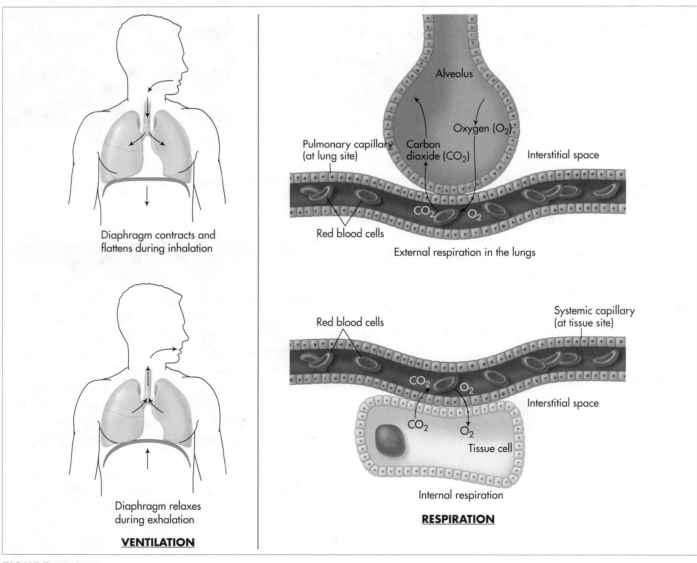

FIGURE 14–2 ■

Contrast of ventilation and external and internal respiration.

The respiratory system is responsible for providing all the body's oxygen needs and removing carbon dioxide. In fact, the body's oxygen reserve lasts only about 4 to 6 minutes. If that reserve is used up and additional oxygen is unavailable, then death is the obvious outcome. Therefore, the body must continually replenish its oxygen by bringing in the oxygen molecules from the atmosphere.

In a general sense, the respiratory system is a series of branching tubes called **bronchi** and **bronchioles** that transport the atmospheric gas deep within our lungs to the small air sacs called **alveoli**, which represent the terminal end of the respiratory system. To better visualize this system, look at a stalk of broccoli held upside down. The stalk and its branches represent the airways, and the green bumpy stuff on the end is like the terminal alveoli. See? Not only is broccoli good for you but it can also be a learning tool!

Each alveolus is surrounded by a network of small blood vessels called **capillaries**. This combination of the alveolar wall and the capillary wall is called the *alveolar–capillary membrane* and represents the connection, or for you computer buffs, the interface, between the respiratory and cardiovascular systems. This is where the vital process of gas exchange takes place. Before getting deeper into this process, let's trace the journey that oxygen molecules must take to arrive at the alveolar–capillary membrane.

THE UPPER RESPIRATORY TRACT

The upper airway is responsible for initially conditioning the inhaled air. It consists of the nose, mouth, pharynx, and larynx and performs several other important functions.

The upper airway begins at the two openings of the nose, called **nares**, or *nostrils,* and ends at the **vocal cords** (see **FIGURE 14–3 ■**). The functions of the upper airway include:

- Heating or cooling inspired (inhaled) gases to body temperature (37 degrees Celsius)
- Filtering particles from the inspired gases
- Humidifying inspired gases to a relative humidity of 100 percent
- Providing for the sense of smell, or **olfaction**
- Producing sounds, or **phonation**
- Ventilating, or conducting, the gas down to the lower airways

The Nose

Although some people do breathe in through their mouths, under normal circumstances we were meant to breathe in through the nose for reasons that will become clear as this discussion progresses. The nose is a semirigid structure made of cartilage and bone. Three main regions are contained within the space behind the nose, called the **nasal cavity**. The nasal cavity is separated into right and left halves by a wall called the *nasal septum* (or septal cartilage), made of bone and cartilage.

FOCUS ON PROFESSIONS

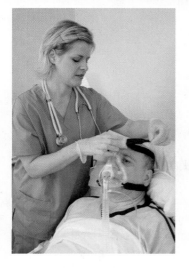

The **respiratory therapist's** main job is to ensure proper ventilation of the respiratory system through a variety of treatment modalities. **Perfusionists**, on the other hand, run a machine that actually performs gas exchange. For example, during a heart or lung transplant, the blood supply is temporarily rerouted through a respirator until the new heart or lung is transplanted. Because this procedure requires a lot of time, the rerouted blood must be oxygenated and carbon dioxide removed via a special mechanical membrane. Learn more about these two related and exciting professions by visiting the websites of national organizations, including the American Association for Respiratory Care (AARC), the National Board for Respiratory Care (NBRC), the American Society of Extracorporeal Technology (AmSECT), and the National Association for Medical Direction of Respiratory Care (NAMDRC).

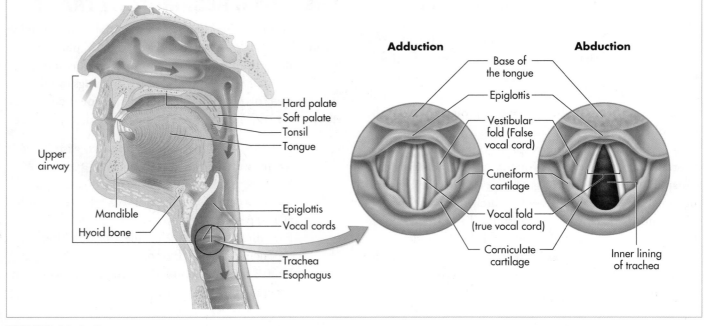

FIGURE 14–3 ■

The upper airway and vocal cords.

The regions contained within each nasal cavity are the vestibular, olfactory, and respiratory regions. See **FIGURE 14–4** ■.

The vestibular region is located inside the nostrils and contains the coarse nasal hairs that act as the first line of defense for the respiratory system. These hairs, called **vibrissae**, are covered with sebum, a greasy substance secreted by the sebaceous glands of the nose. Sebum helps trap large particles and also keeps the nose hairs soft and pliable—those unwanted nose hairs really do have a role as a gross particle filter. (By the way, "gross" in this case means *large*.) The vestibular region helps filter out large particles so they do not enter the lungs, where they could irritate and clog the airways.

The air from the atmosphere must be warmed to body temperature and must also be moistened so the airways and the lungs do not dry out. This is a job for the respiratory region of the nasal cavity, which is lined with mucous membranes that are richly supplied with blood. The respiratory region possesses three scroll-like bones known as **turbinates**, or **conchae** (again see Figure 14–4). These split the cavity into three channels, thereby providing more surface area for incoming air to make contact with the warm moist nasal mucosa. Whereas the respiratory region has a small volume of 20 milliliters, if you could unfold the turbinates, you would have a surface area of *106 square centimeters* (about the size of a 3x5 index card).

Amazing Facts

Breath Test May Detect Cancer

In the past, people have reported dogs that were able to sniff out cancerous (malignant) growths. Recent research by Israeli scientists is proving this to be not to be so "far-fetched." They are developing an electronic sensor that samples the breath and can detect lung, breast, bowel, and prostrate cancers by chemical variations related to the specific tumors.

The olfactory region is strategically placed on the roof of the nasal cavity. The advantage to this is that sniffing inspired gas into this region keeps it there and

does not allow the gas to reach deeper into your lungs. This is a relatively safe way to sample a potentially noxious or dangerous gas without taking a deep breath into the lungs, where it could cause severe damage. It is interesting to note that your ability to taste is related to your sense of smell. If you have ever had a nasty head cold and could not taste your food, now you know why. (Remember that we can only sense five different tastes, but recent research indicates we may be able to differentiate up to a trillion different odors.)

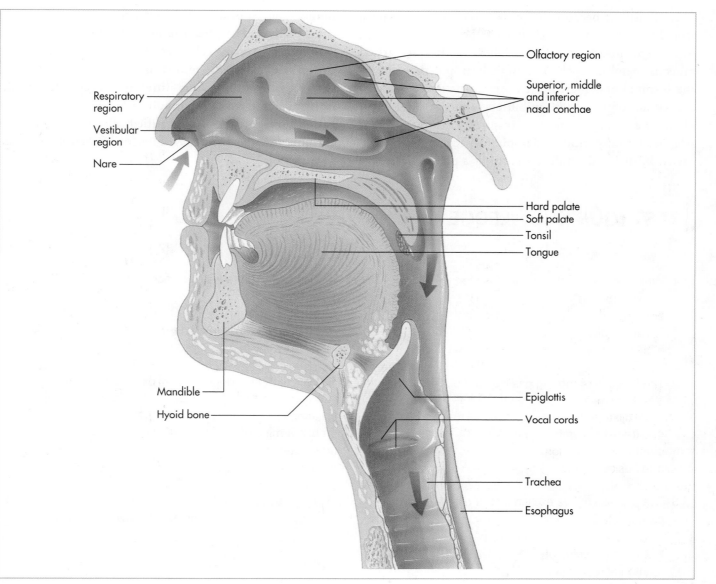

FIGURE 14–4 ■

The nasal regions.

Amazing Facts

Why Do We Breathe through Our Mouths?

You may have seen your favorite football player wearing an odd-looking strip of plastic across the nose. This is to help make breathing easier by increasing the diameter of the nostrils. The nose is responsible for one-half to two-thirds of the total airway resistance in breathing. Airway resistance represents the work required to move the gas down the tube. The larger the tube, the less resistance and therefore less work involved in breathing. Therefore, mouth breathing predominates during stress and exercise because it is easier for the gas to travel through the larger oral opening, due to less resistance. Of course, when you get a head cold and your nasal passages become blocked by secretions, it becomes necessary to breathe through the easier, open route of the mouth. On your journey, you must always be ready for detours.

In addition, because the nasal cavity is no longer a straight passageway, the air current becomes turbulent, so more air makes contact with these richly vascularized mucous membranes that transmit heat and moisture to the inspired gas. Incredibly, these moist mucous membranes add 650 to 1,000 milliliters (almost 3 to 4 cups) of water *each day* to moisten inspired air to 80 percent relative humidity within the respiratory region of the nasal cavity. In such a short distance, this is a pretty impressive humidification process. When the furnace in your house turns on in cold weather, this may dry the inspired air significantly and make it harder for your respiratory region to work. Therefore, humidifying this dry gas with water, such as from a room humidifier, may keep added stress off your body's natural humidification system. The nasal cavity is lined with pseudostratified ciliated columnar epithelium. (See the discussion of mucociliary escalator in the next section.)

TEST YOUR KNOWLEDGE 14–1

Answer the following:

1. Which gas is found in the atmosphere?
   a. oxygen
   b. nitrogen
   c. carbon dioxide
   d. all the above

2. The process of moving gas into and out of the respiratory system is
   a. ventilation.
   b. external respiration.
   c. internal respiration.
   d. diffusion.

3. The process of gas exchange at the body tissues is called
   a. ventilation.
   b. external respiration.
   c. internal respiration.
   d. osmosis.

4. Gas exchange takes place across the
   a. bronchi.
   b. bronchioles.
   c. alveolar–capillary membrane.
   d. nasal cavity.

5. Which of the following takes place in the upper airways?
   a. olfaction
   b. warming of air
   c. filtering of air
   d. all of the above

6. The medical term for the sense of smell is _____, and for producing sound is _____.

Going to Ride the Mucociliary Escalator

The epithelial lining of the nasal cavity plays a very important role in keeping the respiratory system clean and free of debris. Cells in the epithelial layer (or respiratory mucosa) are *pseudostratified* (*pseudo* = false, *stratified* = layered) *ciliated columnar cells* and are found not only in the respiratory region of the nasal cavity but also throughout most of the airways. See **FIGURE 14–5** ■. Remember that the pseudostratified epithelium is a single layer of tall, columnlike cells with nuclei located at different heights, giving the false appearance of two layers of cells, when in fact there is only one—hence the term *pseudostratified columnar*. Now all we need to add is the cilia. Each columnar cell has 200 to 250 cilia on its surface. **Cilia** are hairlike projections that can beat at a fantastic rate. Think of them as super rowers in a boat.

Goblet cells and submucosal glands are interspersed in the respiratory mucosa and produce about 100 milliliters (about 3 ounces) of **mucus** per day. The mucus actually resides as two layers. The cilia reside in the *sol layer*, which contains thin, watery fluid that allows them to beat freely. The *gel layer* is on top of the sol layer; as its name suggests, it is more viscous or gelatinous in nature. This sticky gel layer traps small particles, such as dust or pathogens, on the mucous blanket, much like flypaper. Once the debris is trapped on the mucous blanket, it must be removed from the respiratory system.

So how does this layer of mucus actually work? The microscopic, hairlike cilia act as tiny "oars," and in Figure 14–5, you can see that these oars rest in the watery sol layer. They beat at an incredible rate of 1,000 to 1,500 times per minute and propel the gel layer and its trapped debris onward and

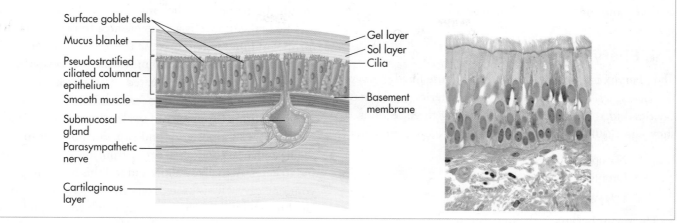

FIGURE 14–5 ■

The mucociliary escalator with corresponding micrograph.

upward about 1 inch per minute to be expelled from the body. The pseudostratified ciliated columnar epithelium, located in the airways of the lungs, propels the gel layer toward the oral cavity to be either expectorated with a cough or swallowed into the stomach. Some texts refer to this epithelial layer as the *mucociliary escalator*, which gives a better picture of what it does. This escalator works 24/7, unless something paralyzes it, such as smoking.

The Sinuses

Have you ever heard of someone being called an airhead? Technically, we are all airheads because the skull contains hollow, air-filled cavities (commonly called **sinuses**) that connect with the nasal cavity via small passageways. Because these are located around the nose, they are called *paranasal* sinuses. They are lined with a respiratory mucosa layer that continually drains its secretions into the nasal cavity. The sinuses are named for the specific facial bones in which they are located: the ethmoid, sphenoid, maxilla, and frontal bones (see **FIGURE 14–6** ■).

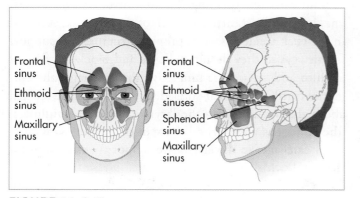

FIGURE 14–6 ■

The paranasal sinuses.

Clinical Application

EXCESSIVE MUCUS PRODUCTION

In some diseases—for example, chronic bronchitis and cystic fibrosis—excess mucus is produced that will need to be expectorated or swallowed. The color of the expectorant is clinically useful. In general, clear mucus is usually normal unless there is an excessive amount that may indicate irritation or the beginning of an inflammatory process. Look if there are other symptoms that may indicate infections. Yellow and green sputum indicates an infection but also indicates that the immune system is helping to fight an infection. Mucus turns green when enzymes (from the defense cells) that fight bacteria are activated. Mucus that is red or brown could indicate the presence of fresh or old blood and tends to indicate that bleeding has occurred, which is often seen in lung cancer or advanced tuberculosis. Cystic fibrosis is an inherited disease that affects the glands and causes them to secrete very thick mucus. This blocks the airways and increases the susceptibility to bacterial infections.

These cavities of air in the bones of the cranium are believed to help in the prolongation and intensification of sound produced by the voice. If you ever shouted inside a cave, you noticed a more resonant quality to the sound. In addition, it is theorized the air-filled sinuses help to lighten the heavy head that sits atop the neck. Not all of the sinuses exist at birth; rather, they develop as you grow and influence facial changes as you mature. Sinuses also provide further warming and moisturizing of inhaled air.

The Pharynx

The pharynx is a hollow, muscular structure lined with epithelial tissues. The **pharynx** begins posterior to the nasal cavities and is divided into the following three sections, as shown in **FIGURE 14–7** ■ by the different colored segments.

- Nasopharynx
- Oropharynx
- Laryngopharynx

The **nasopharynx** is the uppermost section of the pharynx and begins just posterior to the two nasal cavities. Air that is breathed through the nose passes through the nasopharynx. This section also contains lymphatic tissue of the immune system, called the **adenoids**, and passageways to the middle ear, called **eustachian tubes** (or *auditory tubes*). You can understand how an infection located in the nasal cavities can lead to an ear infection, and vice versa. The nasopharynx is lined with respiratory mucosa.

The **oropharynx** is the next region and is located posterior to the oral (buccal) cavity. Air that is breathed through the mouth as well as air that is breathed through the nose passes through here. It is important to note that anything that is swallowed also passes through this section. Therefore, the oropharynx conducts not only air but also food and liquid. For added protection, the oropharynx is lined with stratified squamous epithelium.

The oral entrance is a strategic area to place "guardians" for the immune system because this is where pathogens can easily enter the body. Lymphoid tissue, or **tonsils**, such as the **palatine tonsils**, are located in this area. Another set of tonsils, the **lingual tonsils**, are found at the back of the tongue. During the process of swallowing, the uvula and soft palate move in a posterior and superior position to protect the nasopharynx and nasal cavity from allowing food or liquid to enter. Actually swallow and feel this happening within your oral cavity. This protection can be overcome by forceful laughter, and that is why when you laugh with liquid or food in your mouth, the food or liquid can sometimes come up through your nose.

The **laryngopharynx** is the lowermost portion of the pharynx; an older term for it was the hypopharynx because of its position. Air that is breathed and anything that is swallowed passes through the laryngopharynx. Swallowed materials pass through the **esophagus** to get to the stomach, and air travels through the **larynx** (the next part of the respiratory system) and then the trachea on its way to the lungs. What directs the flow of "traffic" (air to the lungs and food and liquid to the stomach)? Is it a tiny highway worker directing traffic? No, it is directed by the swallowing reflex, which will be discussed shortly.

The Larynx

The larynx, located in the neck, is a triangular chamber inferior to the pharynx that houses the important structures needed for speech. Commonly known as the *voice box*, the larynx is a semirigid structure composed of several types of cartilage connected by muscles and ligaments that provide for movement of the vocal cords to control speech. The "Adam's apple," or thyroid cartilage, is the largest of the cartilages found in the larynx. Inferior to the thyroid cartilage, forming the inferior border of the larynx, is the cricoid cartilage. Both of these cartilages found in the neck are necessary to provide structure and support for airways so they do not collapse and block the flow of air into and out of the lungs. A third cartilage, the epiglottal cartilage, is a leaf-shaped, flaplike structure located above the opening into the larynx called the **epiglottis**. The epiglottis covers the larynx during swallowing. The other cartilages in the larynx are supportive structures for the vocal cords.

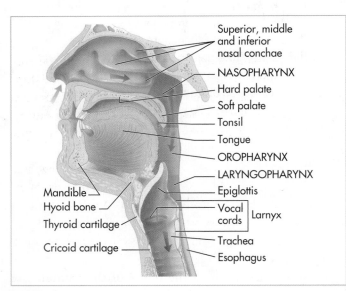

Superior, middle and inferior nasal conchae
NASOPHARYNX
Hard palate
Soft palate
Tonsil
Tongue
OROPHARYNX
LARYNGOPHARYNX
Epiglottis
Vocal cords } Larnyx
Trachea
Esophagus
Mandible
Hyoid bone
Thyroid cartilage
Cricoid cartilage

FIGURE 14–7 ■

The nasopharynx, oropharynx, and laryngopharynx and related structures.

Clinical Application

KEEPING THE VITAL AIRWAY OPEN

Just like any vital highway, the airway needs to remain open to a flow of traffic, or the oxygen molecules will cease to flow into the alveoli and therefore not get into the bloodstream to supply the tissues. Whereas a traffic jam can last for hours, oxygen flow can be disrupted for only a few minutes without tragic results. For example, if the upper airway swells shut from a severe allergic reaction to a bee sting, an emergency airway must be established. Remember, we only have 4 to 6 minutes of oxygen reserve. Review Figure 14–7, and you will see a space between the thyroid and cricoid cartilages. This is where an emergency cricoidthyroidotomy is performed. This space has few blood vessels or nerves, which makes it ideal in an emergency situation to place a temporary breathing tube.

Sometimes a longer-term breathing tube must be inserted into the lungs via a technique called *intubation.* This tube passes through the vocal cords and sits above the juncture (carina) between the right and left lung. A machine called a *ventilator* can move air into and out of the damaged lungs at this juncture.

The tube has an inflatable cuff to seal the airway once it is in place. Knowledge that the vocal cords open and close during breathing becomes clinically significant when intubating a patient. Adduction partially seals the vocal cords and occurs during expiration, whereas abduction opens the cords, increasing the size of the glottic opening during inspiration. If the patient is breathing, it is better to pass the tube with the deflated cuff through the narrow opening of the vocal cords during an inhalation when the cords are maximally open. Conversely, when removing the tube (extubation), the health care professional must always remember to deflate the cuff so it doesn't damage the cords as the tube is pulled back through them. It should go without saying (no pun intended) that a patient cannot talk when properly intubated because the vocal cords cannot function. If you ever see a TV soap opera or movie where someone is plainly talking with a tube going down his or her mouth into the lungs, you will know it is impossible. More permanent airways, called *tracheostomy tubes*, are placed in the neck. Some patients can learn to talk with a specialized tracheostomy tube in place.

The vocal cords are paired membranes located inside the larynx. The **glottis** is the sound-producing structure containing the vocal cords. The space between the vocal cords is called the **rima glottidis**. The glottis allows gas to travel to the trachea and eventually the lungs. Your voice is produced when air is forced past the partially closed vocal cords, causing them to vibrate. You normally speak during an exhalation.

Air that is breathed and anything that is swallowed passes through the laryngopharynx. Then a choice must be made. Swallowed materials *should* pass through the esophagus to get to the stomach, and air *should* travel through the larynx and then the trachea on its way to the lungs. Food and air are directed by a mechanism termed the *glottic mechanism* (swallowing reflex). The epiglottis closes over the opening to the larynx when you swallow and opens up when you breathe. This selective closure is called the *glottic* or

sphincter mechanism and facilitates the closing of the epiglottis over the glottic opening, thus sealing it so food does not enter the lungs. In addition, the soft palate blocks the nasal cavity, and the tongue blocks the oral cavity during swallowing so food can only travel in one direction, into the esophagus.

Thus, the lungs are closed to traffic when you swallow, and the food and liquid travel down the only open tube or route, the esophagus, leading into the stomach. When we breathe in, the gas preferentially travels into the lungs through a process that actually draws it into the lungs because of pressure differences. More on this later.

The vocal cords are the area of division between the upper and lower airways. The lower airways start inferior to the vocal cords. Now we continue our journey down the lower airways all the way down to the end point, or alveoli.

TEST YOUR KNOWLEDGE 14–2

Complete the following:

1. The hairlike structures that propel mucus in the airways are
   a. sol layer.
   b. gel layer.
   c. pathogens.
   d. cilia.

2. Which of the following is *not* true about the sinuses?
   a. air-filled cavities
   b. located in the skull and around the nose
   c. help to lighten the head
   d. gas exchange occurs there

3. Food is prevented from entering the _____ when eating by the closure of the _____.
   a. esophagus; glottis
   b. esophagus; epiglottis
   c. trachea; epiglottis
   d. epiglottis; glottis

4. The vocal cords are found in the
   a. laryngopharynx.
   b. nasopharynx.
   c. oropharynx.
   d. larynx.

5. The oropharynx is lined with _____, whereas the nasopharynx is lined with _____.
   a. respiratory mucosa; stratified squamous epithelium
   b. stratified squamous epithelium; respiratory mucosa
   c. respiratory mucosa; pseudostratified ciliated epithelium
   d. simple cuboidal epithelium; pseudostratified ciliated epithelium

6. Voice is normally produced by vibration of the closed vocal cords during
   a. inspiration.
   b. exhalation.
   c. internal respiration.
   d. external respiration.

7. The upper airway begins at the _____ and ends at the _____.
   a. tonsils, alveoli
   b. nares, bronchi
   c. nares, vocal cords
   d. vocal cords, alveoli

THE LOWER RESPIRATORY TRACT

The airway network that leads to the lungs and then branches out into the various lung segments resembles an upside-down tree and is sometimes called the *tracheobronchial tree*. See **FIGURE 14–8** ■.

Trachea and Bronchi

After leaving the larynx, the inspired air enters the **trachea**, also known by the lay term *windpipe*. The trachea extends from the cricoid cartilage of the larynx to the fifth thoracic vertebrae (approximately to the midpoint of the chest). The cartilage found in the anterior portion of the trachea is in the form of C-shaped structures to provide rigidity and protection for the exposed airway in the neck. The posterior parts of the rings are smooth muscle. This C shape also serves another important purpose. The esophagus lies in the area where the C opens up posteriorly. Without the cartilage, there is some "give" in the posterior aspect of the larynx and trachea, so the

esophagus can expand when you swallow larger chunks of food, and the food won't get stuck against the rigid cartilage of the trachea. The trachea is lined with respiratory mucosa.

The trachea is the largest bronchus and can be thought of as the trunk of the tracheobronchial tree. Once the trachea reaches the center of the chest approximately at the level of vertebrae T5, it begins its first branching, or bifurcates, into two bronchi (bronchus is the singular form), the right mainstem and the left mainstem. The site of bifurcation into the right and left lung is called the **carina** (again, see Figure 14–8). One bronchus goes to the right lung and the other bronchus goes to the left lung. The mainstem bronchi are sometimes also referred to as the *primary bronchi*. Now the bronchi must branch into the five lobar bronchi, one in each of the five lobes of the lungs.

Each lung lobe is further divided into specific segments, and the next branching of bronchi is called the *segmental bronchi*. At the point from the trachea down to the *segmental bronchi*, the tissue layers of the bronchial walls are all the same, only smaller,

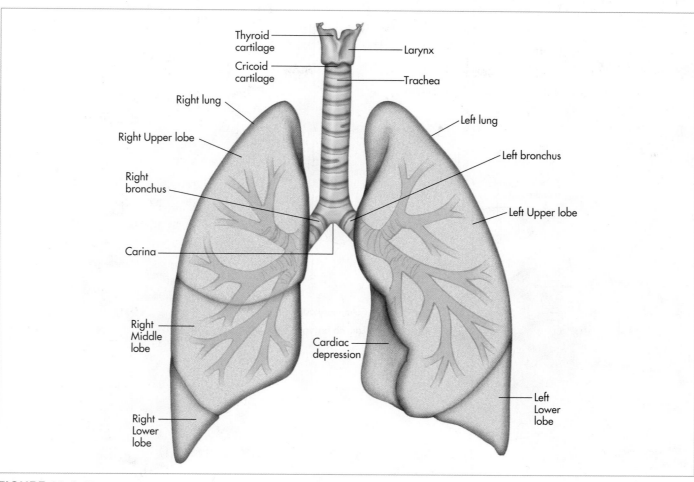

FIGURE 14–8 ▦

The tracheobronchial tree.

Clinical Application

THE ANGLE MAKES A DIFFERENCE

The angle of branching is not the same for both sides of the tracheobronchial tree. The right mainstem branches off at a 20- to 30-degree angle from the midline of the chest. The left mainstem branches off at a more pronounced 40- to 60-degree angle. This is important because the lesser angle of the right mainstem branching allows foreign bodies that are accidentally breathed in to more often lodge in the right lung. This is useful to know if a child has aspirated (taken into the lung) an object, and the physician must enter the lung with a bronchoscope to remove the object. Time may be critical, and it may make a difference if the search is begun immediately in the right lung because its structure increases the probability that the object has lodged there. In addition, a breathing tube or endotracheal tube may be placed too far into the lung, and instead of sitting above the carina so both lungs are ventilated, the tube most likely will pass into and ventilate only the right lung. This is why an x-ray for proper tube placement is so important.

as they branch downward. The first layer is the epithelial layer (remember the mucociliary escalator?) that keeps the area clean of debris. A middle **lamina propria** layer contains smooth muscle, lymph, and nerve tracts. The third layer is the protective and supportive cartilaginous layer (see **FIGURE 14–9** ▦).

The branching becomes more numerous with tiny subsegmental bronchi branching deep within each lung segment. The diameter of subsegmental bronchi ranges from 1 to 6 millimeters. Cartilaginous rings are now irregular pieces of cartilage and will soon fade away completely. Notice as we move toward

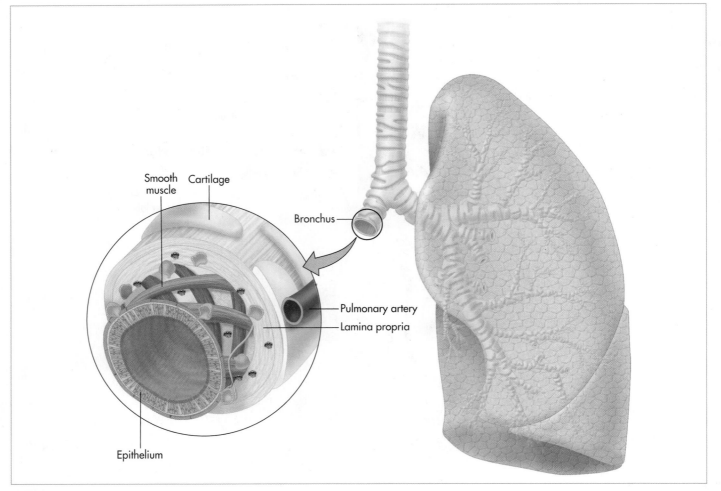

Smooth muscle Cartilage

Bronchus

Pulmonary artery

Lamina propria

Epithelium

FIGURE 14–9 ■

Tissue layers in the bronchi.

the gas exchange regions that the airways simplify to make it easier for gas molecules to pass through. Now we reach the very tiny airways called *bronchioles*; they average only 1 millimeter in diameter. They have no cartilage layer, and the epithelial lining becomes ciliated cuboidal. The bronchioles have smooth muscle in their walls. The cilia, goblet cells, and submucosal gland are almost all gone at his point. There is no gas exchange yet—just simple conduction of the gas mixture containing the oxygen molecules down the tree. Now we reach the terminal bronchioles, which have an average diameter of 0.5 millimeter, no goblet cells, no cartilage, no cilia, and no submucosal glands. This marks the end of the conducting zone. We now journey into the gas exchange or respiratory zone of the lung.

The next airway beyond the terminal bronchiole is called the respiratory bronchiole because a small portion of gas exchange takes place here. The epithelial lining is simple cuboidal cells interspersed with actual alveoli-type cells, which are flat, pancakelike cells called **simple squamous pneumocytes**. Alveolar ducts originate from the respiratory bronchioles wherein the walls of the alveolar ducts are completely made up

of simple squamous cells arranged in a tubular configuration. The alveolar ducts give way to the grape bunchlike structures of several connected alveoli, better known as the *alveolar sacs*. See **FIGURE 14–10** ■. At this point, the walls are simple squamous epithelium—no muscle, no cartilage, no cilia, no mucus; in other words, as simple as possible to allow for gas exchanges.

Clinical Application

THERAPEUTIC OXYGEN

Often, a distressed respiratory system and sometimes the cardiac system need supplemental oxygen to assist its function and meet its needs. There are many ways to deliver an enriched oxygen supply to the lungs, including an oxygen mask, nasal cannula (prongs), and specialized devices to deliver both oxygen and extra humidity to the lungs to assist their function.

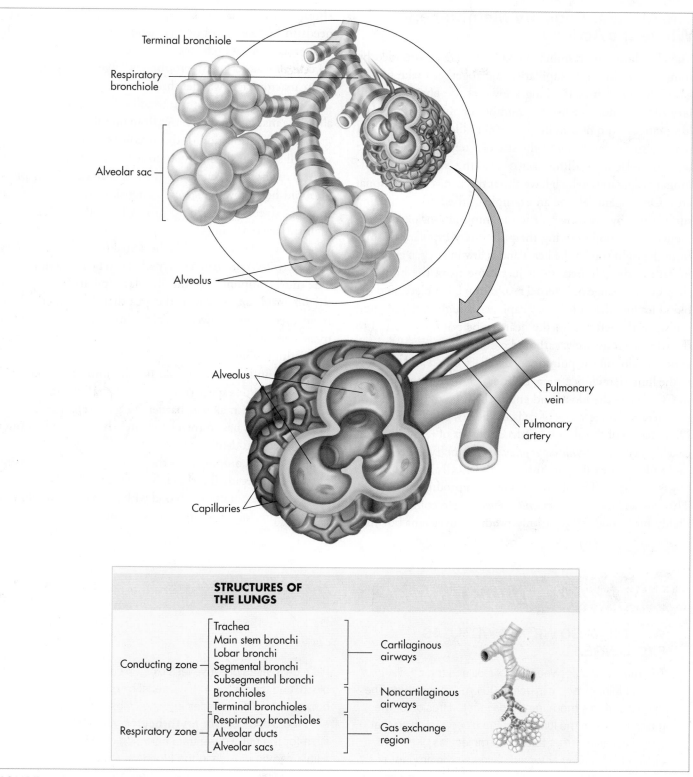

FIGURE 14–10 ■

Conduction and gas exchange structures and functions.

The Alveolar Capillary Membrane: Where the Action Is

The alveoli are the terminal air sacs that are surrounded by numerous pulmonary capillaries and together make up the gas exchange unit of the lung known as the **alveolar capillary membrane**. The average number of alveoli in an adult lung ranges from 300 million to 600 million. This gives it a massive surface area (about the size of a tennis court) for the oxygen molecule to diffuse across into the surrounding pulmonary capillaries, which have about the same cross-sectional area. Once again, we see an example of the body increasing surface area by dividing a structure into millions of tiny segments. The blood entering the pulmonary capillaries comes from the right side of the heart and is low in oxygen and high in carbon dioxide because it just came from the body tissues. Gas exchange or external respiration takes place, and the blood leaving the pulmonary capillary is high in oxygen and travels to the left side of the heart to be pumped around to the tissues. Conversely, carbon dioxide molecules are in high concentration in the pulmonary capillary blood and very low in the lung (remember, there is little CO_2 in the atmosphere), so CO_2 leaves the blood and enters the lung to be exhaled.

There are three types of cells in the alveoli. The majority (95 percent) of the alveolar surface consists of flat, thin, pancakelike cells called *squamous pneumocytes*, or Type I cells. Gas molecules can easily pass through these cells in the process of gas exchange. The alveoli also need to produce surfactant. This is where the Type II *granular pneumocytes* come in. These highly metabolic cells not only produce surfactant but they also aid in cellular repair responsibilities. Finally, this area needs to be free of debris that would act as barriers to the vital process of gas exchange. The "cleanup" cells, called Type III cells or wandering **macrophages**, ingest foreign particles as the macrophages wander throughout the alveoli. There are even small holes between the alveoli called *pores of Kohn* that allow the macrophages to move from one alveolus to another.

On closer inspection of the alveolar capillary membrane, you will see four distinct components. The first layer is the liquid **surfactant** layer that lines the alveoli. This phospholipid helps lower the surface tension in these very tiny spheres (alveoli) that would otherwise collapse due to the high surface tension.

The second component is the actual tissue layer, or *alveolar epithelium*, comprised of type I and type II pneumocytes. The third component of the alveolar capillary membrane is the *interstitial space*. This is the area that separates the basement membrane of alveolar epithelium from the basement membrane of the capillary endothelium and contains interstitial fluid. This space is so small that the membranes of the alveoli and capillary appear fused. However, if too much fluid gets into this space (interstitial edema), the membranes separate, which makes it harder for gas exchange to occur because the gas has to travel a greater distance and through a congested, fluid-filled space.

The fourth component is the *capillary endothelium* (simple squamous epithelium) that forms the wall of the capillary. The capillary contains the blood with the red blood cells that carry the precious gas cargo to its destination.

Clinical Application

WHAT CAN GO WRONG WITH GAS EXCHANGE?

The membrane between the alveoli and the capillaries is quite thin. In fact, it is only 0.004 millimeter thick. The thinness of this membrane aids in the diffusion of the gases between the lungs and the blood. Anything that would act as a barrier to oxygen molecules getting to or through this barrier would decrease the amount of oxygen that gets into the blood. For example, excessive secretions and fluid such as in pneumonia act as a barrier and reduce the oxygen levels in the blood, which can be measured by sampling arterial blood and analyzing the amount of each gas dissolved in it. This is called an *arterial blood gas*, or *ABG*. In the case of severe pneumonia, the level of arterial oxygen known as the PaO_2 decreases because less oxygen can get into the blood, and the $PaCO_2$ in the arterial blood increases because less CO_2 crosses into the lungs to be exhaled.

Red blood cells, or **erythrocytes**, are responsible for the bulk of the transportation of oxygen and a little carbon dioxide in the blood via a protein- and iron-containing molecule called **hemoglobin**, which performs the actual transportation. It is estimated that there are about *280 million* hemoglobin molecules found in *each* erythrocyte. Carbon dioxide is mainly carried in your blood as bicarbonate ions. For more information on the bicarbonate buffering system of your blood see the urinary chapter (Chapter 17).

Clinical Application

ASSESSING VENTILATION AND BLOOD pH

Carbon dioxide levels are the best indicator of ventilation. Due to the rapid diffusion of carbon dioxide to the lungs and its subsequent exhalation, it can be used as a measure of the efficiency of ventilation. In many lung diseases, carbon dioxide levels can rise in the blood and initially form carbonic acid (H_2CO_3). This acid quickly breaks down into its ionic parts, H^+ (hydronium ion) and HCO_3^- (bicarbonate ion.) To prevent too much acidity from building up in the blood, H^+ will be excreted by the kidneys, and more bicarbonate (base) will be formed to buffer the blood to maintain normal pH.

In general, if the hemoglobin is carrying large amounts of oxygen, the blood will be bright red. If there is less oxygen and more carbon dioxide being carried, then the blood will be darker in color. Venous blood has lower levels of oxygen and higher levels of carbon dioxide. As a result, venous blood has a dark red tint. Low levels of red blood cells or anemia would limit the number of hemoglobin molecules that could transport oxygen and thus greatly reduce the amount in the blood available for the tissues. Therefore, the number of red blood cells and the amount of hemoglobin in your blood (both of which can be measured) is important in oxygen delivery to your tissues.

Your body can attempt to respond to low oxygen levels by producing more red blood cells by a process called **erythropoiesis**. This process begins when the kidneys detect low levels of oxygen coming to them from the blood. The kidneys release into the bloodstream a hormone called **erythropoietin**. This substance travels through the blood and eventually reaches specialized cells found in the red bone marrow. When stimulated, these specialized cells begin to increase their production of erythrocytes until demand is met. Having too little iron in the body can also affect oxygen delivery because the iron in the hemoglobin is what holds on to the oxygen molecules. The terms *iron-poor* blood and *tired* blood come from the fact that a patient with low levels of iron tires easily due to low oxygen levels.

APPLIED SCIENCE

The Amazing Surfactant

Not only does surfactant lower the surface tension when the alveoli are small (end-expiration), thereby preventing alveoli collapse, but when you take a deep breath (end-inspiration), your alveoli get larger and the surfactant layer thins and becomes less effective, its surface tension increasing because of its thinning. This prevents overexpansion or rupture of the alveoli. Lack of surfactant can cause stiff lungs that resist expansion. Surfactant develops late in fetal development, and premature babies therefore may not have sufficient levels. Without immediate intervention, their tiny lungs would collapse (**atelectasis**) and thus prevent vital gas exchange. If they are given too much volume to re-expand their stiff lungs, the alveoli may rupture, again because surfactant is not there to prevent overexpansion. Surfactant also has an antibacterial property that helps fight harmful pathogens. Fortunately, medical science has developed surfactant replacement therapy that can instill surfactant into the lungs to maintain their function until babies have matured and can produce it on their own.

TEST YOUR KNOWLEDGE 14–3

Complete the following:

1. The largest bronchus or trunk of the tracheobronchial tree is the
   a. right mainstem bronchus.
   b. left mainstem bronchus.
   c. bronchiole.
   d. trachea.

2. The site of bifurcation of the right and left lungs is called the
   a. alveoli.
   b. carina.
   c. trachea.
   d. capillary.

(continued)

TEST YOUR KNOWLEDGE 14–3 *(continued)*

3. If an object is aspirated into the airways, it is most likely to go to
   a. the right lung.
   b. the left lung.
   c. the stomach.
   d. the oropharynx.

4. The first portion of the airway where gas exchange begins is the
   a. terminal bronchiole.
   b. trachea.
   c. mainstem bronchus.
   d. respiratory bronchiole.

5. The alveolar layer that lowers surface tension to keep the alveoli expanded is the
   a. surfactant layer.
   b. capillary layer.
   c. epithelium layer.
   d. macrophage layer.

6. The alveolar cell that allows for gas exchange is the
   a. squamous cell.
   b. granular cell.
   c. macrophage cell.
   d. Kohn cell.

7. The iron-containing molecule responsible for transporting oxygen in the blood is _____.

THE HOUSING OF THE LUNGS AND RELATED STRUCTURES

The lungs reside in the thoracic cavity and are separated by a region called the **mediastinum**, which contains the esophagus, heart, great vessels (superior and inferior vena cava and aorta), and trachea (see **FIGURE 14–11** ■).

Breathing in and out causes the lungs to move within the thoracic cavity. Over time, an irritation could occur as the lungs rub the inside of the thoracic cage. To prevent such damage, each lung is wrapped in a serous membrane called the *pleura*. The inner layer of the pleura covering the lungs is called the **visceral pleura**. The thoracic cavity and the upper side of the diaphragm are lined with the outer layer of this membrane, the **parietal pleura**. Between these two pleural layers is a microscopic intrapleural space (pleural cavity) that contains a slippery liquid called **pleural fluid** that greatly reduces the friction as an individual breathes. Remember that serous membranes have only a *potential* space between them. The visceral and parietal pleura are essentially "layered" together. There is practically no space between them. (This is the second serous membrane we have seen; the *pericardium* is also a serous membrane.)

The Lungs

The right and left lungs are cone-shaped organs; the rounded peak is called the apex of the lung. The apices (plural of *apex*) of the lungs extend 1 to 2 inches above the clavicle. The bases of the lungs rest on the right and left hemidiaphragm. The right lung base is a little higher than the left to accommodate the large liver lying underneath. The medial surface of the lung has a deep, concave cavity that contains the heart and therefore is called the *cardiac impression* and is deeper on the left side. The **hilum** is the area where the two mainstem bronchi and associated structures attach to each lung. This is also referred to as the *root* of each lung. Each root contains the mainstem bronchus, pulmonary artery and vein, nerve tracts, and lymph vessels.

The right lung has three lobes—the upper, middle, and lower lobes—that are divided by the horizontal and oblique fissures. The left lung has only one fissure, the oblique fissure, and therefore only two lobes, called the upper and lower lobes. You may hear the term **lingula**. This is an area of the left lung that corresponds with the right middle lobe. Why only two lobes in the left, you may ask? Remember that the heart is located in a space (cardiac impression) in the left anterior area of the chest and therefore takes up some space of the left

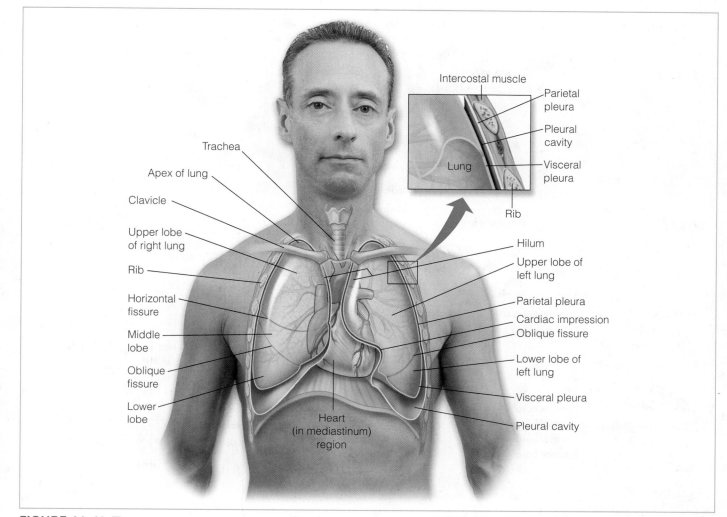

FIGURE 14–11 ■

Structures of the thoracic cavity.

lung. In fact, the right lung is larger, and about 60 percent of gas exchange occurs there. The lobes are even further divided into specific segments related to their anatomical position. For example, the apical segment of the right upper lobe is the top portion or tip of the right upper lobe. Remember, the segmental bronchi enter each lung segment. See **FIGURE 14–12** ■.

The Protective Bony Thorax

The lungs, heart, and great vessels are all protected by the *bony thorax*. This bony and cartilaginous frame provides protection and also movement of the thoracic cage to accommodate breathing. The bony thorax includes the rib cage, the sternum (or breastbone), and the corresponding thoracic vertebrae to which the ribs attach (see **FIGURE 14–13** ■).

The **sternum** is centrally located at the anterior portion of the thoracic cage and is comprised of the manubrium,

body, and xiphoid process. This anatomical landmark is very important for proper hand placement in CPR (cardiopulmonary resuscitation). The hand is placed over the body of the sternum where compressions squeeze the heart between the body of the sternum and the thoracic vertebrae. If the hand placement is too low on the xiphoid process, it can break off and lacerate the internal organs.

The **thoracic cage** consists of 12 pairs of elastic arches of bone called *ribs*. The ribs are attached by cartilage to allow for their movement while breathing. The true ribs are pairs 1 through 7 and are called *vertebrosternal* because they connect anteriorly to the sternum and posteriorly to the thoracic vertebrae of the spinal column. Pairs 8, 9, and 10 are called the false ribs, or *vertebrocostal*, because they connect to the costal cartilage of the superior rib and again posterior to the thoracic vertebrae. Rib pairs 11 and 12 are called the floating ribs because they have no anterior attachment.

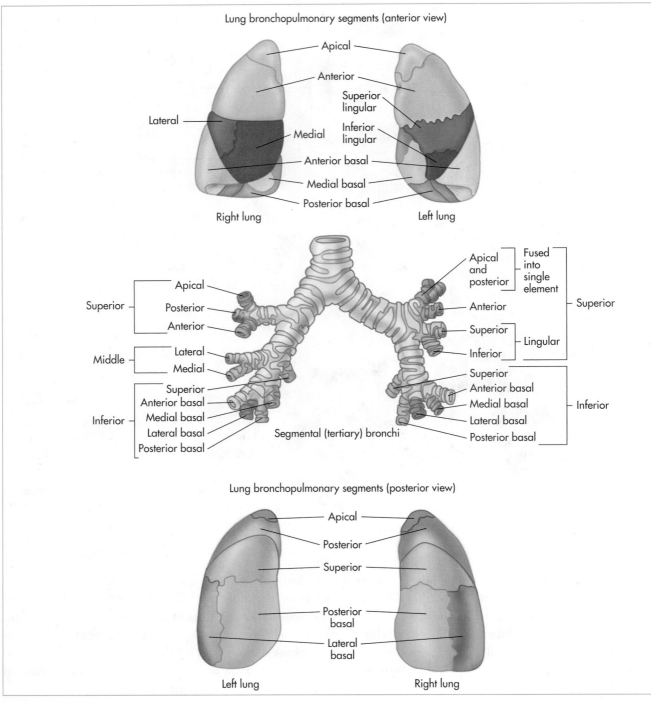

FIGURE 14–12 ■

Bronchopulmonary segments.

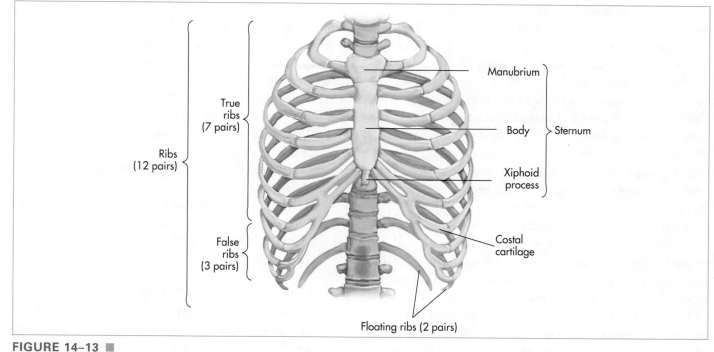

FIGURE 14–13 ■

The thoracic cage.

HOW WE BREATHE

The control center that tells us to breathe is located in the brain, specifically in the **medulla oblongata**. There is also another respiratory area in the pons. *Inspiration* is an active process of ventilation in which the main breathing muscle, the **diaphragm** (a dome-shaped muscle when at rest), is sent a signal via the phrenic nerve, from the cervical plexus of the spinal cord. The diaphragm contracts and flattens, thereby increasing the space in the thoracic cavity (see **FIGURE 14–14** ■). The increase in volume in the thoracic cavity causes a decrease in pressure in the thoracic cavity that is transmitted to the lungs. Keep in mind that volume and pressure are inversely related. Because the pressure in the lungs is now lower than atmospheric pressure, air rushes into the lungs, down the

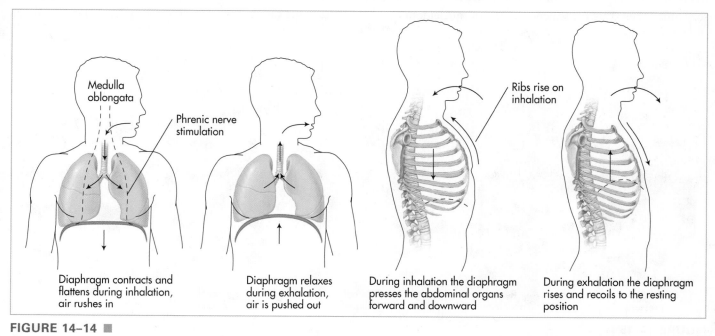

FIGURE 14–14 ■

How we breathe.

pressure gradient (from high to low). The external intercostal muscles also assist by moving the ribs up and outward during inspiration to increase the total volume in the thoracic cavity.

Exhalation, on the other hand, is usually a passive act. As the diaphragm relaxes, it forms a dome shape, which decreases the amount of space in the thoracic cavity. As a result, pressure in the lungs becomes greater than the atmospheric pressure, and the air is pushed out of the lungs. The fact that the lungs are elastic and are stretched during inspiration also aids in expiration because this tissue returns to rest (recoils), much as a stretched rubber band that is released.

What makes the brain tell the lungs how rapidly or how slowly to breathe? Although we can consciously speed up or slow down our breathing, our breathing rate is normally controlled by the level of carbon dioxide in our blood. If blood carbon dioxide levels rise, it means that not enough CO_2 is being ventilated, so the medulla oblongata sends signals to the respiratory muscles to increase the rate and depth of breathing. Sensory receptors in the aorta and carotid arteries and the medulla oblongata constantly monitor blood chemistry. These chemoreceptors actually sense blood pH. As CO_2 levels rise, blood pH falls, as the blood becomes more acidic. So any time blood becomes more acidic, say in untreated diabetes, ventilation rate will increase to "blow off" excess CO_2.

Sometimes the body needs help to breathe beyond resting or normal breathing. For example, during increased physical activity or in disease states in which more oxygen is required, **accessory muscles** are used to help pull up your rib cage to make an even larger space in the thoracic cavity. The accessory muscles used are the scalene and the sternocleidomastoid muscles in the neck and the pectoralis major and pectoralis minor muscles of the chest.

Although exhalation is a passive process, there are times, especially with certain disease states, when exhalation may need to be assisted. Again, the body has accessory muscles of exhalation that assist in a more forceful and active exhalation by increasing abdominal pressure. The main accessory muscles of exhalation are the various abdominal muscles that push up the diaphragm or the back muscles that pull down and thus compress the thoracic cage. The next time you blow out birthday candles, put your hand on your abdomen. You will feel the abdominal muscles tighten to increase the force of expiration to blow out the candles. See **FIGURE 14–15** ■ for the specific accessory muscles of exhalation.

Pulmonary Function Testing

Lung function can be measured in terms of volumes and flows using pulmonary function testing (PFT). First, the various volumes can be measured by having the patient breathe normally and then take a maximum deep breath followed by a maximum exhalation. The tracing is recorded as in **FIGURE 14–16** ■. For example, tidal volume (V_T) is the amount of air moved into or out of the lungs at rest during a single breath. The normal tidal volume is 500 mL, although there is considerable variation depending on age, sex, height, and general fitness. Your inspiratory reserve volume is what you can breathe in beyond a normal inspiration. Likewise, your expiratory reserve volume is what you can exhale beyond a normal exhalation. You can never totally exhale all the air out of your lungs; your residual volume (RV) prevents total lung collapse. We can combine these volumes to get various lung capacities, as shown in Figure 14–16.

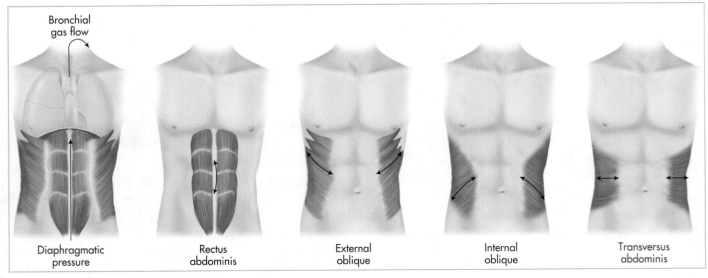

Bronchial gas flow

| Diaphragmatic pressure | Rectus abdominis | External oblique | Internal oblique | Transversus abdominis |

FIGURE 14–15 ■

The accessory muscles of exhalation.

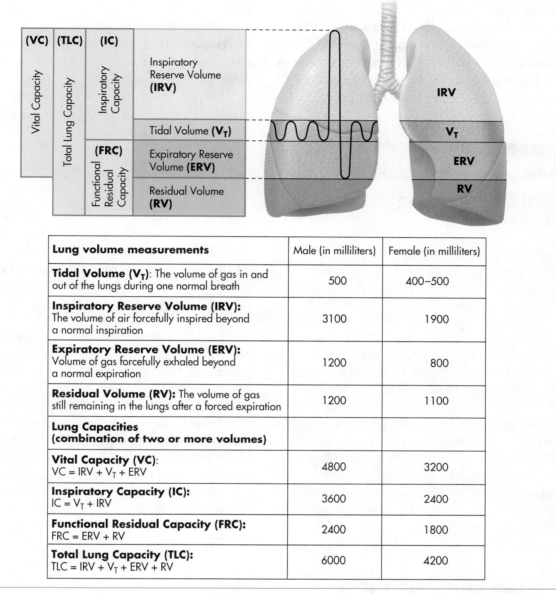

Lung volume measurements	Male (in milliliters)	Female (in milliliters)
Tidal Volume (V_T): The volume of gas in and out of the lungs during one normal breath	500	400–500
Inspiratory Reserve Volume (IRV): The volume of air forcefully inspired beyond a normal inspiration	3100	1900
Expiratory Reserve Volume (ERV): Volume of gas forcefully exhaled beyond a normal expiration	1200	800
Residual Volume (RV): The volume of gas still remaining in the lungs after a forced expiration	1200	1100
Lung Capacities (combination of two or more volumes)		
Vital Capacity (VC): VC = IRV + V_T + ERV	4800	3200
Inspiratory Capacity (IC): IC = V_T + IRV	3600	2400
Functional Residual Capacity (FRC): FRC = ERV + RV	2400	1800
Total Lung Capacity (TLC): TLC = IRV + V_T + ERV + RV	6000	4200

FIGURE 14–16 ■

Normal lung volumes and capacities.

- Function residual capacity (FRC)—the volume of air remaining in the lungs at the end of a normal expiration
- Inspiratory reserve volume (IRV)—the amount of air that can be forcefully inhaled after a normal inspiration
- Expiratory reserve volume (ERV)—the amount of air that can be forcefully exhaled after a normal expiration
- Residual volume (RV)—the volume of air remaining in the lungs after a maximum expiration

- Vital capacity (VC)—the maximum amount of air that can be moved into and out of the respiratory system in a single respiratory cycle

Besides volumes and capacities, we can also measure the flow rates coming out of the lung at various points during a forced (maximum patient effort) vital capacity (FVC). For example, we can measure the forced expiratory volume in 1 second, or (FEV_1). Normally, one can exhale 75 to 85 percent of their FVC in 1 second. However, someone with an obstructive disease would take longer to exhale and get less than 70 percent of their total FVC out in 1 second and therefore have a reduced FEV_1.

Another test that helps establish whether the airways have become "narrower" than normal (as would be seen in an asthma episode) is peak expiratory flow rate, or PEFR, which is the maximum flow rate or speed of air a person can rapidly expel after taking the deepest possible breath. The PEFR test is measured in liters per minute and should be within a predicted range. This a good test to reflect how the larger airways are functioning and to monitor diseases such as asthma that affect these airways.

Amazing Facts

Exhaled CO₂ and Mosquitoes

Mosquitoes are too small to carry flashlights, so how do they find you in the dark? They do it by using carbon dioxide sensors to locate increased concentrations of CO_2 emitted by—you guessed it—your exhaled breath. Once they detect your exhaled CO_2 (which can be up to 164 feet away), they use their heat sensors to find an area of skin on which to begin their banquet. You have an increased chance of being bitten during and right after exercising or doing any strenuous labor. This is because increases of lactic acid and body heat when you are active appear to attract mosquitoes, as does an increase in uric acid. Also, if you have blood type O, you are twice as likely to get bitten as a person with blood type A (type B is somewhere in the middle). Certain skin bacteria also attract mosquitoes; this is why your ankles and feet, which have greater bacterial colonies, seem to be targeted more so than other parts of the body. Finally, pregnant women are twice as likely to be bitten because they exhale about 21 percent more carbon dioxide and their body temperature is approximately 1.26 degrees Fahrenheit warmer than normal.

Another amazing carbon dioxide fact is that many people believe swimmers hyperventilate to get more oxygen in their systems before a sustained underwater dive. In reality, they are "blowing off" CO_2 to get their levels low. Because higher levels of CO_2 cause us to want to breathe, the body is fooled into believing it doesn't need to for a while longer, so swimmers can remain underwater longer. Unfortunately, the body still uses up its oxygen at a regular rate and sometimes uses enough of the reserve that swimmers risk losing consciousness.

TEST YOUR KNOWLEDGE 14–4

Complete the following:

1. The _____ pleura lines the thoracic cavity.
   a. visceral
   b. parietal
   c. mediastinum
   d. chest

2. The portion of the sternum where CPR is performed is the
   a. xiphoid process.
   b. ribs.
   c. manubrium.
   d. body.

3. The _____ nerve innervates the main breathing muscle, called the _____.
   a. thoracic; internal intercostals
   b. thoracic; diaphragm
   c. phrenic; external intercostals
   d. phrenic; diaphragm

4. The amount of air moved during typical resting ventilation is called
   a. inspiratory reserve volume.
   b. vital capacity.
   c. expiratory reserve volume.
   d. tidal volume.

5. As CO_2 rises, chemoreceptors send signals to the
_____ to _____ ventilation.
   a. cerebrum; decrease
   b. heart; increase
   c. medulla oblongata; increase
   d. spinal cord; decrease

6. The process of producing red blood cells is called
_____.

COMMON DISORDERS OF THE RESPIRATORY SYSTEM

Respiratory disease is one of the most common disease groups seen in health care settings. **Atelectasis**, commonly occurring in hospitalized patients, is a condition in which the air sacs of the lungs are either partially or totally collapsed. Atelectasis usually occurs in patients who cannot or will not take deep breaths to fully expand the lungs and keep the passageways open. Surgery or an injury of the thoracic cage (such as broken ribs) often makes deep breathing painful. Taking periodic deep breaths is important not only to expand the lungs but also to stimulate the production of surfactant, which helps keep the small alveolar sacs open between breaths.

Patients with large amounts of secretions who cannot cough them up are also at risk for atelectasis because the secretions block airways and lead to areas of collapse. Quite often, if atelectasis is not corrected and secretions are retained, **pneumonia** can develop within 72 hours. Pneumonia is a lung infection that can be caused by either viruses, fungi, protists, or bacteria. Inflammation occurs in the infected areas, with an accumulation of cell debris and fluid. In certain pneumonias, lung tissue is destroyed. Pneumonias, if severe enough, can lead to death.

Chronic obstructive pulmonary disease (COPD) is a group of diseases in which patients have difficulty getting all the air out of their lungs. Often, large amounts of secretions and lung damage are involved. The diseases involved in COPD are **emphysema** and **chronic bronchitis**. **Asthma**, formerly considered a COPD type disease, is now separated into its own category due to its special characteristics such as its reversibility with proper treatment.

Asthma is a potentially life-threatening lung condition in which the body reacts to an allergy by causing constriction of the airways of the lungs, known as **bronchospasm** (see **FIGURE 14–17** ■). It is difficult to get air in and even more difficult to get air out of the lungs. The inability to get air out of the lungs is known as *gas trapping*. As a result of gas trapping, fresh air cannot get into the lungs, so the victim breathes the same air over and over. This lowers the amount of oxygen in the blood and increases the blood levels of carbon dioxide. Because this is an inflammatory process of the airways, there is also an increase in the amount of mucus that the airways produce. These increased secretions can block the airways (a phenomenon known as *mucus plugging*) and further reduce the flow of fresh air to the lungs. Although asthma can be a life-threatening disease, it can be controlled with the use of medication.

Emphysema is a nonreversible lung condition in which the alveolar air sacs are destroyed and the lung itself becomes "floppy" (see Figure 14–17), much like a balloon that has been inflated and deflated too many times. As the alveoli are destroyed, it becomes more difficult for gases to diffuse between the lungs and the blood. The lung tissue becomes fragile and can easily rupture (much like a worn tire), causing air to escape into the thoracic cavity and further inhibit gas exchange. This causes a pneumothorax, which will be discussed below.

Chronic bronchitis is a lung disease in which there are inflamed airways and large amounts of sputum are being produced. As inflammation occurs, the airways swell, and the inner diameter of the airways become smaller. As they get smaller, it becomes difficult to move air in and out, which increases the work of breathing. Because of this increased work level, more oxygen is used, and more carbon dioxide is produced.

A **pneumothorax** is a condition in which there is air inside the thoracic cavity and outside the lungs, often in the pleural cavity. Remember that the pleural cavity is a *potential* space. Gas or fluid may be forced into the cavity, separating the layers of the membrane. Air can enter the thoracic cavity from two directions. A stab wound or gunshot wound to the chest would allow air to rush into the thoracic cavity from the outside. The lung might develop a leak as a result of either a structural deformity or a disease process (such as in emphysema). In this situation, air would enter the thoracic

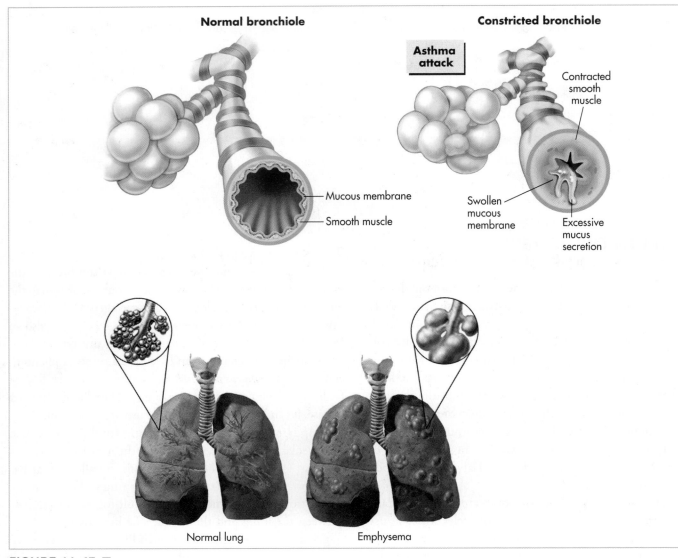

FIGURE 14–17 ■

Asthma and emphysema.

cavity from the lung as air is breathed in. In either case, if the gas cannot escape, it will continue to fill a space in the thoracic cavity and provide less space for the lung or lungs to expand when breathing. If the lungs are too greatly restricted to expand, a life-threatening situation may occur.

A **pleural effusion** is a condition in which an excessive buildup of fluid develops in the pleural cavity between the parietal and the visceral pleura. This fluid may be pus (in which case it is known as **empyema**), serum from the blood (called a **hydrothorax**), or blood (called a **hemothorax**). Because fluids are affected by gravity, pleural effusions tend to move to the lowest point in the pleural space. If a pleural effusion is large enough, it can have the same effect as a large pneumothorax. It can restrict the amount of expansion of a lung or lungs. Because less air can flow into and out of the lungs, the patient has to work harder by breathing in and out more rapidly to meet the body's demands for more oxygen and the removal of carbon dioxide. This additional work of breathing may exhaust an individual to the point that he or she can no longer breathe without intervention. These conditions may progress to atelectasis.

Tuberculosis (TB) is a bacterial infection that has seen a recent rise in occurrence. It thrives in areas of the body that have high oxygen content such as the lung. Tuberculosis bacilli can remain dormant in the body for years before beginning to multiply. If it continues unchecked, vast lung damage can occur. There has been recent concern about a multidrug-resistant form of tuberculosis that is very resistant to the antibiotics that are normally used to treat TB, and this strain has a high mortality rate.

Patients with lung disease may exhibit signs and symptoms such as dyspnea, tachypnea, cyanosis due to low oxygen levels, and use of accessory muscles of ventilation to assist normal breathing. In addition, the cardiac system may exhibit tachycardia to speed up oxygen delivery and may increase the number of red blood cells that carry oxygen.

The major preventable cause of many respiratory diseases is smoking. The annual number of smoking-related deaths in the United States is equivalent to one jumbo jet filled with passengers crashing every day with no survivors, or 450,000 deaths per year.

SUMMARY: Points of Interest

- Moving approximately 12,000 quarts of air each day, the respiratory system is responsible for providing oxygen for the blood to take to the body's tissues and removing carbon dioxide, one of the waste products of cellular metabolism.

- Ventilation is the movement of gases into and out of the lungs; during respiration, oxygen is added to the blood, and carbon dioxide is removed.

- The lungs contain continually branching airways called bronchi and bronchioles.

- At the end of bronchioles are alveolar sacs.

- Each alveolar sac is surrounded by a capillary network where gas exchange occurs with the blood.

- The purpose of the upper airway is to filter, warm, and moisten inhaled air for its journey to the lungs.

- In addition, the upper airway provides for *olfaction* (sense of smell) and *phonation* (speech).

- The mucociliary escalator captures foreign particles, and the hairlike cilia constantly move a layer of mucus up to the upper airway to be swallowed or expelled.

- Adenoids and tonsils aid in preventing pathogens from entering the body.

- Because activities of breathing and swallowing share a common pathway, the epiglottis protects the airway to the lungs from accidental aspiration of food and liquids.

- Vocal cords are the gateway between the upper and lower airways.

- The tracheobronchial tree is like an upside-down tree with ever-branching airways, where the trunk of the tree is represented by the trachea and the leaves by the alveoli.

- The alveolar capillary membrane is where external respiration or gas exchange occurs.

- The bony thorax provides support and protection for the respiratory system.

- The main muscle of breathing is the diaphragm, and accessory muscles assist in times of need such as exercise and disease.

- The medulla oblongata in the brain is the control center for breathing and sends impulses via the phrenic nerve to the diaphragm.

CASE STUDY

A patient comes to the emergency department with wheezing and thick secretions. His heart rate, breathing rate, and blood pressure are all increased. He is using accessory muscles of ventilation to breathe and has peripheral cyanosis. He has a history of allergies and has had a "bad cold" for several days.

a. What are two possible respiratory conditions he may have?

_____

_____

b. Can you think of some recommended treatments for this patient?

_____

_____

c. What would be some positive indicators that your treatment is working? For example, after the treatment, you notice less accessory muscle use. Can you think of at least two more?

_____

_____

Multiple Choice

1. The process of gas exchange between the alveolar area and capillary is
   a. external ventilation.
   b. internal ventilation.
   c. internal respiration.
   d. external respiration.

2. The bulk movement of gas into and out of the lung is called
   a. internal respiration.
   b. ventilation.
   c. diffusion.
   d. gas exchange.

3. Which of the following is *not* a function of the upper airway?
   a. humidification
   b. gas exchange
   c. filtration
   d. heating or cooling gases

4. The largest cartilage in the upper airway is the
   a. cricoid.
   b. eustachian.
   c. mega cartilage.
   d. thyroid.

5. Which structure controls the opening to the trachea?
   a. esophagus
   b. hypoglottis
   c. epiglottis
   d. hyperglottis

6. Cells need oxygen to
   a. make ATP.
   b. get rid of CO_2.
   c. use gasoline.
   d. breathe.

7. The lung capacity that includes tidal volume, inspiratory reserve volume, and expiratory reserve volume is called your
   a. total lung capacity.
   b. functional residual capacity.
   c. inspiratory capacity.
   d. vital capacity.

Fill in the Blank

1. Small bronchi are called _____.

2. The sense of smell is termed _____, and the act of speech is called _____.

3. The hairlike projections called _____ beat within the _____ layer and propel the _____ layer toward the oral cavity to be expectorated.

4. The _____ are thought to lighten the head and provide resonance for the voice.

5. When the diaphragm contracts, lung volume _____ and air flows _____.

Short Answer

1. Describe the tissue layers in the bronchi.

   _____

   _____

   _____

   _____

2. Explain how gas exchange takes place in the lungs.

   _____

   _____

   _____

   _____

3. Discuss the importance of surfactant.

_____

_____

_____

_____

4. Describe the process of normal breathing beginning with the brain.

_____

_____

_____

_____

5. Explain the changes in the wall of the tracheobronchial tree as you move from conducting zone to respiratory zone.

_____

_____

_____

_____

Visit our new **MyHealthProfessions Lab** to accompany *Anatomy & Physiology for Health Professions.* Here you'll find a rich collection of quizzes, case studies, and animations for deeper understanding and application.

15

The Lymphatic and Immune Systems

YOUR DEFENSE SYSTEMS

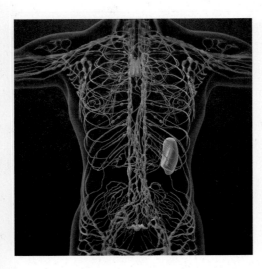

So far in our travels, we have visited control systems, transport systems, and infrastructure, to name just a few. We have seen how each separate system works together to allow the body to function as an integrated unit. However, like all cities, the body must be protected. Cities have police and fire departments. On a larger scale, countries have armies and military bases. Similarly, your body has the immune and lymphatic systems with a variety of protective mechanisms and cells, each performing specific duties. These systems help protect the body from pathogens that can produce disease. Without your immune and lymphatic systems, your journey would be a very short one—the first exposure to a potential pathogenic organism would wreak havoc in your body and literally stop the journey before it began.

LEARNING OUTCOMES

Upon completion of your journey through this chapter, you will be able to:

- List and describe the major components of the lymphatic system and their functions.
- List and describe the major components of the immune system and their functions.
- Explain the antigen–antibody relationship.
- Discuss the different barriers that help prevent infection.
- Name and describe the functions of the white blood cells responsible for protecting the body from invasion.
- Describe the chemicals that assist in the immune response.
- Discuss how inflammatory responses and fevers relate to infection.
- Compare innate immunity to adaptive immunity.
- Describe the function of lymphocytes in the immune response.
- Discuss the ways in which the lymphatic system, innate immunity, and adaptive immunity work together to fight infection.
- List and describe several common diseases of the immune system.

Pronunciation Guide

Correct pronunciation is important in any journey so that you and others are completely understood. Here is a "see and say" Pronunciation Guide for the more difficult terms to pronounce in this chapter. Please note that even though there are standard pronunciations, regional variations of the pronunciations can occur.

basophils (BAY soh filz)
cytokines (SIGH toe kines)
cytotoxic T cells (SIGH toe TOX ick)
dendritic cells (DEN drit ick)
eosinophils (EE oh SIN oh filz)
histamine (HISS tuh meen)
interferon (in ter FEAR on)
interleukins (IN ter LOO kinz)

leukocytes (LOO koh sights)
lymph nodes (LIMF nohdz)
lymphocytes (LIMF oh sights)
macrophages (MAC roh fage ez)
neutrophil (NOO troh fill)
thoracic duct (thoh RASS ik)
thymus (THIGH mus)
tumor necrosis factor (neh KROH sis)

THE DEFENSE ZONE

Although war may seem a harsh analogy to use, it is the reality of what happens when a potentially dangerous threat invades the body. Suppose a nasty army of pathogens attempts to invade your body. First, it must get past your barriers. Many invaders will be repelled simply by your intact skin or the secretions of your mucous membranes. If the invader does get inside your body, it is recognized as *not* belonging in your body. This recognition stimulates a series of responses to neutralize the foreign invader. Weapons in the form of specialized cells are engaged by the immune and lymphatic systems to fend off the pathogens. In addition, the immune and lymphatic systems release powerful chemicals to help to fight off the invaders.

These chemicals also stimulate the inflammatory response and leave a chemical mess to clean up. The "war" also leaves behind an area of neutralized pathogens and excessive debris and fluid that has collected around the battlefield that must be cleaned up. This again is accomplished by the combined and integrated efforts of the immune and lymphatic systems until the danger is over and your body can return to normal functioning. Let's begin the discussion with the lymphatic system, then bring in the immune system, and finally show how the two work in concert to defend your body against infection.

THE LYMPHATIC SYSTEM

The **lymphatic system** is both the transport system and the barracks of your immune system. It is a second circulatory system parallel to the cardiovascular system. As you will soon see, it works closely with the cardiovascular system, and their close proximity is necessary for optimal function of the immune system. The lymphatic system has the following four functions:

- Recycling fluids lost from the cardiovascular system
- Transporting **pathogens** to the lymph nodes, where they can be destroyed
- Storing and developing some types of white blood cells
- Absorbing glycerol and fatty acids from food

Given that the lymphatic system is intimately connected to the function of the cardiovascular system, it should come as no surprise that the smallest tubes of the lymphatic system, called *lymph capillaries*, run near blood capillaries. Lymph capillaries, tubes that form a network around the cells of connective tissues, are so named because they are structurally similar to blood capillaries, but unlike blood capillaries, lymph capillaries terminate at their dead ends and have more permeable walls than blood capillaries. Proteins and fluids are lost from the cardiovascular capillaries and enter the interstitial space. This interstitial fluid lies between the cells and is normally returned to the blood by way of the lymphatic system. The fluid filling the lymph capillaries is known as **lymphatic fluid**, or simply **lymph**. Lymph is a straw-colored clear fluid similar to plasma; its primary component is water, but it also contains digested nutrients, gases, proteins, and white blood cells called lymphocytes and macrophages. (For the relationship between blood capillaries and lymphatic capillaries, see **FIGURE 15–1** ■)

Lymphatic Vessels

Several lymph capillary networks empty into **lymphatic vessels**, which are structurally similar to veins, including having valves to direct flow. Lymphatic vessels are located in almost all tissues and organs that have blood vessels.

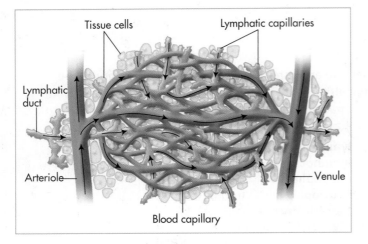

FIGURE 15–1 ■

Relationship between blood and lymph capillaries.

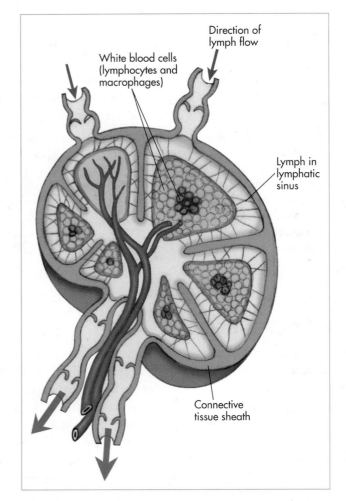

FIGURE 15–2 ■

The lymph node structure.

Body movement and contraction of smooth muscle in the vessel walls propel lymph through the system. Small lymphatic vessels empty into larger lymphatic vessels. Larger lymphatic vessels empty into **lymph nodes**. Ranging in size from a pinhead to an olive, the lymph nodes can be thought of as purification plants strategically placed all along the pathways or vessels of the lymphatic system. Think about a water system for a city where a system of pipes (vessels) brings the dirty water into a plant with a purification system (node) that then recycles clean water back into the system.

Lymph nodes are small, encapsulated bodies divided into sections (see **FIGURE 15–2** ■). Inside the nodes are sections of lymphatic tissue containing white blood cells known as **lymphocytes**. The lymphatic tissue is surrounded by *lymphatic sinuses* (channels) filled with lymph fluid. A number of lymphatic vessels enter or exit each lymph node. This ensures that all lymph fluid must pass through a lymph node for filtration and destruction of pathogens by the white blood cells; it also ensures that the flow slows enough to allow the lymphocytes and macrophages to destroy pathogens.

Lymph nodes are concentrated in several areas around the body and are identified by their regional location: cervical, axillary, inguinal, pelvic, abdominal, thoracic, and supratrochlear. Notice that the lymph nodes are concentrated to catch pathogens where they are most likely to enter the body, such as in the lungs, digestive system, and reproductive system. Lymphatic tissue is also found in the pharynx (throat), in patches commonly known as tonsils and adenoids, in the thymus and spleen (more on these lymphatic structures later), and in Peyer's patches associated with the digestive system. **Tonsils** are masses of lymphocyte-producing lymphatic tissues located in the rear of the pharynx. The three sets of tonsils include the *palatine tonsils*,

located on either side of the oropharynx; the *pharyngeal tonsils* (*adenoids*), located at the posterior nasopharynx; and the *lingual tonsils*, located at the base of the tongue.

Lymphatic vessels leaving lymph nodes empty into one of several **lymphatic trunks**. These trunks, named for their location, are the lumbar, intestinal, bronchomediastinal, subclavian, and jugular. Lymphatic trunks empty into one of two ducts. The lumbar (right and left), intestinal, left bronchomediastinal, left subclavian, and left jugular trunks all empty into the **thoracic duct**, a large duct that runs from the abdomen up through the diaphragm and into the left subclavian vein. More than two-thirds of the lymphatic system drains into the thoracic duct. The right bronchomediastinal, right subclavian, and right jugular trunks empty into the **right lymphatic duct**, a smaller duct within the right thorax that empties into the right subclavian vein (see **FIGURE 15–3** ■).

So what we have is a major recycling plant within the body. The circulation of lymphatic fluid, then, follows this pattern: blood to tissue to lymphatic capillaries to lymphatic vessels

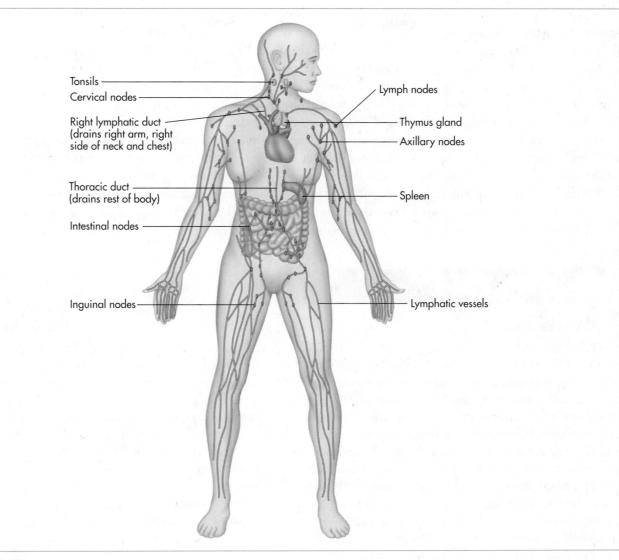

Tonsils

Cervical nodes

Right lymphatic duct
(drains right arm, right
side of neck and chest)

Thoracic duct
(drains rest of body)

Intestinal nodes

Inguinal nodes

Lymph nodes

Thymus gland

Axillary nodes

Spleen

Lymphatic vessels

FIGURE 15–3 ■

The lymphatic system.

to lymph nodes to lymphatic vessels to lymphatic trunks to lymphatic ducts to subclavian veins and then back to the blood. The fluid that moves from blood capillaries into tissues is exposed to the white blood cells in the lymph nodes, where pathogens are removed and destroyed and the fluid is then recycled back to the cardiovascular system. If pathogens are not removed, the nodes can become enlarged and inflamed. For example, in tonsillitis, which can be viral or bacterial in nature, the symptoms include sore throat, fever, difficulty swallowing, swollen tonsils, and swollen lymph nodes.

Lymph Organs

There are two larger collections of lymphatic tissue, known as lymph organs. These lymph organs are the spleen and the thymus. Although they are not strictly lymph nodes and are

not part of lymph circulation, they are so similar to lymph nodes that they are classified as part of the lymph system.

The **spleen** (see Figure 15–3) is a spongy organ in the upper left quadrant of the abdomen. It is structurally similar to lymph nodes, but instead of having lymphatic sinuses, the spleen has blood sinuses. The spleen is also much larger than individual lymph nodes. Islands of white pulp (the soft part of an organ) containing lymphocytes and islands of red pulp containing both red blood cells and white blood cells are surrounded by these blood sinuses. One of the functions of the spleen is to remove and destroy old, damaged, or fragile red blood cells. Can you guess the second function of the spleen, given its anatomy? Because it is similar to a lymph node, the spleen also destroys pathogens in the bloodstream in the same way that lymph nodes destroy pathogens in the lymph.

Although the spleen is a very important organ, it is not one of the vital organs and in some cases, such as trauma, it may need to be surgically removed. Spleen removal in children can severely compromise their ability to ward off disease, so it is rarely done, but in an adult it has much less effect. You'll soon see one reason for this is that as we age, the body becomes better at fighting off infections that it has seen in the past, but new invaders present more of a challenge when we are first exposed to them as children. However, in adults there is an increased risk of septicemia (blood stream infection) if the entire spleen is removed, and therefore to decrease this risk every effort is made to leave at least some of the spleen intact when removal is indicated. Because of the spleen's rich supply of blood vessels, injury to the spleen can often cause serious internal bleeding.

The **thymus** is a soft organ located between the aortic arch and sternum (again, see Figure 15–3). The thymus is very large in children because of all the new infections it must be ready to fend off. It gets smaller or even disappears in adults as the immune system fully matures in its ability to fight infection. The thymus is packed with lymphocytes, which mature into a type of white blood cell called a **T lymphocyte**. The thymus also secretes hormones called *thymosins* that stimulate the maturation of T lymphocytes in lymph nodes. Although thymosins are found in other tissues, they are named for the thymus where they were first found.

Clinical Application

CANCER STAGES

When patients are diagnosed with cancer, they are often told they have a certain "stage" of cancer. Cancer is staged and prognosis is determined by the amount of metastasis (spread). The lymphatic system is amazingly efficient at capturing and transporting pathogens from connective tissue to lymph nodes for destruction. Unfortunately, this ability can also be a liability when cancerous cells develop in one part of the body and use the lymphatic system to hitch a ride to distant areas of the body. The cancerous cells can make their way from their point of origin into lymphatic capillaries, and if the white blood cells in the lymph nodes do not overpower the tumor cells, cancer cells can move around the body, invading many different areas simultaneously and forming new tumors.

Cancers that are diagnosed after they have already spread are much more likely to be fatal than cancer that is treated before cells have a chance to spread. This is why screening for certain types of cancer is so important and often why lymph nodes near tumor sites are removed for study. The earlier a patient is diagnosed, the better the chances of beating the disease. Although most types of cancer have specific staging criteria, cancer stages generally follow this pattern:

- Stage 1: No spread from point of origin
- Stage 2: Spread to nearby tissues
- Stage 3: Spread to nearby lymph nodes
- Stage 4: Spread to distant tissues and organs

Stage 4 cancers are much more difficult to treat.

FOCUS ON PROFESSIONS

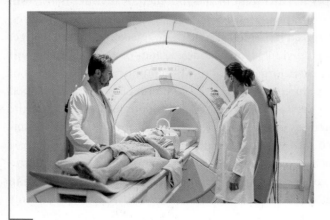

Nuclear medicine deals with the treatment of various types of cancer and attempts to prevent the spread of the cancer through the lymphatic system. Learn more about nuclear medicine and the related professional profiles of opportunities that exist in this field by visiting the websites of national organizations, including the Society of Nuclear Medicine and Molecular Imaging (SNMMI) or the Joint Review Committee on Educational Programs in Nuclear Medicine Technology (JRCNMT).

TEST YOUR KNOWLEDGE 15–1

Choose the best answer:

1. Any organism that invades your body and causes disease is known as a
   a. bacteria.
   b. fungus.
   c. virus.
   d. pathogen.

2. Which of the following areas does *not* have a large number of lymph nodes?
   a. cervical
   b. axillary
   c. abdominal
   d. adrenal

3. Cancer that has entered the lymph nodes is in this stage:
   a. first
   b. second
   c. third
   d. center

4. Which cells are housed in lymph nodes?
   a. red blood cells
   b. white blood cells
   c. platelets
   d. lymph nodules

5. The thoracic duct of the lymphatic system empties into this blood vessel.
   a. right subclavian vein
   b. left subclavian vein
   c. aorta
   d. hepatic portal vein

6. The function of the thymus is to
   a. remove pathogens from blood.
   b. destroy damaged red blood cells.
   c. both a & b
   d. none of the above

7. Swelling of lymph nodes indicates increased number of white blood cells in the nodes. Why would this happen?
   a. injury
   b. infection
   c. anemia
   d. bleeding

THE IMMUNE SYSTEM

If the lymphatic system can be considered a transport and storage system for the body's defense systems, then the components of the **immune system** are the weapons and the actual troops, much like the National Guard, which can be called in to protect a city in times of crisis or disaster. The immune system is a series of cells, chemicals, and barriers that protect the body from invasion by pathogens. Some of the weapons are active, some are passive, some are inborn, and others are acquired. Together they form a system that is remarkably good at keeping the body free of infection.

Antigens and Antibodies

As you should remember from our discussion of blood types in Chapter 13, cells have molecules on the outer surface of their membranes that can be used to identify them. These molecules are called **antigens**. Each human being has unique cell surface antigens, as do all other living things, including bacteria, viruses, animals, and plants. The presence of these unique fingerprints, or antigens, allows the immune system to distinguish between cells that are naturally yours and cells that are not. This ability, called **self-recognition** and **non–self-recognition**, is at the heart of immune system function.

Antigens are like the identity codes sent out by airplanes. Air traffic controllers and fighter jets on patrol over a no-fly zone depend on the identity codes to tell which aircraft are friendly. Antigens do the same for your immune system. A well-functioning immune system ignores your antigens (self) and attacks other antigens (non-self). We will discuss this in more depth later in this chapter.

As part of its defense system, your body can make proteins that bind to antigens, eventually leading to their destruction. Do you remember these proteins from the discussion of blood types? They are **antibodies**, one of the most potent weapons in the body's defensive arsenal. Antibodies are called into action when a foreign antigen invades the body.

Innate versus Adaptive Immunity

The immune system defends the body on two fronts, by *innate (inborn) immunity* and *adaptive (acquired) immunity*. **Innate (inborn) immunity** is the first line of defense against invasion. As the name suggests, innate immunity is the body's inborn ability to fight infection. It prevents invasion, or if pathogens do get inside, innate immunity recognizes the invasion and takes steps to stop the infection from spreading. However, innate immunity can recognize only a general type of pathogen, such as virus versus fungus, or patterns of similarity among pathogens, but it cannot recognize specific pathogens. Innate immunity *cannot* improve with experience, and because it does not recognize specific pathogens, it cannot "remember" an infection the body has encountered before.

Innate immunity consists of a collection of relatively crude mechanisms for defending the body from infection, sort of like building a wall around a city or having metal detectors at the airport. Walls can keep out some invaders, and metal detectors can tell if someone might be carrying a metallic weapon, but neither can respond to specific threats. There is a world of difference between car keys and pocket knives, but metal detectors cannot tell them apart. That's why you have to take your keys out of your pocket when you go through a metal detector. Other parts of innate immunity are like weapons of mass destruction, indiscriminately killing pathogens and healthy tissue alike.

The back-up for innate immunity consists of a different platoon of mechanisms that specifically target invaders, remember invaders from previous encounters and therefore prepare for future invasions, and improve their responses with experience. These mechanisms are known as **adaptive (or acquired) immunity** because the mechanisms can recognize specific invaders and can "learn" and change each time they are engaged. The components of adaptive immunity can be trained as an elite fighting force for particular pathogens. Their goals are "surgical strikes," targeting particular invaders and sparing as much of the healthy body tissue as possible. *Vaccinations* work because of adaptive immunity.

It is tempting to think of these two parts of immunity as separate entities. However, the two work closely together. Innate immunity prepares the way for adaptive immunity, weakening some pathogens and stimulating components of adaptive immunity. Adaptive immunity in turn further stimulates innate immunity. It is through the mutual cooperation of both innate and adaptive immunity attacking the pathogen on two fronts that invaders can be removed from the body.

TEST YOUR KNOWLEDGE 15–2

Choose the best answer:

1. Cell surface molecules that can be used to identify cells are called
   a. antibodies.
   b. antigens.
   c. antihistamines.
   d. antibiotics.

2. Proteins that bind to antigens are called
   a. binding proteins.
   b. receptors.
   c. hormones.
   d. antibodies.

3. This type of immunity has no memory and is not specific:
   a. adaptive.
   b. acquired.
   c. innate.
   d. nonspecific.

4. Smallpox has been wiped out and polio nearly so due to large-scale vaccination programs. Vaccinations work by triggering _____ immunity.
   a. inborn
   b. natural
   c. adaptive
   d. innate

Components of the Immune System

We often think the immune system begins in the blood with the white blood cells. However, physical barriers exist to act as a first line of defense to attempt to stop the infective agents from getting into the body in the first place. This is much like concrete traffic barriers you see in front of public buildings.

Barriers

Anything that prevents invaders from getting inside your body prevents infection. Therefore, your body has many barriers located in the places where invaders are most likely to gain entrance. Physical barriers include skin and the mucous membranes of the eyes, digestive system, respiratory system, and reproductive system. Not only are these surfaces difficult to penetrate, but they are also packed with white blood cells and lymph capillaries to trap any invaders that might get through. The fluids associated with these physical barriers contain chemicals that act as chemical barriers. These chemicals are contained in tears, saliva, digestive juices, urine, mucous secretions, and sweat. One example is the oil secreted by the sebaceous glands of your integumentary system, which can be antibacterial. These barriers, both chemical and physical, prevent some invaders from ever getting inside the body. They are the "fortress" of the body, part of your innate immunity. After reading this information, can you see why wounds are frequent sources of infection?

White Blood Cells

If an invader has an opportunity to enter the body, white blood cells (**leukocytes**) are responsible for defending the body against invaders. You learned about red blood cells and platelets in Chapter 13. Red blood cells are responsible for carrying oxygen throughout the body, and platelets are responsible for the blood's ability to clot. White blood cells, on the other hand, are the mobile units of the immune system. White blood cells, which form in the bone marrow like red blood cells and platelets, move to other parts of the body to grow and mature until they are needed during an invasion. They are generally not released into the bloodstream in large numbers unless an infection is present.

Leukocytes can be divided into two groups. *Polymorphonuclear granulocytes* are cells with granules or spots in their cytoplasm. *Mononuclear agranulocytes* have no granules in their cytoplasm. These two groups contain several different types of cells that play a role in the body's defense against infection. **FIGURE 15–4** ■ shows the major white blood cells found in the plasma.

In a police department of a large city, several types of jobs are needed for the entire department to function: traffic control officers, homicide detectives, forensic crime scene technicians, evidence control officers, internal affairs investigators, and more. Each has a specific duty and is called on as needed, but in essence they all have the same goal—fighting crime. Similarly, the body has various types of white blood cells that are required to protect the body in varying circumstances. The following categories describe the major white blood cells in the plasma and the additional specialized white blood cells of the lymphatic system.

Neutrophils Neutrophils are granulocytes whose function is phagocytosis. Phagocytic cells ingest pathogens and cellular debris. Neutrophils originate in the bone marrow and are the most common leukocyte in the bloodstream. Neutrophils are the first cells to arrive at the site of damage. They immediately begin to clean up the area by ingesting pathogens, and they release chemicals that increase tissue damage and inflammation, stimulating the immune response. Neutrophils are part of innate immunity.

Macrophages Macrophages are modified monocytes, a type of agranulocyte, that leave the bloodstream and enter tissues. They are also phagocytic cells, which are active in the later stages of an infection. In addition to phagocytosis, these cells release chemicals to stimulate the immune system. Macrophages also act as antigen-presenting cells, wearing the antigens of pathogens on the outside to stimulate adaptive immunity. (More details will be seen later.) Macrophages are also part of innate immunity. Macrophages, monocytes, and several other types of phagocytic cells found in organs and tissues are part of the **mononuclear phagocyte system** (or **reticuloendothelial system**). Organs or tissues that are part of the system are the spleen, lymph nodes, liver, lungs, adipose tissue, and mucosa. Osteoclasts, which destroy bone, for example, are cellular parts of the system, as are the macrophages in the alveoli of the lungs.

Basophils and Mast Cells Basophils and mast cells release chemicals to promote inflammation. **Basophils** are granulocytes that enter infected tissues from the bloodstream. Basophil numbers are very low unless an active infection is present. **Mast cells** are found stationed throughout the body. They are always found in connective tissue. For example, when the mast cells in the connective tissue of the nose are stimulated, chemicals are released that lead to rhinitis, more commonly called "runny nose." Mast cell stimulation in the lungs can trigger an asthmatic attack. Both basophils and mast cells are part of innate immunity.

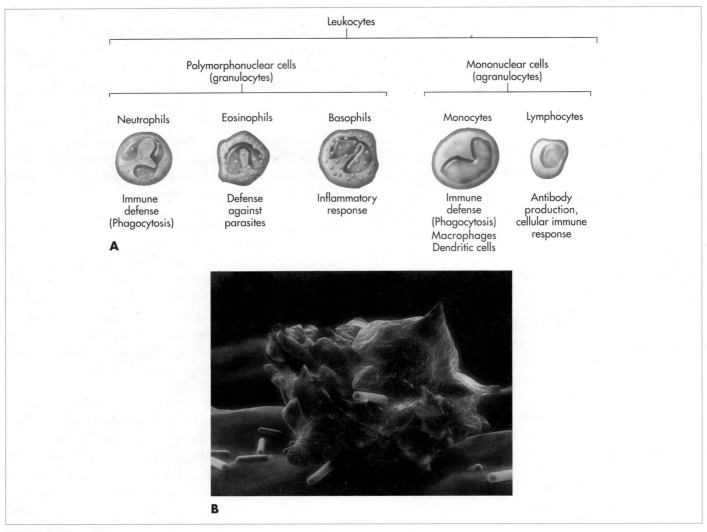

FIGURE 15–4 ■

(A) Major leukocytes. (B) Enhanced color photograph from a scanning electron microscope of a macrophage ingesting rod-shaped bacteria.

Eosinophils **Eosinophils** are granulocytes that move to inflamed areas, participate in allergic reactions, kill parasites, and modulate inflammatory response. Eosinophil numbers are generally low in the bloodstream unless active infection or allergies are present. Eosinophils are part of innate immunity.

Dendritic Cells **Dendritic cells** are another member of a group of cells that are modified monocytes (part of the mononuclear phagocyte system). Their most important job is as **antigen-presenting cells** (APCs). These cells are able to ingest foreign antigens and place the foreign antigens into their own cell membrane. Then the dendritic cells display the foreign antigens and look for the lymphocytes that match the antigen. This is an important trigger of adaptive immunity. These APCs are the red flags or "all points bulletins" that alert your adaptive immune system to respond. They are

an important bridge between innate and adaptive immunity. **FIGURE 15–5** ■ shows the antigen-presenting process.

Natural Killer Cells **Natural killer (NK) cells** are a type of lymphocyte. These lymphocytes are part of innate immunity. They are crude weapons, releasing chemicals to kill any cells displaying foreign antigens, whether they are pathogens or the body's own infected cells. Natural killer cells take out the neighborhood. These cells patrol the body, wiping out any infected cell they encounter. Some early symptoms of a cold or flu are actually due to the action of the NK cells damaging tissues, not from the infection.

T Lymphocytes **T lymphocytes** (*T cells*) are lymphocytes responsible for a portion of adaptive immunity known as **cell-mediated immunity**. There are several different types of T cells,

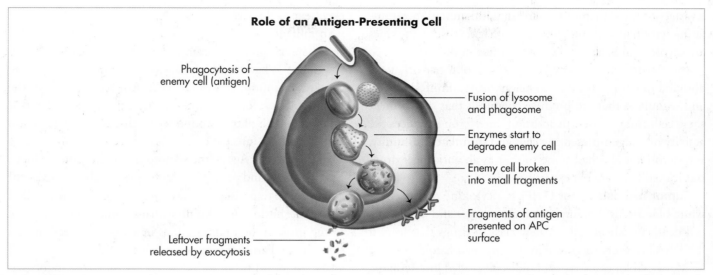

Role of an Antigen-Presenting Cell

Phagocytosis of enemy cell (antigen)

Fusion of lysosome and phagosome

Enzymes start to degrade enemy cell

Enemy cell broken into small fragments

Fragments of antigen presented on APC surface

Leftover fragments released by exocytosis

FIGURE 15–5 ■

The role of antigen-presenting cell (APC).

including **cytotoxic T cells** (literally "cell poison"), which kill infected cells and release immune stimulating chemicals; **helper T cells**, which help activate other parts of adaptive immunity; **regulatory T cells**, which regulate immune response; and **memory T cells**, which remember pathogens after exposure.

B Lymphocytes B lymphocytes (*B cells*) are lymphocytes responsible for the part of adaptive immunity known as **antibody-mediated immunity**. There are two types of B cells: **plasma cells**, which produce antibodies to non–self-antigens, and **memory B cells**, which remember pathogens. TABLE 15–1 ■ gives a synopsis of the white blood cells involved in the immune response.

Chemicals

Not only do blood cells fight invaders, but chemicals found in the body can also assist in neutralizing and destroying invaders. **Cytokines** are proteins produced by damaged tissues and white blood cells that stimulate immune response in

TABLE 15–1 WHITE BLOOD CELLS INVOLVED IN IMMUNE RESPONSE

CELL TYPE	FUNCTION	INNATE OR ADAPTIVE
Neutrophils	Phagocytosis early in infection.	Innate.
Macrophages	Phagocytosis later in infection, stimulate immune system, antigen-presenting cell.	Innate but stimulate adaptive immunity.
Basophils and mast cells	Release inflammatory chemicals. Basophils are mobile; mast cells are found in connective tissue.	Innate.
Eosinophils	Fight parasites and contributes to allergic reactions.	Innate.
Dendritic cells	Antigen-presenting cells.	Innate but stimulate adaptive immunity.
Natural killer cells	Kill cells displaying foreign antigens.	Innate.
T cells (lymphocytes)	Kill pathogens directly, regulate immune response, activate other lymphocytes, remember past infections.	Adaptive.
B cells (lymphocytes)	Release antibodies to foreign antigens, remember past infections.	Adaptive.

a variety of ways, including increasing inflammation, stimulating lymphocytes, and enhancing phagocytosis. Cytokines are involved in both innate and adaptive immunity.

Interferon refers to any group of glycoproteins that are antiviral in nature. It binds to neighboring, uninfected cells and stimulates them to produce chemicals that may protect these cells from viruses. In addition, interferon enhances the activity of antigen-presenting cells and stimulates immunity. Interferon has also had some success as an anticancer drug, but it is still considered experimental.

Tumor necrosis factor (TNF) is a cytokine produced by white blood cells. It stimulates macrophages and also causes cell death in cancer cells. A new class of drugs that inhibit TNF has been very successful in treating rheumatoid arthritis.

Many cytokines are types of molecules called **interleukins**. There are at least 10 different interleukins. They are involved in nearly every aspect of innate and adaptive immunity. Interleukins also have been used with moderate success in treating some forms of cancer.

Complement cascade is a complex series of reactions that activate more than 20 proteins that are usually inactive in the blood unless activated by a pathogen invasion. When these proteins are activated, they have a variety of effects, including **lysis** (*to break down or destroy*) of bacterial cell membranes, stimulation of phagocytosis, and attraction of white blood cells to the site of infection. Complement cascade is part of *both* innate and adaptive immunity. It is innate, but the adaptive immune response can trigger complement cascade.

Inflammation

Inflammation, or the inflammatory response, is one of the most familiar weapons in the body's arsenal. Everyone has experienced the swelling, pain, heat, and redness associated with inflammation at one time or another. Think back several chapters ago to our example of hitting your thumb with a hammer. What would happen to your thumb within a few minutes of injury? It would swell, turn red, get hot to the touch, and hurt for some time after the injury. Remember that inflammation is part of wound repair, discussed in Chapter 5. What about an infected cut? Or a sore throat when you have a cold or the flu? Again, the symptoms are the same: redness, heat, swelling, and pain. This reaction is a deliberate action of your body in response to tissue damage, whether a mechanical injury, like hitting your thumb with a hammer, or damage due to the invasion of a pathogen, as in a wound infection or a strep throat. Part of this response helps to wall off the infected area to prevent further spread and allow the battle to focus at this site. This process, called **margination**, is an attempt to isolate the problem. Recent research has demonstrated a link between chronic stress and inflammation. This is yet another reason to try to learn to properly manage your stress.

When tissue is damaged, the cells send out chemicals such as **histamine**, a cytokine, which have several effects. These chemicals attract white blood cells to the site of the injury, increase the permeability of capillaries, and cause local vasodilation. Extra fluid moves from the capillaries into the damaged tissue, causing swelling. More blood comes to the site, increasing the temperature of the tissue. White blood cells enter the area, destroying pathogens and clearing away dead and dying cells. The increase in fluid and cells coming to the area increases the pressure and is part of the reason the area remains painful, even as the damage is being repaired. Inflammation is an innate immune mechanism, but it is also an important player in adaptive immunity. Please see **FIGURE 15–6** ■.

Clinical Application

INFLAMMATION: A DOUBLE-EDGED SWORD

Inflammation, like many of the body's weapons, has a positive feedback loop. Once inflammation starts, it continues until turned off. This kind of runaway positive feedback can cause problems if localized swelling increases pressure, causing more tissue damage. One of the reasons you "ice" a sprained ankle is to decrease inflammation to prevent further damage. Inflammation is a particular problem in enclosed or small spaces like the cranium, spinal column, thoracic cage, and extremities where a small buildup of pressure can cause serious damage. Even more dangerous is inflammation that becomes systemic, spreading throughout the whole body. A type of hypersensitive inflammation due to allergies is called **anaphylaxis**, which often causes blood pressure to plummet due to widespread vasodilation. Some people who are allergic to insect stings may experience this kind of inflammation. Anaphylaxis can be fatal unless treated by a medical professional immediately.

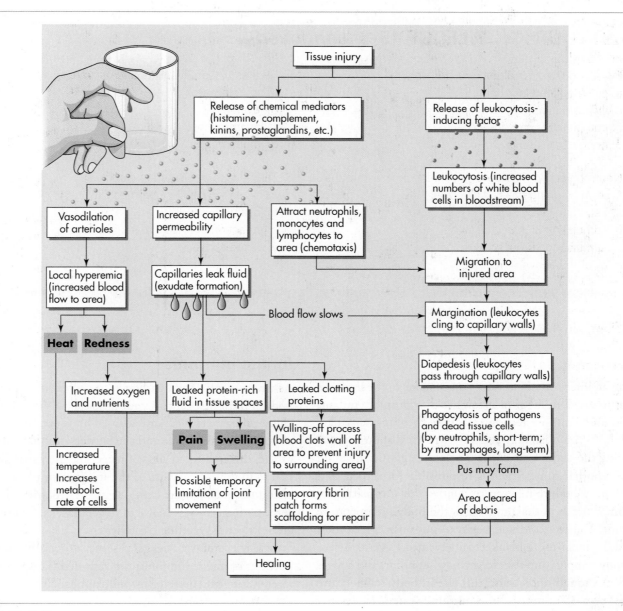

FIGURE 15–6 ■

Inflammatory response.

TEST YOUR KNOWLEDGE 15–3

Choose the best answer:

1. Which of the following is *not* a function of complement cascade?
   a. lysis of bacterial cell membrane
   b. stimulation of macrophages
   c. chemotaxis
   d. swelling

2. These chemicals may protect the body against viruses and some cancers:
   a. complement.
   b. cytokines.
   c. interferons.
   d. immunoglobulins.

(continued)

TEST YOUR KNOWLEDGE 15–3 *(continued)*

3. B lymphocytes are directly responsible for
   a. cell-mediated immunity.
   b. inflammation.
   c. complement cascade.
   d. none of the above

4. Neutrophils and macrophages aid the innate immune system by doing this:
   a. secreting cytokines.
   b. stimulating phagocytosis.
   c. stimulating immune response.
   d. all of the above

5. Redness, heat, swelling, and pain are all symptoms of
   a. complement.
   b. fever.
   c. inflammation.
   d. infection.

6. The release of histamine can cause
   a. increased capillary permeability.
   b. localized vasodilation.
   c. attraction of WBC's to injury site.
   d. all the above

Fever

During an infection, tissues and components of the immune system release a number of cytokines that promote inflammation and immune responses. These cytokines circulate through the bloodstream and often reach distant targets, including the brain. One of the cytokine targets in the brain is the hypothalamus, which is responsible for setting and maintaining body temperature. Under the stimulation of cytokines, the hypothalamus raises the body's temperature set point. You feel cold and begin to put on more clothes, to huddle under more blankets and even to shiver. Eventually, body temperature rises to the new set point, and a fever results. Although unpleasant, this rise in body temperature is a deliberate attempt by the immune system to destroy the pathogens that have invaded the body. Like the rest of the innate response system, fever is a crude weapon against invaders. It might help fight off the infection, but it also causes overall discomfort.

HOW THE IMMUNE SYSTEM WORKS

Pathogens are all around you. Every breath you take, every surface you touch, everything you put into your mouth has potential pathogens. It's enough to make you run for the disinfectant. The potential for infection is all around you, *but* if your immune system is working as it should, most of these potential pathogens are prevented from entering your body. If some pathogens do get in, most are defeated by the powerful armies of your immune system. Let's look at your defense systems in closer detail.

Innate Immunity

As we have seen, for a pathogen to successfully invade your body, it must first get past your physical (i.e., intact skin) and chemical barriers (i.e., antibacterial body secretions). Think of your body as a castle and the barriers of innate immunity as the alligator-filled moat protecting the castle from the marauding hoards. Most of the millions of pathogens you encounter each day are kept out by these barriers. However, some pathogens—influenza or the cold virus, for example—are very good at getting past barriers.

When a pathogen does get past the barriers, the more active portions of innate immunity are activated. The presence of a foreign antigen is detected by **neutrophils**. Neutrophils ingest the foreign antigen, destroy it, and release chemicals (cytokines, for example) that attract other white blood cells to the site of infection and stimulate inflammation. Continuing our castle analogy, the neutrophils are the guards who greet any marauders who manage to slip past the alligators.

The release of cytokines and stimulation of inflammation attract **macrophages** and **natural killer (NK) cells** to the infection site. Macrophages destroy more infected cells by phagocytosis. The NK cells use chemicals to destroy infected cells. Both cells release chemicals that further stimulate inflammation, activate more immune cells, and trigger the complement cascade. Back to our analogy, the castle guards sound the alarm that the castle has been breached, summoning more troops to fight the invaders.

At this point, the infected cells, or the pathogens themselves, are under attack on several fronts: phagocytosis, noxious chemicals, membrane rupture, clumping, and inflammation. Chemicals have signaled your hypothalamus to raise your body temperature, and you run a fever. You feel like…, well you know how you feel. There is no question in your mind that you are ill. Finishing our analogy, even though the guards are protecting the castle, the castle will be damaged.

You would think this would be enough to fight off most pathogens. But keep in mind that this is crude warfare. Innate immunity simply destroys anything that is non-self. It does not use surgical strikes or specific weapons. Innate immunity lays waste to the infected area with almost indiscriminate attacks. Defending the castle is warfare in the crudest sense— no specialized weapons, just desperate attempts to defeat the invaders. Uninfected cells can be destroyed in the process.

In some cases, these mechanisms are enough, but often the innate immune system is buying time for adaptive immunity to ready the "big guns"—the B and T cells of adaptive immunity. Indeed, the activities of innate immunity stimulate adaptive immunity. Chemicals released by NK cells, neutrophils, and other cells help activate adaptive immunity. When antigen-presenting cells ingest pathogens, they display the foreign antigen on their cell membranes. *This ability to display foreign antigens without being infected is absolutely necessary for activation of B and T cells.*

Adaptive Immunity

Remember how many sore throats and colds you suffered through back in grade school? Chances are, they do not happen as frequently now that you're an adult. This is because your immune system can adapt. Fighting specific pathogens is the job of adaptive immunity. This part of the immune system, because it is acquired, has memory, "learns" with experience, and recognizes specific pathogens. It is because of adaptive immunity that most people get the chicken pox only once. (Thank goodness for that!) Although the chicken pox was considered close to eradication, an increasing number of unvaccinated children are leading to an increase of chicken pox cases. The cells responsible for the adaptive immune system, B and T lymphocytes, remember pathogens and mount specific responses to those pathogens if they meet again. It is because of adaptive immunity that immunizations are able to prevent illness. When was the last time you heard of somebody in the United States getting polio? Just 60 years ago, polio was an epidemic in the United States. Keep in mind that innate and adaptive immunity work hand in hand. One cannot do its job without the other.

Lymphocyte Selection

To function, lymphocytes must be able to destroy pathogens and not destroy the body's own tissues. Think of these cells as members of the local fire company. They have a very specific job—putting out fires. Like any professional firefighter, lymphocytes must be *selected*. During **positive selection**, lymphocytes that can actually recognize and bind to antigens (any antigens) are allowed to survive. Lymphocytes that fail to do their job do not survive, much like a firefighter who cannot carry a hose or climb a ladder will not become part of the company. Unfortunately, some of these selected lymphocytes actually recognize and bind to your antigens. If not destroyed, they will attack and destroy your own tissues. By the same token, fire companies take care not to hire arsonists to work for the fire department. The destruction of lymphocytes that destroy the body's own tissue is known as **negative selection**. Both positive and negative selection must work for your immune system to function appropriately. You must have lymphocytes that attack invaders but don't attack you.

Lymphocyte Activation

Lymphocytes develop and mature when you are a baby or a very young child. Just like you, they begin as an undifferentiated cell, meaning they have the potential to become anything. They must then undergo a maturation process to become **differentiated**—in other words, to grow up to be a specialized cell with a specialized function. Undifferentiated lymphocytes are produced in the bone marrow, but some migrate to the thymus and are destined to become T cells. Others stay, develop, and mature in the bone marrow to become B cells.

After they are specialized, lymphocytes can go into suspended animation. For the lymphocytes to fight off the pathogen, they must have a wake-up call. Picture the fire company sleeping in the middle of the night and the alarm going off. This kind of wake-up call for lymphocytes is called **lymphocyte activation**. See **FIGURE 15–7** ■ to see how the immune system activates lymphocytes.

LEARNING HINT

Lymphocyte Names

Remember that **T** cells come from the **T**hymus and **B** cells come from the **B**one marrow.

Let's go back to innate immune response for a minute. When a pathogen invades your tissues, your innate immunity mounts a response to the pathogen. One part of innate immunity is phagocytosis of infected cells or bits of pathogen. When these cells—macrophages, dendritic cells, and others—eat the pathogen, the pathogen's antigens are displayed on the outside of the phagocytic cells, kind of like little "Wanted" posters.

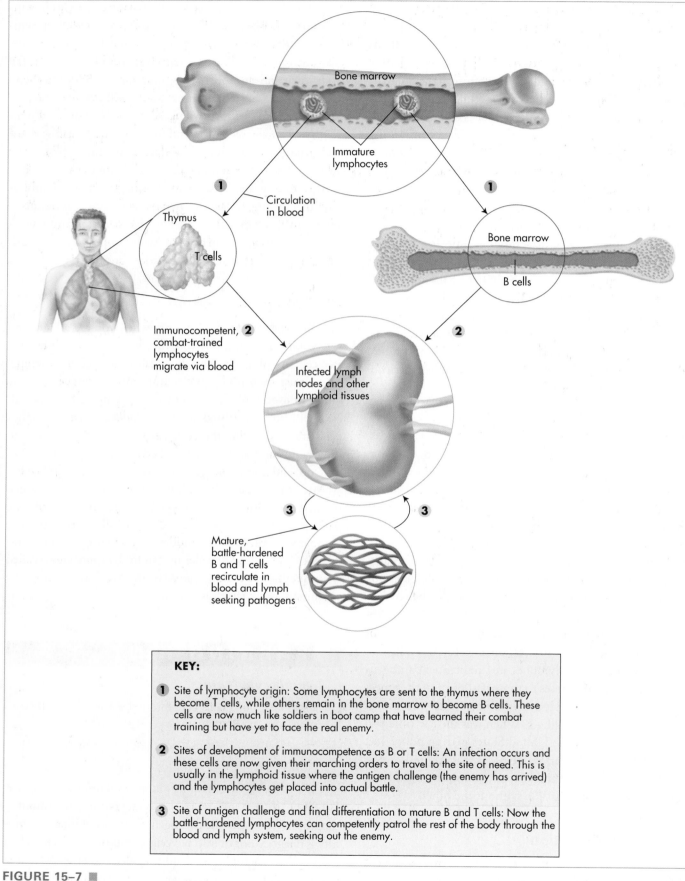

Bone marrow

Immature
lymphocytes

1

Circulation
in blood

1

Thymus

T cells

Bone marrow

B cells

Immunocompetent, **2**
combat-trained
lymphocytes
migrate via blood

2

Infected lymph
nodes and other
lymphoid tissues

3

3

Mature,
battle-hardened
B and T cells
recirculate in
blood and lymph
seeking pathogens

KEY:

1 Site of lymphocyte origin: Some lymphocytes are sent to the thymus where they become T cells, while others remain in the bone marrow to become B cells. These cells are now much like soldiers in boot camp that have learned their combat training but have yet to face the real enemy.

2 Sites of development of immunocompetence as B or T cells: An infection occurs and these cells are now given their marching orders to travel to the site of need. This is usually in the lymphoid tissue where the antigen challenge (the enemy has arrived) and the lymphocytes get placed into actual battle.

3 Site of antigen challenge and final differentiation to mature B and T cells: Now the battle-hardened lymphocytes can competently patrol the rest of the body through the blood and lymph system, seeking out the enemy.

FIGURE 15–7 ■

Lymphocyte differentiation and activation.

These cells then prowl the body, displaying these tiny bits of pathogen, searching for the lymphocytes that can recognize the pathogen. When the right lymphocytes meet the right antigen display, the lymphocytes are activated (their wake-up call for battle). This activation is the beginning of adaptive immunity.

Lymphocyte Proliferation

The body has only a few lymphocytes that recognize each invader to which it has been exposed. But to fight off an infection, hundreds of thousands of lymphocytes are needed to attack the infection. Simple activation of lymphocytes is not enough. The activated lymphocytes must make thousands of copies of themselves to fight off the thousands of pathogens reproducing in the body. This reproduction of lymphocytes is called **lymphocyte proliferation** (see **FIGURE 15–8** ■). Just like one platoon would not be enough to repel a full-scale invasion of a country, or one fire company enough to save a city block from burning down, a few lymphocytes are not enough to defend the entire body.

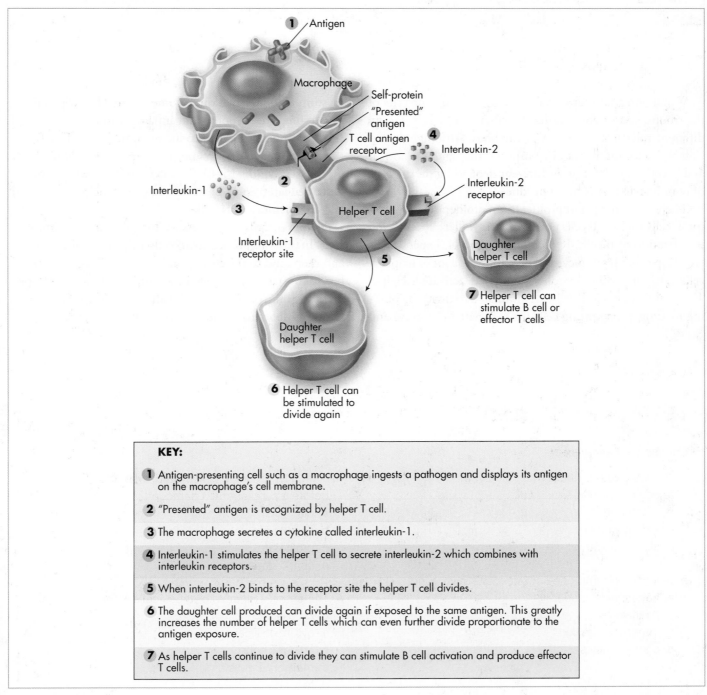

KEY:

1 Antigen-presenting cell such as a macrophage ingests a pathogen and displays its antigen on the macrophage's cell membrane.

2 "Presented" antigen is recognized by helper T cell.

3 The macrophage secretes a cytokine called interleukin-1.

4 Interleukin-1 stimulates the helper T cell to secrete interleukin-2 which combines with interleukin receptors.

5 When interleukin-2 binds to the receptor site the helper T cell divides.

6 The daughter cell produced can divide again if exposed to the same antigen. This greatly increases the number of helper T cells which can even further divide proportionate to the antigen exposure.

7 As helper T cells continue to divide they can stimulate B cell activation and produce effector T cells.

FIGURE 15–8 ■

Activation and proliferation of helper T cells.

Clinical Application

AIDS

The acquired immune deficiency syndrome (AIDS) is caused by infection with the human immunodeficiency virus (HIV), a virus that specifically targets and destroys a type of helper T cell called CD-4. CD-4 cells are necessary for the proliferation of B cells. As helper T cells are infected with HIV and begin to die, their numbers decrease dramatically, so B cell and T cell proliferation is too slow to respond to an infection. Patients with full-blown AIDS often die from massive infections that they would otherwise be able to fight easily. These same infections are also found in patients with other types of immune deficiency diseases or who are taking immunosuppressant drugs to prevent post-transplant organ rejection or to treat autoimmune diseases.

When you first met lymphocytes, earlier in our tour of the troops, you discovered that B cells and T cells have very different roles in the defense of the body. Although activation and selection is, for our purposes, the same for both B and T cells, proliferation is different depending on the type of lymphocyte that is being produced.

There are two types of proliferation: proliferation of effector T cells (helper T cells and cytotoxic [killer] T cells) and proliferation of B cells. Remember, the job of helper T cells is to help other lymphocytes. There must be a lot of helper T cells before any other lymphocytes can be activated. Helper T cells and cytotoxic T cells are stimulated to divide by binding to antigen-presenting cells (from innate immunity) and by stimulation by cytokines (some secreted by cells from the innate immune response and inflammation). The helper T cells continue to divide, producing more helper T cells, and then help (hence their name) in the proliferation of B cells (again, see Figure 15–8). The cytotoxic T cell function is described later. Some of the cytotoxic and helper T cells will become memory cells.

Helper T cells are necessary for the reproduction of B cells. In order to proliferate, B cells are primed by an antigen and then bind to the corresponding helper T cell, which has been activated by an antigen-presenting cell, in order to proliferate. Some of these B cells will become plasma cells and release antibodies, whereas others will become memory cells.

TEST YOUR KNOWLEDGE 15–4

Choose the best answer:

1. To be activated, T cells must bind with
   a. an antigen-presenting cell.
   b. a pathogen.
   c. a damaged cell.
   d. all of the above

2. Selection for immune-competent cells is called
   a. negative selection.
   b. positive selection.
   c. immune selection.
   d. competency selection.

3. After a lymphocyte is activated, what must it do before it can fight off a pathogen?
   a. die
   b. agglutinate
   c. proliferate
   d. congregate

4. The primary function of these cells is the activation of B cells:
   a. cytotoxic T cells.
   b. helper T cells.
   c. memory T cells.
   d. regulatory T cells.

B and T Cell Action

So, let's get back to the body's response to invasion. The innate immune system has been attacking the pathogen or cells infected with the pathogen on a number of fronts, using phagocytic cells, NK cells, fever, and a variety of noxious chemicals. A number of the body's own cells have been destroyed in the process, but the pathogen has not been defeated. However, while innate immunity has been holding down the fort, antigen-presenting cells (APCs) have sent out a signal calling on the weapons of adaptive immunity: B cells and T cells.

B Cells

B cells are responsible for a type of adaptive immunity known as **humoral**, or **antibody-mediated immunity**. B cells fight pathogens by making and releasing antibodies to attack a specific pathogen. These B cells develop into **plasma cells** and **memory B cells**. Antibodies are made by plasma cells and released into the bloodstream. Antibodies bind to the antigens of infected cells or the antigens on the surface of freely floating pathogens. They are missiles programmed to home in on a specific target. Antibodies destroy pathogens using several methods, including inactivating the antigen, causing antigens to clump together, activating complement cascade, causing the release of chemicals to stimulate the immune system, and enhancing phagocytosis. This response to the pathogen is called the **primary response**.

All of these antibody-mediated mechanisms not only destroy pathogens specifically, but they also further stimulate both adaptive and innate immune response, continually increasing response to the pathogen. Remember that immune response is a positive feedback loop that must be deliberately turned off. It will not stop on its own. This makes sense if you think in terms of protection. Your protective systems should not give up until the danger is passed. Smoke alarms keep wailing until there is no more smoke.

Other B cells, memory B cells, are stored in lymph nodes until they are needed at some future date. If the body is exposed to the same pathogen in the future, memory cells allow it to mount a much faster response to the invasion. This response is known as **secondary response** and is responsible for the ability of adaptive immunity to improve with experience (see **FIGURE 15–9** ■).

T Cells

There are at least four types of T cells: helper T cells, cytotoxic T cells, regulatory T cells (formerly known as suppressor T cells), and memory T cells. We have already seen the action of helper T cells.

Cytotoxic T cells are responsible for a part of adaptive immune response known as **cell-mediated immunity**, so called because the cytotoxic T cells are directly responsible for the death of pathogens or pathogen-infected cells. Cytotoxic T cells release a cytokine called **perforin**, which causes

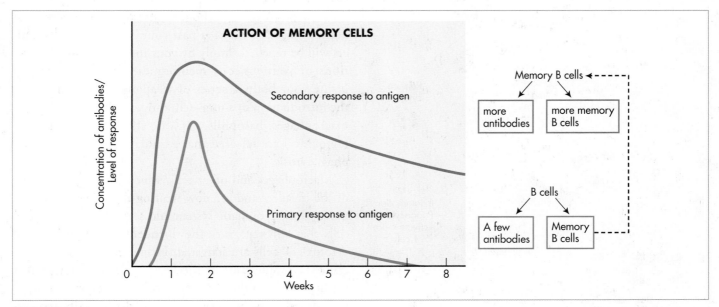

FIGURE 15–9 ■

The primary response causes B cells to produce *memory* B cells and a few antibodies. The second exposure causes the secondary response to produce more memory B cells and even more antibodies to fight the invaders. Now that the body has antibodies and more memory B cells, the secondary response begins more rapidly after exposure, produces more antibodies, and lasts a longer time.

infected cells to develop holes in their membranes and die. Cytotoxic T cells also release other cytokines that stimulate both innate and adaptive immunity, especially attracting macrophages to the site of infection to dispose of cellular debris. The response of cytotoxic T cells is the primary response of cell-mediated immunity. Some T cells, rather than becoming cytotoxic T cells, give rise to memory T cells. Like memory B cells, memory T cells are responsible for secondary response, storing the recognition of the pathogen until the next encounter (see **FIGURE 15–10** ■). This memory of the pathogen is responsible for the secondary response.

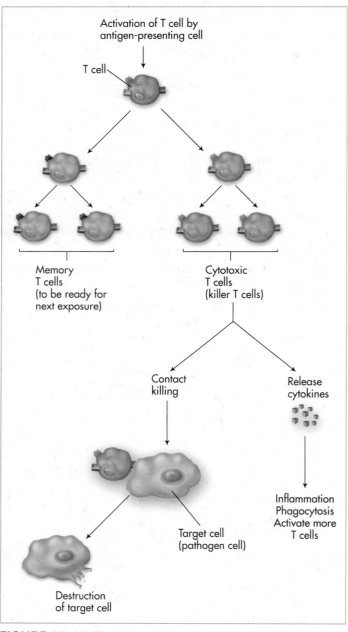

FIGURE 15–10 ■

Cell-mediated immunity, primary and secondary response.

Regulatory T cells are the off-switch for the immune system. Immunity is controlled largely by positive feedback. Tissue damage causes the release of stimulatory chemicals that cause inflammation and increased immune response. Increased immune response results in the release of more chemicals, which causes more stimulation, which causes more chemicals to be released, and so on. Something must actively work to turn off the response when the threat is over or the immune response could become rampant and out of control and thus cause damage. This is the job of the regulatory T cells.

A bit of mystery surrounds regulatory T cells. For years, scientists suspected their existence, but these cells have only been found in the last 25 years. These cells can shut off cytotoxic T cells, helper T cells, and antigen-presenting cells. A malfunction of regulatory T cells may be implicated in some types of allergies, asthma, and autoimmune disease.

THE BIG PICTURE

At this point we have talked about the lymphatic system, innate immunity, and adaptive immunity as separate means to the same end: ridding the body of invading pathogens. We have mentioned repeatedly that the divisions are *not* separate but are intimately connected. Now that we have inspected them separately, it is time to put the entire defense system back together as a single, integrated fighting force (see **FIGURE 15–11** ■).

A nasty army of pathogens attempts to invade your body. First, they must get past your barriers. Many invaders will be repelled simply by your intact skin or the secretions of your mucous membranes. If the invaders get inside your body, a series of weapons are stimulated by the introduction of a non–self-antigen. Cells (neutrophils, macrophages, basophils, etc.) are stimulated. Chemicals (cytokines) are released that stimulate inflammation and phagocytosis.

Macrophages and other cells, which have ingested some of the invaders and are now wearing the foreign antigens, move to the lymphatic system and search for the T and B cells that will recognize the intruder. Helper T cells and cytotoxic T cells are activated. Helper T cells activate and cause the proliferation of B cells and release chemicals that further stimulate the phagocytic cells and inflammation. B cells produce antibodies that destroy the invaders and further stimulate immune response. Cytotoxic T cells destroy invaders directly and release chemicals that further stimulate immune response.

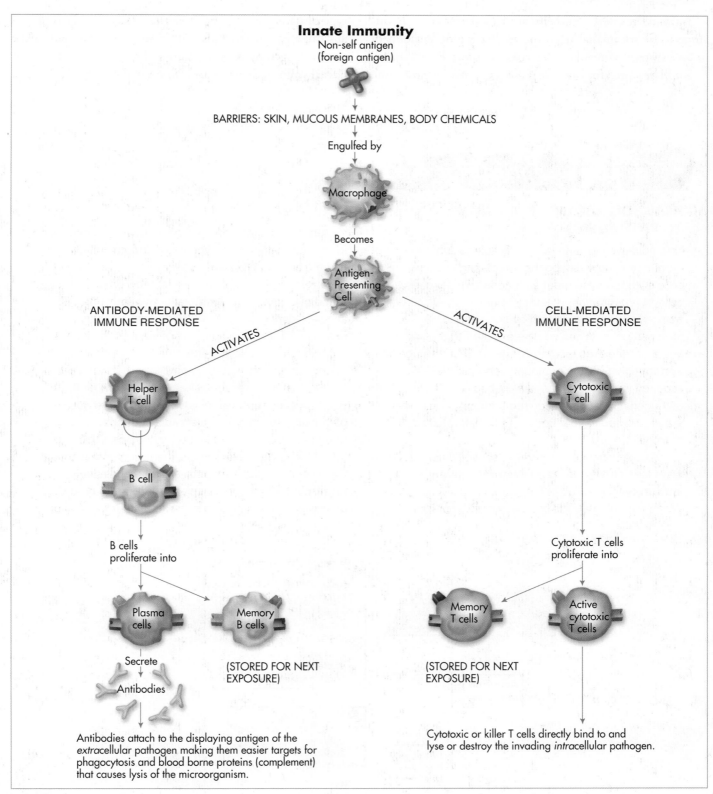

Innate Immunity
Non-self antigen
(foreign antigen)

BARRIERS: SKIN, MUCOUS MEMBRANES, BODY CHEMICALS

Engulfed by

Macrophage

Becomes

Antigen-
Presenting
Cell

ANTIBODY-MEDIATED
IMMUNE RESPONSE

ACTIVATES

ACTIVATES

CELL-MEDIATED
IMMUNE RESPONSE

Helper
T cell

Cytotoxic
T cell

B cell

B cells
proliferate into

Cytotoxic T cells
proliferate into

Plasma
cells

Memory
B cells

Memory
T cells

Active
cytotoxic
T cells

Secrete

(STORED FOR NEXT
EXPOSURE)

(STORED FOR NEXT
EXPOSURE)

Antibodies

Antibodies attach to the displaying antigen of the
*extra*cellular pathogen making them easier targets for
phagocytosis and blood borne proteins (complement)
that causes lysis of the microorganism.

Cytotoxic or killer T cells directly bind to and
lyse or destroy the invading *intra*cellular pathogen.

FIGURE 15–11 ■

The battle plan of the body's defenses.

Immune response, both innate and adaptive, will continue to be stimulated until the feedback loop is stopped, at least in part by regulatory T cells. Memory B cells and T cells will be stored for later use if another army of those same type of pathogens attempts another invasion. Macrophages and other phagocytic cells will clean up the debris left by the warfare waged by your immune system. Once the danger is passed, your body will return to normal.

Clinical Application

HOW YOU ACQUIRE IMMUNITY TO PATHOGENS

Your adaptive immune system is able to acquire immunity to new pathogens by creating memory cells each time you meet a pathogen. This process, called *immunization*, whether natural or medical, trains your immune system by creating memory cells for a pathogen. When you are exposed to the pathogen a second time, you do not get ill. Your immune system fights off the pathogen very quickly. In active acquired immunity, *you make* antibodies to fight the pathogens. In passive acquired immunity, antibodies *are introduced* to your body, and therefore you don't make your own.

You can acquire immunity in several different ways (see **FIGURE 15–12** ■). **Natural active immunity** is acquired in the course of daily life. When you catch a virus or a bacterium, your immune system fights it off, and memory cells are created for the next meeting. Anybody old enough to have had the chicken pox as a child (before the vaccine became available) is usually protected from a second round of chicken pox. **Artificial active immunity** is acquired during vaccinations. Getting a measles shot exposes you to small amounts of weakened virus, not enough to make you sick, but enough for your immune system to create memory cells. If you meet the virus later in life, you will be able to fight it off. Babies acquire **natural passive immunity** to many pathogens via antibodies passed across the placenta or during breast-feeding. These antibodies, which babies can't yet make, protect them from infection for several months after birth. **Artificial passive immunity** is acquired when antibodies from one person are injected into another to help fight infection.

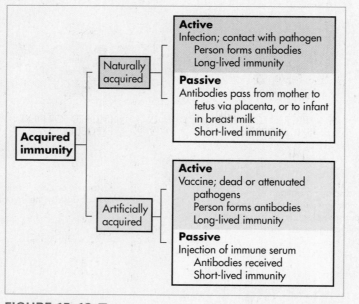

FIGURE 15–12 ■
Types of immunities.

TEST YOUR KNOWLEDGE 15–5

Choose the best answer:

1. B cells, once activated, can become two different kinds of cells: memory B cells and
   a. cytotoxic T cells.
   b. natural killers.
   c. plasma cells.
   d. macrophages.

2. Secondary response is mediated by
   a. cytotoxic T cells.
   b. macrophages.
   c. memory cells.
   d. all of the above

3. _____ cells are responsible for antibody-mediated immunity, whereas cell mediated immunity is performed by _____ cells.
   a. B cells; cytotoxic T cells
   b. B cells; cytotoxic B cells
   c. B cells; plasma cells
   d. Plasma cells; memory cells

4. These cells, which were only discovered recently, are part of the "off switch" for the immune system.
   a. cytotoxic T cells
   b. memory T cells
   c. regulatory T cells
   d. helper T cells

5. This type of immunity is acquired as a result of vaccinations:
   a. artificial active immunity
   b. natural active immunity
   c. artificial passive immunity
   d. natural passive immunity

COMMON DISORDERS OF THE IMMUNE SYSTEM

Immune disorders can be life threatening because of a weakened or compromised body defense system. The system can become compromised by factors outside the body, such as invading viruses or by a situation in which the body attacks itself.

Immunodeficiency Disorders

Patients with any of several types of immunodeficiency disorders have immune systems that are underactive. Their immune systems do not respond adequately to the invasion of pathogens and therefore do not protect them from infection. Patients who are immune deficient get sick very easily and do not recover quickly. Minor infections can be fatal. Some immune-deficient patients become infected by pathogens that usually don't infect humans. Immune deficiency can be caused by viruses, genetics, chemical or radiation exposure, or even medication.

Immune-compromised patients include those with AIDS, SCID (severe combined immune deficiency, a genetic disorder), leukemia (cancer of the white blood cells), some forms of anemia, and patients undergoing chemotherapy or taking immunosuppressant drugs after organ transplant.

Autoimmune Disorders

Autoimmune disorders are the opposite of immunodeficiency disorders, exactly what you would expect, given their name. Autoimmune disorders occur when the immune system attacks some part of the body. For some reason, the body fails to recognize "self" and destroys its own tissues as if they were foreign tissues. There are literally hundreds of autoimmune disorders. Any part of the body can come under attack by mistake. Some of the more common disorders (and what they attack) are as follows:

- Rheumatoid arthritis (joint linings)
- Multiple sclerosis (myelin sheath in central nervous system)
- Lupus erythematosus (every tissue, perhaps DNA)
- Type 1 diabetes (beta cells in pancreas)
- Myasthenia gravis (acetylcholine receptors in skeletal muscle)
- Graves' disease (thyroid gland)
- Addison's disease (adrenal gland)

Just this short list illustrates how devastating an auto-immune disorder can be. Imagine the full power of your immune system turning against your thyroid gland or myelin sheath. The effects are devastating. Most autoimmune disorders can be treated with immunosuppressant drugs, but treatment may not be spectacularly successful, and side effects are often severe.

Allergies

During an allergic reaction the immune system mounts a hyperactive response to a foreign antigen, often treating a harmless antigen, such as grass or mold or insect bite, as an invading pathogen. Local reactions—such as hay fever, hives, skin rashes, and asthma—are generally mild and not life threatening. Asthma can be an exception depending on its severity because it interferes with ventilation. Systemic reactions, known as anaphylaxis, are life threatening. During anaphylaxis, mast cells and basophils release immune-stimulating chemicals throughout the body. The chemicals cause widespread vasodilation, which leads to dangerously low blood pressure and heart failure. Hives and asthma may also accompany an anaphylactic reaction. FIGURE 15–13 ■ shows stimulation of the mast cells within the nose due to an allergen, which causes allergic rhinitis. Note that mast cells are found throughout the body. If overstimulated in the eyes, mast cells cause red and runny eyes; if overstimulated in the lungs, they can cause allergic asthma.

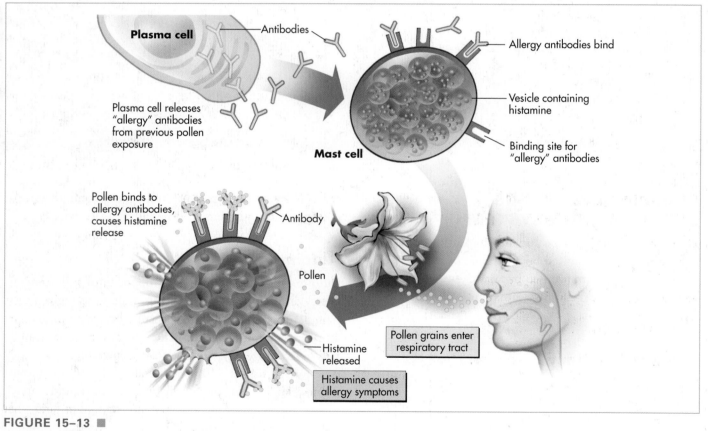

FIGURE 15–13 ■

Allergic rhinitis.

- The lymphatic system is the transport system for the immune system and houses the lymphocytes. It consists of lymph capillaries, vessels, trunks, and ducts containing lymphatic fluid and lymph nodes, which house white blood cells.

- Lymph nodes are concentrated in several regions of the body: cervical, axillary, inguinal, pelvic, abdominal, thoracic, and supratrochlear. These patches are in areas where pathogens are most likely to enter. Tonsils, adenoids, spleen, and thymus all contain lymphatic tissue.

- Fluid leaking from blood capillaries enters tissue fluid and flows into lymph capillaries. The fluid is carried through lymph capillaries to lymph vessels to lymph nodes. In the nodes, any pathogens are destroyed by white blood cells. Fluid then flows from nodes to vessels to lymphatic trunks to collecting ducts and into either the right or left subclavian vein, returning the fluid to the bloodstream.

- The thymus and spleen are lymphatic organs. The spleen contains blood sinuses and removes dead and dying red blood cells as well as pathogens. The thymus is the birthplace of T lymphocytes.

- Immune system function is based on its ability to recognize cell surface molecules called antigens. The immune system must tolerate self-antigens (the body's antigens) and destroy non–self-antigens (foreign cells).

- The immune system is divided into two separate but extremely interdependent parts: innate immunity and adaptive immunity. Innate immunity is nonspecific, has no memory, and cannot improve performance with experience. Adaptive immunity is specific, has memory, and can improve performance with experience.

- Barriers prevent pathogens from getting into the body. Barriers can be either physical or chemical. Intact skin and formation of tears from your eyes are examples of barriers.

- The immune system uses a dozen or more different types of cells to combat pathogens. All these cells are leukocytes or modified leukocytes. Some are part of innate immunity, and some are part of adaptive immunity. Their functions range from phagocytosis, chemical stimulation of other cells, and antigen display to antibody secretion and direct destruction of pathogens.

- Immune response is stimulated by a variety of chemicals, including the cytokines and complement.

- Inflammation, the familiar redness, heat, swelling, and pain associated with infection, is a powerful tool in the immune system's arsenal. During inflammation, white blood cells are stimulated and attracted to the site of infection to destroy pathogens and clean up cellular debris. Inflammation, like much of immune response, is a two-edged sword. Too much inflammation may be more damaging than the infection itself.

- Similar to inflammation, fever is a deliberate attempt by the body to destroy a pathogen. Chemicals can cause the hypothalamus to raise the temperature set point in an attempt to make the body temperature too hot for pathogens.

- Innate immune mechanisms are triggered by the presence of foreign antigens in the body. These mechanisms hold off the infection and stimulate adaptive immune mechanisms.

- Adaptive immunity uses T and B lymphocytes to fight specific pathogens. Lymphocytes must be selected during development to recognize foreign antigens but to ignore the body's own antigens. To fight a pathogen, lymphocytes must be activated by binding with antigen-displaying cells. Once activated, lymphocytes must proliferate, making thousands of copies of themselves. Helper T cells are required for proliferation of B cells.

- B cells are mediators of antibody-mediated immunity. They are activated after being primed by an antigen and by binding to helper T cells. When B cells begin to proliferate, they become either plasma cells or memory B cells. Plasma cells secrete antibodies during the primary response. Antibodies help destroy pathogens by binding to antigens on infected cells. Memory B cells are stored for the next time the pathogen is encountered. They mediate secondary response.

- Cytotoxic T cells mediate cell-mediated immunity by directly killing infected cells. This is the primary T cell response. Like B cells, cytotoxic T cells are activated by helper T cells. Some T cells become memory T cells and mediate secondary response if the pathogen is encountered again.

- Regulatory T cells are one of the off-switches for the immune system.

- Keep in mind that innate and adaptive immunity do not work separately. They work together. One stimulates the other in a huge positive feedback loop. If either innate or adaptive immunity stops working, the whole system breaks down.

John has made big changes in his life. An IV drug user for more than 5 years, he recently completed an inpatient rehabilitation program and got serious about staying off drugs. His cousin, Bill, suggested that John move west to a quiet rural area and work on Bill's farm. John had lived in the city all his life so he took Bill up on his offer, figuring it will be a true fresh start.

John loved the peace and quiet and adjusted to the physical labor. Things went well for a few weeks, and then John fell ill. His head was stuffy, his nose ran, he had a cough, ran a low-grade fever, and his glands (actually his cervical lymph nodes) swelled. No matter how much John slept, it was never enough. The mystery illness would hang around for a few days and then seem to go away, only to come back in a few days. Frustrated and a little scared, John finally went to see Bill's doctor.

1. Given John's history and symptoms, what might the doctor suspect?

_____

_____

2. The doctor ran some blood tests, including a differential white cell count, and found that John's T cell count was normal, and there were no signs of HIV antibodies. However, John's eosinophil, basophil, and neutrophil counts were elevated. What do the symptoms suggest now that AIDS has been ruled out?

_____

_____

Multiple Choice

1. Lymphocytes are selected for their ability to
   a. recognize antigens.
   b. ignore self-antigens.
   c. carry oxygen.
   d. both a and b

2. Mounting an excessive immune response to a harmless antigen is called a(n)
   a. autoimmune disorder.
   b. allergy.
   c. immunodeficiency.
   d. AIDS infection.

3. Which of the following is an innate immune cell?
   a. neutrophil
   b. memory cell
   c. helper T cell
   d. plasma cell

4. Lymphocytes are activated by binding with antigens on
   a. bacteria.
   b. antigen-presenting cells.
   c. viruses.
   d. lymph nodes.

5. Innate immunity is not stimulated by foreign antigens.
   a. true
   b. false
   c. it depends
   d. all of the above

6. Fever and inflammation are both part of what kind of immunity?
   a. auto
   b. adaptive
   c. acquired
   d. innate

7. What do inflammation and fever have in common?
   a. They are part of homeostasis.
   b. They are both vicious cycles.
   c. They are both part of adaptive immunity.
   d. all of the above

8. Match the following cells and description of function

a. B lymphocytes   _____ release chemicals to promote inflammation

b. T lymphocytes   _____ cell-mediated immunity

c. eosinophils   _____ antibody-mediated immunity

d. natural killer cells   _____ act as antigen presenting cells

e. mast cells   _____ participate in allergic reaction/kills parasites

f. macrophages   _____ releases chemicals to kill infected cells

Fill in the Blank

1. Vaccinations stimulate _____ immunity.

2. Lymphocytes are part of adaptive immunity except for _____ cells.

3. B cell count will eventually drop in a person with AIDS because of decreased _____ cells.

4. Antihistamines block the effects of these cells: _____.

5. _____ selection selects for immune competent cells.

6. A patient presents with chronic upper respiratory symptoms of sneezing, runny nose, and postnasal drip but no fever, muscle aches, or any other symptoms. What is your initial diagnosis?

_____

Short Answer

1. List the regions of the body containing many lymph nodes.

_____

_____

_____

2. Trace the circulation of lymph from the cardiovascular system through the lymphatic system and back to the cardiovascular system.

_____

_____

_____

_____

3. List four types of cells and their functions in immunity.

_____

_____

_____

_____

4. Explain the differences between innate and adaptive immunity.

_____

_____

_____

5. Steroids or other potent anti-inflammatory medications often leave patients more susceptible to infection. Why?

_____

_____

_____

_____

6. Cancers such as leukemia and lymphoma often leave patients susceptible to infection, as do some chemotherapy treatments for other types of cancer. Explain.

_____

_____

_____

_____

Visit our new **MyHealthProfessions** Lab to accompany *Anatomy & Physiology for Health Professions*. Here you'll find a rich collection of quizzes, case studies, and animations for deeper understanding and application.

16

The Gastrointestinal System

FUEL FOR THE TRIP

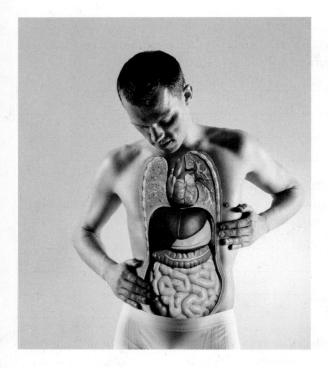

So far, we have discussed a variety of body systems and learned how they are put together and how they function. All the systems of the body need to function together to create a smooth-running machine. But just like a Ferrari, no matter how well it is designed nor how precisely it is put together, the body cannot function without fuel. This chapter focuses on the **gastrointestinal (GI) system** and how it:

- *Takes in (ingests)* raw materials
- *Breaks them down (digests)* both physically and chemically to usable elements
- *Absorbs* those elements
- *Eliminates* what isn't usable

These processes are accomplished through an amazing array of main and accessory organs and substances. Here is a concept to ponder as we travel through the digestive system: the food that enters your mouth, travels through your digestive system, and is eventually eliminated is never once *inside* your body, but basically remains in a tube-like "highway," with materials contained within the food exiting the highway ramps in specific areas.

LEARNING OUTCOMES

At the end of your journey through this chapter, you will be able to:
- Locate and describe the functions of the main organs of the digestive system.
- Differentiate between ingestion and digestion and between mechanical and chemical processing of food.
- Trace the journey of a bolus of food from the mouth to the anus.
- Discuss the structure of teeth.
- Identify the layers that make up the walls of the alimentary tract.
- Describe the various enzymes and chemicals needed for digestion.
- Locate and describe the function of the accessory organs for digestion.
- Describe common disorders of the gastrointestinal system.

Pronunciation Guide

Correct pronunciation is important in any journey so that you and others are completely understood. Here is a "see and say" Pronunciation Guide for the more difficult terms to pronounce in this chapter. Please note that even though there are standard pronunciations, regional variations of the pronunciations can occur.

adventitia (ADD ven TISH ah)
alimentary tract (AL ah MEN tar ee)
anus (AY nus)
appendicitis (ah PEN dih SIGH tiss)
appendix (ah PEN dicks)
bolus (BOW lus)
buccal (BUCK all)
cecum (SEE kum)
cementum (see MEN tum)
cholecystitis (KOH lee sis TYE tiss)
cholecystokinin (CCK) (KOH lee SIS toe KINE in)
cholelithiasis (KOH lee lih THY ah sis)
chyle (KILE)
chyme (KIME)
deciduous teeth (dee SID you us)
defecation (def eh CAY shun)
duodenum (DOO oh DEE num)
emulsification (ee MULL sih fih KAY shun)
epiglottis (ep ih GLAH tiss)
esophagus (eh SOFF ah gus)
frenulum (FREN you lum)
fundus (FUN dus)
gastrin (GAS trin)
gingiva (JIN jih vuh)
ileum (ILL ee um)
jejunum (jee JOO num)

labia (LAY bee ah)
lacteal (LACK tee al)
mastication (MASS tih CAY shun)
mesentery (MEZ in TARE ee)
palate (PAL at)
pancreas (PAN kree ass)
pancreatitis (PAN kree ah TYE tiss)
parotid salivary gland
  (pah ROT id SAHL ih vair ee gland)
periodontal (PAIR ee oh DON tal)
peristalsis (pair ih STALL sis)
pharyngoesophageal sphincter
  (fah RING goh ee SOFF uh JEE al SFINK ter)
pharynx (FAIR inks)
plicae circulares (PLY kay sir cue LAIR es)
ptyalin (TYE ah lin)
pyloric sphincter (pye LOR ik SFINK ter)
pylorus (pye LOR us)
rugae (ROO gay)
serosa (seh ROSE ah)
sublingual salivary glands
  (sub LING gwall SAHL ih vair ee)
submandibular salivary glands
  (SUB man DIB you lar SAHL ih vair ee)
uvula (YEW view lah)
villi (VILL eye)

SYSTEM OVERVIEW

The digestive tract (often called the **alimentary tract** or **alimentary canal**), is a muscular tube consisting of the organs of the digestive system. This tube begins at the mouth and ends at the **anus**. Between these two points are the pharynx, esophagus, stomach, and small and large intestines. In addition, *accessory organs*, such as teeth, salivary glands, liver, pancreas, and gallbladder, are necessary for processing materials into usable substances. Refer to **FIGURE 16–1** ■ as we journey through the digestive system.

The components of the digestive system work together to perform the following general steps:

1. Ingestion
2. Mastication
3. Digestion
4. Secretion
5. Absorption
6. Excretion (defecation)

Food first enters the mouth, an activity called **ingestion**. Once food is ingested, it is *mechanically processed* by the actions of the teeth and tongue, which *physically* break down the food by chewing. The chewing action is called **mastication**. This mechanical mixing process also continues in the movement of the digestive tract, as you will soon see. **Digestion** is the *chemical process* of breaking down food into small molecules. This is necessary so nutrients can be absorbed by the lining of the digestive tract.

The **secretion** of acids, buffers, enzymes, and water aid in the breakdown of food. Once the food is broken down both physically and chemically, it is ready for **absorption** through the lining of the digestive tract for use by the body. Finally, waste products and unusable materials are prepared for **excretion** and are eliminated by the body through **defecation**.

Now that you have a general idea of what's going on, let's begin the journey through the digestive system from beginning to end as a slice of double cheese, pepperoni pizza would!

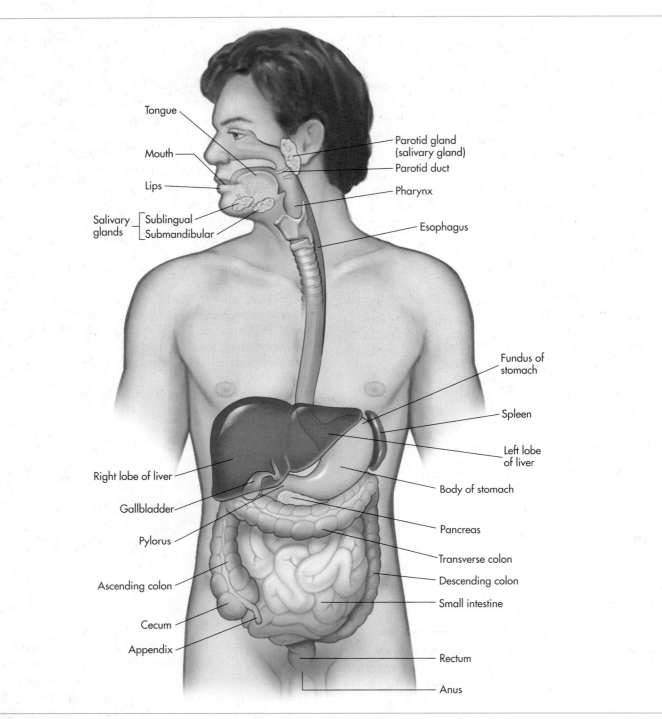

FIGURE 16–1 ■
The digestive system.

THE ORAL CAVITY

Your mouth is the opening that leads to the oral cavity, which is also called the **buccal** cavity. Your lips, or **labia**, act as a door to this chamber. The *hard* and *soft* **palates** create the roof of the chamber, whereas the **tongue** acts as the floor. The sides of the cavity are created by your cheeks. The tongue's base (area of attachment) and the **uvula** ("little grape"), that punching bag–shaped object dangling down from the soft palate, act as the boundary between the oral cavity and the next part of the digestive system, the **pharynx**. As we discovered in our travels through the respiratory system, the soft palate and uvula aid in swallowing because they help direct food toward the pharynx and help block food from coming out your nose. A pair of lingual tonsils is back there, too. As we learned in the immune system chapter, the tonsils help in fighting infection as part of the lymphatic system. Your oral cavity receives, or *ingests*, food. The food is tasted, *mechanically* broken down into smaller pieces, and *chemically* broken down to some degree. Liquid is added to make it easier to swallow. See **FIGURE 16–2** ■ to view the oral cavity.

Tongue

Your tongue is a muscular structure that performs many duties. It provides taste stimuli to your brain, senses temperature and texture, manipulates food while chewing, and aids in swallowing. As the tongue moves the food around in the oral cavity, saliva is added to moisten and soften the food, while teeth continue to crush the food until it reaches the right consistency. The tongue pushes the food into a ball-like mass called a **bolus** so it can be passed on to the pharynx. If you can push that bolus into the pharynx with your tongue, why don't you swallow your tongue too? A membrane under your tongue, called the lingual **frenulum**, which you can see when you lift up your tongue, prevents this from happening. Not only is the frenulum important for swallowing, but it also aids in proper speaking. An abnormally short frenulum prevents clear speech, hence the term "tongue-tied."

Salivary Glands

As you can see in **FIGURE 16–3** ■, there are three pairs of salivary glands, all of which are controlled by the autonomic nervous system. A large **parotid salivary gland** is found slightly inferior and anterior to each ear. These are the ones that swell up and make you look like a chipmunk if you get the mumps, which was common in the author's childhood

but now is rare due to immunizations. The ducts from these glands empty into the upper portion of the oral cavity. The smallest of the salivary glands, the **sublingual salivary glands**, are located under the tongue. The **submandibular salivary glands** are located on both sides along the inner surfaces of the mandible, or lower jaw.

On average, these glands collectively produce *1 to 1.5 liters of saliva daily!* Small amounts of saliva are continuously produced to keep your mouth moist, but once you smell food, start eating, or even think about eating, look out! The flood gates open! Although saliva is mostly water (99.4 percent), it also contains some antibodies, buffers, ions, waste products, and **enzymes**. Salivary amylase (also known as **ptyalin**) is one of the digestive enzymes that speeds up the chemical activity that breaks down carbohydrates. Starches are broken down into smaller molecules, such as glucose, that are more easily absorbed further down in the digestive tract. So, before you even swallow a bite of pizza, amylase is breaking down the starch in the crust. Saliva plays an important role even *after* you eat. As the saliva is continuously secreted in small amounts, it cleans the oral surfaces and also aids in reducing the amount of bacteria that grows in your mouth. Just remember, that action is *not* a substitute for brushing your teeth!

Teeth

The final important components of the mechanical aspect of digestion in the oral cavity are the teeth. It is unfortunate that we get only two sets of them in a lifetime and this is why it is so important to take good care of your teeth.

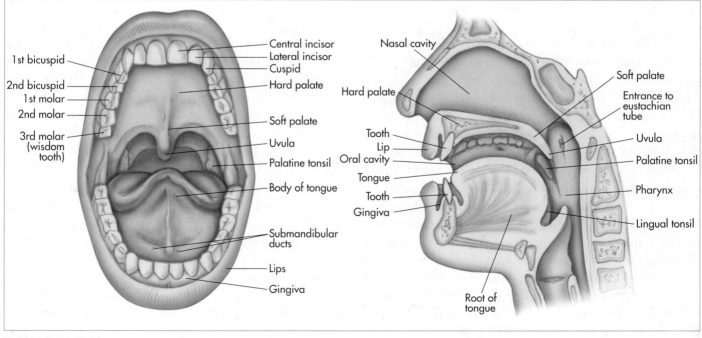

FIGURE 16–2 ■

The mouth and oral cavity.

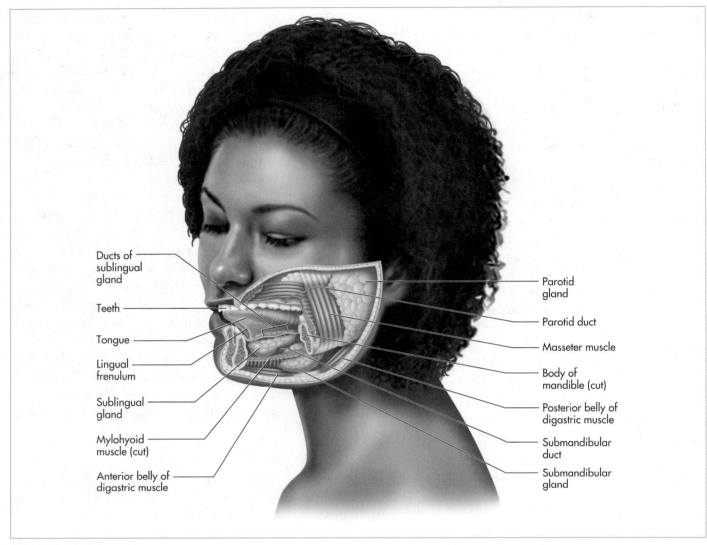

FIGURE 16–3 ■

The salivary glands and related structures of the oral cavity.

The first set of teeth are called *baby teeth*, or more properly, **deciduous teeth**. Like the leaves on a deciduous tree, they fall away in time. They appear beginning at around 6 months of age, starting with the lower central incisors, and all 20 teeth are usually in place by 2½ years of age. Between the ages of 6 and 12 years the Tooth Fairy is kept busy, as these teeth are pushed out and replaced by the 32 larger *permanent teeth*. The exception to this is the *wisdom teeth*, which may not appear until an individual is as old as 21 years.

Not all teeth are the same, as you can see by their shapes and locations. Each has special responsibilities. Look at **FIGURE 16–4** ■ as we discuss the various types of teeth. The first tooth type is the **incisor**, which is located at the front of your mouth, unless you are an aggressive hockey player. Incisors are blade-shaped teeth used to cut food. **Canine teeth** are for holding, tearing, or slashing food. Canine teeth are also known as eyeteeth, or **cuspids**, and are located next to the incisors. Next in line are the **bicuspids**, or premolars, which are transitional teeth. **Molars**

are the final type of teeth and have flattened tops. Both the bicuspids and molars are responsible for crushing and grinding.

Regardless of its type, the structure of each tooth is pretty much the same. As you can see in Figure 16–4, each tooth has a *crown, neck,* and *root*. The **crown** is the visible part of the tooth. It is covered by the hardest biologically manufactured substance in the body, **enamel**. The **neck** is a transitional section that leads to the *root*.

Internally, most teeth are made up of a mineralized, bone-like substance called **dentin**. The next internal layer is a connective tissue called **pulp**, which is located in the *pulp cavity*. The pulp cavity also contains blood vessels and nerves that provide nutrients and sensations. The nerves and blood vessels get to the pulp cavity via the infamous root canal.

The **root** is nestled in a bony socket and is held in place by fibers of the **periodontal** ligament. In addition, **cementum** covers the dentin of the root, aiding in securing the *periodontal ligament*. Cementun is a soft version of bone.

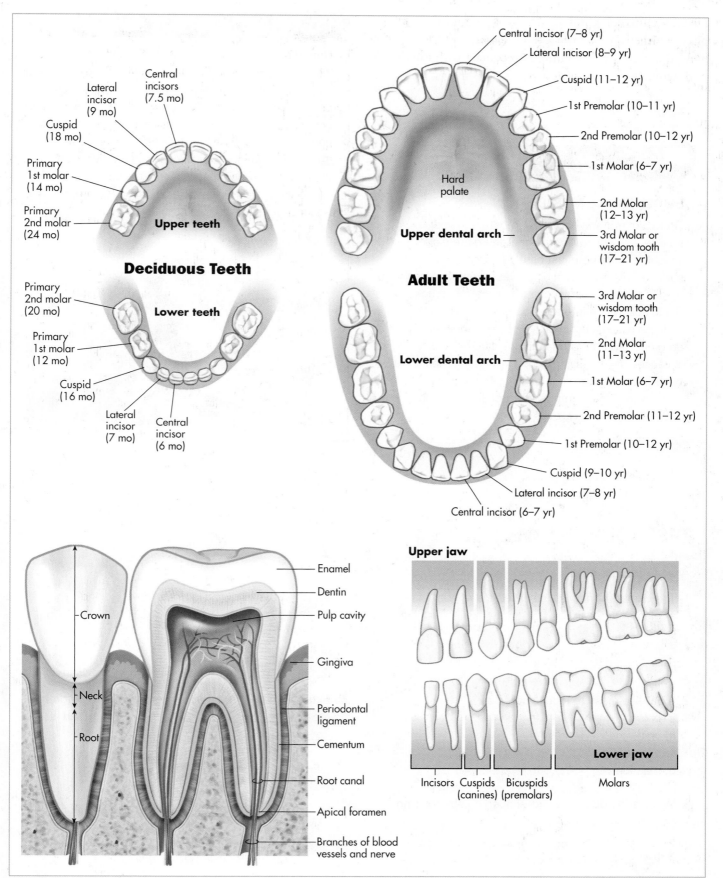

FIGURE 16–4 ◼

Types, location, and structures of teeth.

Healthy gums, or **gingiva**, also help to hold the teeth in place. Epithelial cells form a tight seal around the tooth to prevent bacteria from coming into contact with the tooth's cementum.

Clinical Application

SUBLINGUAL MEDICATION

Go to a mirror and open your mouth. Lift your tongue, and you will notice that there are blood vessels everywhere just barely underneath the surface. This sublingual blood vessel network can readily absorb substances such as certain drugs. Rapid absorption into the blood system is vital in some cases, such as for those who need the drug nitroglycerin to treat angina quickly. Angina is caused by insufficient blood flow to the heart, which decreases oxygen delivery to coronary tissues. Nitroglycerin improves coronary blood flow and in most cases relieves angina.

FOCUS ON PROFESSIONS

Dental assistants and **hygienists** are dedicated to keeping the teeth and surrounding structures clean and free of disease. In addition, they assist in taking x-rays and making impressions for dental cosmetics. Learn more about these professions by visiting the websites of national organizations, including the American Dental Assistant Association (ADAA), the National Dental Assistant Association (NDA), the National Association of Dental Assistants (NADA), the American Dental Hygienists Association (ADHA), and the National Dental Hygienists Association (NDHA).

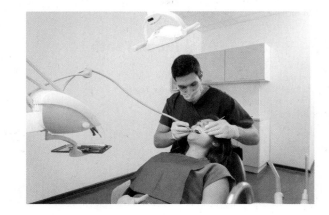

TEST YOUR KNOWLEDGE 16–1

Answer the following:

1. The digestive tract is also called the
   a. elementary canal.
   b. integumentary canal.
   c. alimentary canal.
   d. panama canal.

2. A ball-like mass of food is called a
   a. bolus.
   b. wad.
   c. chyme.
   d. mastion.

3. What is the punching bag–shaped object dangling from the soft palate?
   a. tonsil
   b. uvula
   c. labia
   d. incisor

4. Which of the following is *not* a salivary gland?
   a. parotid
   b. sublingual
   c. submandibular
   d. substernal

5. Externally, the three main structural parts of a tooth are the _____, _____, and _____.

PHARYNX

The pharynx brings us to the next part of the journey. As explained in the respiratory system chapter, the pharynx is a common passageway not only for food but also for water and air. It has three parts: the *nasopharynx*, the *oropharynx*, and the *laryngopharynx*. The nasopharynx is primarily a part of the respiratory system. The oropharynx and the laryngopharynx serve double duty as a passageway for food, water, and air. During swallowing, passageways to the nasal and respiratory regions are protected from the accidental introduction of food and liquids. The nasopharynx is blocked by the soft palate, and a flap of tissue, called the **epiglottis**, covers the airway to the lungs as the trachea rises during swallowing. These actions force the food to enter the only possible route, the esophagus.

ESOPHAGUS

Measuring approximately 10 inches (25 centimeters) long, the **esophagus** is responsible for transporting food from the pharynx to the stomach. It extends from the pharynx, through the thoracic cavity and diaphragm, to the stomach, which is located in the abdominal cavity (see **FIGURE 16–5** ■).

The esophagus is normally a collapsed tube, much like a deflated balloon, until a bolus of food is swallowed. As this bolus moves to the esophagus, a muscular ring at the beginning of this structure, known as the **pharyngoesophageal sphincter**, relaxes. This is like opening the door to the esophagus so food can enter. We can't rely on gravity to move food through the esophagus, so the muscles of the esophagus begin rhythmic contractions that work the food down to the stomach. This rhythmic muscular contraction is known as **peristalsis**. When the bolus reaches the end of the esophagus, a second door must be opened to allow entry to the stomach. This is the **lower esophageal sphincter (LES)**, also known as the *cardiac sphincter*, which relaxes to let food into the stomach and then closes to prevent acidic gastric juices from squirting up into the esophagus. Heartburn (pyrosis) is what happens if that door inadvertently opens.

The esophagus also helps move the bolus by excreting mucus so its walls are slippery. The esophageal walls are lined with stratified squamous epithelium, which makes the esophagus resistant to abrasion, temperature extremes, and irritation by chemicals.

The whole process of swallowing food takes about 9 seconds on average. Dry or "sticky" food may take longer with repeated attempts to work it down. (Did you ever try to swallow too large a bite of a peanut butter sandwich and have it stick, pounding on the LES door?) Fluids take only a few seconds to get to the stomach.

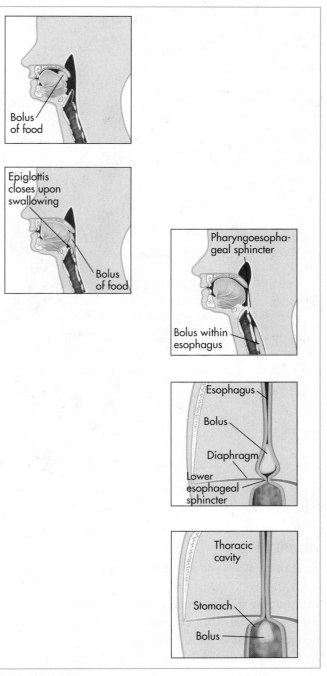

FIGURE 16–5 ■

The movement of a bolus of food from the mouth to the stomach via the esophagus.

THE WALLS OF THE ALIMENTARY CANAL

It is interesting to note that the same four basic tissue types form the wall of the entire alimentary canal from the esophagus onward (see **FIGURE 16–6** ■). The innermost layer that lines the lumen of the canal is the **mucosa** (mucous membrane). This layer is composed mostly of surface epithelium with some connective tissue and a thin smooth muscle layer

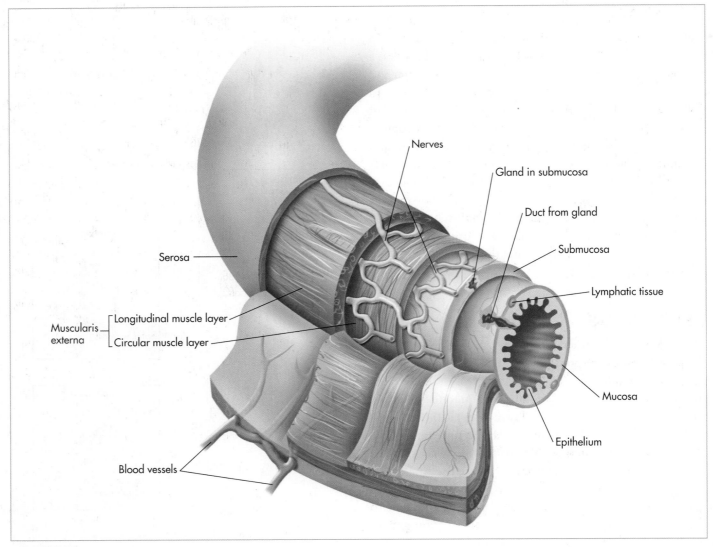

FIGURE 16–6 ■

Basic tissue types and structures of the alimentary canal.

surrounding it. The mucosa also possesses cells that secrete *digestive enzymes* to break down foodstuffs and *goblet cells* that secrete *mucus* for lubrication.

The **submucosa** is the next layer and is composed of soft connective tissue. This layer contains blood and lymph vessels, lymphatic tissue, similar to your tonsils, called Peyer patches, and nerve endings. The next layer is the **muscularis** externa, composed of two layers of smooth muscle. The innermost layer encircles the canal, whereas the outer layer is longitudinal in nature so it lies in the direction of the canal. There is an additional third layer of oblique smooth muscle, but it is only found surrounding the stomach.

The outermost layer is the **serosa**, composed of a single thin layer of flat serous fluid-producing cells supported by connective tissue. For most of the canal, the serosa is the *visceral peritoneum*. The peritoneum is a **serous membrane**

in the abdominopelvic cavity (see **FIGURE 16–7** ■). Like all serous membranes, it has two layers. The visceral peritoneum covers the organs, and the parietal peritoneum lines the wall of the abdominopelvic cavity. Between the layers is a fluid-filled potential space called the peritoneal cavity. This fluid is important for both keeping the outer surface of the intestines moist and allowing friction-free movement of the digestive organs against the abdominopelvic cavity. The peritoneum is different from the other serous membranes, the pericardium and the pleura, for two reasons. First, some abdominal organs such as the urinary bladder and the duodenum are not surrounded by peritoneum and are called *retroperitoneal organs*. Second, the peritoneum has several extensions called **mesentery** that drape over the abdominal organs. The esophagus differs from the rest of the alimentary canal in that it possesses only a loose layer of connective tissue called the **adventitia**.

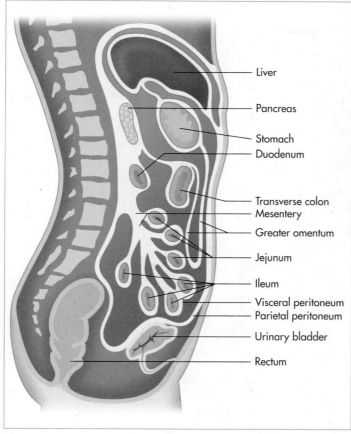

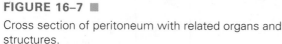

Liver

Pancreas

Stomach
Duodenum

Transverse colon
Mesentery

Greater omentum

Jejunum

Ileum

Visceral peritoneum
Parietal peritoneum

Urinary bladder

Rectum

FIGURE 16–7 ■

Cross section of peritoneum with related organs and structures.

STOMACH

The stomach is located in the left side of the abdominal cavity under the diaphragm and is covered almost completely by the liver. This J-shaped organ is approximately 10 inches (25 centimeters) long with a diameter that varies, depending on how much you eat at any given time. Although the stomach can hold up to 4 liters (about a gallon) when totally filled, it can expand or decrease in diameter thanks to deep folds, called **rugae**, in the stomach wall that allow for these size changes. As the stomach receives food from the esophagus, it performs several functions:

- Acts as a temporary holding area for the ingested food
- Secretes gastric acid and enzymes, which it mixes with the food, causing chemical digestion
- Regulates the rate at which the now partially digested food (a thick, heavy, creamlike liquid called **chyme**) enters the small intestine
- Absorbs small amounts of water and substances on a very limited basis (although the stomach does absorb alcohol)

It takes about four hours for the stomach to empty after a meal. Liquids and carbohydrates pass through fairly quickly. Protein takes a little more time, and fats take even longer, usually between 4 to 6 hours.

The stomach is divided into four regions. The **cardiac region** of the stomach (closest to the heart) surrounds the lower esophageal sphincter (see **FIGURE 16–8** ■). The **fundus**, a dome-shaped region, which is actually lateral and slightly superior to the cardiac region, temporarily holds the food as it first enters the stomach. The **body** is the midportion and largest region of the stomach. The funnel-shaped, terminal end of the stomach is called the **pylorus**. Most of the digestive work of the stomach is performed in the pyloric region. This is also the region where chyme must pass through another door, the **pyloric sphincter**, to travel to the small intestine. Two other points of interest are the concave curve called the *lesser curvature* and the larger convex curve to the left of the lesser curve called the *greater curvature*.

The muscular action of the stomach works much like a cement mixer and is achieved by the three layers of muscle found in its walls. One layer is *longitudinal*, one is *circular*, and the third is *oblique* in orientation. This arrangement of muscles enables the stomach to churn food as it mixes with gastric juices excreted by *gastric glands* from *gastric pits* in the columnar epithelial lining of the stomach as well as to work the food toward the pyloric sphincter through peristalsis. With the combined efforts of muscle action and gastric juices, both physical and chemical digestion occur in the stomach.

Gastric juice is a general term for a combination of *hydrochloric acid (HCl)*, *pepsinogen*, and *mucus*. About 1,500 milliliters of gastric juice is produced each day by gastric glands. Pepsinogen is secreted by the *chief cells*, and HCl is secreted by *parietal cells*. These two cell types have a special relationship in that once pepsinogen makes contact with HCl, the chief digestive enzyme, **pepsin**, is formed. Pepsin is needed to break down proteins, like the ones found in our pepperoni pizza topping. Even though it doesn't actually digest food by itself, HCl does break down connective tissue in meat (our pepperoni, again). HCl must be very strong to work. Normally, it has a very acidic pH of 1.5 to 2. This highly acidic environment plays another important role: killing off most pathogens that enter the stomach. Why doesn't the stomach digest itself, you may wonder. A healthy stomach is protected by **mucous** cells, which generate a thick layer of mucus to shield the stomach lining from the effects of HCl. Parietal cells also secrete a protein that is known as *intrinsic factor*, which is needed for absorption of vitamin B_{12}. Vitamin B_{12} is needed for the formation and growth of red blood cells. In some people, this important protein is not produced in sufficient amounts or they may have a

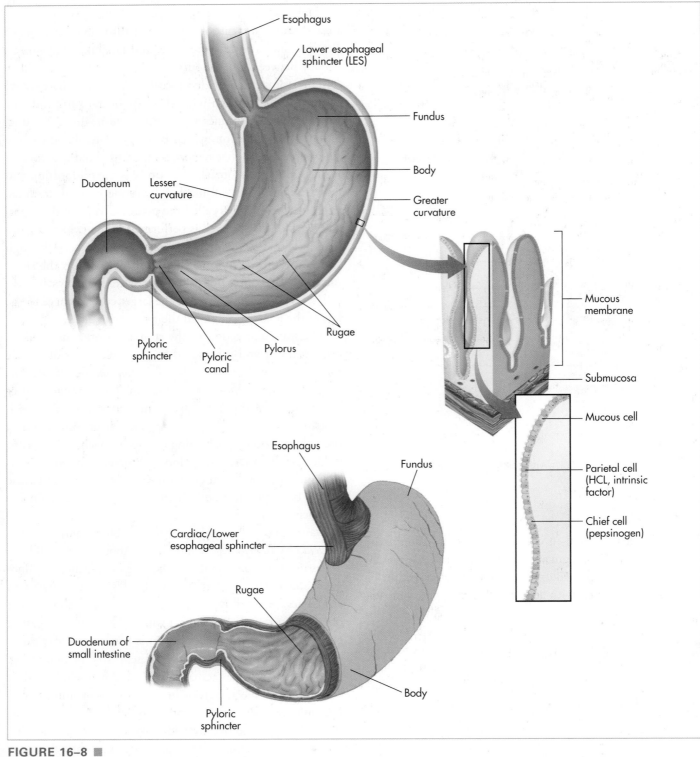

FIGURE 16–8 ■

The stomach.

condition that destroys intrinsic factor. Regardless of the cause, insufficient intrinsic factor can lead to a vitamin B_{12} deficiency called pernicious anemia. **TABLE 16–1** ■ describes gastric glands and their functions.

The stomach's activity is controlled by the parasympathetic nervous system, particularly the *vagus nerve*. When the vagus nerve is stimulated, the stomach's *motility* (churning action) increases, as does the secretory rates of the gastric glands.

The three distinct phases of gastric juice production are illustrated in **FIGURE 16–9** ■. The *cephalic phase* occurs as a result of sensory stimulation, such as the sight or smell of food. This sensory input stimulates the parasympathetic

TABLE 16–1 GASTRIC GLANDS AND THEIR FUNCTIONS

DIGESTIVE CELLS	SECRETION TYPE	FUNCTION
Chief cells	Pepsinogen	Begins digestion of protein
Parietal cells	HCl	Kills pathogens, activates pepsinogen, breaks down connective tissue in meat
	Intrinsic factor	Aids in absorption of vitamin B_{12}
Mucous cells	Alkaline mucus	Protects stomach lining
Endocrine cells	The hormone gastrin	Stimulates gastric gland secretion

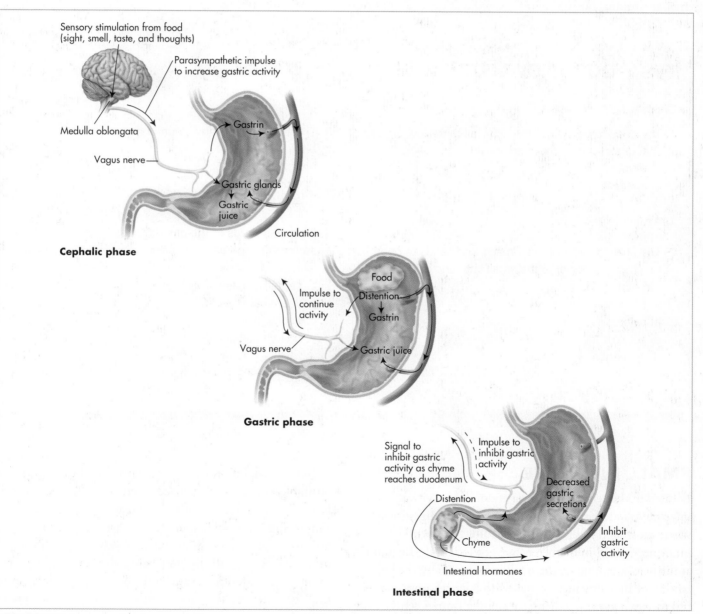

FIGURE 16–9 ∎

Phases of gastric secretions.

nervous system via the medulla oblongata, and the release of the hormone **gastrin** is increased. When gastrin travels through the blood and reaches the stomach, gastric gland activity is increased. So, the sight or smell of that pizza literally does get your gastric juices flowing.

This leads us to the *gastric phase*, in which over two-thirds of the gastric juices are secreted as the food moves into the stomach. As the food moves in, the stomach begins to distend. As the stomach distends, it sends signals back to the brain, which fires a reply to the gastric glands to step up their work.

As chyme is formed, it is passed through the pyloric sphincter to the first part of the small intestine, the duodenum. This begins the *intestinal phase* of gastric juice regulation. As the duodenum distends and senses the acidity of chyme, intestinal hormones are released that cause the gastric glands in the stomach to decrease gastric juice production. The brain is also signaled and sends a message to inhibit gastric juice secretion because it is no longer needed now that the food bolus (now called chyme) has left the stomach. When the chyme begins its movement through the duodenum and on to the rest of the small intestine, those inhibitory responses are halted so gastric juice production can continue once again when a new bolus of food enters the stomach.

Interestingly, the rate of the movement of chyme is very important. If chyme passes too quickly through the stomach, the food particles may not be sufficiently mixed with gastric juices, leading to insufficient digestion. Chyme that is not given time to be neutralized may lead to acidic erosion of the intestinal lining.

TEST YOUR KNOWLEDGE 16–2

Choose the best answer:

1. The deep folds of the stomach wall that allow for size changes of the stomach are called
   a. rugby.
   b. sphincter.
   c. rugae.
   d. glottal folds.

2. The final "door" of the stomach that needs to open for chyme to travel to the small intestine is located at the end of the
   a. fundus.
   b. pylorus.
   c. epiglottis.
   d. adventitia.

3. The inner wall of the alimentary canal is the
   a. serosa.
   b. muscular.
   c. mucosa.
   d. submucosa.

4. A full two-thirds of the gastric juices secreted in the stomach happen as food passes through this gastric juice production phase:
   a. cephalic phase.
   b. intestinal phase.
   c. gastric phase.
   d. pharyngeal phase.

5. The stomach's activity is controlled by the
   _____ nervous system.

SMALL INTESTINE

Located in the central and lower abdominal cavity, the small intestine is, surprisingly, *the* major organ of digestion. It is where most food is digested (see **FIGURE 16–10** ■). The small intestine is small in diameter, but not in length. Beginning at the pyloric sphincter, the small intestine is also the longest section of the alimentary canal, with a length up to 20 feet (up to 6 meters) and a diameter ranging from 4 centimeters where it connects with the stomach to 2.5 centimeters where it meets the large intestine.

In the small intestine, almost 80 percent of the absorption of usable nutrients takes place when chyme comes in contact with the mucosal walls. Amino acids, fatty acids, ions, simple sugars, vitamins, and water are all absorbed here. Some of the remaining 20 percent was already absorbed by the stomach, with the rest being absorbed by the large intestine. Any residue that cannot be utilized is sent on to the large intestine for removal from the body. Two types of muscular action occur in the small intestine. **Segmentation** is the muscle action that mixes chyme and digestive juices,

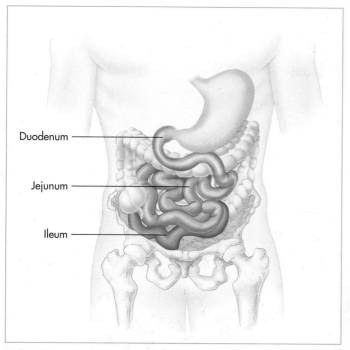

Duodenum

Jejunum

Ileum

FIGURE 16–10 ■
The small intestine.

again working much like a cement mixer. The second action is **peristalsis**, moving undigested food remains toward the large intestine.

There are three regions of the small intestine. The **duodenum** is approximately 25 centimeters long and is located near the head of the **pancreas**. The duodenum gets its name from *duo* (two) and *denum* (ten), which equal 12, because the organ is 12 finger widths (10 inches) long. The **jejunum** is the middle section and is approximately 2.5 meters (8 feet) long. The terminal end of the small intestine is the **ileum**, a 2-meter (6 to 7 feet) section that attaches to the large intestine at the *ileocecal valve*.

The structure of the wall of the small intestine is rather interesting. The wall possesses circular folds called **plicae circulares** and fingerlike protrusions into the lumen called **villi** (see **FIGURE 16–11** ■). The villi also have outer layers of columnar epithelial cells, which possess microscopic extensions known as *microvilli*. These villi are tightly packed, giving the mucosa a velvety texture and appearance. The purpose of the microvilli, villi, and circular folds is to provide an incredible increase in the surface area of the small intestine. This area, almost the surface area of a tennis court, increases the efficiency of the absorption of nutrients.

Each villus (singular form of villi) contains a network of capillaries and a lymphatic capillary called a **lacteal**. Intestinal glands are located between villi. The capillaries absorb and transport sugars (the result of carbohydrate digestion) and amino acids (the result of protein digestion) to the liver for further processing before they are sent throughout the body. Glycerol and fatty acids (obtained from the digestion of fat) are absorbed by the villi and converted into a lipoprotein that travels on to the lacteal, where it is now a white, milky substance called **chyle**. Chyle goes directly into lymphatic vessels that then deposit it into the blood stream via the left subclavian vein for distribution throughout the body.

The previously discussed pyloric valve is important in allowing small portions of chyme to enter the duodenum because the small intestine can process only small amounts of food at a time. To control the amount of food and rate of digestion of food in the duodenum, the walls of the small intestine secrete several digestive enzymes important for the final stages of chemical digestion and two hormones that control the activity of the pancreas, gallbladder, and stomach. The pancreas is stimulated to secrete as a result of the hormone **secretin** that is produced by the small intestine. Gallbladder activity is stimulated by the hormone **cholecystokinin (CCK)**, which is also produced by the small intestine. See **TABLE 16–2** ■ for the hormones active in the digestive process.

At the duodenum, additional secretions are added from the pancreas and gallbladder. The pancreas provides pancreatic juices, and the gallbladder provides bile. Bile *emulsifies* fat; that is, it makes fat able to disperse in water, making the fat found in the cheese of the pizza easier to break down. Pancreatic juice contains enzymes and sodium bicarbonate, which neutralizes the acidic chyme. The small intestine also produces digestive enzymes that are needed to complete chemical digestion. These enzymes (and mucus) are produced by exocrine cells. *Lactase*, *maltase*, and *sucrase* are needed for the digestion of double sugars called *disaccharides* that are contained in starches (such as in the pizza crust). *Peptidase* is needed to digest portions of the protein structure called peptides. Intestinal *lipase* is needed for digestion of certain fats. It is interesting to note that the secretion of these substances is mainly due to the presence of chyme in the small intestine. Because of the acidity of chyme, both chemical and mechanical irritation occur. This irritation, plus the distention of the intestinal wall, cause the localized reflex action that results in the release of the enzymes and the two hormones.

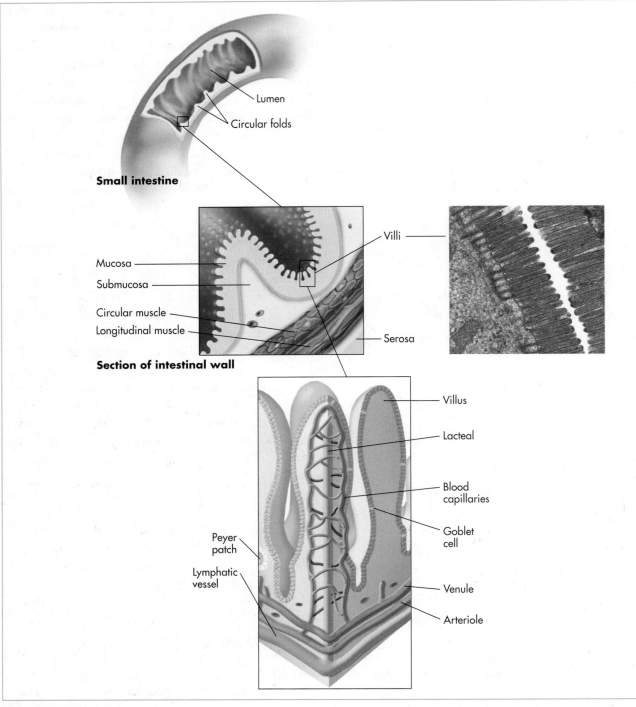

Small intestine

Lumen

Circular folds

Villi

Mucosa

Submucosa

Circular muscle

Longitudinal muscle

Serosa

Section of intestinal wall

Villus

Lacteal

Blood capillaries

Goblet cell

Peyer patch

Lymphatic vessel

Venule

Arteriole

FIGURE 16–11 ■

Illustration of villi with corresponding micrograph.

TABLE 16–2 HORMONES IN THE DIGESTIVE PROCESS

HORMONE	SECRETING ORGAN	ACTION
Gastrin	Stomach	Stimulates release of gastric juice
Secretin	Duodenum	Stimulates release of bicarbonate and water from pancreas and bile from liver; slows stomach activity
Cholecystokinin (CCK)	Duodenum	Stimulates digestive enzyme release from pancreas and bile release from gallbladder; slows stomach activity

LEARNING HINT

Emulsifiers

Think about what Italian salad dressing is like before you shake it. Emulsifiers allow the oil, water, and vinegar to blend together.

FOCUS ON PROFESSIONS

Dieticians provide valuable information on nutrition and specialized diets. These experts are intensively involved in the design of specialized diets for diabetes and many other illnesses. Learn more about this important profession by visiting the websites of national organizations such as the American Dietetic Association, the Academy of Nutrition and Dietetics, and the Canadian Institute of Food Science and Technology.

LARGE INTESTINE

Beginning at the junction with the end of the small intestine (*ileocecal orifice*) and extending to the **anus**, the **large intestine** almost totally borders the small intestine (see FIGURE 16–12 ■).

The large intestine is responsible for

- Water reabsorption
- Absorption of vitamins produced by normal bacteria in the large intestine
- Packaging and compacting waste products for elimination from the body

Because there are no villi in the walls of the large intestine, little nutrient absorption occurs here.

Approximately 1.5 meters (5 feet) long and 7.5 centimeters (2.5 inches) in diameter, the large intestine is divided into three main regions: the *cecum, colon,* and *rectum.* The large intestine is large in diameter, but not in length.

A pouch-shaped structure, the **cecum** receives any undigested food, such as cellulose, and water from the ileum of the small intestine. The infamous **appendix** is attached to the cecum. About 9 centimeters (3 inches) long, the appendix is a slender, hollow, dead-end tube lined with lymphatic tissue. Because it is wormlike in appearance, it is often called the *vermiform* appendix. The appendix has long been considered a *vestigial organ*—an organ whose size and function seem to have been reduced as humans evolved. Evidence suggests that because it possesses lymphatic tissue, it somehow fights infection. More recently, researchers have theorized that the appendix may replenish the beneficial bacteria in our digestive tract when they are destroyed by disease. If the appendix becomes blocked, inflammation can occur, causing **appendicitis**. Treatment for appendicitis is surgical removal of the appendix (*appendectomy*) along with antibiotic treatment.

The **colon** can further be divided into four sections: ascending, transverse, descending, and sigmoid. The *ascending* colon travels up the right side of the body to the level of the liver. The *transverse* colon travels across the abdomen just below the liver and the stomach. Bending downward near the spleen, the *descending* colon goes down the left side, where it becomes the *sigmoid* colon. The sigmoid ("S"-shaped) colon extends to the **rectum**. The rectum opens to the anal canal, which leads to the anus, which relaxes and opens to allow the passage of solid waste or feces.

Peristalsis continues in the large intestine but at a slower rate. As these slower, intermittent waves move fecal matter toward the rectum, water is removed, turning feces from a watery soup to a semisolid mass. Some of the water (used in digestion) and electrolytes are reabsorbed by the cecum and the ascending colon. Although this is a relatively small amount of water reabsorption, it is crucial in maintaining the proper fluid balance in the body.

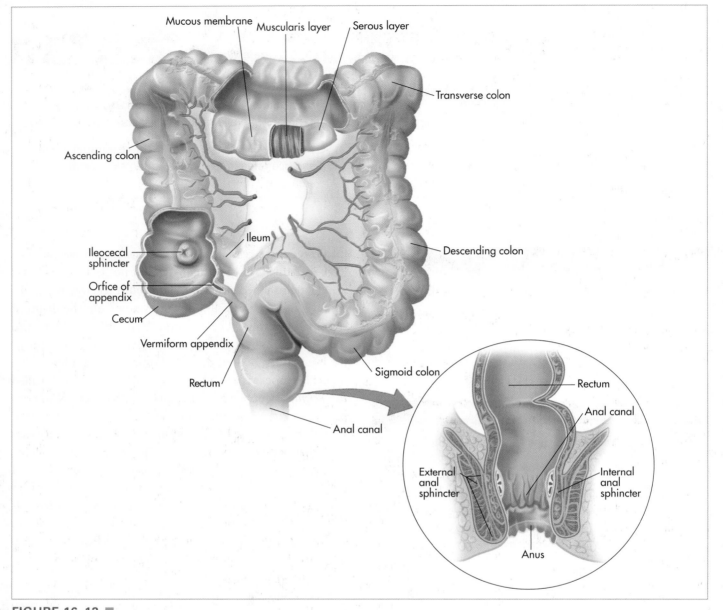

FIGURE 16–12 ■
The large intestine.

As the rectum fills with feces, a **defecation** reflex occurs, which causes rectal muscles to contract and the anal sphincters to relax. If fecal material moves through the large intestine too rapidly, not enough water is adequately reabsorbed, and **diarrhea** occurs. Conversely, if fecal matter remains too long in the large intestine, too much water is removed, and **constipation** occurs.

Defecation, like urination (discussed in the next chapter), is controlled by a combination of voluntary control and reflexes. Two sphincters surround the anal opening, the internal anal sphincter, which is involuntary, and the external anal sphincter, which is voluntary. When feces enter the rectum, the wall stretches, triggering the defecation reflex. The walls contract, and the internal sphincter relaxes and opens. The external sphincter relaxes only when you decide to open it. You have control, within limits, of when and how often you defecate.

Bacteria found in the large intestine play two important roles: the bacteria help to (1) further break down indigestible materials and (2) produce B complex vitamins as well as most of the vitamin K that we need for proper blood clotting. Here is a case where bacteria in the right place keep us healthy. If those same bacteria left the intestinal wall and entered the bloodstream, it could be fatal.

Clinical Application

COLOSTOMY

Sometimes a portion of the colon must be bypassed because of disease to allow for healing and/or surgical repair. A new opening needs to be made, and this procedure is called a *colostomy*. A colostomy can be temporary or permanent, depending on the condition. The sites where this procedure is formed are shown in **FIGURE 16–13** ▪.

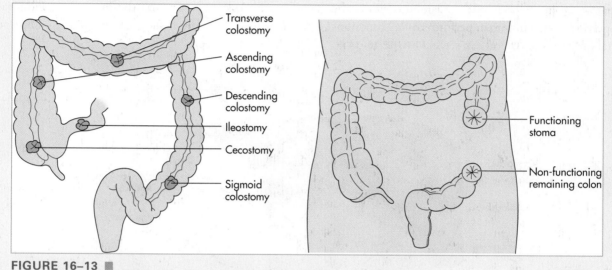

FIGURE 16–13 ▪
Colostomy sites.

TEST YOUR KNOWLEDGE 16–3

Choose the best answer:

1. The fingerlike projections of the wall of the small intestine are called
   a. microvilli.
   b. villi.
   c. lacteals.
   d. rugae.

2. This structure may be considered vestigial.
   a. cecum
   b. fundus
   c. appendix
   d. lacteal

3. The duodenum releases this hormone to decrease gastric activity.
   a. CCK
   b. gastrin
   c. secretin
   d. both a & c

4. This organ does most of the digestion and absorption in your digestive tract.
   a. small intestine
   b. large intestine
   c. pancreas
   d. liver

5. The muscle action that mixes chyme and digestive juices is called:
   a. peristalsis
   b. lacteal action
   c. segmentation
   d. gastrospasm

ACCESSORY ORGANS

In addition to the salivary glands of the mouth, other accessory organs are necessary for digestion: the liver, gallbladder, and pancreas.

Liver

Weighing in at approximately 1.5 kilograms (3.3 pounds) and located inferior to the diaphragm, the liver is the largest glandular organ in the body *and* the largest organ in the abdominopelvic cavity. This organ performs many functions that are vital for survival. As you can see in **FIGURE 16–14** ■,

the liver is divided into a larger right lobe and a smaller left lobe. The right lobe also has two smaller, inferior lobes.

The liver receives about 1.5 quarts of blood *every minute* from the hepatic portal vein (carrying blood full of the end products of digestion) and the hepatic artery (providing oxygen-rich blood). This blood flows past the hepatocytes (liver cells), which process the substances in that blood. Blood then leaves each lobule via a central vein, which drains into the hepatic vein. The hepatic vein then drains into the inferior vena cava, returning the processed blood back to circulation. Thus, the liver is a giant blood-filled sponge, much like the spleen.

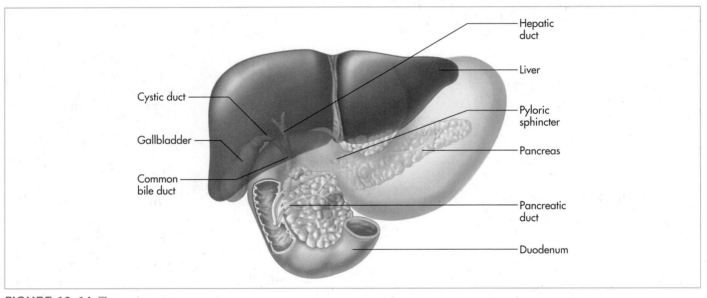

FIGURE 16–14 ■

The liver.

Clinical Application

LACTOSE INTOLERANCE

This unfortunate condition is the inability to digest the sugar (lactose) found in milk and dairy products such as cheese and ice cream. A person with lactose intolerance has a deficiency of lactase, an intestinal enzyme. As a result, lactose is not sufficiently digested. Normal bacteria found in the intestine utilize those undigested sugars with gas production as a by-product. This is what causes that "bloated feeling" you see on TV advertisements. In addition, the undigested lactose prevents normal water absorption by the small intestine, so diarrhea is formed. Thus, the cheese on the pepperoni pizza in our example would not be the meal of choice for individuals who are lactose intolerant.

Interestingly, it seems that there is a genetic basis for this condition. In some populations, lactase production continues throughout their entire lives. Approximately 16 percent of the Caucasian population develops lactose intolerance, whereas 80 to 90 percent of the African American and Asian American populations develop this condition to some degree.

To avoid this situation, individuals must either avoid milk and other dairy products or take an oral form of the enzyme lactase before consuming such products.

Although this chapter is about the digestive system, the liver plays a central role in regulating the metabolism of the body. It is important to understand *all* the functions that this amazing organ performs. Here is a list of what the liver does.

- Detoxifies (removes poisons) the body of harmful substances such as certain drugs and alcohol.
- Creates body heat.
- Destroys old blood cells and recycles their usable parts while eliminating unneeded parts such as the pigment *bilirubin*. Bilirubin is eliminated in bile and gives feces its distinctive color.
- Forms blood plasma proteins, such as *albumin* and *globulins*.
- Produces the clotting factors *fibrinogen* and *prothrombin*.
- Creates the anticoagulant *heparin*.
- Manufactures *bile*, which is needed for the digestion of fats.
- Stores and modifies fats for more efficient usage by the body's cells.
- Synthesizes *urea*, a by-product of protein metabolism, so it can be eliminated by the body.
- Stores the simple sugar *glucose* as *glycogen*. When the blood sugar level falls below normal, the liver reconverts glycogen to glucose and releases enough of it into the bloodstream to bring blood sugar back to an acceptable concentration.
- Stores iron and vitamins A, B_{12}, D, E, and K.
- Produces cholesterol.

Stimulated into action by the duodenum's secretion of the hormone *secretin*, bile production is a critical liver digestive function. The salts found in bile act like a detergent to break up fat into tiny droplets that make the work of digestive enzymes easier. This mechanical action of breaking up fat into smaller particles is called **emulsification**, and it provides more surface area for the enzymes to do their job of chemically digesting fat.

In addition, bile helps in the absorption of fat from the small intestine and transports bilirubin and excess cholesterol to the intestine for elimination. Once produced by the liver's cells, bile leaves the liver via the **hepatic duct** and travels through the cystic duct to the gallbladder, where it is stored until needed by the small intestine.

Gallbladder

The gallbladder is a sac-shaped organ approximately 7.5 to 10 centimeters (3 to 4 inches) long, located inferior to the liver's right lobe. Again, please refer to Figure 16–14.

While it is storing the bile, your gallbladder also concentrates it by reabsorbing much of its water content. This makes the bile 6 to 10 times more concentrated than it was in the liver. This is a bit of a balancing act: If too much water is reabsorbed and the bile is constantly too concentrated, bile salts may solidify into gallstones.

When fatty foods enter the duodenum, the duodenum releases the hormone CCK (cholecystokinin). This release causes the smooth muscle walls of the gallbladder to contract and squeeze bile into the **cystic duct** and on through the **common bile duct** and then into the duodenum.

Pancreas

Although discussed in Chapter 12, "The Endocrine System," your pancreas also plays an extremely important role in digestion. This organ of 15 centimeters (6 to 9 inches) long is located posterior to the stomach and extends laterally from the duodenum to the spleen (see **FIGURE 16–15** ■). The exocrine portion of this organ secretes buffers and digestive enzymes through the *pancreatic duct* to the duodenum. The buffers are needed to neutralize the acidity of the chyme in the small intestine. With the buffer pH ranging from 7.5 to 8.8, the acidic chyme is neutralized, saving the intestinal wall from damage. This secretory action is activated by the release of hormones by the duodenum.

The general digestive enzymes excreted by the pancreas are *carbohydrases* that work on sugars and starches, *lipases* that work on lipids (fats), *proteinases* that break down proteins, and *nucleases* that break down nucleic acids.

COMMON DISORDERS OF THE DIGESTIVE SYSTEM

Symptoms of digestive disorders generally include one or more of the following:

- Vomiting
- Diarrhea
- Constipation
- Abdominal pain

Vomiting is a protective means of ridding the digestive tract of an irritant or overload of food. Sensory fibers are stimulated by the irritant or overdistention and send signals to the vomiting center (yes, you have a vomiting center) in the medulla oblongata. Motor impulses are then sent to the diaphragm and abdominal muscles to contract, which opens the sphincter at the esophageal opening, and the contents are *regurgitated*.

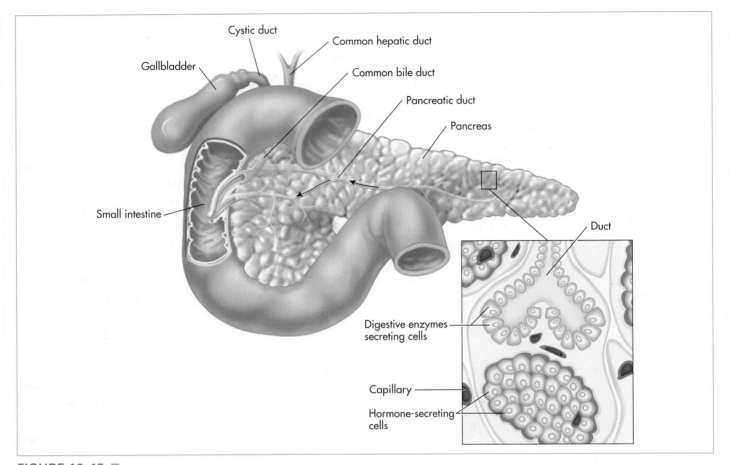

FIGURE 16–15 ■

The pancreas.

Diarrhea results when the fluid contents from the small intestine are rushed through the large intestine before water can be adequately reabsorbed, creating watery feces. Proper absorption of electrolytes and nutrients is also prevented, which can cause serious problems.

Constipation is the opposite of diarrhea; the feces travel so slowly through the colon that too much water is reabsorbed and the stool becomes hard and dry and difficult to push through the system.

One of the more common diseases sometimes blamed on our fast-paced society is **peptic ulcer disease (PUD)**, which can affect the lining of the esophagus, stomach, or duodenum. The most commonly affected region is the upper part of the small intestine, or duodenum. It is caused by an imbalance in the juices of the stomach that produce excess acid and erodes the mucosal lining of the digestive tract. Once thought to be mainly caused by stress, it is now believed the majority of the ulcers are caused by the bacteria *Helicobacter pylori*, which opens a wound in the lining that is made worse by exposure to digestive juices and stomach acids. The current thought is that stress is a contributing factor, increasing gastric acidity and facilitating the colonization of a damaged stomach wall. See **FIGURE 16–16** ■.

A host of diseases are associated with the digestive system. **TABLE 16–3** ■ lists some of the more common ones.

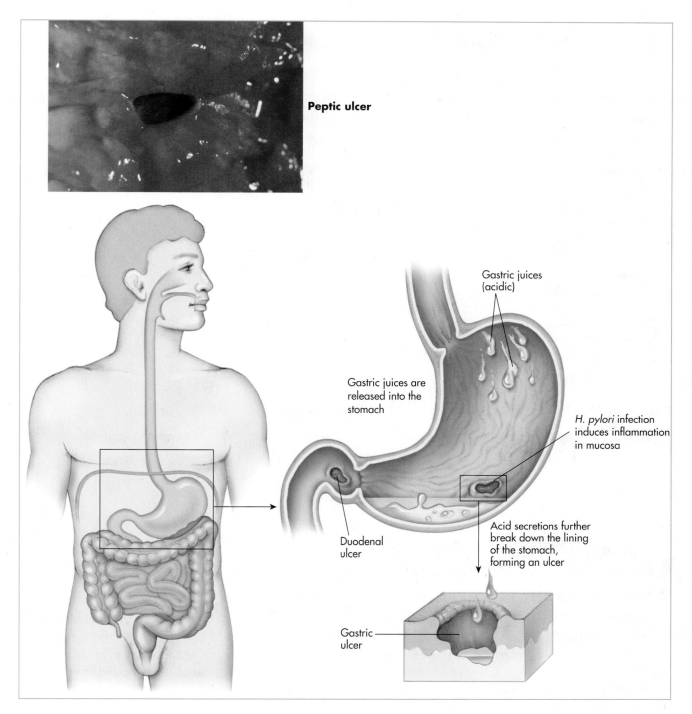

Peptic ulcer

Gastric juices (acidic)

Gastric juices are released into the stomach

H. pylori infection induces inflammation in mucosa

Duodenal ulcer

Acid secretions further break down the lining of the stomach, forming an ulcer

Gastric ulcer

FIGURE 16–16 ■

Peptic ulcer disease (PUD).

TEST YOUR KNOWLEDGE 16–4

Choose the best answer:

1. The chief function of the gallbladder is
   a. to make bile.
   b. to store bile.
   c. to make cholesterol.
   d. to store cholesterol.

2. Which of the following is one of the functions of the liver?
   a. maintaining fluid balance
   b. making digestive enzymes
   c. detoxification
   d. digesting protein

3. The pancreas releases the following into the duodenum:
   a. bile
   b. digestive enzymes.
   c. secretin.
   d. CCK.

4. The liver receives 1.5 quarts of blood every minute from which blood vessel(s)?
   a. hepatic portal vein
   b. hepatic aorta
   c. hepatic artery
   d. a & c

5. This hormone released from the duodenum causes smooth muscle contraction of the gallbladder to release bile.
   a. HGF
   b. CCK
   c. intrinsic factor
   d. lipase

Clinical Application

CHOLECYSTITIS AND PANCREATITIS

As we previously discussed, stones can form from substances in the bile while it is stored in the gall-bladder. This condition is called **cholelithiasis**. These stones, which are most often formed from choles-terol, can range in size from grains of sand to marble-size and larger. This condition can worsen if the stones lodge in the bile ducts, causing extreme pain, which, surprisingly, often radiates to the right shoul-der. If inflammation develops, the condition is called **cholecystitis**.

If the bile backs up into the liver, the disease *obstructive jaundice* can occur. In this scenario, bilirubin is reabsorbed back into the blood, giving the victim a yellowish tint to the skin and eyes.

The problem must be resolved by unblocking the bile ducts. This can be done by dissolving the stone through medication, using shock waves to smash the stones (*lithotripsy*), or surgically removing them.

Problems can also occur with the pancreas when the bile duct becomes blocked. In some cases, the pancreatic enzymes back up into the pancreas. As a result, those enzymes begin to inflame and destroy the pancreas. This condition is known as **pancreatitis** and can be caused by excessive alcohol consumption, gallbladder disease, or some irritation that causes an abnormally high rate of pancreatic enzyme activation. If this situation is not stopped, death can eventually occur.

TABLE 16–3 PATHOLOGY OF THE DIGESTIVE SYSTEM

DISEASE	DESCRIPTION
abscess (AB sess)	Swelling of soft tissues and the release of pus as a result of infection.
anorexia (an oh REK see ah)	Loss of appetite that can accompany other conditions such as a gastrointestinal (GI) upset; also eating disorder anorexia nervosa.
bulimia (boo LEE me ah)	Eating disorder that is characterized by recurrent binge eating and then purging of the food with laxatives and vomiting.
caries (KAIR eez)	Also known as a dental cavity, this is the gradual decay of teeth.
cholecystitis (KOH lee sis TYE tiss)	Inflammation of the gallbladder.
cholelithiasis (KOH lee lih THY ah sis)	Formation or presence of stones, or calculi, in the gallbladder or common bile duct.
cirrhosis (sih ROH sis)	Chronic disease of the liver; causes scarring.
cleft lip	Congenital anomaly in which the upper lip fails to come together. Often seen along with a cleft palate. Corrected with surgery.
cleft palate	Congenital anomaly in which the roof of the mouth has a split or fissure. Corrected with surgery.
Crohn's disease (KROHNZ)	Form of chronic inflammatory bowel disease affecting the ileum and/or colon. Also called *regional ileitis*. Named for Burrill Crohn, an American gastroenterologist.
diverticulitis (DYE ver TICK yoo LYE tiss)	Inflammation of a diverticulum or sac in the intestinal tract, especially in the colon.
enteritis (en ter EYE tiss)	Inflammation of only the small intestine.
esophageal stricture (eh soff ah JEE al STRIK chur)	Narrowing of the esophagus that makes the flow of fluids and food difficult.
esophageal varices (eh soff ah JEE al VAIR ih seez)	Enlarged and swollen veins in the lower end of the esophagus; they can rupture and result in serious hemorrhage.
fissure (FISH er)	Cracklike split in the rectum or anal canal.
gastritis (gas RYE tiss)	Inflammation of the stomach that can result in pain, tenderness, nausea, and vomiting.
gastroenteritis (GAS troh en ter EYE tiss)	Inflammation of the stomach and small intestine.
gingivitis (JIN jih VIGH tiss)	Inflammation of the gums, characterized by swelling, redness, and a tendency to bleed.
gum disease	Inflammation of the gums, leading to tooth loss; generally due to poor dental hygiene.
hemorrhoids (HEM oh roydz)	Varicose veins in the rectum.

DISEASE	DESCRIPTION
hepatitis (HEP ah tie tiss)	Inflammation of the liver.
hiatal hernia (high AY tal)	Protrusion of the stomach through the diaphragm and extending into the thoracic cavity; reflux esophagitis is a common symptom.
ileitis (ill ee EYE tiss)	Inflammation of the ileum.
impacted wisdom tooth	Wisdom tooth that cannot erupt because it is tightly wedged into the jaw bone.
inguinal hernia (IN gwin nal)	Hernia or outpouching of intestines into the inguinal region of the body.
intussusception (IN tuh suh SEP shun)	Result of the intestine slipping or telescoping into another section of intestine just below it. More common in children.
irritable bowel syndrome (IBS)	Disturbance in the functions of the intestine from unknown causes. Symptoms generally include abdominal discomfort and alteration in bowel activity.
malabsorption syndrome	Inadequate absorption of nutrients from the intestinal tract. May be caused by a variety of diseases and disorders, such as infections and pancreatic deficiency.
peptic ulcer	Ulcer occurring in the lower portion of the esophagus, stomach, and duodenum thought to be caused by the acid of gastric juices, possibly initiated by bacterial infection.
periodontal disease (PAIR ee oh DON tal)	Disease of the supporting structures of the teeth, including the gums and bones.
polyposis (pall ee POH sis)	Small tumors that contain a pedicle or footlike attachment in the mucous membranes of the large intestine (colon).
pyorrhea (PYE oh REE ah)	Discharge of purulent material from dental tissue.
reflux esophagitis	Acid from the stomach backs up into the esophagus causing inflammation and pain.
ulcerative colitis	Ulceration of the mucous membranes of the colon of unknown origin. Also known as *inflammatory bowel disease (IBD)*.
volvulus (VOL vyoo lus)	Condition in which the bowel twists on itself and causes an obstruction. Painful and requires immediate surgery.

- The digestive tract is a hollow tube extending from the mouth to the anus. It utilizes a variety of accessory organs that allow the digestion of food and the absorption of nutrients necessary for life.

- Food is processed mechanically and chemically to efficiently break it down to usable substances.

- Following are the main components of the alimentary canal and their functions:

ORGAN	DIGESTIVE ACTIVITY	SUBSTANCE DIGESTED	REQUIRED DIGESTIVE SECRETIONS
Mouth, oral cavity, and pharynx	Chews food and mixes it with saliva; forms food into a *bolus*, and swallows	Starch	Salivary amylase
Esophagus	Moves bolus to the stomach through *peristalsis*	Not applicable	Not applicable
Stomach	Stores food, also churns food while mixing in digestive juices	Proteins	Hydrochloric acid, pepsin
Small intestine	Secretes enzymes, receives secretions from the pancreas and liver, neutralizes the acidity in chyme, absorbs nutrients into the bloodstream and lymphatic system	Carbohydrates, fats, amino acid, proteins	Intestinal and pancreatic enzymes, bile from the liver
Large intestine	Creates and absorbs fat-soluble vitamins, reabsorbs water, forms and eliminates feces	No digestion but produces vitamin K for clotting	Not applicable

- The bulk of the digestive process and the absorption of most nutrients occur in the small intestine.

- Although not *directly* a part of the alimentary canal, the accessory organs (liver, gallbladder, and pancreas) are needed for proper and efficient functioning of the digestive process.

- The rate of speed that food travels through the gastrointestinal system affects the acidity of the digesting food, the absorption of nutrients, and the quality of the feces.

- Diseases of the alimentary canal can be a result of heredity, the type and amount of food consumed, substance abuse, or emotional issues.

CASE STUDY

A patient arrives in the emergency department around 3:00 a.m. with a severe burning sensation in his chest. The patient is anxious and thinks he is having a heart attack. All vital signs are within normal limits, and no other pain or discomfort is noted in other regions of the body. He states he ate a large bowl of spicy spaghetti around 11:30 p.m. Before falling asleep, he was uncomfortable and felt his large volume of food hadn't digested. He also states this burning sensation has happened in the past after eating, especially at night and when lying on his right side.

a. Do you think this is a heart attack? How would the emergency department rule out a heart attack?

_____

_____

b. What do you think the problem is?

_____

_____

c. What physiological process is malfunctioning?

_____

_____

d. Why is the position of the patient important?

_____

_____

e. What suggestions would you make to the patient to prevent future episodes?

_____

_____

REVIEW QUESTIONS

Multiple Choice

1. Which of the following is not a responsibility of the large intestine?
   a. production of vitamin K
   b. absorption of water
   c. digestion of carbohydrates
   d. elimination of feces

2. Starches begin to be digested in the
   a. oral cavity.
   b. esophagus.
   c. stomach.
   d. large intestine.

3. This structure prevents food and liquid from entering the lungs:
   a. uvula.
   b. pharynx.
   c. epiglottis.
   d. glottis.

4. What is the purpose of the ileum?
   a. It is where the small intestineand large intestine connect
   b. It is a crucial part of the pelvis
   c. It is important in the digestion of fats
   d. It allows blood flow to the villi for proper nutrient absorption

5. Which of the following is *not* a colon segment?
   a. transverse
   b. ascending
   c. descending
   d. absorbing

Fill in the Blank

1. _____ is the muscle action that mixes chyme with digestive juices, whereas _____ is the muscular action that moves food through the digestive system.

2. This vermiform structure is attached to the large intestine and is considered a vestigial organ: _____.

3. The exocrine portion of this important organ secretes buffers needed to neutralize the acidity of chyme and also secretes several digestive enzymes: _____.

4. _____ is the mechanical and chemical breaking up of fat into smaller particles that can more readily be acted upon by digestive enzymes.

5. The end result of fecal matter remaining in the large intestine too long, with too much water being removed from it, is _____.

Short Answer

1. Explain the difference between *chyme* and *chyle*.

_____

_____

_____

_____

2. Explain the importance of bacteria in the large intestine.

_____

_____

_____

_____

3. Discuss the importance of the liver in the digestive process.

_____

_____

_____

_____

4. Could you live without a gallbladder? Defend your answer.

_____

_____

_____

_____

5. List the changes in the anatomy of the walls of the alimentary canal from esophagus to anus.

_____

_____

_____

_____

Visit our new **MyHealthProfessions Lab** to accompany *Anatomy & Physiology for Health Professions.* Here you'll find a rich collection of quizzes, case studies, and animations for deeper understanding and application.

The Urinary System

FILTRATION AND FLUID BALANCE

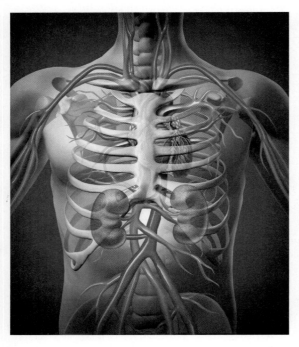

A city must have a safe, reliable water supply, usually obtained by pumping water from a reservoir or diverting a river. Sometimes cities have a series of wells to supply drinkable water. In desert areas, there are even special water treatment plants to remove salt from seawater to make fresh water for human consumption. In any case, there must be a way to clean the water. Water purification plants remove chemicals and debris and disinfect the water before it ever gets to your faucet. You are completely unaware of the activities of your city's water purification plant, but if it stopped working, you would be extremely unhappy. Imagine a glass full of muddy, bacteria-laden water. Yum!

Your body also must have a purification plant for its major fluid: blood. Your liver does some of the purification, but your urinary system is responsible for controlling the electrolyte (ion) and fluid balance of your body. The kidneys filter blood, reabsorb and secrete ions, and produce urine. Without your kidneys, fluid and ion imbalance, blood pressure irregularities, and nitrogen waste buildup would cause death in a matter of days.

LEARNING OUTCOMES

At the end of your journey through this chapter, you will be able to:

- Present an overview of the organs and functions of the urinary system.
- Describe the external and internal anatomy and physiology of the kidneys.
- Discuss the microscopic anatomy of the kidney and the importance of renal blood flow.
- Describe the process of urine formation.
- Trace the pathway of tubular reabsorption or secretion of electrolytes and other chemicals.
- List and discuss the importance of hormones for proper kidney function.
- Describe the anatomy and physiology of the bladder and urine removal from the body.
- Discuss several common disorders of the urinary system.

Pronunciation Guide

Correct pronunciation is important in any journey so that you and others are completely understood. Here is a "see and say" Pronunciation Guide for the more difficult terms to pronounce in this chapter. Please note that even though there are standard pronunciations, regional variations of the pronunciations can occur.

afferent arterioles (AFF er ent ahr TEE ree ohlz)
aldosterone (al DOSS ter ohn)
antidiuretic hormone (ADH) (AN tih dye yoo RET ick)
atrial natriuretic hormone
  (AY tree al NAY tree your ET ick)
calyx, calyces (KAY licks, KAY leh seez)
efferent arterioles (EFF er ent ahr TEE ree ohlz)
external urethral sphincter (yoo REE thral SFINK ter)
glomerulus (gloh MAIR you lus)
glomerular capsule (gloh MAIR you ler)
glomerulonephritis (gloh MAIR you loh neh FRY tiss)

glomerulosclerosis (gloh MAIR you loh skleh ROH sis)
ischemia (iss KEE me uh)
juxtaglomerular apparatus
  (JUX tuh gloh MAIR you ler)
renal hilum (REE nal HIGH lum)
renal medulla (REE nal meh DULL lah)
renin-angiotensin-aldosterone
  (RIN en-an gee oh TEN sen-al DOSS ter ohn)
ureter (yoo REE ter)
urethra (yoo REE thrah)

SYSTEM OVERVIEW

The urinary system (see **FIGURE 17–1** ▓) consists of two *kidneys*, bean-shaped organs located in the superior dorsal abdominal cavity; two *ureters*, tubes that carry urine from each kidney to the single *urinary bladder*, located in the inferior ventral pelvic cavity; and the *urethra*, the tubing that transports urine from the bladder to the outside of the body. The kidneys are retroperitoneal (situated behind the peritoneum [which is the membrane that lines the cavity of the abdomen]), and the right kidney is a bit inferior to the left because the liver takes up so much room.

The job of the urinary system is to make urine, thereby controlling the body's fluid and electrolyte balance, and eliminating waste products. To make urine, three processes are necessary: *filtration, reabsorption,* and *secretion*. **Filtration** is the movement of substances through a porous membrane under pressure. In this case, the blood is filtered and some substances pass through the filter. What passes through the filter is called a *filtrate*. Through **reabsorption**, this filtrate can then reenter into the bloodstream, or, through **secretion**, leave the body as urine. Keep in mind that the part of the filtrate that is reabsorbed is conserved and brought back into the bloodstream, whereas the part that is secreted is eliminated from the body. You'll learn how this process occurs as you travel through this chapter.

THE ANATOMY OF THE KIDNEY

The **kidney** is a very intricate filtration system. Although you have two kidneys, you can actually function well with only one healthy kidney. That is why someone can donate a kidney while he or she is alive.

External Anatomy

The external anatomy of the kidney is relatively simple. The kidney is covered by a fibrous layer of connective tissue called the **renal capsule**. The indentation that gives the kidney its bean-shaped appearance is called the **renal hilum** (*hilum* = root). At the hilum, the renal artery brings blood into the kidney to be filtered. Once filtered, the blood leaves the kidney via the renal vein. The **ureter** is also attached at the hilum. The ureter transports the urine away from the kidney to the bladder (see **FIGURE 17–2** ▓).

Internal Anatomy

The internal anatomy of the kidney (Figure 17–2) is considerably more complicated than its external anatomy. The kidney can be divided into three regions. The outer region is the **renal cortex** (*cortex* is Latin for "rind," or outer layer, like the rind of a watermelon); the middle region is the **renal medulla** (*medulla* = inner portion); and the innermost region is the **renal pelvis**. Adding the word *renal* is important here.

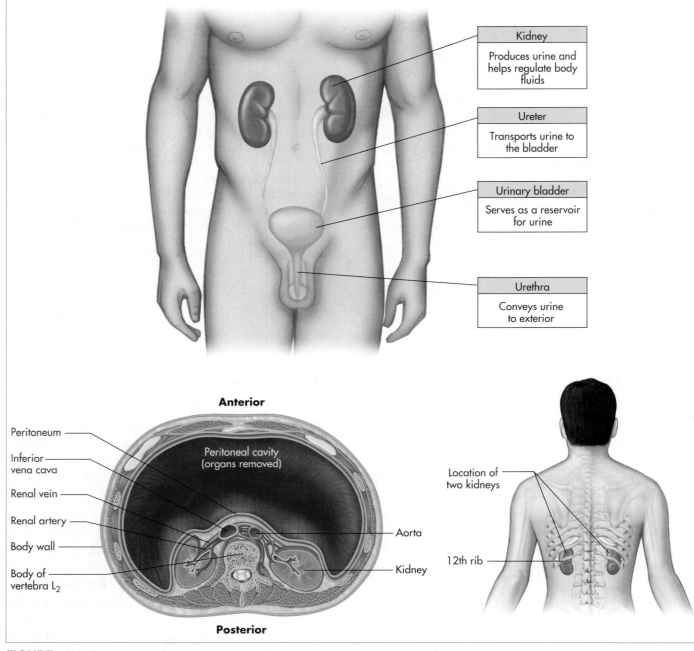

FIGURE 17–1 ■

Anatomy of the urinary system.

Remember that the brain and the adrenal gland both have a medulla and a cortex. Also keep in mind that the body also has more than one pelvis, as in the bony pelvis. The renal cortex is grainy in appearance and has very little obvious structure to the naked eye. The renal cortex is where the blood is actually filtered.

The renal medulla contains a number of triangle-shaped striped areas called **renal pyramids**. The renal pyramids are composed of collecting tubules for the urine that is formed in the kidney. Adjacent pyramids are separated by narrow **renal columns**, which are extensions of the cortical tissue.

The renal pelvis is a funnel. The funnel is divided into two or three large collecting cups, called **major calyces** (*calyces* = cup or cup-shaped). Each major **calyx** is divided into several **minor calyces**. The calyces form cup-shaped areas around the tips of the pyramids to collect the urine that continually drains through the pyramids. The kidney is essentially a combination of a filtration and collection system. The blood

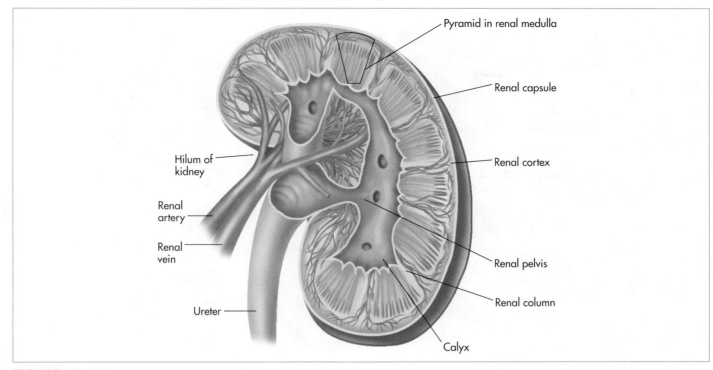

FIGURE 17–2 ■
The internal and external anatomy of the kidney.

is filtered by millions of tiny filters in the cortex, the filtered material flows through tiny tubes in the medulla, and the resulting urine is collected in the renal pelvis. The renal pelvis, which is simply the enlarged proximal portion of the ureter, empties into the ureter. The ureter then carries the urine to the **urinary bladder**, where it is stored and eventually eliminated from the body (again, see Figure 17–2).

Blood Vessels

Because the kidney's job is to filter blood, the blood must reach every part of the kidney. A single **renal artery** enters each kidney at the hilum (see **FIGURE 17–3** ■). The renal artery then branches into five segmental arteries. The segmental arteries branch into lobar arteries. The lobar arteries branch into interlobar arteries, which pass through the renal columns. Arcuate arteries originate from the interlobar arteries. The *arcuate* arteries are so named because they arch around the base of the pyramids in the renal medulla. Many tiny cortical radiate (interlobular) arteries branch from the arcuate arteries, supplying blood to the renal cortex. These cortical radiate arteries give rise to numerous **afferent arterioles** (*afferent* = to carry toward).

Each afferent arteriole leads to a ball of capillaries called a **glomerulus**. **Efferent arterioles** (*efferent* = to carry away

from) then leave from the glomerulus and travel to a specialized series of capillaries called the **peritubular capillaries** and **vasa recta** (straight, collecting tubes) that are associated with the **renal nephron**, the functional unit of the kidney. The peritubular capillaries wrap around the tubules of the nephron. You have seen a situation like this in the lungs, where the pulmonary capillaries surround the alveoli. Having blood vessels close to the nephron allows efficient movement of ions between blood and the fluid in the nephron, just as having pulmonary capillaries near the alveoli allows efficient diffusion of respiratory gases between the alveoli and the bloodstream.

From each set of peritubular capillaries, blood flows out the cortical radiate veins. From there, the blood flows out a series of veins that are the direct reverse of the arteries, with one exception. There are no segmental veins. The blood finally leaves the kidney via the **renal vein**. Please refer to Figure 17–3 for a diagram of the renal blood vessels.

Microscopic Anatomy of the Kidney: The Nephron

So far we have looked at an overview of the kidneys' structure and function. Now let's take a closer look at what actually happens within the kidneys. The business end

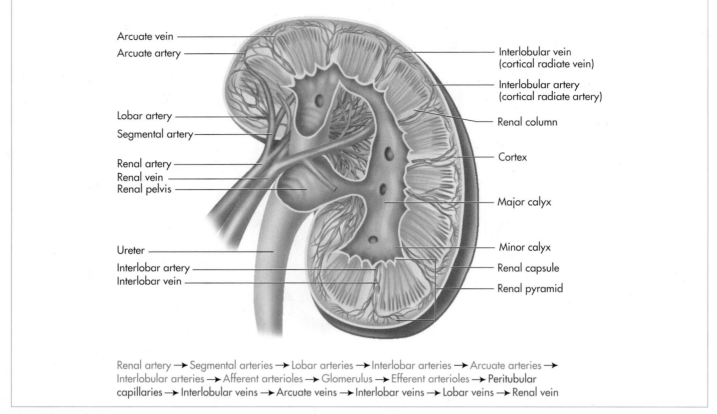

Arcuate vein
Arcuate artery
Interlobular vein (cortical radiate vein)
Interlobular artery (cortical radiate artery)
Lobar artery
Segmental artery
Renal column
Renal artery
Renal vein
Renal pelvis
Cortex
Major calyx
Ureter
Interlobar artery
Interlobar vein
Minor calyx
Renal capsule
Renal pyramid

Renal artery → Segmental arteries → Lobar arteries → Interlobar arteries → Arcuate arteries → Interlobular arteries → Afferent arterioles → Glomerulus → Efferent arterioles → Peritubular capillaries → Interlobular veins → Arcuate veins → Interlobar veins → Lobar veins → Renal vein

FIGURE 17–3 ▪
Renal blood vessels and the pathway of blood through the renal system.

of the kidney, the part that performs its real functions, consists of millions of microscopic funnels and tubules. These fundamental functional units of the kidney are called **nephrons** (see **FIGURE 17–4** ▪). Here is another example of anatomy that increases surface area. Millions of tiny nephrons have much more surface area than several large nephrons. The nephron is divided into two distinct parts: the **renal corpuscle** and the **renal tubule**. The renal corpuscle is a filter, much like a window screen or coffee filter.

LEARNING HINT

Visualizing the Peritubular System

Think of the peritubular capillaries as blue yarn wrapped around plastic pipe, which represents the actual tubular system. You will soon learn that the filtrate that stays in the pipe eventually becomes urine, and the filtrate that is reabsorbed into the blue yarn (peritubular capillaries) is brought back into the body.

Blood enters the renal corpuscle via the **glomerulus**, a ball of capillaries. Surrounding the glomerulus is a double-layered membrane called the **glomerular capsule** (Bowman's capsule). The layers of the glomerular capsule are similar to the layers of a serous membrane like the pleura or pericardium. The inner layer of the glomerular capsule, the visceral layer, surrounds the glomerular capillaries. The visceral layer is made of specialized squamous epithelial cells called **podocytes**. The combination of podocytes and the simple squamous epithelium making up the walls of the glomerular capillaries makes a very effective filter.

The outer, or parietal, layer of the glomerular capsule is simple squamous epithelium and completes the container for the filter. Blood flows into the glomerulus and everything *but* blood cells and a few large molecules, mainly proteins, are pushed from the capillaries across the filter and into the glomerular capsule. The material filtered from the blood into the glomerular capsule is called **glomerular filtrate**. Can you see why blood cells or excessive protein found in urine may indicate a kidney filtration problem?

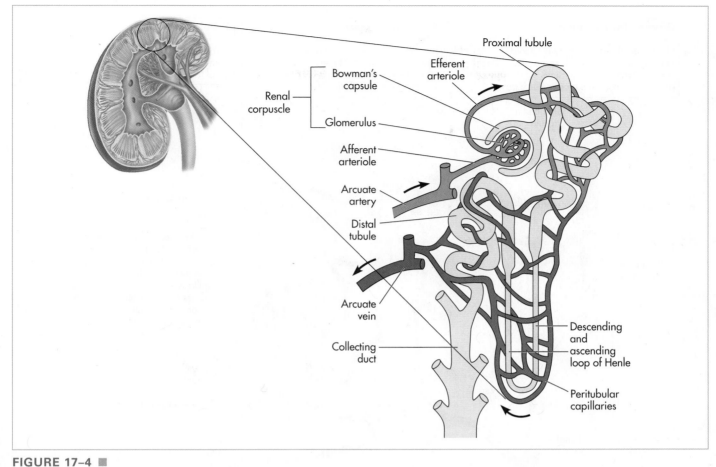

FIGURE 17–4 ■
The nephron.

The rest of the nephron is a series of tubes known as the **renal tubule**, sort of like a Habitrail system for a gerbil or hamster (see **FIGURE 17–5** ■). Just like the water filtration system in our towns and cities, the water (glomerular filtrate) travels through a network of pipes (tubules), where the impurities remain in the pipes to be discharged while the filtered water is collected (peritubular capillaries) and recycled back into the city's water supply.

Now back to the kidney. Glomerular filtrate flows from the glomerular capsule into the first part of the renal tubule, the **proximal tubule**. The wall of the proximal tubule is made of cuboidal epithelium with microvilli. From the proximal tubule, glomerular filtrate flows into the **nephron loop** (also called the loop of Henle). The nephron loop consists of two segments, the **descending loop**, with a structure similar to the proximal tubule, and the **ascending loop**, with a wall made of simple cuboidal epithelium without microvilli. From the nephron loop, the glomerular filtrate flows into the **distal tubule**. The wall of the distal tubule is like that of the ascending branch of the nephron loop.

From the distal tubule, glomerular filtrate flows into one of several **collecting ducts**, also made of cuboidal epithelium. The collecting ducts lead to the minor calyces, then to the major calyces, renal pelvis, and ureter. At this point, the glomerular filtrate is urine. Again, if you refer to our previous learning hint, what stays in the tubular system (plastic pipe) eventually gets eliminated as urine.

As you might expect, blood vessels are in close proximity to the nephrons because certain substances within the filtrate must be brought back into the bloodstream. Blood approaches the nephron via the afferent arteriole. Blood flows from the afferent arteriole into the glomerulus, a capillary ball surrounded by the glomerular capsule. Blood flows from the glomerulus via the efferent arteriole into the peritubular capillaries and vasa recta, a series of blood vessels surrounding the renal tubules (or the "blue yarn" from the Learning Hint). These surrounding blood vessels allow for reabsorption back into the bloodstream from the filtrate that is within the tubular system. Blood then leaves the area of the nephron via the cortical radiate veins.

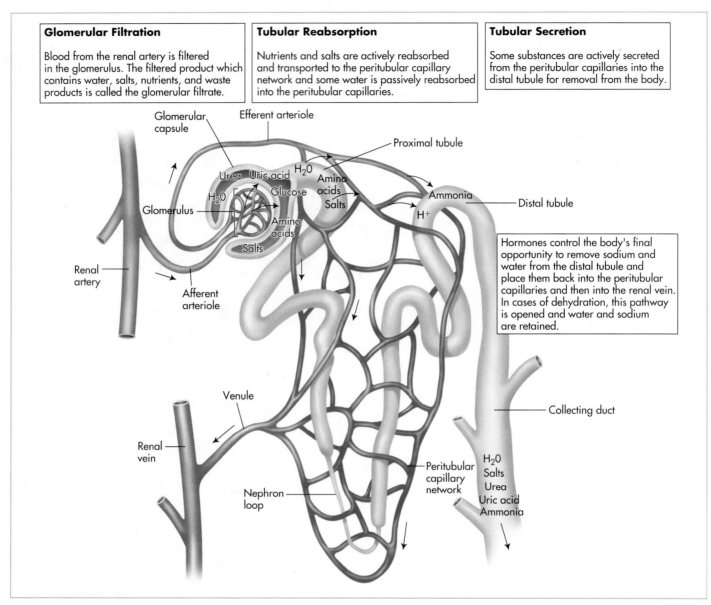

Glomerular Filtration

Blood from the renal artery is filtered in the glomerulus. The filtered product which contains water, salts, nutrients, and waste products is called the glomerular filtrate.

Tubular Reabsorption

Nutrients and salts are actively reabsorbed and transported to the peritubular capillary network and some water is passively reabsorbed into the peritubular capillaries.

Tubular Secretion

Some substances are actively secreted from the peritubular capillaries into the distal tubule for removal from the body.

Hormones control the body's final opportunity to remove sodium and water from the distal tubule and place them back into the peritubular capillaries and then into the renal vein. In cases of dehydration, this pathway is opened and water and sodium are retained.

FIGURE 17–5 ■

A functional renal unit.

Clinical Application

TRAUMA, ISCHEMIA, AND KIDNEY DAMAGE

The kidney is obviously very well vascularized. Each nephron is literally surrounded by blood vessels, and the flow of blood around the nephron is controlled by flow through the afferent arteriole. **Ischemia** is a condition of tissue injury resulting from too little oxygen delivery to tissues, usually caused by decreased blood flow. When blood flow to the nephrons decreases for a period of time, oxygen delivery to the nephron decreases, and ischemia can result. Decreased blood flow to the kidneys results from anything that causes prolonged constriction of the afferent arterioles. Probably the most common cause of prolonged vasoconstriction in the kidney is any number of hormonal mechanisms used to increase blood pressure—for example, after severe blood loss.

For example, a young boy runs into a storm door, puncturing his femoral artery, which begins to bleed profusely. As his blood volume falls, so does his blood pressure. His body fights desperately to bring his blood pressure back to normal, causing widespread vasoconstriction. The afferent arterioles,

under the influence of sympathetic hormones and other vasoconstrictors, get smaller and smaller, greatly decreasing blood supply to the nephrons. If the situation continues long enough, the tissues will become ischemic and eventually begin to die. Even if the boy survives the initial blood loss from the wound, his kidneys may be damaged, resulting in temporary or permanent renal failure. It is not uncommon for a trauma patient to survive the initial trauma only to become the victim of organ damage due to tissue death.

TEST YOUR KNOWLEDGE 17–1

Choose the best answer:

1. What carries urine from the kidneys to the bladder?
   a. urethra
   b. ureter
   c. vagina
   d. uterus

2. The renal _____ is the outer region of the kidney.
   a. medulla
   b. pelvis
   c. hilum
   d. cortex

3. These vessels carry blood into the glomerulus:
   a. peritubular capillaries.
   b. afferent arterioles.
   c. segmental arteries.
   d. none of the above

4. The fundamental functional unit of the kidney is the
   a. renal corpuscle.
   b. renal pelvis.
   c. nephron.
   d. pyramid.

5. Glomerular filtrate flows from the _____ into the _____.
   a. proximal tubule; distal tubule
   b. ascending loop; descending loop
   c. glomerular capsule; proximal tubule
   d. proximal tubule; collecting duct

URINE FORMATION

As the body's blood purification system, the job of the kidneys is to control fluid and electrolyte balance by carefully controlling urine volume and composition. The kidneys also remove nitrogen-containing waste and other impurities from blood. To form urine, the nephron must perform three processes: *glomerular filtration, tubular reabsorption,* and *tubular secretion*. Please see **FIGURE 17–6** ■ for a diagram of these three processes.

During **glomerular filtration**, fluid and molecules pass from the glomerular capillaries into the glomerular capsule, across a filter composed of the wall of the capillaries and the podocytes of the glomerular capsule. The filtrate flows into the renal tubule, where the composition of the filtrate is controlled by **tubular reabsorption** and **tubular secretion**. Substances that are reabsorbed pass from the renal tubule into the peritubular capillaries and will not end up in urine but stay within the body. Substances that are secreted pass

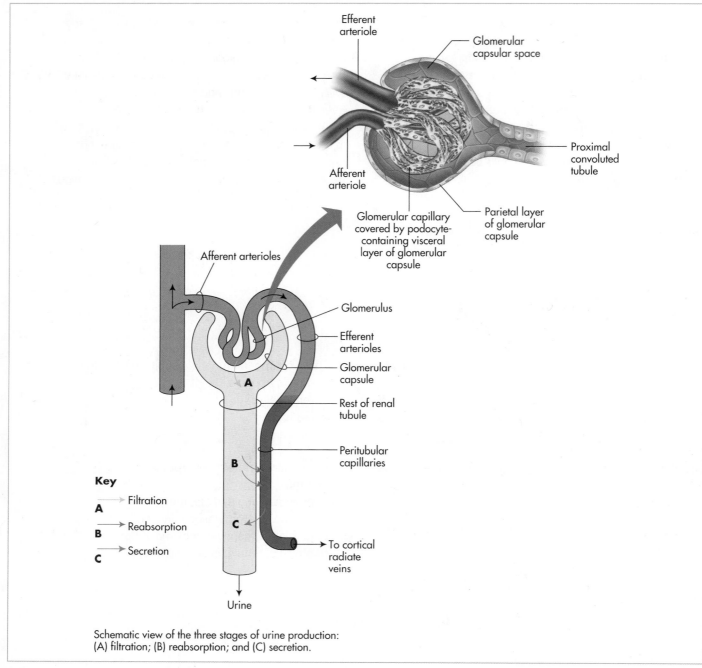

Schematic view of the three stages of urine production: (A) filtration; (B) reabsorption; and (C) secretion.

FIGURE 17–6 ■

The processes involved in urine formation.

from the peritubular capillaries into the renal tubule and eventually leave the body via the urine. The combination of all three processes is necessary for the formation of urine. *Filtration* moves fluid and chemicals into the nephron from blood, and *reabsorption* and *secretion* control the chemistry and volume of urine. **Glomerular filtrate** is chemically similar to blood, whereas urine is chemically very different. Some substances, like glucose, are normally completely reabsorbed, and other substances, such as the metabolic waste products urea and creatinine, are secreted such that urea and creatinine are much more concentrated in urine

than in blood. See **TABLE 17–1** ■ for a comparison of normal plasma, glomerular filtrate, and urine chemistry.

Control of Filtration

Think for a moment about filters with which you are familiar. What controls these filters? What force drives filtration? What determines whether a substance passes through the filter or stays on one side? The example you are likely most familiar with is a window screen. Why do you have window screens in your windows? To keep out the bugs. Without screens, every insect in the neighborhood would be in

TABLE 17–1 KIDNEY FLUID CHEMISTRY

SUBSTANCE	PLASMA	GLOMERULAR FILTRATE	URINE
Protein	3,900–5,000	None	None
Glucose	100	100	None
Sodium	142	142	128
Potassium	5	5	60
Urea	26	26	1,820
Creatinine	1.1	1.1	140

All concentrations in mg/100 mL

your bedroom eating you alive, right? So what determines whether something gets through the screen? The most obvious answer is the size of the mesh in the screen. Dust gets through the screen, but most bugs don't. Imagine a screen with holes twice the size of a typical screen. You would spend all night swatting mosquitoes! The screens would be pretty much useless. Filter size determines what gets through the filter. All filters are *selective*: Only some substances pass through, mainly due to the size of the openings in the filter (see FIGURE 17–7 ■).

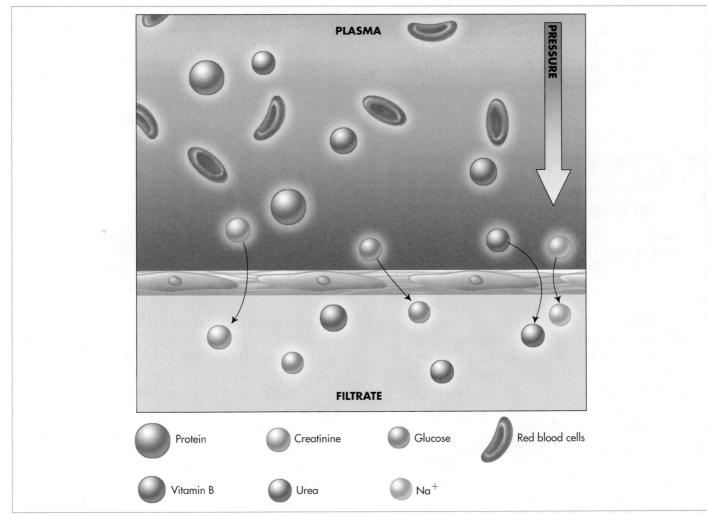

FIGURE 17–7 ■
Filter selectivity.

Can you think of a situation in which something might get through a window screen? Leaving behind the bugs, let's think about a screened-in porch. During a gentle snowstorm, snow doesn't come through the screen. But if that snowstorm has a high wind, the inside of the porch is covered in snow. The high winds force the snow through the screen. Substances are moved through a filter by differences in pressure across the filter. Pressure pushes stuff through the holes. The higher the pressure on one side of the filter compared to the other side, the faster substances are filtered.

Amazing Facts

Glomerular Filtration

The millions of tiny filters in your kidneys perform a truly Herculean task. Average glomerular filtration rate is 110 milliliters per minute, or 160 liters per day. That's more than 40 gallons filtered every 24 hours.

This combination works great in coffeemakers. The filters have holes too small to let any but the tiniest coffee grounds pass through. The pressure of the water on top of the filter pushes the water and the chemicals that make coffee grounds into drinkable coffee through the filter, but the grounds stay on the other side.

The renal filter works in much the same way. Like most filters, the podocytes and capillary walls of the renal corpuscle create a filter with fixed openings. Plasma and many of the substances dissolved in plasma pass through the filter, but red and white blood cells, platelets, and some large molecules, such as proteins, do not pass through the filter in a healthy kidney, but remain in the bloodstream. What passes through the filter is predetermined by the size of the openings. This explains why protein in urine is a sign of kidney damage. Under normal circumstances, protein molecules are too large to fit through the glomerular filter, so proteins do not get into the renal tubule or into the urine. Only when the filter is damaged can protein pass into the filtrate and then into the urine (see FIGURE 17–8 ■).

Filtration Rate

Filtration rate, however, can be controlled by changing the pressure difference across the filter. The most obvious way to control the pressure is to change the pressure of the blood in the glomerular capillaries. Higher pressure in the glomerulus will increase filtration; lower pressure will decrease filtration. You might think that every minor change in systemic blood

Clinical Application

DIABETIC NEPHROPATHY

Diabetes mellitus is a condition characterized by abnormally high blood glucose. This hyperglycemia, caused by production of too little insulin or by insensitivity to insulin, wreaks havoc with blood chemistry, including osmotic balance. One of the functions of your kidneys is to remove all that extra glucose from your blood. When the blood glucose level is high, the kidneys must work that much harder to remove it. Patients with elevated glucose eliminate a much greater volume of urine than do patients with healthy levels of blood glucose because the kidneys try to excrete the excess blood glucose.

Prolonged high blood glucose causes a type of kidney damage known as **diabetic nephropathy**. It begins with a thickening of the filter surface of the glomerular capsule and eventually leads to a complete breakdown of that tissue. Once the tissue is damaged, the selectivity of the filter is destroyed. Substances that usually would not pass through the filter and into glomerular filtrate, such as proteins and blood cells, begin to appear in urine. The efficiency of filtration is compromised, and kidney function begins to deteriorate. Protein and blood cells in the urine are early indicators of renal failure. Diabetics can help prevent the onset of kidney damage by keeping blood sugar levels as tightly controlled as possible, preventing high blood pressure, and reducing blood cholesterol to safe levels. Diabetes is one of the leading causes of kidney failure in the United States. (The other is hypertension.)

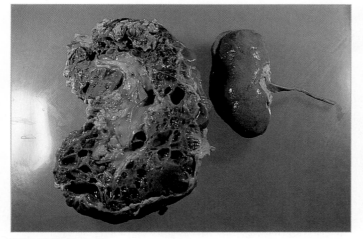

FIGURE 17–8 ■

Comparison of damaged and healthy kidneys.

Clinical Application

POLYCYSTIC KIDNEY DISEASE

Polycystic kidney disease (PKD) is a genetic disorder in which large cysts form in the kidneys. One form of PKD is so serious that some patients die in infancy. The more common form is an adult-onset disorder characterized by decreasing kidney function as normal nephrons are displaced by the cysts. As more and more cysts develop, kidneys get very large. In fact, one polycystic kidney has gone on record with a weight of 22 pounds! There is no cure for PKD except kidney transplantation. About half a million people in the United States have PKD.

pressure would affect glomerular filtration rate. That would be the logical conclusion. However, the glomerulus is protected from minor changes in blood pressure by a mechanism called **autoregulation**. As systemic blood pressure increases, the afferent arterioles leading into the glomerulus constrict, decreasing the amount of blood getting into the glomerulus. If less blood gets into the glomerulus, the pressure doesn't rise. Autoregulation protects the delicate filter from repeated rapid changes in blood pressure caused, for example, by walking up steps.

Autoregulation can be overridden in situations when blood pressure must be regulated. Because the kidney controls fluid volume, it is often part of mechanisms, along with the cardiovascular system, that regulate systemic blood pressure. For example, if there is a decrease in systemic blood pressure or volume, such as during severe blood loss, glomerular filtration decreases dramatically in an attempt to conserve fluid volume by producing less urine.

Remember that the fight-or-flight response (changes in the body in response to stress) includes decreased urine production. The sympathetic nervous system and the hormones of the adrenal medulla, epinephrine and norepinephrine, decrease glomerular filtration by causing dramatic vasoconstriction of the afferent arterioles. This prevents blood from flowing to the glomerulus, decreasing glomerular filtration rate. Small changes in systemic blood pressure do not affect glomerular filtration because autoregulation keeps glomerular pressure relatively constant, but during shock, for example, glomerular filtration decreases significantly. This is one of the reasons that urine output is monitored in trauma and surgery patients.

One serious complication of severe blood loss is permanent kidney damage due to decreased blood flow and subsequent death of kidney tissue.

The reverse is also true: If blood volume is elevated, sympathetic output to the afferent arterioles decreases, the arterioles dilate, and glomerular filtration rate increases, allowing the kidneys to get rid of excess fluid.

Control of Tubular Reabsorption and Secretion

Regulation of glomerular filtration controls the speed of filtration and ultimately the amount of urine formed. Regulation of **tubular reabsorption** and **tubular secretion** controls the chemistry and volume of the urine. Substances that are reabsorbed move from the tubule back to the bloodstream via the peritubular capillaries and stay in the body. Substances that are secreted stay in the tubule and eventually leave the body via the urine. Thus, anything that affects reabsorption and secretion affects urine chemistry.

The first thing that affects tubular reabsorption and secretion is tubule permeability. Each portion of the tubule can reabsorb and secrete different substances. Remember that molecules can move across membranes via several different methods. *Diffusion* is the movement of molecules from high to low concentration. *Osmosis* is the movement of water across a semipermeable membrane. Some molecules can only move across membranes by being carried across by proteins. This type of movement is called *carrier-mediated transport*, which may be *active* or *passive*. For review of transport methods, see Chapter 4. Differences in tubule permeability result

Clinical Application

KIDNEY STONES

Kidney stones are exactly what their name implies: hard bodies (stones) in the kidney. Kidney stones result when substances in the urine crystallize in the renal tubule, often because the concentration of the molecule is higher than normal in the renal tubule. However, sometimes the cause of kidney stones is a mystery. Stones can be made of many different chemicals, including calcium or uric acid, or can be caused by kidney infection. Some individuals appear to be more susceptible to stones than others, and once you have had a kidney stone, you are more susceptible to kidney stones in the future. Many kidney stones pass through the kidney unnoticed. However, larger or irregularly shaped stones may lodge in the kidney tubules, obstructing flow and irritating nearby tissues. Most patients diagnosed with kidney stones are driven to seek treatment because of blood in their urine (hematuria) or excruciating lower back or pelvic pain. Patients with kidney stones often describe the pain as the worst they have ever felt. Even painful stones will often pass on their own without medical intervention.

Patients are treated for pain and sent home with instructions to drink lots of water and wait for the stone to pass. Often, they are asked to save the stone as it passes so it can be sent for chemical analysis. Twenty years ago, the only treatment for a stone too large to pass on its own was surgery to remove the stone. Today, however, a noninvasive technique called **lithotripsy**, which uses shock waves applied to the outside of the body, can often break up the stone so it is small enough to pass through the kidney, decreasing the need for surgery.

FOCUS ON PROFESSIONS

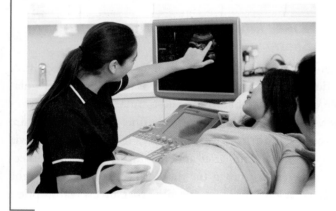

Ultrasound technicians help to view the kidneys for diagnostic purposes. They also perform diagnostic images on other body organs. Learn more about this profession by visiting the websites of national organizations, including the Society of Diagnostic Medical Sonography (SDMS), the American Registry for Diagnostic Medical Sonography (ARDMS), and the American Institute of Ultrasound in Medicine (AIUM).

TEST YOUR KNOWLEDGE 17–2

Choose the best answer:

1. Glomerular filtrate is most similar in composition to
   a. blood.
   b. lymph.
   c. urine.
   d. none of the above

2. When substances move from the tubule into the bloodstream, this is known as
   a. secretion.
   b. reabsorption.
   c. filtration.
   d. all of the above

3. If blood pressure increases beyond normal range, what happens to glomerular filtration rate?
   a. It increases.
   b. It decreases.
   c. It stays the same.
   d. none of the above

4. Which of the following is not typically found in urine?
   a. glucose
   b. protein
   c. blood cells
   d. all of the above

5. What controls the selectivity of the kidney filter?
   a. blood pressure
   b. the size of the holes in the filter
   c. the charge of the molecules
   d. time of day

in dramatic differences in which molecules are reabsorbed or secreted in each part of the tubule. See **TABLE 17–2** ■ for a list of substances reabsorbed or secreted in each part of the tubule.

Amazing Facts

Tubular Reabsorption

You already know about the amazing ability of your kidneys to filter blood. However, the ability of your renal tubule to reabsorb the fluid filtered by the glomerulus is just as incredible. Your kidneys filter 160 liters (40 gallons) per day, yet you only produce between 1 and 3 liters (less than 1 gallon) of urine per day.

The second factor that affects tubular reabsorption and secretion is a special type of circulation around the nephron loop, called **countercurrent circulation**. When ions move across cell membranes, they move from areas of high to low concentration. They are said to move down their concentration gradient. In a solution, if there is a lot of solvent (water), there is less solute (dissolved substances), and vice versa, so you would expect that solute and solvent would move in opposite directions down their concentration gradients.

The characteristics of the nephron that make the countercurrent circulation work include the concentration gradient in the fluid surrounding the nephron, with low ion concentration at the beginning of the descending loop and high concentration at the tip of the loop, and the differences in permeability between the descending loop (water) and ascending loop (ions).

As filtrate flows into the *descending loop*, *water* is reabsorbed, and the concentration of ions in the loop increases

TABLE 17–2 INDIVIDUAL TUBULE FUNCTIONS

TUBULE	SUBSTANCES REABSORBED OR SECRETED
Proximal tubule	Potassium, chloride, sodium*, magnesium, bicarbonate, phosphate, amino acids, glucose, fructose, galactose, lactate, citric acid, water, hydrogen (H^+), neurotransmitters, bile, uric acid, drugs, toxins, ammonia, urea
Descending loop	Water**, urea
Ascending loop	Sodium, potassium, chloride, urea
Distal tubule	Sodium, potassium, chloride, hydrogen (H^+), water
Collecting duct	Sodium, potassium, chloride, water, urea

*(80% of sodium is normally reabsorbed in the proximal tubule)
**(90% of water is normally reabsorbed in the descending loop)

as water leaves the tubule. As the filtrate turns the corner and enters the *ascending loop*, much of the water has left, and the fluid is extremely concentrated. The ascending loop is permeable only to ions, so *ions* are reabsorbed from the ascending loop. Water and ions that leave the renal tubule enter the capillaries and go back to the bloodstream (see **FIGURE 17–9** ■).

The third set of factors that affect reabsorption and secretion are several hormones that regulate blood pressure (see Chapter 13), "The Cardiovascular System." You were introduced briefly to these mechanisms when you learned about regulation of blood pressure. It should come as no surprise that these mechanisms affect kidney function because the kidneys control ion and fluid balance. The hormones that affect the kidneys perform a variety of functions. You met some of these hormones during your visit to the cardiovascular and endocrine systems.

- **Antidiuretic hormone** (ADH) is made by the hypothalamus and secreted from the posterior pituitary when blood pressure decreases or blood ionic concentration increases. This hormone increases the permeability of the collecting ducts and distal tubules so that more water is reabsorbed, thereby increasing the blood volume and blood pressure and diluting the ionic concentration. Less urine is produced as more water is reabsorbed, hence the name *antidiuretic hormone*. Alcohol actually inhibits ADH from working and thus prevents the distal tubules and collecting ducts from becoming more permeable to water. The water then stays in the renal

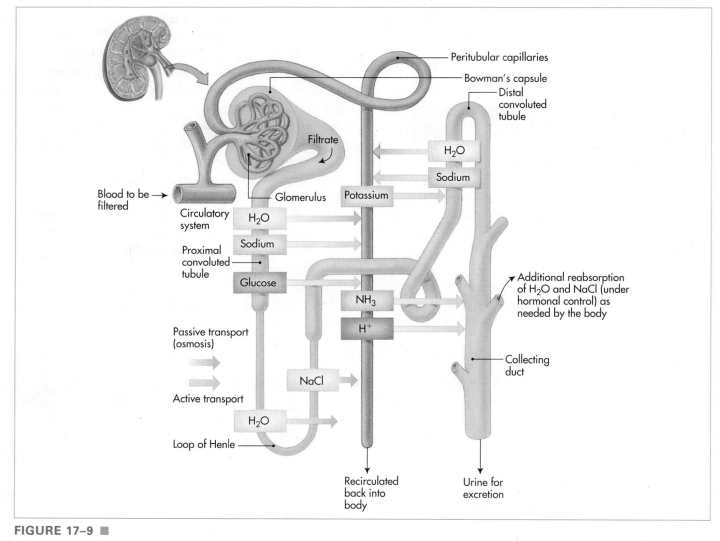

FIGURE 17–9 ■

Sites of tubular reabsorption and secretion.

tubule and is sent to the bladder, thereby increasing urination. The more alcohol you drink, the more dehydrated you become.

- **Aldosterone** is an adrenocorticosteroid, a steroid secreted by the adrenal cortex. When plasma sodium decreases or plasma potassium increases, aldosterone is secreted. It increases the reabsorption of sodium ions (thus bringing more back into the blood) and secretion of potassium ions (thus decreasing the plasma levels) by the distal tubule and ascending limb of the nephron loop. Because sodium is reabsorbed back into the bloodstream, so is more water, and urine volume therefore decreases under the influence of aldosterone.

- **Atrial natriuretic hormone (ANH)** is secreted by the atria of the heart when blood volume increases, due to atrial stretch. This hormone decreases sodium reabsorption and therefore increases urination. Does this make sense? If blood volume has increased dramatically, how would you keep blood pressure constant? Would you get rid of water or keep more water? Atrial natriuretic hormone is the antagonist of aldosterone and inhibits antidiuretic hormone (ADH) secretion. It also increases glomerular filtration rate by dilating the afferent arterioles. All of these effects increase urination and therefore decrease blood volume.

- **Renin-angiotensin-aldosterone** system is a series of chemical reactions that regulate blood pressure in several different ways. When there is a decrease in blood flow to the kidney, a special group of cells near the glomerulus called the **juxtaglomerular apparatus** (*juxta* = near) secretes renin into the bloodstream. Renin converts **angiotensinogen**, a protein made by the liver, into angiotensin I. An enzyme made by the lungs, **angiotensin-converting enzyme (ACE)**, converts angiotensin I to angiotensin II. Angiotensin II (active angiotensin) has several different effects. It increases thirst, increases ADH secretion, increases aldosterone secretion, and causes vasoconstriction. Blood pressure is therefore increased either by increased fluid volume due to higher water intake or decreased urination caused by increased levels of ADH or aldosterone. Notice how the kidneys, lungs, and liver work together to regulate blood pressure. Many patients with high blood pressure may be given an ACE inhibitor, which inhibits all the previous effects and therefore lowers blood pressure.

The Urinary Bladder and Urination Reflex

Glomerular filtrate flows out the collecting ducts into the minor calyces and then into the major calyces that form the renal pelvis. Once the glomerular filtrate leaves the collecting ducts, its concentration cannot be changed. At this point, filtrate is urine. Urine collects in the renal pelvis and flows down the ureters to the urinary bladder, where it is stored.

The urinary bladder (see **FIGURE 17–10** ■) is a small, hollow organ posterior to the pubic symphysis and behind the peritoneum. It is lined with transitional epithelium, the only

---

APPLIED SCIENCE

Electrolytes and Acid–Base Balance

Remember in Chapter 14 that we described the role of the lungs in maintaining acid–base balance by controlling levels of carbon dioxide within the blood and mentioned the fact that the kidneys also play a major role. The kidneys maintain electrolyte balance by selectively excreting or reabsorbing the electrolytes within the tubular system. One very important interaction is the relationship of hydrogen ions (H^+) and bicarbonate ions (HCO_3^-). The relationship between these ions determines the blood's pH (level of acidity or alkalinity). CO_2 levels in the blood are also involved in acid–base balance, as most CO_2 is carried in the blood as bicarbonate ions. This is referred to as the *acid–base relationship*. If too much acid is present in the blood, H^+, which increases acidity and causes the pH to drop, will be excreted to a greater level in the urine. At the same time, more bicarbonate ions (base that neutralizes acids) will be reabsorbed back into the acidic blood to bring the pH value back toward normal. The respiratory system's role in maintaining the acid–base balance is by increasing ventilation to "blow off" more acid in the form of exhaled carbon dioxide (carbonic acid) if the blood is too acidic.

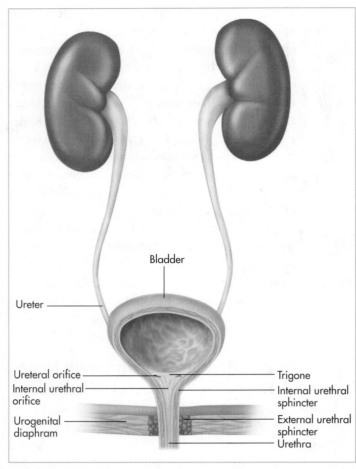

Bladder

Ureter

Ureteral orifice

Internal urethral orifice

Urogenital diaphram

Trigone

Internal urethral sphincter

External urethral sphincter

Urethra

FIGURE 17–10 ■

The urinary bladder.

epithelium stretchy enough to expand as the bladder fills. The stretchiness of the bladder is enhanced by a series of pleats called *rugae*. The bladder has a muscular wall consisting of several layers of circular and longitudinal smooth muscle, called the *detrusor muscle*, and is covered by connective tissue and parietal peritoneum.

As urine accumulates, the bladder fills and stretches. At some point, this stretch triggers urination, or voiding—the emptying of the bladder. The stretch of the bladder triggers a reflex in the sacral spinal cord that increases contractions of the detrusor muscle. However, the pons (in the brain) has inhibitory control over the spinal cord reflex, allowing voluntary control of urination.

Urine leaves the bladder via the **urethra**, a thin muscular tube lined with several different types of epithelium along its length. For details on the anatomy of the urethra, including sexual differences, see Chapter 18. Parts of the brain can inhibit urination by controlling the **internal urethral sphincter**, a valve at the junction of the bladder and the urethra, and the **external urethral sphincter**, a valve that is part of the muscles of the pelvic floor. The internal urethral sphincter is involuntary, whereas you have voluntary control of the external sphincter. Sympathetic stimulation of these sphincters prevents urine from leaving the body (see **FIGURE 17–11** ■). Fortunately, although you have little control over contractions of the bladder wall, you have very good control over the sphincters.

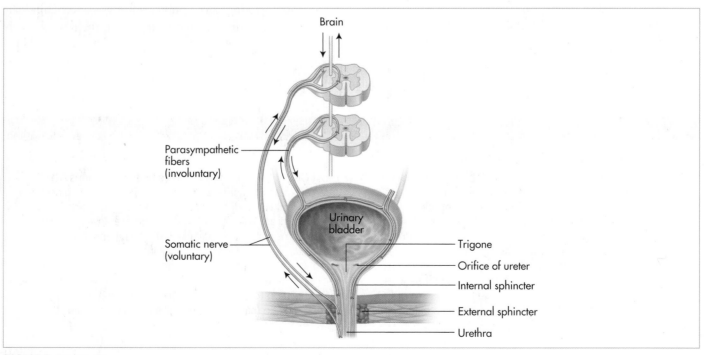

Brain

Parasympathetic fibers (involuntary)

Somatic nerve (voluntary)

Urinary bladder

Trigone

Orifice of ureter

Internal sphincter

External sphincter

Urethra

FIGURE 17–11 ■

Control of urination.

TEST YOUR KNOWLEDGE 17–3

Choose the best answer:

1. Which of the following is usually completely reabsorbed in the proximal tubule?
   a. sodium
   b. urea
   c. glucose
   d. water

2. The descending nephron loop is permeable to _____, whereas the ascending is permeable to _____.
   a. water; ions
   b. ions; water
   c. water; water
   d. ions; ions
   e. all of the above

3. If blood pressure falls dramatically, what happens to urine output?
   a. It increases.
   b. It decreases.
   c. It stays the same.
   d. not enough information

4. Which hormone increases urine output?
   a. ADH
   b. aldosterone
   c. ANP
   d. erythropoietin

5. The series of pleats found in the bladder to enhance stretching are called:
   a. sphincters
   b. rugae
   c. gyri
   d. ureters

COMMON DISORDERS OF THE URINARY SYSTEM

Overuse or abuse of drugs can severely affect renal function. **Analgesic nephropathy** is caused by long-term use of pain relievers, particularly nonsteroidal anti-inflammatory drugs (NSAIDs) such as ibuprofen and naproxyn, particularly when combined with caffeine, codeine, or acetaminophen. Even over-the-counter dosages can cause chronic kidney damage leading to kidney failure.

Chronic renal failure is an ongoing, progressive kidney disease. Often, its progression can be controlled by treating the underlying cause of the damage or controlling blood pressure and blood cholesterol. Chronic kidney failure may lead to **end-stage renal failure**, or the final stage of renal failure. Patients in end-stage renal failure can be treated only with kidney dialysis or transplantation.

Diabetes insipidus is an endocrine disorder characterized by too little antidiuretic hormone (ADH) or insensitivity of the kidney to ADH. Without normal ADH activity, copious amounts of urine are produced. Even as the patient becomes dehydrated, the production of urine cannot be slowed. A rarer form of the disorder is caused by abnormalities of the thirst mechanism, in which patients drink uncontrollably. Patients with uncontrollable thirst can actually drink so much water that they have water toxicity (dangerously low blood sodium because of dilution), which can cause brain damage or death. *Diabetes mellitus* also causes excessive urination, but because of the increase in blood glucose, urination is the body's attempt to excrete excess glucose. *Diabetes*, which means "passing through," refers to the excess urination seen in both diabetes insipidus and diabetes mellitus, although they are very different disorders.

Glomerulonephritis is an inflammation of the glomerulus. **Glomerulosclerosis** is scarring of the glomerulus. Both cause damage to the delicate filter apparatus. When the filter is damaged, blood cells and blood proteins enter the filtrate and eventually appear in the urine. Removal of waste products is decreased, and electrolyte balance is generally abnormal because of the change in urine chemistry. There are many causes of glomerulonephritis and glomerulosclerosis, including bacterial infection, diabetic nephropathy, systemic lupus erythematosus, and genetic disorders such as Alport's syndrome and Goodpasture's syndrome.

Clinical Application

URINARY TRACT INFECTION

Urinary tract infection (UTI) is often caused by the movement of fecal bacteria into the urinary tract. It can also be caused by viruses, fungi, and various sexually transmitted diseases (STDs). Symptoms include frequent, painful urination. Sometimes the urine is bloody or cloudy or has an unusual odor. This type of infection must be treated promptly because it can cause damage to the kidneys if the infection moves from the bladder up the ureter and into the kidneys. Urinary tract infections are more common in women than in men, probably because women's urethras are shorter than men's. These infections may be prevented in susceptible individuals by drinking plenty of water, which helps to "flush out" pathogens.

Hemolytic uremic syndrome is a disorder caused by an infection with specific types of the bacteria *E. coli*, typically from eating undercooked meat. The bacteria infect the digestive tract and release toxins that destroy red blood cells. The damaged red blood cells lodge in the blood vessels in the kidney, blocking them and preventing blood flow to the nephrons. Without treatment, permanent kidney damage may result.

Amazing Facts

Urine

In a healthy renal system, the urine produced is sterile. The urea found in urine is the same substance that is used to melt ice in the winter. Urea is also a component in plant fertilizer; although nitrogen is a waste product for humans, it is an essential product for plant growth.

SUMMARY: Points of Interest

- The urinary system consists of paired kidneys and paired ureters, which carry urine to the single urinary bladder. The urethra transports urine from the bladder to outside the body. The function of the urinary system is control of fluid and electrolyte balance and elimination of nitrogen-containing waste.

- The kidney is bean-shaped and covered in a capsule. It has an indentation known as the renal hilum and an interior cavity known as the renal sinus. The kidney can be divided into three regions: renal cortex, renal medulla, and renal pelvis. The renal pelvis is a funnel that is divided into large pipes, the major calyces. Each major calyx is divided into several minor calyces. The renal pelvis empties into the ureter.

- The kidney is very well vascularized. Blood is supplied to each kidney by a renal artery. The blood vessels split into smaller and smaller branches until there are millions of tiny arterioles, called the afferent arterioles. The afferent arterioles supply millions of nephrons, the functional unit of the kidney, with blood. Blood leaves the kidney by a series of veins and ultimately returns to circulation via the renal vein.

- The nephron is the functional unit of the kidney. There are millions of nephrons in each kidney. The nephron is divided into two parts. The renal corpuscle, consisting of the glomerulus (capillaries), and the glomerular capsule, filters blood and produces glomerular filtrate. The renal tubule—consisting of the proximal tubule, nephron loop, distal tubule, and collecting ducts—controls the concentration and volume of urine by reabsorbing and secreting water, electrolytes, and other molecules. The walls of the nephron are made of epithelium. The type of epithelium changes depending on the specific function of each part of the nephron.

- Urine is formed by a combination of three processes: glomerular filtration, tubular reabsorption, and tubular secretion. The selectivity of the glomerular filter is determined by the size of the openings in the filter and the difference between the blood pressure of the glomerulus and the pressure in the glomerular capsule. The size of the filter does not change unless the glomerulus is damaged. Protein, for example, cannot pass through the filter. However, the filtration rate will change if the pressure in the glomerulus changes. Most of the time, autoregulation, which is control of the diameter of the afferent arteriole, keeps glomerular pressure and the glomerular filtration rate constant. But sympathetic stimulation can regulate (in this case decrease) glomerular filtration and urine output due to constriction of afferent arterioles.

- Tubular reabsorption and secretion are controlled by differences in tubular permeability. The proximal tubule is the most versatile, reabsorbing dozens of different molecules. The nephron loop is part of an elaborate countercurrent mechanism, with the descending loop permeable to water and ascending loop permeable to ions. The distal tubule and collecting ducts reabsorb water. The permeability of the renal tubule can be regulated by a number of hormones that control blood pressure. These hormones—aldosterone, ADH, atrial natriuretic hormone, and others—regulate blood pressure by regulating urine volume and ion secretion. Changes in urine volume change total body fluid volume and thereby change blood pressure.

- The urinary bladder is a collecting and storage structure for urine and is located in the pelvic cavity. It has a muscular wall. Contractions of the muscle result in voiding (urination); in other words, emptying the bladder. Urination is a reflex controlled by sacral spinal cord neurons, but ultimately controlled by parasympathetic neurons in the pons. Signals from a full bladder reach the spinal cord and then the pons. Sympathetic neurons control two valves, the internal and external urethral sphincters, both of which allow significant control of the urination reflex.

CASE STUDY

Jane has recently developed very annoying symptoms. She has to urinate several times a day and plans her activities based on how close she will be to a restroom. Sometimes it seems that she spends every waking moment in there. She hasn't slept through the night in more than a week. She goes to see her doctor, who orders a series of tests to differentiate between several disorders that cause frequent urination: diabetes mellitus, overactive bladder, and urinary tract infection.

Jane's urinalysis results:

Urine bacteria	no
Blood	no
Leukocytes	no
Glucose	elevated
Proteins	No

a. What is your diagnosis and why?

_____

_____

b. What do you think are possible medical treatments?

_____

_____

c. Research and list suggested lifestyle changes.

_____

_____

Multiple Choice

1. The function of this part of the renal nephron is filtration of blood:
   a. renal calyx.
   b. renal corpuscle.
   c. renal cortex.
   d. renal columns.

2. The collecting ducts are found in this part of the kidney:
   a. renal cortex.
   b. renal capsule.
   c. renal pelvis.
   d. renal pyramids.

3. This tube leads from the urinary bladder to the outside:
   a. collecting ducts.
   b. distal tubule.
   c. ureter.
   d. none of the above

4. The ion responsible for causing acidic blood is
   a. Na^+.
   b. H^+.
   c. K^+.
   d. HCO_3^-.

5. The renal hormone secreted by the hypothalamus when blood pressure decreases to promote the reabsorption of water is
   a. aldosterone.
   b. atrial natriuretic hormone.
   c. antidiuretic hormone.
   d. epinephrine.

6. Why do the cells in the proximal tubule have microvilli?
   a. to increase surface area
   b. to move particles along the mucociliary escalator
   c. to differentiate it from the distal tubule
   d. to increase filtration rate

7. Which of the following is a possible cause of blood in the urine?
   a. decreased filtration
   b. UTI
   c. decreased tubular reabsorption
   d. decreased blood pressure

8. If a patient experiences severe dehydration, what would you expect to happen to urine volume?
   a. It would increase.
   b. It would decrease.
   c. It would stay the same as usual.
   d. not enough information

Fill in the Blank

1. Most substances are reabsorbed or secreted in this part of the renal tubule: _____.

2. This part of the renal tubule has an elaborate countercurrent mechanism for reabsorption of sodium and water: _____.

3. This hormone is released by the heart when fluid volume increases: _____.

4. Urination reflex is mediated by this part of the CNS: _____.

5. As blood sodium levels decrease, this hormone is released by the adrenal cortex: _____.

6. The _____ is the funnel-shaped end of the ureter.

Short Answer

1. List and explain the activity of three regulators of kidney function.

_____

_____

_____

_____

2. Explain the three processes that are necessary for urine formation. In which part of the nephron are these functions performed?

_____

_____

_____

_____

3. Describe the structure of the wall of the urinary bladder.

_____

_____

_____

4. Explain the control of the urination reflex.

_____

_____

_____

5. Trace the flow of blood into, through, and out of the kidney.

_____

_____

_____

_____

6. Explain the symptoms of one kidney disorder. Relate the symptoms to kidney function.

_____

_____

_____

_____

Visit our new **MyHealthProfessions Lab** to accompany *Anatomy & Physiology for Health Professions.* Here you'll find a rich collection of quizzes, case studies, and animations for deeper understanding and application.

18

The Reproductive System

REPLACEMENT AND REPAIR

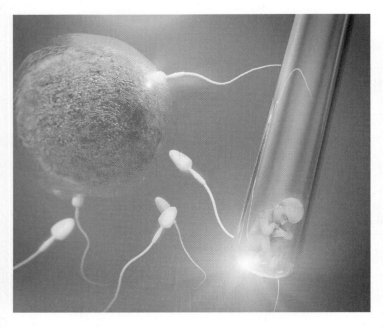

For a city to run smoothly, it must have an infrastructure, buildings, roads, playgrounds, schools, and more. All these structures must be repaired on a regular basis, or if damaged beyond repair, they must be replaced. As a city grows along with its population, it needs the resources and means to expand. The same is true of your body. Cells and tissues are damaged or simply wear out. Damaged or worn-out cells and tissues must be repaired or replaced. Asexual reproduction, or *mitosis*, the process by which cells make exact copies of themselves, is absolutely necessary to maintain a healthy body. Mitosis was discussed in Chapter 4. Ultimately, cellular reproduction is needed for the complicated process by which humans produce new humans: sexual reproduction. Without this ability, the human species would die out, and the journey would end for the human race. Thankfully, all the splendid diversity of the human race is passed on for generations to come—to enjoy this amazing journey called "life."

LEARNING OUTCOMES

At the end of your journey through this chapter, you will be able to:

- Differentiate mitosis from meiosis and the role of each in the human life cycle.
- Locate and describe the functions of the female reproductive organs.
- Discuss female reproductive physiology, including the phases of the menstrual cycle, oogenesis, follicle development, and ovulation.
- Discuss the effects of hormonal control on the female reproductive system.
- Locate and describe the functions of the male reproductive organs.
- Discuss male reproductive physiology, including spermatogenesis.
- Discuss the effects of hormonal control on the male reproductive system.
- Describe pregnancy and the stages of labor and delivery.
- Explain common disorders of the female and male reproductive systems.

Pronunciation Guide

Correct pronunciation is important in any journey so that you and others are completely understood. Here is a "see and say" Pronunciation Guide for the more difficult terms to pronounce in this chapter. Please note that even though there are standard pronunciations, regional variations of the pronunciations can occur.

abruptio placentia (ah BRUP tee oh plah sen shah)
amenorrhea (ah MEN oh REE ah)
bulbourethral gland (BUHL boh yoo REE thral)
clitoris (KLIT oh ris)
corpus luteum (KOR pus LOU tee um)
cryptorchidism (kript OR kid izm)
endometrium (EHN doh MEE tree um)
epididymis (ep ih DID ih mis)
eukaryotic cell (you CARE ee AH tic)
fimbria (FIM bree ah)
follicle-stimulating hormone
   (FALL ih kle STIM you LAY ting)
gamete (GAM eet)
genitalia (jen ih TAIL ee uh)
gonadotropin-releasing hormone
   (GON uh doh TROH pin)
human chorionic gonadotropin
   (KOH ree ON ick GON uh doh TROH pin)
hydrocele (HIGH droh seel)
labia majora (LAY bee ah mah JOR ah)
labia minora (LAY bee ah mih NOR ah)
luteal phase (LOO tee al faze)
luteinizing hormone (LOO tee ah NIZE ing)
meiosis (my OH sis)
menses (MEN seez)

menstruation (MEN stroo AY shun)
mitosis (my TOE sis)
myometrium (MY oh MEE tree um)
oocyte (OH oh site)
oogenesis (OH oh JEN eh sis)
perimetrium (pair ee MEE tree um)
primordial follicles (pry MORE dee all FALL ih kulz)
progesterone (proh JESS ter ohn)
pudendal cleft (pew DEN dall)
seminal vesicles (SEM ih nal VESS ih kulz)
seminiferous tubules (SEM ih NIF er us TOO byoolz)
sertoli cells (sir TOW lee)
spermatids (SPER mah tidz)
spermatocytes (sper MAT oh sites)
spermatogonia (SPER mat oh GO nee uh)
spermatozoa (sper MAT oh ZOE ah)
testis, testes (TESS tis, TESS teez)
testicles (TESS tih kulz)
testosterone (tess TOSS ter ohn)
urethra (yoo REE thrah)
uterus (YOO ter us)
vagina (vah JYE nah)
vas deferens (VAS DEFF er enz)
vulva (VULL vah)
zygote (ZIGH goht)

TISSUE GROWTH AND REPLACEMENT

Although mitosis was discussed in the Chapter 4, we will briefly review that form of cellular reproduction in this chapter. Cellular reproduction is the basis for *all* more complex reproduction, so this is a good starting point.

Mitosis

Cellular reproduction is the process of making a new cell. It is also known as **cell division** because one cell divides into two cells when it reproduces. Remember, cells can only come from other cells. When cells make *identical* copies of themselves *without the involvement* of another cell, the process is called **asexual reproduction**. Most cells can reproduce themselves asexually, whether they are animal cells, plant cells, or bacteria.

The cells that make up the human body are a type of cell known as a **eukaryotic cell**. Eukaryotic cells have a nucleus, cellular organelles, and usually several chromosomes in the nucleus. The genetic material of the cell, DNA, is bundled into "packages" of chromatin, known as *chromosomes*. Because chromosomes carry all the instructions for the cells, all cells must have a complete set after reproduction. These instructions include how the cell is to function within the body and blueprints for reproduction. No matter whether a cell has one chromosome, such as bacteria, or 46 chromosomes, such as humans, all the chromosomes must be copied before the cell can divide. As we saw in Chapter 4, bacteria, because they have only one chromosome, no nucleus, and few organelles, can divide very easily via the process of binary fission.

Eukaryotic cells like yours, on the other hand, must go through a more complicated set of maneuvers to reproduce. Not only do your cells have to duplicate all 46 of their chromosomes, but they also have to make sure that each cell gets all the chromosomes and all the right organelles. The process of sorting the chromosomes so that each new cell gets the right number of copies of all the genetic material is called **mitosis**. Mitosis is the only way that eukaryotic cells can reproduce asexually. For a quick review of mitosis, return to Chapter 4.

Mitosis in the Body

Mitosis, asexual cellular reproduction, serves many purposes in your body. Any time your cells must be replaced, mitosis is the method used to replace them. Many of your tissues, such as bone, epithelium, skin, and blood cells, are replaced on a regular basis. Repair and regeneration of damaged tissue is accomplished by mitosis as well. If you cut your hand, the skin is replaced, first by collagen, but eventually by the original tissue type. Mitosis increases in cells near the injury so that the damaged or destroyed cells can be replaced. A broken bone is replaced in much the same way.

Growth is also accomplished by mitosis. Lengthening of bones as you grow—indeed, most ways that tissue gets bigger—is due to mitosis of cells in the tissues or organs. Without mitosis, your body would not be able to grow or replace old or damaged cells.

SEXUAL REPRODUCTION

Thus far we have discussed cell division for growth and repair, but we must also be able to perpetuate the species. For humans, this requires sexual reproduction.

Reduction Division: Meiosis

Many animals reproduce sexually; that is, they produce, with the aid of another individual, offspring that are not identical to themselves. Sexual reproduction involves the union of a cell from one organism with a cell from another organism of the same species, combining DNA from both cells. In animals, females produce **eggs** and males produce **sperm** for the purpose of reproducing sexually. These special cells are known as **gametes**.

Gametes are produced by a specialized type of cell division known as **meiosis**, or **reduction division**. Meiosis is called reduction division because the daughter cells produced at the end of meiosis have half as many chromosomes as the original mother cell. These daughter cells must have half as many chromosomes because they will fuse with another gamete during sexual reproduction. In humans, the total number of chromosomes in a cell is 46. If the gametes did not lose half of their chromosomes somewhere along the way, then the cell that resulted from sexual reproduction would have twice as many chromosomes (92 chromosomes) than is normal for human cells. It is absolutely necessary to control the number of chromosomes in a cell. Cells with too few or too many chromosomes often die.

LEARNING HINT

Mitosis versus Meiosis

These words sound and look alike and are therefore often confused. Remember, *mei*osis produces ga*me*tes or sexual cells, which contain half of the chromosomes because the sexual union of male and female will contribute the other half. M*i*tosis (*I* reproduce myself) is asexual and produces exact copies of the cell and the full complement of chromosomes because no union is needed.

The fact that you were produced by the fusion of an egg from your mother and a sperm from your father means that your 46 chromosomes can be thought of as being 23 *pairs* of chromosomes. Each pair of chromosomes consists of one from your father and one from your mother. They can be thought of as pairs because they can be matched based on size, shape, and which genes they carry. For example, you get a chromosome 1 from your father and a chromosome 1 from your mother, the same for chromosome 2, 3, 4, and up to 22.

The 23rd "pair" of chromosomes is a set of sex chromosomes. These are called *sex chromosomes* because their identity determines the sex of an individual. XX is female, and XY is male (see **FIGURE 18–1** ■). The female always contributes an X, but the male can contribute either an X or Y chromosome. The male actually determines the sex of the baby by either contributing an X chromosome for a girl or a Y chromosome for a boy.

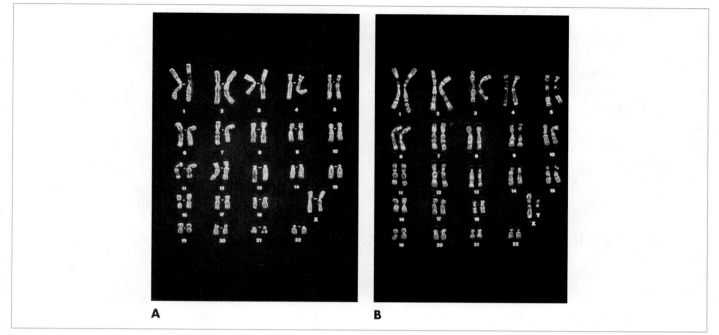

FIGURE 18–1 ■

Human chromosomes. (A) Female. (B) Male.

Clinical Application

DOWN SYNDROME

Down syndrome is a relatively common birth defect that causes short stature, heart defects, increased risk of leukemia, Alzheimer's disease, and intellectual disability. Down syndrome is caused by the presence of an extra chromosome (trisomy-21) in a person's cells. At some time during meiosis, usually in the mother, chromosomes fail to separate, leaving some daughter cells without a chromosome 21 and others with two copies of chromosome 21. If the egg with the extra chromosome is fertilized, the resulting fetus will have three copies of chromosome 21 instead of two.

In general, the possibility of having a baby with Down syndrome increases dramatically in women over 35 years old but can occur at any child-bearing age. Down syndrome is one of very few disorders resulting from abnormal chromosome numbers, probably because most fertilized eggs with abnormal numbers of chromosomes do not develop normally enough to survive (see **FIGURE 18–2** ■).

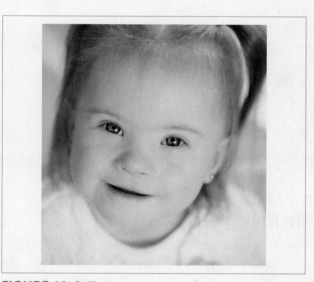

FIGURE 18–2 ■

A child with Down syndrome.

THE HUMAN LIFE CYCLE

Both mitosis and meiosis are absolutely necessary parts of human life. Without them, cells could not be replaced, injuries could not be repaired, and new humans could not be produced. The relationship between mitosis and meiosis and their importance can be easily explained by looking at human life as a cycle (see **FIGURE 18–3** ■). Eggs and sperm, with only half as many chromosomes as other cells, are produced by meiosis in specialized organs known as the **gonads**. The male gonads are called **testes**. The female gonads are the **ovaries**. During sexual reproduction, the gametes (egg and sperm) unite and combine their genetic material. This union and combination of genetic material is called **fertilization**. The fertilized egg is known as a **zygote**. Unlike gametes, which have only 23 chromosomes, the zygote has the typical number of chromosomes for a human cell: 46. The zygote undergoes millions of rounds of mitosis and development within the female to change from an *embryo* to a *fetus* (the infant that is not born yet). The rest of this chapter is devoted to describing sexual reproduction in humans.

TEST YOUR KNOWLEDGE 18–1

Choose the best answer:

1. Cells with half the number of chromosomes used for sexual reproduction are known as
   a. zygotes.
   b. sister cells.
   c. gametes.
   d. half cells.

2. Organs that produce sperm and egg are called
   a. gametes.
   b. gonads.
   c. zygotes.
   d. chromosomes.

3. After _____, the egg is called a _____ and has 46 chromosomes.
   a. reproduction; gamete
   b. meiosis; daughter cell
   c. mitosis; zygote
   d. fertilization; zygote

4. After fertilization, development from embryo to fetus to baby to adult is accomplished by
   a. meiosis.
   b. binary fission.
   c. mitosis.
   d. cellular respiration.

5. The union of egg and sperm is called
   a. zygote.
   b. fertilization.
   c. reproduction.
   d. mitosis.

THE HUMAN REPRODUCTIVE SYSTEM

Reproductive organs are called **genitalia**. The general term *primary genitalia* refers to the gonads, which produce the gametes. The *accessory genitalia* are all the other structures that aid in the reproductive process. In this section, we will first discuss female anatomy and physiology and then male anatomy and physiology.

Female Anatomy

In females, the gonads are the ovaries. The other genitalia are the uterine tubes (also known as oviducts or fallopian tubes), the uterus, the vagina, and the external genitalia, called the vulva.

The Ovary

The primary genitalia, or **ovaries**, are oval-shaped paired structures, about 3 centimeters long, in the peritoneal cavity. There is one ovary on each side of the uterus. Several ligaments suspend or anchor each ovary. The **mesovarium** suspends the ovary, the *suspensory ligament* attaches the ovary to lateral pelvic wall, and the *ovarian ligament* anchors the ovary to the uterine wall. Blood vessels, the ovarian artery, and the ovarian branch of the uterine artery travel through the mesovarium and suspensory ligament and supply the ovary with oxygenated blood. Please see **FIGURE 18–4** ■ for a diagram of internal reproductive anatomy. The ovary is covered by a fibrous capsule called the **tunica albuginea** made of cuboidal epithelium.

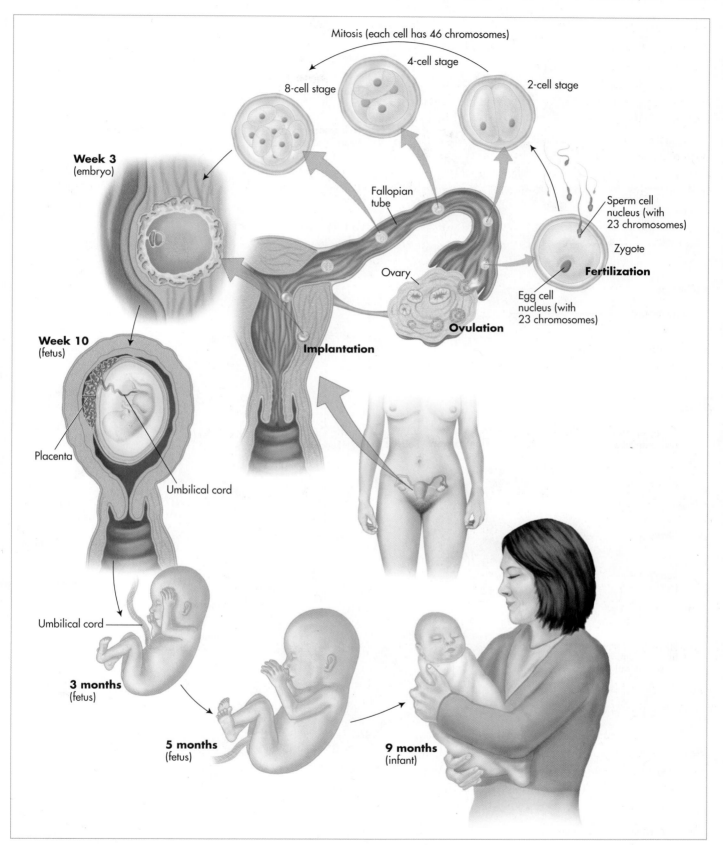

FIGURE 18–3 ■

The early stages of the human life cycle.

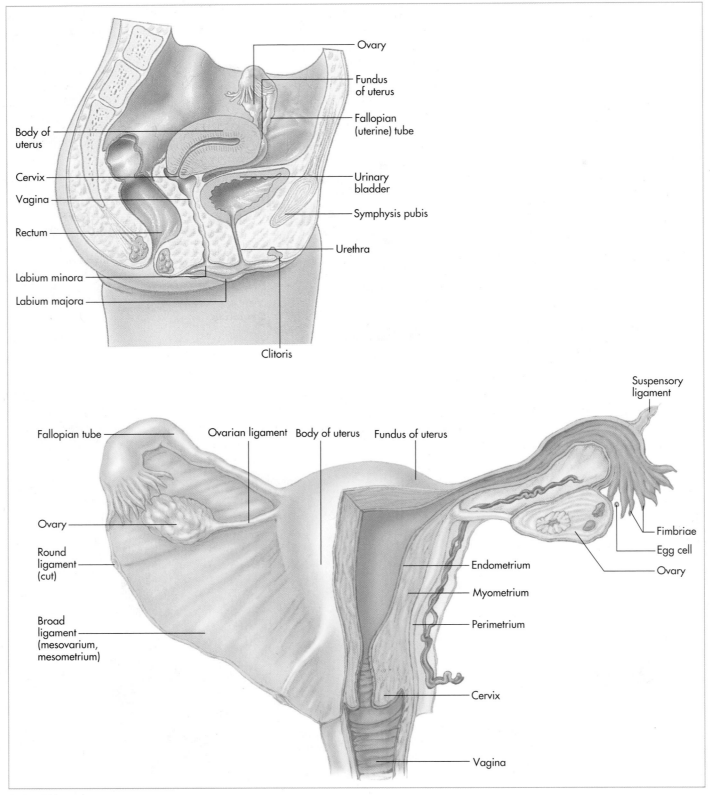

FIGURE 18–4 ■

Internal female reproductive organs.

The interior of the ovary is divided into the cortex, which contains the eggs, and the medulla, which contains blood vessels, nerves, and lymphatic tissue surrounded by loose connective tissue. The anatomy of the cortex is relatively complicated and will be described during our discussion of physiology.

The Uterine Tubes

The **uterine tubes**, also known as **oviducts** or **fallopian tubes**, are the passageways for the egg to get to the uterus. The uterine tubes begin as a large funnel, the **infundibulum**, surrounded by ciliated projections, the **fimbria**. The infundibulum leads to a widened area, the **ampulla**, followed by a longer, narrower portion known as the **isthmus**. The uterine tubes are connected to the superior portion of the uterus. The tube is constructed of sheets of smooth muscle lined with highly folded, ciliated, simple columnar epithelium. The outside of the tube is covered by the visceral peritoneum and suspended by a mesentery known as the **mesosalpinx**.

The Uterus

The thick-walled and pear-shaped **uterus** is in the pelvic cavity, posterior and superior to the urinary bladder and anterior to the rectum. The major portion of the uterus is called the *body*. The rounded superior portion between the uterine tubes is the *fundus*, and the narrow inferior part is the *isthmus*. The **cervix** is a valvelike portion of the uterus that protrudes into the vagina, where the cervical canal connects with the vagina. Like the ovaries, the uterus is suspended and anchored by a series of ligaments. The **mesometrium** attaches the uterus to the lateral pelvic walls. (The combination of the mesometrium and mesovarium is called the *broad ligament*.) The lateral cervical ligaments attach the cervix and vagina to the lateral pelvic walls. The uterus is anchored to the anterior wall of the pelvic cavity by the round ligaments.

Like most of the hollow organs or tubes we have visited, the walls of the uterus consist of three layers. The **perimetrium**, the outermost layer, is also the *visceral peritoneum*. (Just like the outermost layer of the heart is the visceral pericardium.) The middle layer, **myometrium**, consists of smooth muscle, and the **endometrium**, or inner lining, is a mucosa layer of columnar epithelium and secretory cells. The mucosa has two divisions. The *basal layer* is responsible for regenerating the uterine lining each month. The *functional layer* sheds about every 28 days when a woman has her period.

The endometrium is highly vascularized, which is no big surprise to any woman of child-bearing age. Blood is supplied by the uterine arteries that branch from the internal iliac arteries on each side. The uterine arteries split into arcuate arteries, which supply the myometrium, and radial arteries, which supply blood to the endometrium. As you might expect, because the endometrium has two separate divisions, there are two different types of radial arteries. Straight radial arteries supply the basal layer. Spiral radial arteries supply the functional layer. The spiral arteries actually degenerate and regenerate every month, as part of the menstrual cycle, and undergo spasms that contribute to the shedding of the endometrium each month. Blood returns to circulation via a network of venous sinuses. For more on control of the menstrual cycle, see the section titled "Hormonal Control of Female Reproduction," later in this chapter.

The Vagina

The **vagina** is a smooth muscular tube with a mucous membrane lining, approximately 10 centimeters long, that runs from the uterus to the outside of the body. The vagina has

---

Clinical Application

ENDOMETRIOSIS

Each month, women of child-bearing age shed and replace the endometrium, the lining of the uterus. In many women, this endometrial tissue escapes from the uterus and implants in unexpected locations within the abdominal and pelvic cavities. There, the tissue responds to the woman's hormonal cycles, continuing to build up and degenerate each month. Unfortunately, the continued proliferation, degeneration, and bleeding of endometrial tissue within the abdominal and pelvic cavities can cause scarring and damage to the organs. Many women who have endometriosis have no noticeable symptoms, whereas other women experience severe abdominal and back pain around the time of their periods. Untreated, endometriosis can cause adhesions on the intestines and urinary bladder, which can be extremely painful and must be removed surgically. Endometriosis is the most common cause of infertility because it blocks the uterine tubes and therefore blocks the journey of the egg, and scars the ovaries and uterus.

several purposes, including receiving the penis during inter-course, allowing for the passage of menstrual fluid out of the uterus, and functioning as the birth canal, allowing the movement of the baby out of the uterus during childbirth. The external opening of the vagina may be covered by a perforated membrane called the **hymen**. A torn hymen was once thought to "prove" that a woman had had intercourse. However, many hymens are highly perforated and easily ruptured by day-to-day activities such as riding a bicycle or jogging. An intact hymen is no longer considered a litmus test for virginity; however, some cultures still hold this erroneous belief to be true.

The External Genitalia

The external genitalia (FIGURE 18–5 ■), collectively known as the **vulva**, although not perhaps as obvious as the male external genitalia, are a complex and important part of reproduction. The **vulva** is surrounded on each side by two prominences called the **labia majora**. The labia majora are rounded fat deposits that meet and protect the rest of the external genitalia. The labia majora meet anteriorly to form the **mons pubis**. Both the mons pubis and the labia majora are covered by pubic hair. The **perineum** is the area between the vagina and the anus.

Between the two halves of the labia majora is an opening known as the **pudendal cleft**. Within the pudendal cleft lies the **vestibule**, a space into which the urethra (anterior) and vagina (posterior) empty. Unlike the male reproductive system, the female reproductive system is completely separate from the urinary system. The lateral border of the vestibule is formed by the thin **labia minora**, which meet anteriorly to form the **prepuce**. Several glands, such as Bartholin's gland, surround the vestibule, helping to keep it moist.

Just posterior to the prepuce, and anterior to the vestibule, is the **clitoris**. It is a small erectile structure, 2 centimeters in diameter. Like the penis, the clitoris has a shaft, or body, and a glans (tip), and it becomes engorged with blood during sexual arousal. However, the clitoris increases in diameter, not in length.

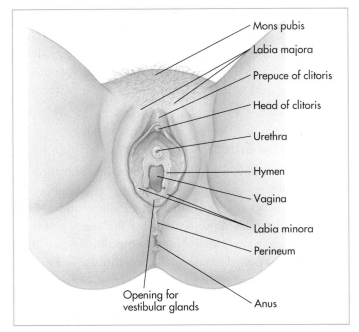

FIGURE 18–5 ■
The external female genitalia (vulva).

Mammary Glands

The **mammary glands** are another set of external accessory sexual organs in the female, far removed from the pubic area. The mammary glands are milk-production glands housed in the breasts (see FIGURE 18–6 ■). In young children, mammary tissue is virtually identical in boys and girls. At puberty, estrogen and progesterone stimulate breast development in girls. In adult females, the breasts consist of 15 to 20 lobes, which are glandular, and large amounts of adipose tissue. Each lobe is divided into smaller lobules, which house milk-secreting sacs called *alveoli*, when a woman is **lactating** (producing milk). Milk, made in the alveoli, travels through a series of ducts and sinuses, eventually reaching the *nipple*. The **areola** is the darkened area that surrounds the nipple. Milk production is controlled by the hormone prolactin.

TEST YOUR KNOWLEDGE 18–2

Choose the best answer:

1. The _____ is also known as the birth canal.
   a. ovary
   b. uterus
   c. uterine tubes
   d. vagina

2. The inner lining of the uterus that is shed each month is the
   a. perimetrium.
   b. endometrium.
   c. myometrium.
   d. all of the above

3. This part of the female reproductive system is erectile.
   a. ovary
   b. labia majora
   c. clitoris
   d. penis

4. The female external genitalia are collectively known as the
   a. uvula.
   b. vulva.
   c. vomer.
   d. valvular.

5. The sacs that secrete milk in lactating women are called
   a. mammary glands.
   b. alveoli.
   c. lobules.
   d. breasts.

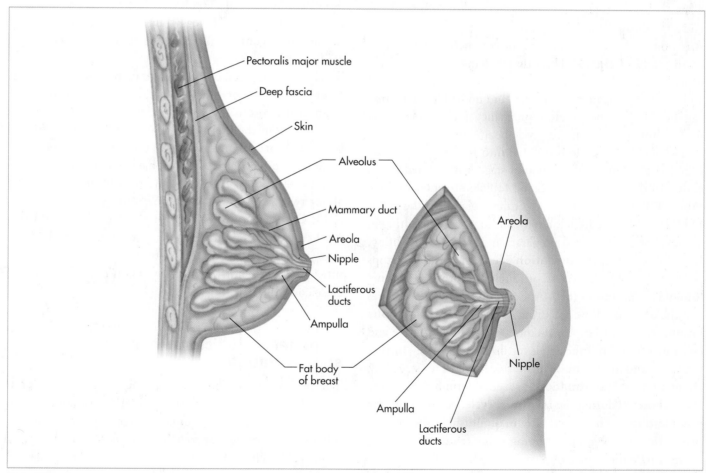

FIGURE 18–6 ■
The mammary glands.

REPRODUCTIVE PHYSIOLOGY: FEMALE

Female reproductive physiology is closely tied to a regulated cycle. This cycle is normally regulated by hormonal control.

The Menstrual Cycle

Female reproduction is organized around an approximately 28-day cycle involving both the ovaries and the uterus, collectively known as the *menstrual cycle*. This cycle can range from 25 to 35 days in duration and involves the ovaries, uterus, pituitary gland, and hypothalamus. The **ovarian cycle** involves the monthly maturation and release of eggs from the ovary. The **uterine cycle** consists of the monthly buildup, degeneration, and shedding of the uterine lining. These cycles begin during a woman's teen years at the beginning of puberty, with **menarche**, or the first menstrual cycle. These cycles normally end during her 40s or 50s, with the end of **menopause**. Menopause is the cessation of menstruation as characterized by symptoms such as hot flashes, dizziness, headaches, and emotional changes. The ultimate goal of these cycles is to release an egg that might be fertilized and to prepare the uterus to receive and nourish the fertilized egg should pregnancy result. If pregnancy does not occur, the uterine lining sheds, and the cycle begins again.

The menstrual cycle is divided into four stages, usually over 28 days. During the **follicular** stage, which usually lasts about 10 days, a hormone called **follicle-stimulating hormone (FSH)** is released by the pituitary gland. At the ovary, FSH stimulates the follicle and ovum to mature, resulting in a release of estrogen and preparation of the uterine lining. In the next stage, the **ovulation** stage, the pituitary stops producing FSH and starts producing another hormone, **luteinizing hormone (LH)**. At day 14, the follicle ruptures and the ovum is released. During the third stage, the **corpus luteum** stage, the corpus luteum secretes progesterone and continues to do so if the egg is fertilized, preventing further ovulation and maintaining the uterine lining. This stage lasts about 14 days. **Menstruation**, the actual term for the bleeding that occurs during the menstrual cycle, occurs if the egg is not fertilized. The corpus luteum diminishes progesterone production and the uterine lining is broken down and discharged over the course of 3 to 6 days. You will learn more about these stages and the structures and hormones involved as you read this chapter.

The menstrual cycle, occurring approximately every 28 days in sexually mature women who are not pregnant, begins with the first day of **menses**. Menses is the time period when the uterine lining is shed. You are probably more familiar with the term *menstruation*. Menstruation is the actual shedding of the endometrium, whereas menses is the time during which a woman is menstruating. In more common terms, menses is the time during which a woman is having her "period," and menstruation is the "period" itself. Menses typically lasts 4 to 5 days but can be longer or shorter in different women and can even vary month to month in the same woman.

After menses is over, the endometrium begins to proliferate, or build up, readying itself for the egg that is about to be released from the ovary, during ovulation. From day 1 to day 14, the ovary is also busy. In the ovary, an egg cell, or **oocyte**, is undergoing a number of developmental changes getting ready for ovulation on day 14 (can vary from day 11 to 21). The time between the end of menses and ovulation is known as the **follicular** or **proliferative phase** because the endometrium is proliferating and the follicles are maturing in the ovary. **Follicle** is the term used to refer to an egg and associated helper cells. **Ovulation** is the release of a mature egg from the ovary. The egg travels from the ovary to the uterus, by way of the Fallopian tube, which has been getting ready to receive the egg.

The time between ovulation and menses is known as the **luteal phase**, or **secretory phase**, because of the development of the corpus luteum in the ovary and the beginning of secretion in the uterus. If the oocyte has been fertilized by a sperm, it will implant in the thickened endometrium. If the egg does not implant within a few days, the endometrium will begin to degenerate and menstruation will occur about two weeks after ovulation. Sounds simple enough, right? The cycle is deceptively simple when described without details or information about control of the cycle. Now that you understand the cycle itself, let's get down to the nitty-gritty. Just how does an egg mature, and how is the cycle controlled?

Oogenesis, Follicle Development, and Ovulation

The process by which eggs are produced is called **oogenesis**. Oogenesis begins with the birth of *oogonia*, or egg stem cells, in the ovary. The oogonia undergo mitosis, producing millions of **primary oocytes**. This happens very early in a woman's life. There are millions of primary oocytes produced in a fetus. That's right: Women have all the eggs they will ever have five months before they are born.

Primary oocytes, because they are born via mitosis, still have all 46 chromosomes. To become gametes, they must undergo meiosis to cut their chromosome number to 23. Remember, gametes must have only 23 chromosomes for fertilization (successful combining of sperm and egg) to produce a cell with the normal number of 46 chromosomes. So, primary oocytes begin meiosis. However, they do not fully complete this process. The primary oocytes stay in a "suspended animation" until puberty when they finish developing. That's at least a 10-year time period!

These primary oocytes eventually are surrounded by helper cells, called **granulosa cells**. Once surrounded by granulosa cells, the primary oocyte and surrounding cells are known as **primordial follicles**. These primordial follicles stay dormant until puberty. Hormonal signals during puberty cause some primordial follicles to enlarge and increase the number of granulosa cells. These enlarged cells are then called *primary follicles* and form thousands of microscopic sacs within the ovary (see **FIGURE 18–7** ■).

Once a girl reaches puberty, each month one primary follicle will become a *secondary follicle*. The secondary follicle will not complete its development unless it is ovulated and fertilized. Just before ovulation, the secondary follicle matures, fills with fluid, and moves toward the surface of the ovary, where it becomes a visible lump. The mature follicle in its sac is also called a **graafian follicle**. The fimbria of the uterine tubes brush the surface of the ovary, causing the follicle to rupture. When the follicle ruptures, the egg is released into the peritoneal cavity. The fimbria then pulls the egg toward the funnel, drawing it into the uterine tube.

As the egg travels down the uterine tube (also called the **oviduct** or **fallopian tube**), it either will or will not be fertilized. The egg is viable for 12 to 24 hours after ovulation and sperm, once they reach the uterus, are viable for 24 to 72 hours. If sperm are present in the uterine tube and all the conditions are right, the sperm will penetrate the egg, fertilizing it and triggering the rest of the egg development. The successfully fertilized egg has 46 chromosomes and is now called a **zygote**. The zygote starts out as a single cell, but the cell divides, and subsequent cell divisions multiply the number of cells in the zygote as it travels down the fallopian tube to implant in the uterus. When the zygote enters the uterus, the newly proliferated endometrium is ready for it. If the zygote successfully implants in the uterus, pregnancy will result, and the woman will not menstruate. The ruptured follicle left behind in the ovary during ovulation will become the **corpus luteum** (remember the *luteal* phase?) and secrete hormones to help maintain the thickened endometrium, which will now serve to nourish the growing fetus.

If there are no sperm in the uterine tube, conditions are not right, or something goes wrong after fertilization, the zygote will not implant in the uterus. If there is no implantation within a few days, the uterine lining will begin to degenerate, and the woman will have her period. The corpus luteum will become a corpus albicans and eventually disappear (see **FIGURE 18–8** ■).

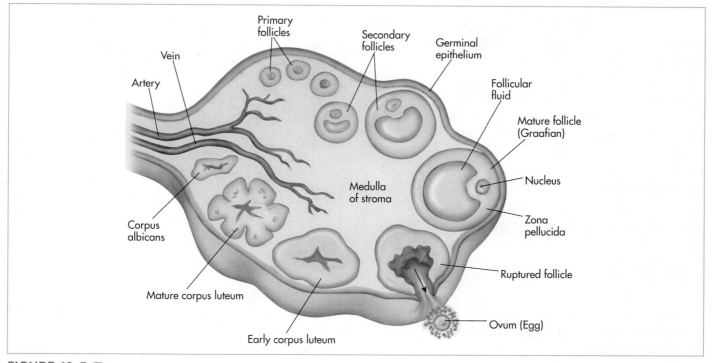

FIGURE 18–7 ■

Maturation of a follicle and release of egg.

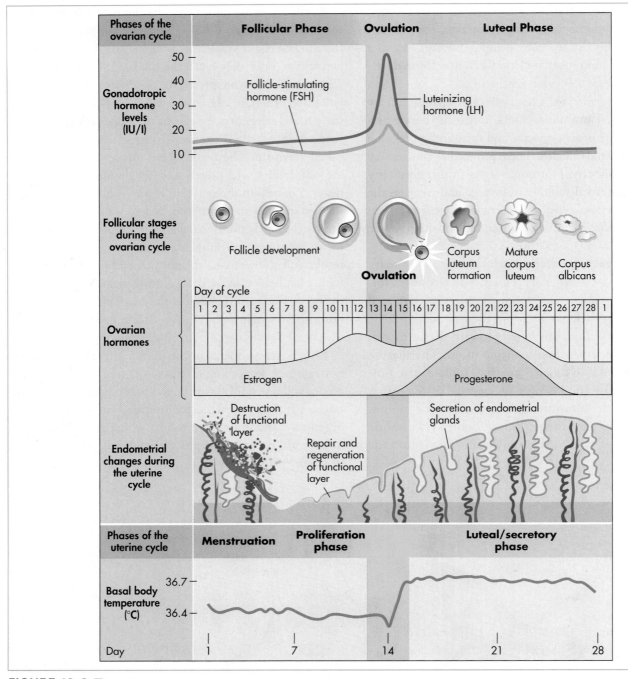

FIGURE 18–8 ■

The menstrual cycle.

TEST YOUR KNOWLEDGE 18–3

Choose the best answer:

1. The time from the end of menses to ovulation is what phase?
   a. luteal phase
   b. follicular phase
   c. mitotic phase
   d. ovarian phase

2. This structure, formed after ovulation, secretes a hormone that helps maintain the endometrium.
   a. secondary follicle
   b. primary oocyte
   c. corpus luteum
   d. tunica albuginea

3. The act of the egg being expelled from the ovary is called
   a. oogenesis.
   b. ovulation.
   c. puberty.
   d. pregnancy.

4. If _____ does not occur, the endometrium will degenerate, and a woman will menstruate.
   a. sex
   b. ovulation
   c. fertilization
   d. oogenesis

5. A woman's eggs do not complete meiosis until
   a. she is born.
   b. they are fertilized.
   c. they implant in the endometrium.
   d. she reaches puberty.

Hormonal Control of Female Reproduction

It seems obvious that something must control the complex cyclic changes in the female reproductive system. The control system that keeps the uterus and ovaries in synch is the endocrine system, specifically hypothalamic, pituitary, and ovarian hormones.

Remember that hormones are chemical signals released by one organ into the bloodstream to control another organ or tissue some distance away. Hormone levels are generally controlled by negative feedback. As hormone levels rise, the organ releasing the hormone decreases the amount of hormone released. Hormones are often released as part of a hierarchy, with the hypothalamus releasing a hormone that controls the pituitary, which then releases a hormone that controls another organ.

The hormones controlling female reproduction are no exception. The menstrual cycle is controlled by a combination of four hormones: **estrogen** and **progesterone** from the ovaries, and **luteinizing hormone (LH)** and **follicle-stimulating hormone (FSH)** from the pituitary gland. At the beginning of puberty, estrogen and progesterone secretion from the ovaries increases greatly, increasing the secretion of LH and FSH.

The release of **gonadotropin-releasing hormone (GnRH)** from the hypothalamus causes an increase in the secretion of LH and FSH from the pituitary. Follicle-stimulating hormone initiates the development of primary follicles each month, and luteinizing hormone triggers ovulation. During this part of the cycle (the follicular or proliferative phase), estrogen levels continue to rise as more and more is secreted by the developing follicle. Estrogen exerts a positive influence on the hypothalamus, increasing secretion of GnRH and thus increasing LH and FSH secretion. This positive feedback loop increases the levels of LH and FSH, stimulating follicle development and triggering ovulation. Rising estrogen levels also stimulate proliferation of the uterine lining (endometrium).

Once ovulation occurs, the feedback loop actually reverses itself. The leftover ruptured follicle, now the corpus luteum, begins to secrete progesterone and secretes a little estrogen. Under the influence of progesterone, estrogen exerts negative feedback on the hypothalamus and pituitary, decreasing GnRH, LH, and FSH secretion. Progesterone also exerts negative feedback on the hypothalamus and pituitary. Thus, during the luteal, or secretory, phase, LH, FSH, and estrogen levels drop while progesterone levels rise. These hormonal changes prevent another egg from maturing.

For about 10 days after ovulation, progesterone levels remain high as the corpus luteum continues to secrete the hormone. Progesterone's effect on the uterus is to *maintain* the buildup of the endometrium and to decrease uterine contractions. If no pregnancy results, then the corpus luteum will degenerate and stop producing progesterone. Decreased progesterone causes degeneration of the endometrium, followed by menstruation. Decreased progesterone also releases the hypothalamus and pituitary from inhibition. The FSH and LH levels rise, and the cycle begins again (please reexamine Figure 18–8).

If pregnancy does result, the implanted fertilized egg secretes a hormone called **human chorionic gonadotropin (HCG)**. This hormone stimulates the corpus luteum, which keeps secreting progesterone and a little estrogen to maintain the uterine lining. At about three months' gestation (pregnancy), the placenta begins to secrete its own progesterone and estrogen, thereby becoming an endocrine organ. For a list of hormones and functions related to pregnancy, please see **TABLE 18–1** ∎.

TABLE 18–1 HORMONES CONTROLLING PREGNANCY

HORMONE	WHERE SECRETED	CAUSES
Human chorionic gonadotropin	Implanted fertilized egg	Maintains the function of corpus luteum; this is what gives a positive pregnancy test
Estrogen and progesterone	Corpus luteum for first two months of pregnancy; then by the placenta	Both stimulate development of uterine lining and mammary glands; progesterone prohibits uterine contractions during pregnancy; estrogen relaxes the pelvic joints; once labor begins, estrogen negates the effects of progesterone on uterine contractions and makes the myometrium sensitive to oxytocin
Prolactin	Anterior pituitary gland	Stimulates milk production by breasts
Oxytocin	Posterior pituitary gland	Uterine contractions to begin labor; stimulates the release of milk from the breasts (see **FIGURE 18–9** ■)

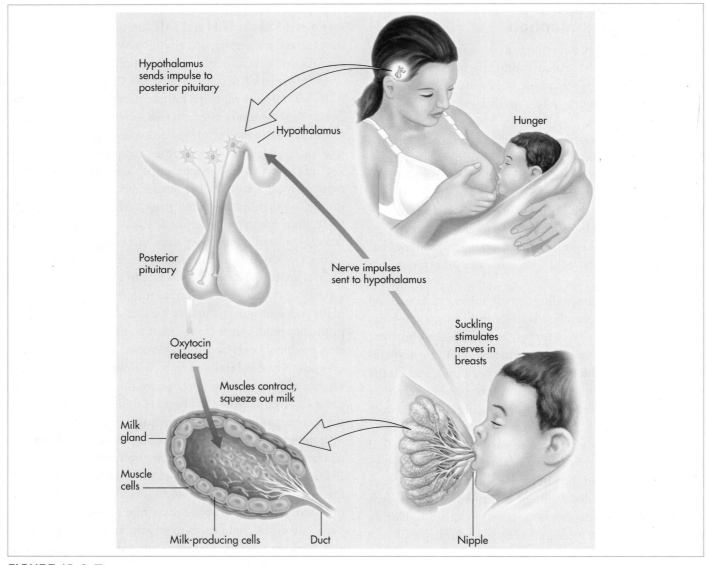

FIGURE 18–9 ■

Oxytocin and breast-feeding.

TEST YOUR KNOWLEDGE 18–4

Choose the best answer:

1. At puberty, the ovaries begin to secrete
   a. FSH.
   b. LH.
   c. estrogen.
   d. all of the above

2. These hormones stimulate follicle maturation and ovulation:
   a. estrogen and progesterone.
   b. estrogen and GnRH.
   c. LH and FSH.
   d. FSH and progesterone.

3. Before ovulation, estrogen _____ the secretion of FSH and LH.
   a. decreases
   b. increases
   c. stops
   d. maintains the same level of

4. The role of progesterone is to
   a. promote ovulation.
   b. keep the endometrium from shedding.
   c. enhance fertilization.
   d. increase FSH and LH levels.

5. The fertilized egg secretes this hormone, which helps maintain the endometrium.
   a. prolactin
   b. oxytocin
   c. FSH
   d. HCG

Male Anatomy

Like the female reproductive system, the male reproductive system has a pair of gonads. In the male, these gonads are called the *testes*. The testes produce the male gamete or sperm that must travel along its journey to find the egg. Unlike the female, the male gonads are external. In addition, the male has many accessory genitalia—the penis, which is an external sperm-delivery organ; several sperm ducts; the epididymis; the vas deferens; and the urethra. The urethra performs dual roles, as a channel for both excreting urine and expelling semen. Males also have several accessory glands: the prostate gland, the seminal vesicles, and the bulbourethral glands. Please see **FIGURE 18–10** ■ for the anatomy of the male reproductive system.

The Testes (Testicles)

The gonads, the **testes** (or **testicles**), are paired glands suspended in a sac called the **scrotum**. The testicles form in the abdomen during the last three months of embryonic development and migrate into the scrotum. The testicles are external genitalia, one hanging on either side of the penis. The failure of the testes to descend into the scrotal sac is termed **cryptorchidism** and may require surgical intervention. If the testes remain undescended, the male may become sterile because of the body's heat destroying the sperm. Viable sperm cannot be made at normal human body temperature.

Each small, walnut-shaped testis is surrounded by a serous membrane, called the **tunica vaginalis**, which originates from the peritoneum. The inside of the testes are divided into 250 to 300 wedges called *lobules*, each of which contain one to four **seminiferous tubules**. The seminiferous tubules, which are made of epithelium and areolar tissue, contain sperm stem cells and sperm helper cells (**sertoli cells**, or nurse cells).

The Penis

The other part of the external genitalia in males is the penis. The **penis**, from the Latin word for "tail," is a sperm-delivery organ that transfers sperm to outside of the body. The attached portion of the penis is called the *root*, whereas the freely moving portion is the *shaft* or *body*. The tip of the penis, the **glans penis**, is covered by a loose section of skin called the *foreskin*, unless a man has been circumcised. Internally, the penis contains the **urethra**, which is a transport passage for both sperm and urine. (But not at the same time!) In addition, the penis has three erectile bodies, all of which are tubes with a spongelike network of blood sinuses.

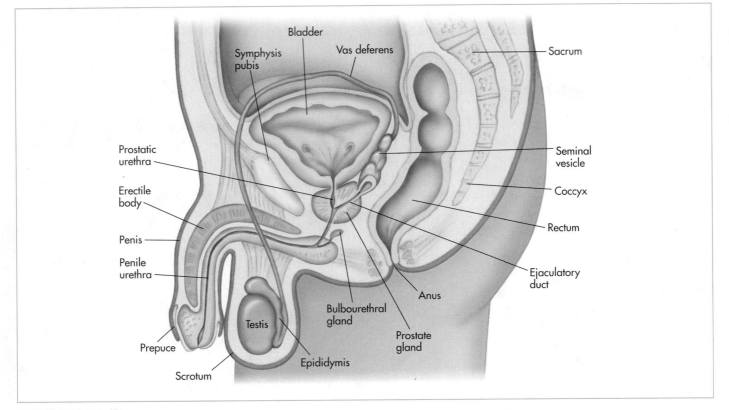

FIGURE 18–10 ■

Male reproductive anatomy.

Boxers or Briefs?

Normal human body temperature is too warm for healthy sperm development. The testes are on the outside of the body because sperm development is extremely temperature sensitive, and sperm could not develop normally inside the pelvic cavity. Indeed, there is some speculation that very tight clothing might contribute to male infertility by holding the gonads too close to the body and raising their temperature. In addition, there is a testes–blood barrier to prevent the immune system from destroying sperm, which the white blood cells would recognize as invaders.

The Epididymis

There are several ducts in the male reproductive system. The **epididymus** is a comma-shaped duct on the posterior and lateral part of the testes. It looks something like a stocking cap for each testis. It contains a highly coiled tube that connects the testes to the vas deferens. If unraveled, the epididymis would be 6 meters long. It is made of pseudostratified ciliated epithelium and smooth muscle. Sperm mature here.

The Vas Deferens

The **vas deferens** is a tube approximately 30 centimeters long that transports sperm. It is lined with ciliated pseudostratified epithelium, like the epididymis, but it has a thick smooth muscle layer and is surrounded by a connective tissue layer called the *adventitia*. The vas deferens runs from the scrotum to the penis via a relatively complicated pathway: from the anterior part of the scrotum as a pair of tubes, one on each side, through the abdominal wall (via the inguinal canal) and into the pelvic cavity, and along the posterior bladder wall. Posterior to the bladder, the vas deferens joins the seminal vesicle to form the **ejaculatory duct**. The ejaculatory duct then passes through the prostate gland and empties into the urethra. Remember, the urethra carries both sperm and urine in males. Between the scrotum and the inguinal canal, the vas deferens runs through a tube, with blood vessels and nerves, collectively called the *spermatic cord*.

Accessory Glands

There are three accessory glands in the male reproductive system. The **seminal vesicles** are highly coiled glands posterior to the bladder, made of pseudostratified epithelium, smooth muscle, and connective tissue. The **prostate** gland is a chestnut-sized gland surrounding the urethra just inferior to the bladder. It is a dense mass of connective tissue and smooth muscle with embedded glands. The **bulbourethral glands** are pea-sized glands inferior to the prostate.

TEST YOUR KNOWLEDGE 18–5

Choose the best answer:

1. The _____ are the gonads, where sperm are made.
   a. vas deferens
   b. testes
   c. scrotum
   d. penis

2. After passing the seminal vesicles, the vas deferens becomes the
   a. prostate gland.
   b. urethra.
   c. penis.
   d. none of the above

3. Sperm mature in the
   a. epididymis.
   b. testes.
   c. scrotum.
   d. penis.

4. Enlargement of the prostate gland can cause difficult urination if it becomes enlarged. Why?
   a. It presses on the bladder.
   b. It squeezes the urethra.
   c. It blocks the seminal vesicles.
   d. It causes a hernia.

REPRODUCTIVE PHYSIOLOGY: MALE

Unlike female reproduction, male reproductive physiology is not organized around a tightly controlled monthly cycle. Let's explore the physiological processes of the male reproductive system.

Spermatogenesis

Sperm production, in the testes, is a continuous process beginning when a boy reaches puberty and usually continuing until death. As such, the control of **spermatogenesis**, sperm production, is much less complicated than the control of oogenesis. Spermatogenesis occurs in the seminiferous tubules.

The **spermatogonia**, sperm stem cells, undergo mitosis to form primary **spermatocytes**. Unlike primary oocytes, the *primary spermatocytes* do not wait to go through meiosis. Primary spermatocytes form two *secondary spermatocytes*. Secondary spermatocytes complete meiosis to form **spermatids**, and spermatids go through a period of development to form immature **spermatozoa (sperm)**. All of this takes place in the testes inside the seminiferous tubules. The distribution of the different stages of sperm development is predictable. Spermatogonia line up against the walls of the tubules, and mature sperm cluster near the lumen of the tubules (see **FIGURE 18–11** ■). Sperm then travel from the seminiferous tubules to the epididymis, where the sperm spend about two weeks maturing and gaining the ability to swim.

Hormonal Control of Male Reproduction

Testosterone is the most important male sex hormone. Before birth, human chorionic gonadotropin (HCG) secreted by the placenta causes the embryonic (still developing) testes to secrete testosterone, masculinizing the fetus. Fetuses not exposed to testosterone or insensitive to testosterone anatomically look female. After birth, there is little testosterone secreted until puberty. At puberty, two hormonal changes occur that signal the beginning of sexual maturity. First, testosterone secretion by the testes increases dramatically.

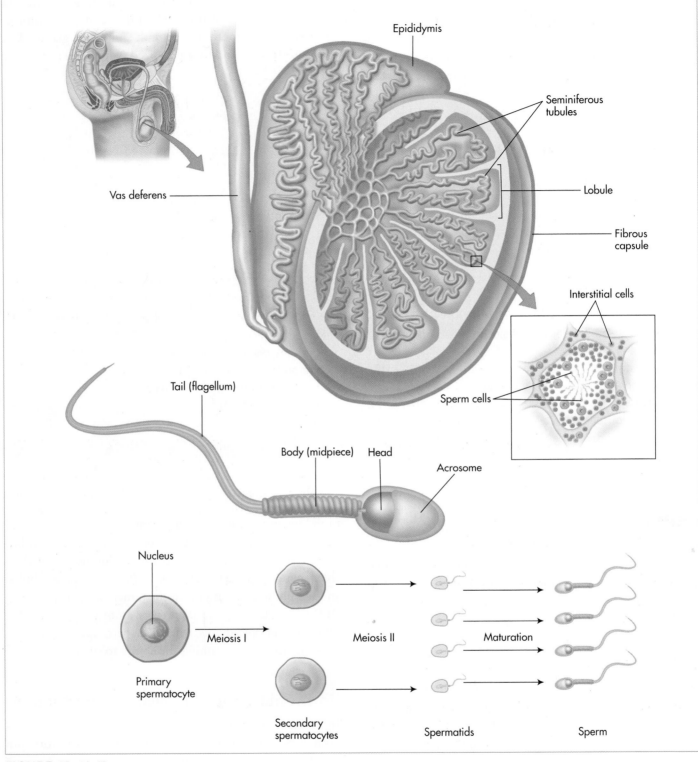

FIGURE 18–11 ▪

Spermatogenesis.

ANDROGEN INSENSITIVITY SYNDROME

Testosterone secretion in utero is important for masculinizing a male fetus. Males who are not sensitive to testosterone will not respond to the masculinizing effects and will not develop normal male reproductive systems. Androgen insensitivity is a genetic disorder that can result in a broad range of malfunctions of the male reproductive system, from complete lack of external or internal male genitalia (testicular feminization—individuals have the anatomical appearance of a female but they are genetically male) to patients with ambiguous genitalia to patients who have typical male genitalia but are sterile.

Second, there is a change in the relationship between testosterone and GnRH, LH, and FSH. (Yes, the same hormones that control female reproduction control male reproduction.) Before puberty, the small amount of testosterone that is secreted by the testes inhibits GnRH secretion. After puberty, testosterone does not inhibit GnRH secretion. So after puberty, GnRH, and therefore FSH and LH, secretion increases. In addition, FSH and LH also enhance testosterone secretion in a major positive feedback loop, but only after the onset of puberty. Testosterone secretion at puberty is also responsible for the obvious physical changes of the male secondary sexual characteristics, including body, facial, and pubic hair growth; deepening of the voice; and increased muscle and bone mass.

Luteinizing hormone and follicle-stimulating hormone have the same functions in males as they do females. They stimulate gamete development. They are controlled the same way in males as in females. Gonadotropin-releasing hormone is released from the hypothalamus, which stimulates LH and FSH secretion from the pituitary.

Erection and Ejaculation

When a man is sexually aroused, the erectile bodies in the penis (remember the spongelike tissue with blood spaces?) become engorged with blood, stiffening and expanding the penis. The change in shape of the penis is called an **erection**.

For sperm to leave the male reproductive system, ejaculation must occur. **Ejaculation** is the expulsion of **semen** (sperm and assorted chemicals) from the urethra. Smooth muscle contracts throughout the ducts and glands of the male reproductive system and propels the sperm from the epididymis into the vas deferens, which then carries the sperm into the pelvic cavity. As the sperm passes the seminal vesicles, sugar and chemicals are added to the sperm. The sperm and chemicals then enter the ejaculatory duct. As the ejaculatory duct passes through the prostate gland, prostatic fluid is added, liquefying the semen and protecting sperm from the acid environment of the vagina by the secretion of an alkaline substance. The semen then passes by the bulbourethral glands, which add mucus to the semen. The semen then enters the urethra and is carried outside the body.

If a man is engaged in sexual intercourse with a woman and ejaculates, the sperm enter the vagina and make their way to the uterus and into the uterine tubes. The female reproductive system is not particularly hospitable to sperm, and many sperm do not survive the journey to the uterine tubes. If there is an egg waiting to be fertilized in the uterine tubes, sperm will find the egg and attempt to penetrate it and fertilize it. The egg is not a passive participant in fertilization, but may actually engulf the sperm and even choose which sperm to allow inside. One sperm and only one sperm will fertilize the egg. If the egg is fertilized, and all other conditions are met, a pregnancy will result.

Amazing Facts

Hormones

Did you know that females have some natural testosterone and males have natural estrogen? It's true. The balance between the hormones—not the presence or absence of the hormones—is what is important.

TEST YOUR KNOWLEDGE 18–6

Choose the best answer:

1. The stiffening and expanding of the penis is known as
   a. ejaculation.
   b. erection.
   c. emulsification.
   d. erectile dysfunction.

2. The combination of sperm, sugars, chemicals, and mucus is
   a. semen.
   b. urine.
   c. spermatozoa.
   d. all of the above

3. Male secondary sexual characteristics, masculinization of the body, and enhancement of FSH and LH levels are caused by
   a. LH.
   b. FSH.
   c. estrogen.
   d. testosterone.

4. How does the relationship between GnRH, LH, FSH, and testosterone change at the onset of puberty?
   a. No hormones are secreted after puberty.
   b. The feedback changes from negative to positive.
   c. There is no relationship between the hormones before puberty.
   d. The body does not respond to testosterone before puberty.

PREGNANCY

Pregnancy occurs when an egg is fertilized by the sperm and implants in the female reproductive system. The period of time during which the developing baby grows within the uterus is called the **gestation period**, which is approximately 40 weeks. A baby born before 37 weeks gestation is termed a *premature infant*.

From the time the egg is fertilized by a sperm and implants in the uterine wall until the eighth week, the developing infant is referred to as an *embryo*. During the embryonic period, the organs and systems are fundamentally formed. Beyond the eight-week period until the birth, the developing infant is called a *fetus*. Between the fourth and sixth months of development, the fetus begins to move. **FIGURE 18–12** ■ shows the stages *in utero* of human development.

The growing fetus is nourished by a spongy structure called the **placenta**, which is attached to the fetus and the mother via the umbilical cord. The fetus is encased in a membranous sac called the **amnion**, which contains the amniotic fluid in which the fetus floats. **Labor** is the actual process whereby the fetus is delivered from the uterus through the vagina and into the outside world.

Labor consists of three stages. In the *dilation stage*, the uterine smooth muscle begins to contract, thereby moving the fetus down the uterus and causing the cervix to begin to dilate.

Clinical Application

CONTRACEPTION

The prevention of pregnancy is termed **contraception** ("against conception") and can be accomplished by a number of means such as intrauterine devices (IUDs), spermicidal agents, birth control pills, skin implants, patches, or condoms.

Sterilization of the male can be accomplished through a **vasectomy**. The vas deferens are the tubes that carry the sperm into the urethra, and tying off these tubes prevents the sperm from traveling out of the penis during sexual intercourse. Females may be sterilized via **tubal ligation**. The fallopian tubes are cut, clipped, or tied off, preventing the egg from traveling from the ovary to the uterus.

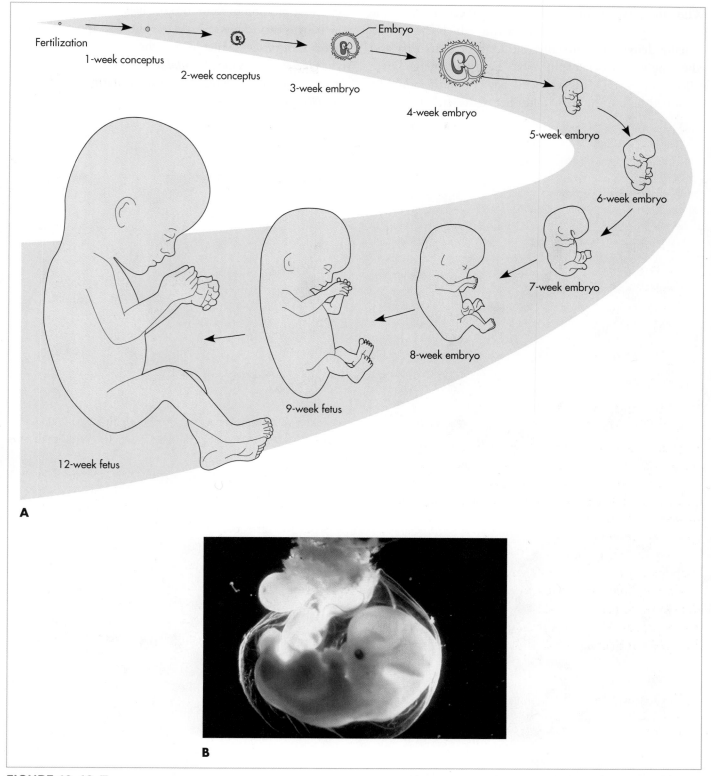

Fertilization

1-week conceptus

2-week conceptus

3-week embryo

Embryo

4-week embryo

5-week embryo

6-week embryo

7-week embryo

8-week embryo

9-week fetus

12-week fetus

A

B

FIGURE 18–12 ■

(A) The stages in utero of human development. (B) Actual photo of fetus at week 9.

When the cervix is completely dilated (10 centimeters), the second stage (*expulsion*) begins, during which the baby is actually delivered. Generally, the head presents first and when the widest part of the baby's head has emerged, it is called *crowning*. This is when the baby's mouth should be suctioned before the baby takes her or his first breath to prevent aspiration of fluid into the baby's lung. Sometimes, the baby is turned around and the buttocks appear first in a *breech presentation*, which makes the delivery difficult. The last stage of labor is the *placental stage*, in which the placenta, or afterbirth, is delivered due to final uterine contractions (see **FIGURE 18–13** ■).

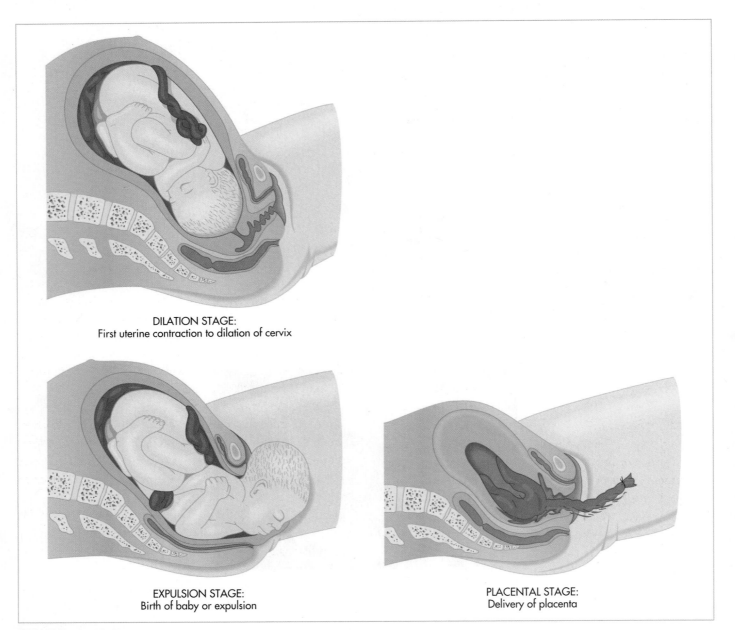

DILATION STAGE:
First uterine contraction to dilation of cervix

EXPULSION STAGE:
Birth of baby or expulsion

PLACENTAL STAGE:
Delivery of placenta

FIGURE 18–13 ■

Stages of labor.

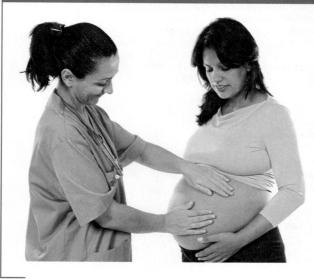

Doulas and **midwives** assist the mother through the labor and delivery process. Learn more about these professionals by visiting the websites of national organizations, including the National Association of Certified Professional Midwives (NACPM), Midwives Alliance of North America (MANA), the American College of Nurse-Midwives, DONA International, and the Childbirth and Postpartum Professional Association (CAPPA).

COMMON DISORDERS OF THE REPRODUCTIVE SYSTEM

Both male and female reproductive systems are susceptible to many disorders. Common to both systems are **sexually transmitted diseases (STDs)**. However, each system has its own specific disorders tied to anatomical and physiological differences of the sexes.

Disorders of the Female Reproductive System

The first menstrual period is referred to as *menarche*, and *menopause* represents the ending of menstrual activity, both of which are normal events in the female reproductive system. However, this normal cycle can be disrupted. **Amenorrhea** is the absence of menstruation and can be a result of pregnancy, menopause, or other factors such as emotional distress, extreme dieting or exercise, or poor health. **Dysmenorrhea** is difficult menstruation, usually resulting in painful cramping.

Premenstrual syndrome (PMS) occurs several days prior to the onset of menstruation. It is characterized by effects on many systems of the body, including emotions. These symptoms vary among individuals and usually subside near the onset of menstruation.

Like any system, the reproductive system can become infected. **Vaginitis** is the inflammation of the vagina that is usually caused by a microorganism such as bacteria or yeast. Vaginitis is sometimes a result of sexually transmitted diseases. Sexually transmitted diseases represent a large number of infections found in both male and female reproductive systems and can be bacterial, viral, or fungal.

The cervix is the area where a *Pap Test* (named after George Papanicolaou) is performed that examines scrapings from the cervical cells to detect the presence of cancer. Regular Pap tests allow for early detection, which increases the likelihood of successful treatment.

In some cases of pregnancy, the fertilized egg implants in the fallopian tubes and does not make the full trip down to the uterus. This is an **ectopic pregnancy**, also referred to as a tubal pregnancy, that requires surgical intervention. **Abruptio placentia** is an emergency situation also requiring surgery in which the placenta tears away from the uterine wall before the twentieth week of pregnancy.

Postpartum depression is a potentially serious psychological state that can occur after childbirth. Mothers should be monitored for signs and symptoms with follow-up treatment/counseling because it can lead to a decrease in the quality of life and possible harm to the mother or baby or both.

Mastitis is inflammation of the breast, which can occur at any age and in both males and females, but is usually associated with lactating females.

Breast cancer is one of the leading causes of death in women between the ages of 32 and 52 and kills about 40,000 women a year. Men can also get breast cancer but at a lower rate. The National Cancer Institute estimates that there will be approximately 2,300 new cases of male breast cancer in 2014, compared to approximately 230,000 new female cases. Cancer of the breast may require a full or partial *mastectomy*, but the earlier it is detected, the better the chance for a positive outcome. **FIGURE 18–14** ■ shows the steps for breast self-examination.

WHY DO THE BREAST SELF-EXAM?

There are many good reasons for doing a breast self-exam each month. One reason is that it is easy to do and the more you do it, the better you will get at it. When you get to know how your breasts normally feel, you will quickly be able to feel any change, and early detection is the key to successful treatment and cure.

REMEMBER: A breast self-exam could save your breast—and save your life. Most breast lumps are found by women themselves, but in fact, most lumps in the breast are not cancer. Be safe, be sure.

WHEN TO DO BREAST SELF-EXAM

The best time to do breast self-exam is right after your period, when breasts are not tender or swollen. If you do not have regular periods or sometimes skip a month, do it on the same day every month.

NOW, HOW TO DO BREAST SELF-EXAM

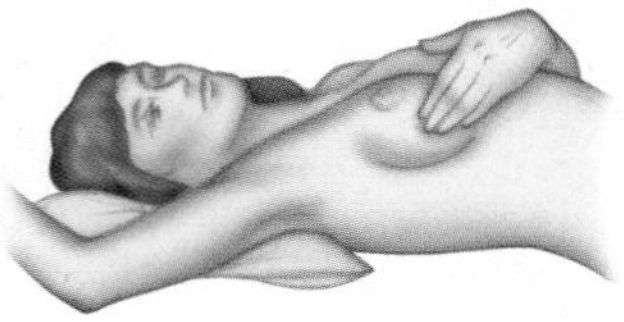

1. Lie down and put a pillow under your right shoulder. Place your right arm behind your head.

2. Use the finger pads of your three middle fingers on your left hand to feel for lumps or thickening. Your finger pads are the top third of each finger.

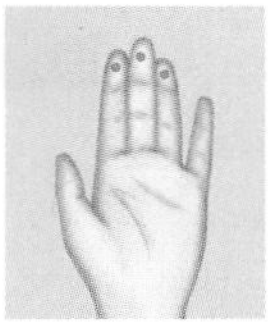

3. Press firmly enough to know how your breast feels. If you're not sure how hard to press, ask your health care provider. Try to copy the way your health care provider uses the finger pads during a breast exam. Learn what your breast feels like most of the time. A firm ridge in the lower curve of each breast is normal.

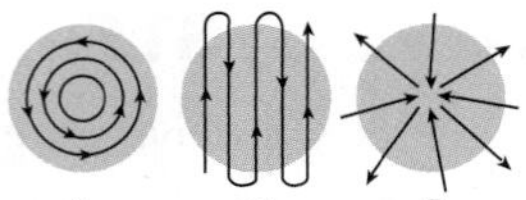

4. Move around the breast in a set way. You can choose either the circle (A), the up and down line (B), or the wedge (C). Do it the same way every time. It will help you to make sure that you've gone over the entire breast area, and to remember how your breast feels.

5. Now examine your left breast using your right hand finger pads.

6. If you find any changes, see your doctor right away.

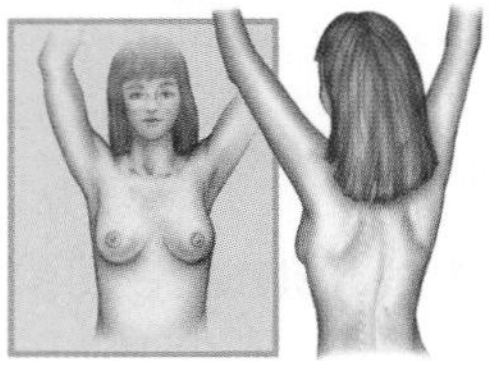

FOR ADDED SAFETY

You should also check your breasts while standing in front of a mirror right after you do your breast self-exam each month. See if there are any changes in the way your breasts look: dimpling of the skin, changes in the nipple, or redness or swelling.

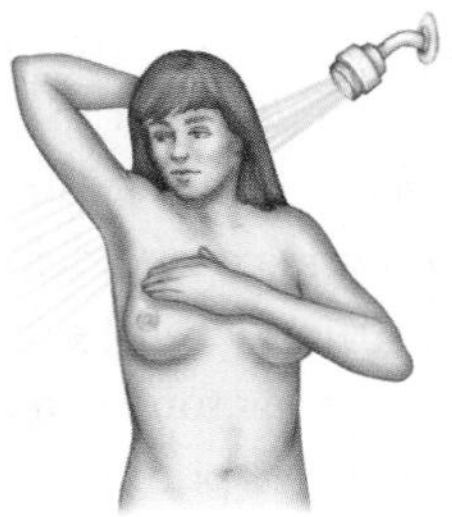

You might also want to do a breast self-exam while you're in the shower. Your soapy hands will glide over the wet skin, making it easy to check how your breasts feel.

FIGURE 18–14 ■

Breast self-examination.

Amazing Facts

A Million-to-One Shot
The adult male produces 200 million sperm daily, but it takes only one sperm to fertilize the egg.

Disorders of the Male Reproductive System

In **erectile dysfunction disorder (EDD)**, the penis cannot attain full erection or maintain an erection. Medication can help increase blood flow to the penis and thus treat some forms of erectile dysfunction. The inability to develop an erection is often referred to as *impotency*. Underlying causes

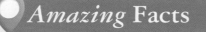

of EDD may be psychological, physiological, or a combination of both.

Impotency is often confused with the inability to conceive children due to low sperm counts. This is incorrect. To determine male fertility, a semen analysis must be performed. Semen is collected 3 to 5 days after abstaining from sexual activity. The semen is analyzed for the shape, number, and swimming strength of the sperm. This is also used to determine the effectiveness of a vasectomy in which the blocking of the vas deferens should result in no sperm in the semen sample 6 weeks postoperatively

The failure of the testes to descend into the scrotal sac is termed **cryptorchidism** and may require surgical intervention. If the testes remain undescended, the male may become sterile because of the body heat destroying the sperm. A **hydrocele** is an abnormal collection of fluid within the testes.

Benign prostatic hyperplasia (BPH) is the enlargement of the prostrate gland and is commonly seen in males over 50 years old (see **FIGURE 18–15** ■). **Prostate cancer** is a slow-growing cancer that also affects males within this age group and can be treated effectively if detected early. A *PSA test (prostate-specific antigen)* can aid in early detection, but there is some controversy concerning its accuracy. The National Cancer Institute estimates that there will be approximately 233,000 new cases of prostate cancer in 2014.

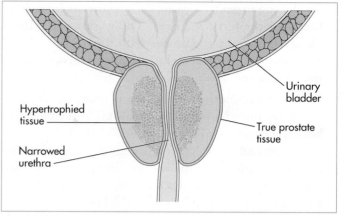

FIGURE 18–15 ■
Benign prostatic hyperplasia.

Testicular cancer is a cancer that starts in the testes. Though it is a relatively rare cancer (estimated 8,800 new cases in 2014), it is important to mention here because it is most common in young or middle-aged men, and it is the most common cancer in men between 15 and 34. Symptoms may include lumps, swelling, or pain in the scrotum or there may be no symptoms at all. Testicular cancer is treatable even if it has spread. Regular testicular exams can help catch testicular cancer early.

SUMMARY: Points of Interest

- Tissues grow, are replaced, and are repaired by asexual reproduction. Cells make identical copies of themselves. Asexual reproduction takes place all over the body as tissues grow or are repaired. Some tissues, such as epidermis, blood, and bone, replace themselves continually, always by asexual reproduction. Asexual reproduction in eukaryotic cells is accomplished by a relatively complex process called mitosis.

- If an organism is going to reproduce sexually, it must use specialized cells called gametes with only half the typical number of chromosomes for that organism. Each gamete must have half as many chromosomes because, during fertilization, the gametes will fuse and combine their genetic material.

- In humans, the gametes are eggs and sperm. Eggs and sperm are produced by a special type of cell division called meiosis, or reduction division. Reduction division produces four daughter cells, each with only

23 chromosomes. These cells are not identical to each other or to the mother cell.

- Cells undergoing meiosis go through two divisions. The chief difference between mitosis and meiosis is the pairing of homologous chromosomes (alike in size, shape, and genetic content) during meiosis.

- Human reproduction can be described as a cycle, known as the human life cycle. Adult humans have specialized organs called gonads (ovaries and testes) that produce gametes via meiosis. Gametes combine during sexual reproduction in a process known as fertilization. The fertilized egg is called a zygote. The zygote undergoes many rounds of mitosis, eventually becoming an embryo, a fetus, a baby, a child, and finally an adult.

- The female reproductive system consists of several internal genitalia. The gonads (ovaries) produce eggs (gametes). The uterine tubes provide a passageway for the egg to get to the uterus. The uterus is an incubator for the fertilized eggs. The vagina is the birth canal, connecting the uterus with the outside world. The external genitalia include the external opening of the vagina and several protective structures.

- Female reproductive physiology is relatively complicated, organized around a monthly cycle of changes in both the ovaries and the uterus, collectively known as the menstrual cycle. The cycle begins with menstruation, the shedding of the uterine lining. After the lining, the endometrium, has finished shedding, it begins to build up again in a process called proliferation. As the endometrium is proliferating, an egg (follicle) is maturing in the ovary. Eventually, the follicle will be released from the ovary (ovulation) and travel to the uterus. If fertilization occurs, then the fertilized egg will implant in the thickened endometrium, and pregnancy will result. If the egg is not fertilized, the endometrium will degenerate, and menstruation will occur.

- Control of the menstrual cycle is accomplished by four hormones: estrogen, progesterone, follicle-stimulating hormone (FSH), and luteinizing hormone (LH). During puberty, the ovaries begin to secrete larger amounts of estrogen and progesterone, which cause the development of female secondary sexual characteristics and set the cycle in motion.

- The cycle works this way: The hypothalamus releases gonadotropin-releasing hormone (GnRH) that causes the pituitary to increase secretion of FSH and LH. The follicle-stimulating hormone and the luteinizing hormone cause follicles to develop and eventually trigger ovulation. Estrogen levels continue to rise as the developing follicles secrete more and more estrogen. Estrogen causes positive feedback to the hypothalamus and pituitary, which increases the levels of FSH and LH. This positive feedback loop continues right up until ovulation.

- At ovulation, the ruptured follicle (left behind after ovulation) begins to secrete progesterone and backs off on estrogen secretion. Under the influence of progesterone, the feedback loop between estrogen and the hypothalamus and pituitary reverses itself, becoming a negative feedback loop. Thus, LH and FSH levels drop. Progesterone levels continue to rise, maintaining the thickened endometrium in case fertilization occurs. If fertilization does not occur, progesterone decreases, the endometrium degenerates, and the cycle begins all over again.

- The male reproductive system has somewhat more obvious external genitalia, the penis, and the testes. Internal genitalia include a series of ducts, the vas deferens, the ejaculatory duct, and the urethra, as well as a series of glands, the seminal vesicles, prostate, and bulbourethral glands.

- Male reproductive physiology is not cyclic and is therefore a bit less complicated than female reproduction. Sperm, like eggs, develop via meiosis under the control of LH and FSH in the testes. Sperm mature in the epididymis. When a man is sexually aroused, the penis becomes engorged with blood, and an erection occurs. If arousal continues, ejaculation, the movement of sperm from the testes to the penis and out of the man's body, may occur. During ejaculation, sperm move from the epididymis through the vas deferens and ejaculatory duct and out the urethra. Along the journey, the seminal vesicles, prostate, and bulbourethral glands add sugar, chemicals, and mucus to the sperm to form semen.

- Testosterone is the chief male hormone. It is secreted by the testes and is responsible for masculinizing male fetuses, triggering LH and FSH production, and the development of male secondary sexual characteristics.

CASE STUDY

Maria and her husband, Trey, have been planning a family for many years. Now that the time seems right, she cannot seem to get pregnant. After two years of trying, they have decided to consult their family physician for a referral to a fertility specialist. Before making the referral, their family doctor runs some tests.

Here are the results: Trey is producing sperm at normal levels, and the sperm are healthy and mobile.

Maria's hormone levels and all other blood tests are normal. She has a more or less regular menstrual cycle, but she has always had cramps during the middle of her cycle. On further questioning, she admits to the doctor that in the last few years, the pain seemed to get worse, but she thought that was just normal for her. She also admits to some low back pain and some urinary disturbances, particularly around the time of her period.

a. To prevent exploratory abdominal surgery, can you think of any other diagnostic tests?

_____

_____

b. What should Maria's doctor be looking for, given the timing of the pain during the cycle and the inability to get pregnant?

_____

_____

REVIEW QUESTIONS

Multiple Choice

1. In each lobule of the testes are several _____, tubes in which the sperm are made and develop.
   a. seminal vesicles
   b. seminiferous tubules
   c. bulbourethral glands
   d. all of the above

2. The female primary genitalia are the
   a. ovaries.
   b. uterus.
   c. vagina.
   d. testes.

3. This division of the endometrium sheds each month:
   a. horny layer.
   b. basal layer.
   c. menstrual layer.
   d. none of the above

4. This hormone stimulates ovulation:
   a. estrogen.
   b. progesterone.
   c. LH.
   d. FSH.

5. Which of the following is *not* a function of asexual reproduction (mitosis)?
   a. making gametes
   b. tissue growth
   c. tissue repair
   d. all are functions of asexual reproduction

6. Which of the following hormones are elevated during pregnancy?
   a. LH
   b. FSH
   c. testosterone
   d. HCG

Fill in the Blank

1. The stiffening of the penis is known as a(n) _____, and the actual movement of sperm out of the penis is _____.

2. In the male reproductive system the _____ are posterior to the bladder, and the _____ gland is inferior to the bladder.

3. _____ is the type of cell division that produces egg and sperm.

4. After ovulation, estrogen and progesterone send _____ (positive or negative) feedback to the pituitary and hypothalamus.

5. The union of sperm and egg is called _____.

6. _____ is the leading cause of female infertility.

Short Answer

1. Trace the journey of a sperm from its birth through fertilization.

_____

_____

2. Explain the role of hormones in controlling the female reproductive cycle.

_____

_____

_____

_____

3. Explain the stages of labor and childbirth.

_____

_____

_____

_____

4. Explain the human life cycle.

_____

_____

_____

_____

5. Explain the development of an oocyte in the ovary through ovulation.

_____

_____

_____

_____

Visit our new **MyHealthProfessions Lab** to accompany *Anatomy & Physiology for Health Professions*. Here you'll find a rich collection of quizzes, case studies, and animations for deeper understanding and application.

19

The Journey's End

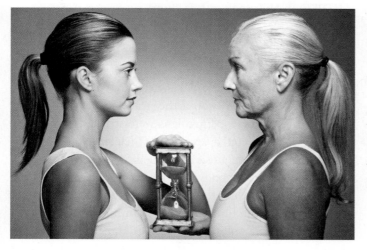

For any of you who have ever taken a memorable journey or have lived through a significant event, you know that you have been changed to some degree forever. We hope that this text has, in some positive ways, also changed you.

The following topics are just a small sampling of how anatomy and physiology play an important role in many areas. We have added a whole section of Amazing Facts so you can impress friends, family, and the old boyfriend or girlfriend who dumped you back in high school. They'll be sorry now! Enjoy the chapter.

LEARNING OUTCOMES

At the end of your journey through this chapter, you will be able to:

- Discuss the relationship between forensic science and anatomy and physiology.
- Relate anatomy and physiology changes to the process of aging.
- Describe the concept of wellness and personal choices.
- List and describe wellness concepts for each body system.
- Discuss cancer prevention and treatment.
- Dazzle your friends with amazing anatomy and physiology facts.

Pronunciation Guide

Correct pronunciation is important in any journey so that you and others are completely understood. Here is a "see and say" Pronunciation Guide for the more difficult terms to pronounce in this chapter. Please note that even though there are standard pronunciations, regional variations of the pronunciations can occur.

anhidrosis (an HIGH droe sis)
bacilli (bah SILL eye)
Chlamydia trachomatis
 (klah MID ee ah tra KOH mah tiss)
forensic science (for IN sik)
geriatric (JAIR ee AT rik)
herpes simplex virus 2 (HER peez)

human papilloma virus (pap ih LOW ma)
incontinence (in KAHN tih nens)
Neisseria gonorrhoeae
 (nye SEE ree ah gon oh REE ah)
spina bifida (SPY nah BIFF ih dah)
thallium (THAL ee um)
Treponema pallidum
 (TREP oh NEE mah PAL ih dum)

FORENSIC SCIENCE

We've all watched movies or TV shows featuring supersleuths solving such crimes as murders or disappearances using some amazing scientific technology. Some of the methods used seem pretty far-fetched, as though invented just for entertainment purposes. Actually, much of the forensic science we see on TV is very close, if not "dead on," to the actual technologies that are applied to solve crimes. It is important to note that this kind of investigation can be extremely tedious and take longer than a 46-minute TV show to solve. Also, most forensic scientists don't look like supermodels or drive $60,000 SUVs. This section deals with just a sampling of how anatomy and physiology are used to help solve crimes and explain historical mysteries.

So what exactly is forensic science? Simply put, **forensic science** is the application of science to law. A forensic scientist often searches for and examines physical traces that can be useful in establishing or excluding some association between a victim and an individual suspected of committing a crime. It is interesting to note that both physical science and social sciences such as psychology are used when solving crime. The natural science of anatomy and physiology often plays a key role in solving a crime or identifying the remains of a victim.

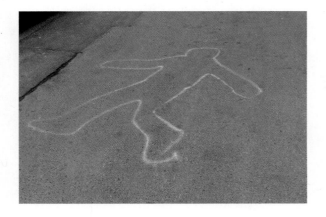

Disease Detection

Forensic science has unlocked ancient mysteries and allowed us to learn something about the health of ancient people. Proof that the ancient Egyptians were stricken with tuberculosis was discovered by examining their skeletons. We normally think of tuberculosis as a lung disease, but tuberculosis thrives in areas of the body that possess high levels of oxygen. These include the lungs, brain, kidneys, and *the ends of long bones!* Because the lungs of most mummies were long ago decomposed, the only thing left to examine are the skeletal remains, particularly the ends of the long bones such as the femur. On examination of these bones, bone scouring that is typically caused by tuberculosis was discovered. This form of bone scouring is from the destruction of the smooth bone surface as a result of colonization by the tuberculosis **bacilli**.

APPLIED SCIENCE

Tomatoes Were Once Thought to Be Poisonous
For several hundred years, it was believed that tomatoes were poisonous. This misconception persisted because during the Middle Ages, the wealthier people ate from pewter plates that contained high levels of lead. The acidic tomatoes leached out the lead, which was consumed and resulted in varying degrees of lead poisoning.

Primitive Surgery

Forensic scientists have discovered evidence of primitive surgery. A skull fragment found in a 400-year-old trash dump at the site of the Jamestown, Virginia, settlement provided evidence that skull surgery had been performed on a patient. The circular marks on the fragment indicated that there was an attempt to drill a hole in the skull, probably to relieve pressure on the brain due to a skull fracture that may have been caused by a war club blow to the head or an accident.

Scientists analyzing the fragment were able to determine that the patient was a European male on the basis of the fragment's shape and thickness *and* because the bone contained traces of lead that was absorbed by the body from using lead-glazed pottery and/or eating from pewter plates.

Remains Identification

Nazi Josef Mengele, the "Angel of Death," was responsible for the deaths of at least 400,000 people during World War II. As the war ended, Mengele escaped to South America and avoided capture. There were numerous reported sightings of him throughout the years, but investigations failed to uncover the war criminal. Then, in 1979, an elderly man named Wolfgang Gerhard drowned and was buried in a Brazilian cemetery. Suspicions that he was Mengele prompted the Brazilian government to exhume the body. Analysis of the bones revealed a right-handed male Caucasian between 60 and 70 years old with a height approximated within a half centimeter of Mengele's. The forensic anthropologists had a pile of bones, a shattered skull, and no current medical information or dental records, so they turned to a technique called *video skull–face superimposition*. After reconstructing the shattered skull, the experts marked it with pins at 30 specific structural landmarks. The same thing was done with a picture of Mengele that was scaled to match the size of the skull. Compared side by side, the pins matched up. Photo images of the skull and picture were then superimposed, and the points again matched up. They had their man. Later, when his old dental records were found, it was again a match, as was a later DNA analysis. More recently, an updated similar procedure was used to determine the actual facial structure of Tutankhamen (King Tut), the boy pharaoh of Egypt.

APPLIED SCIENCE

Forensics and History

Today, DNA fingerprinting techniques are used extensively to clear up mysteries. For example, it is now standard to use this technology to solve rape and murder cases. The uniqueness of the DNA fingerprint has also helped determine that Thomas Jefferson, or a close male relative, did actually father some of the children of his slave Sally Hemmings. In addition, DNA fingerprinting was used to identify many of the victims of the World Trade Center, Pentagon, and Flight 93 near Shanksville, Pennsylvania, after the September 11 attacks.

APPLIED SCIENCE

If Bones Could Speak

Skeletal remains can also assist in determining the sex of an individual. The female pelvis is shaped like a basin and is wider than that of the male to allow for the larger birth canal. In general, it is broader and lighter than the male pelvis, and the pubic angle is 100 degrees or greater (see **FIGURE 19–1** ■). The male pelvis is more funnel shaped and is heavier and stronger, with a pubic angle of 90 degrees or less. In addition, male bones are denser and more heavily sculpted with more obvious muscle attachments than female bones.

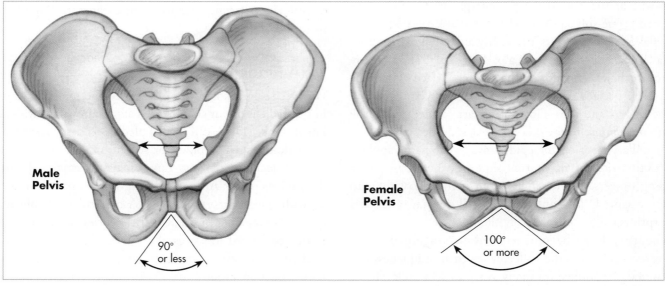

FIGURE 19–1 ■

The male pelvis and female pelvis.

Murder Most Foul!

Although it possesses no vocal chords, your hair speaks volumes about your health and your habits. Hair can reveal the race of an individual, whether the hair was cut or pulled from the body, or if it was dyed. If the hair shaft has its follicle still attached, genetic information such as DNA or blood type can also be discerned. Hair samples can place an individual at the scene of a crime.

Even though hair is technically dead, just like your fingernails and toenails, it acts like a library (as do your nails), storing information about substances to which you have been exposed, or have ingested. Because hair grows relatively slowly, it can contain a *timeline* of exposures to those substances.

In an interesting case of **thallium** poisoning, a woman was convicted of murdering her husband, partially on the basis of hair samples from the victim. The victim's hair was long enough that it provided a record of ingestion of thallium for approximately 330 days. During that period of time, the spikes in concentration of thallium in sections of his hair matched the times the victim was with his wife. Drops in the level of thallium in other sections of his hair coincided with the times he was away from his wife or in the hospital for other illnesses. There was a massive spike in thallium concentration a few days before he died, which was indicative of premeditated poisoning. In a plea bargain, it was revealed that the victim's wife had been feeding him rat poison that contained thallium to collect on a life insurance policy.

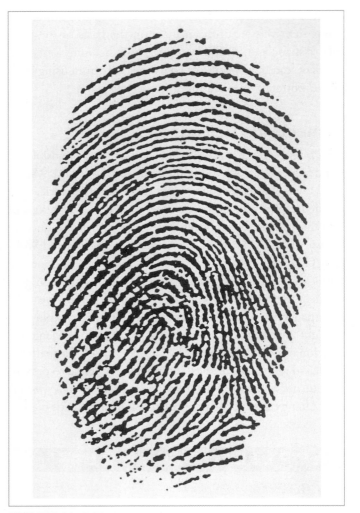

FIGURE 19–2 ■
The fingerprint.

Fingerprints

Even with all the new advances, fingerprints are still a time-honored crime-solving method (see **FIGURE 19–2** ■). Like snowflakes, no two prints are exactly alike. Fingerprints are actual *friction ridges* that form a pattern on the anterior surface of the hands and also on the plantar surface of the feet. They are especially prominent on the skin covering the tips of the fingers and toes. Fingerprints are formed inside the womb in response to the pull of the elastic fibers in the dermal papillary layer on the epidermis. As the name applies, the friction ridges help prevent slippage when grasping or holding objects. Interestingly, even identical twins who have the same DNA configuration will not have identical fingerprints.

Scientists have been interested in fingerprints for centuries—as early as the 1600s, when their uniqueness was discovered and studied for many years. In 1880, Dr. Henry Faulds wrote the first article suggesting that fingerprints could be used to solve crimes. In 1886, Faulds began trying to convince Scotland Yard to adopt a fingerprinting identification system.

DNA Fingerprinting

Forensic scientists may also use DNA, the molecule found in the nucleus of our cells, to identify unknown individuals. For instance, DNA can be sampled at a crime scene from body fluids, such as blood or semen, or can be extracted from skeletal or even very tiny soft tissue remains. During the process of DNA fingerprinting (which has nothing to do with actual fingerprints), DNA molecules are split into pieces and separated using electrical currents. These pieces can be compared to pieces of a known DNA sample from a relative of a victim, from hair samples off a comb or from mouth cells on a toothbrush, or the DNA can be compared to that of a suspect in a criminal case.

TEST YOUR KNOWLEDGE 19-1

Choose the best answer:

1. This part of your body acts as a library and provides a timeline to record substances that you have ingested or have been exposed to:
   a. heart.
   b. lungs.
   c. hair.
   d. spinal cord.

2. This metal has been detected in the bones of medieval skeletons and can be traced to eating from pewter plates:
   a. silver.
   b. gold.
   c. kryptonite.
   d. lead.

3. Proof that ancient Egyptians had tuberculosis was discovered by examining their
   a. tombs.
   b. bones.
   c. hair.
   d. mommies.

4. One difference between male and female skeletal remains can be determined by examining the angle of the
   a. skull.
   b. vertebrae.
   c. sternum.
   d. pelvis.

5. Using DNA fingerprinting technology
   a. isolates DNA from the fingerprints of suspects.
   b. compares unknown samples of DNA to known samples.
   c. makes DNA to cure disease.
   d. clones animals.

GERIATRICS

Many regions in the United States are exhibiting a major change in patient demographics. In general, the nation is experiencing a growth in the older population due to safer workplaces, healthier lifestyles, effective vaccines and medications, and opportunities to access health care. In addition, the large population of baby boomers (born between 1946 and 1964) are now reaching the geriatric age and requiring more medical services. As a result, you probably will deal with a high number of **geriatric** patients in the health care profession that you choose. Even the maternity departments may have 50- to 60-year-old mothers in the future, as witnessed by several recent news reports.

Geriatric patients differ in many ways from other patient age groups, so it is important to recognize these differences to provide the best health care possible for this patient population. Here are some general tidbits to get you started.

The general use of the term *elderly* when describing patients is somewhat misleading. Currently, this patient group can be divided into the following classifications:

- Age 65 to 75: younger old
- Age 76 to 84: older old
- Age 85 and older: elite old

Using the vague term *aging* as a way to generally describe a patient is inaccurate in that an individual's body does not age uniformly. For example, a person might look older due to aging skin but may have the cardiovascular system of someone 10 to 15 years younger than his or her chronological age. With that said, there is the general "1 percent rule" in which we see a 1 percent decrease in the function of most body systems each year beginning around the age of 30.

So what general characteristics or tendencies do health care workers see in an aging patient? The hallmark sign of aging is a decrease in the ability to maintain homeostasis. Older individuals may have normal baselines but will begin exhibiting a decrease in the ability to adapt to stressors. Often, disease processes, along with aging, will accelerate the loss of body reserves that younger patients take for granted, such as recovery time or complications following an accident or surgery. In addition, you

Amazing Facts

You're Not Getting Older, You're Getting Smarter

There are a lot of misconceptions about the brain and aging. In the absence of disease, your brain continues to mature up to the age of 50. Interestingly, we have better overall brain function and decision-making skills at age 60 than at age 30. In general, as we age, we are better at anticipating problems and we can also reason things out better than when we were younger. These advantages may be, in part, a result of our diverse life experiences. Even though an older person may lose up to 1,000 neurons a day, you have to realize that we all started out with several billion. This is why you may not see the beginnings of a decrease in brain function until the age of 75.

---

may have increased difficulties evaluating these patients because of decreases in their vision, hearing, and possibly their mental abilities.

General Body Changes

Let's take a general look at the aging process of the body. There is a decrease in the total body water for both males and females. The clinical significance of this is that older people have a tendency to dehydrate more rapidly, which can potentially affect the excretion rate of medications they are on.

From ages 20 to 70, we see a loss of lean body mass due to a loss (up to 30 percent) in the number of muscle cells, atrophy of remaining muscle cells, and a general decrease in muscle strength. Conversely, we see an increase in total body fat, which slowly increases between the ages of 25 and 45, peaking at 40. This trend of increasing body fat can continue up to age 70. The fat accumulated is a "deeper" fat, meaning that it is more abdominal fat and found more in the viscera than subcutaneously.

Bone density usually reaches its greatest peak around age 35. Contrary to what you see on TV, loss of bone mass occurs both in women *and* men. For women, during the first 5 years postmenopause, 1 to 2 percent bone loss per year can occur. In general, in both sexes there is a 1 percent loss per year between the ages of 55 and 70. After that, it is approximately 0.5 percent per year.

So, in general, as individuals age, they lose muscle mass and bone density, and gain fat. This varies among individuals and can be affected by lifestyle choices. Later in this chapter, we discuss steps that can be taken to slow (or even reverse) these processes.

Gustatory Changes

Sensory changes can also occur with aging. The senses of taste and smell begin to deteriorate as a natural process of aging. The number of taste buds decreases by about 50 percent as the body reaches the geriatric stage. Sweet versus bitter tastes become less discernible. The acuity of salt and bitter tastes declines. Orange juice may taste metallic. Patients on oxygen via a nasal cannula may also have a decrease in their sense of taste. These changes are clinically significant because they may make it more difficult to ensure a properly balanced diet for good health and activity. There is also a concern associated with additional functional and physiological difficulties affecting grocery shopping and food preparation. It is estimated that 33 percent of the geriatric population lives alone. These and other sensory impairments affect activities of daily living (ADLs), and as a result, we see approximately 5 to 15 percent of this population exhibiting protein and calorie malnutrition.

Additional barriers to proper nutrition include tooth loss, ill-fitting dentures, difficulties in swallowing, and decreases in salivary secretion. Also, there are decreases in digestive juices' acidity and secretion, nutrient absorption, and bowel function.

The Brain and Nervous System

The main problem with the aging process and the nervous system is the slower reaction time that occurs. As a result, older patients are more likely to be injured in automobile accidents, falls, burns, and other types of trauma.

Pain is often associated with the aging process. Even though the authors of this book are young in spirit, vibrant, and good looking, they have occasional creaking joints and stiff, sore muscles! Untreated pain can lead to an overall decrease in the quality of a person's life, including impaired sleep, a decrease in socialization, confusion, depression, malnutrition, polypharmacy (use of multiple medications), and impaired ambulation. If any of these conditions were already present before the pain began, the pain may cause these conditions to worsen.

Often, geriatric patients are undermedicated for pain. This may be because patients who are debilitated, cognitively impaired, or have a history of substance abuse are sometimes unable to effectively relate how they feel. Sometimes, it is a result of the ignorance of health care professionals who cannot recognize indicators of pain.

Clinically, these are some of the potential behavioral changes related to pain:

- Changes in personality such as becoming agitated, quiet, withdrawn, sad, confused, depressed, grumpy
- Loss of appetite
- Screaming, swearing, name-calling, grunting, noisy breathing
- Crying, rocking, fidgeting
- Splinting or rubbing a sore area, wincing
- Cold, clammy, and pale skin

The Cardiovascular System

Within the cardiovascular system, we see changes such as calcification of the heart valves, which decreases their efficiency. We also see a decrease in the flexibility of the blood vessels. This makes the vessels less able to deal with blood pressure changes, so increased blood pressure is common. There is also a decrease in cardiac output and an approximate 25 percent decrease in the maximum heart rate.

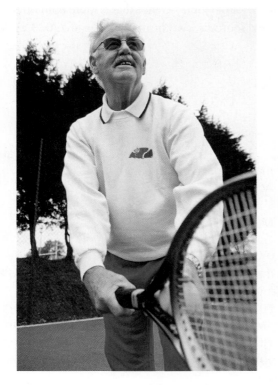

The Genitourinary System

Between the ages of 20 and 80, individuals lose about 50 percent of their renal function. This is clinically significant when one considers the number of drugs used by the geriatric population that are excreted by the kidneys. Therefore, a patient with impaired renal (and/or liver) function can experience decreased metabolism and excretion of medication. This can lead to an accumulation of the drug in the body at harmful or toxic levels. There is also an increase in **incontinence** (loss of bladder control) in this group often due to a loss of muscle tone, effects of surgical procedures, and side effects of some medications.

The Integumentary System

Here, we see a loss in skin elasticity often due to collagen loss, increased skin delicacy, multiple skin lesions, and increased rates of skin cancer. In addition, wound healing may take longer, hair loss or greying of hair, thickening of the nails and drier skin may result. Although many of these problems could have been prevented by limiting sun exposure and not smoking earlier in their lives, the use of medications such as systemic corticosteroids does accelerate many of these conditions.

Polypharmacy

Polypharmacy, the administration of many drugs at the same time, is a major concern for this patient group. Contributing factors to this problem include the fact that these patients typically see several specialists for a variety of diseases, often with one doctor not knowing what the other is prescribing. These multiple diseases have competing therapeutic needs, and the combinations of utilized drugs can cause life-threatening situations. Aging also can affect the rates of drug absorption, drug distribution throughout the body, metabolism of the drugs, as well as their excretion from the body.

Not taking drugs as directed (drug compliance) is often a problem with geriatric patients. This can be either not taking the correct amount of medication or not taking it frequently enough. There are several reasons this can occur, such as not hearing or understanding the directions, a desire to save money, confused mental state, a physical inability to take the medication by themselves, or simply because some individuals dislike taking medications.

As a health care professional, you should always take precautions when working with older patients. Review the drugs that the person is taking, looking for possible drug

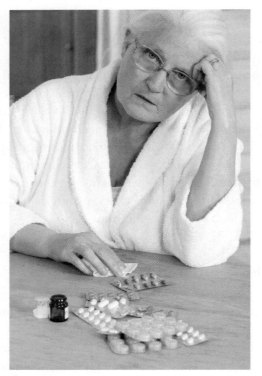

Polypharmacy.

interactions or medications that are no longer needed. Look at your patient's liver and kidney functions. They have the potential to affect the rate of removal of medications from the body and resultant blood drug levels. When medicating with opioids, dose by age, not by body weight. Remember, opioids slow the gastrointestinal tract. In general, when considering an *equal* dose given to a geriatric patient compared to a middle-aged patient, analgesics are stronger and last longer in elderly patients. So, start low and go slow.

WELLNESS

One of the most important personal choices you will ever make will be deciding what kind of lifestyle you want to live. Choices you make now may have a *profound* effect on your future health and life span. Will you eat properly, exercise within reason, smoke, do drugs and/or drink alcohol, live or work in a dangerous environment, or have risky behaviors?

Individual accountability and *informed choices* are two key concepts in deciding your lifestyle. It is amazing that individuals have sued fast-food companies for making their food too appealing and, as a result, making the "victim" get fat. Cigarette companies have been sued for health problems caused by smoking. The cigarette companies may bear some responsibility in that they denied the dangers posed by their product, but in each of these cases, the individual, at some level, made a choice to engage in activities that were unhealthy.

Yes, peer pressure is real, but it is too often looked at from the negative side. What about peers and influential people who promote good, healthy lifestyles? Think about it. Do you know people or have friends who do healthy things? Once again, it is a conscious choice to surround yourself with the type of friends you want.

To make healthy choices, do some research. Read and critically analyze what you read. Utilize multiple *reliable* sources. Although the Internet is a wonderful source of information, it contains a lot of "junk" science that is more opinion than fact. One good source is www.healthypeople.gov/2020, which was

TEST YOUR KNOWLEDGE 19–2

Choose the best answer:

1. Older patients may experience dangerous drug side effects due to
   a. decreased metabolism of the drugs.
   b. polypharmacy leading to drug interactions.
   c. problems in taking medications as directed.
   d. all of the above

2. The hallmark sign of aging is the decrease in the ability to maintain
   a. cardiac enzymes.
   b. exercise potential.
   c. homeostasis.
   d. sense of humor.

3. _____ is a term used for the administration of many drugs at the same time.
   a. Addiction
   b. Polypharmacy
   c. Multimeds
   d. Overdose

4. In the absence of disease, your brain continues to mature up to the age of
   a. 50.
   b. 35.
   c. 75.
   d. 10.

launched in December 2010. This website contains a 10-year agenda for improving our nation's overall health.

Let's take a quick review of the body systems that we covered and briefly discuss some ways to improve your health. Although there are always some controversial issues in wellness, we discuss here the most widely accepted medical information.

The Nervous System

Let's talk a little bit about stress. First of all, stress is a natural part of life. Stress is also good and necessary: It is a motivator and it helps you protect yourself. The problem occurs when stress becomes chronic, and you can no longer effectively deal with it. The high cost of stress is that it can affect your body's systems to varying degrees. A poor stress response can lead to an assortment of problems such as eating and digestive disorders, decreased immune response, decreased memory and work capacities, sleep problems, joint and muscle aches, heart problems, and personality changes. Some of these problems can be life threatening. For an extensive review of a healthful stress management system, remember to consult your Study Companion Guide found in the back of this book.

Often, when dealing with a patient, we focus specifically on the presenting illness and fail to realize we should look at the whole person. The "whole person" includes not only other systems of the body but also the mental and spiritual aspects of the person. Too often in the past, dealing with mental health has had a negative image. We don't hide the fact that we have the flu or a broken arm, so why should we hide the fact that we may be sad for long periods of time (depression) and need help to resolve that condition?

Physically, your brain and spinal cord need protection especially against physical trauma. It is important to always wear the appropriate protective gear for any activity. For example, proper-fitting helmets for bike riding, skateboarding, and sports such as football are critical in preventing or greatly decreasing the risk of brain trauma.

The Skeletal System

Diet is extremely important in the growth and protection of your bones. A diet rich in calcium and vitamins helps maintain good bone growth and development. Weight-bearing exercise has also been shown to be beneficial in maintaining healthy bones over a lifetime.

Even with a good diet and exercise plan, repetitive motion injury is a real possibility. One common occupational condition related to repetitive motion, such as typing on a keyboard, playing a piano, or hammering, is known as **carpal tunnel syndrome**. Although this syndrome is caused by injury to the median nerve, it is the result of the *skeletal* structure of the wrist being too restrictive during extended periods when the wrist is kept in an upward bent position. **FIGURE 19–3** ■ illustrates the structures that affect this repetitive syndrome.

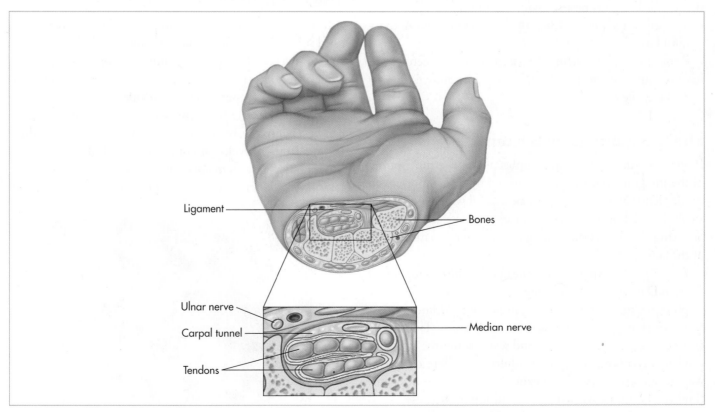

FIGURE 19–3 ■

Anatomical structures affecting carpal tunnel syndrome.

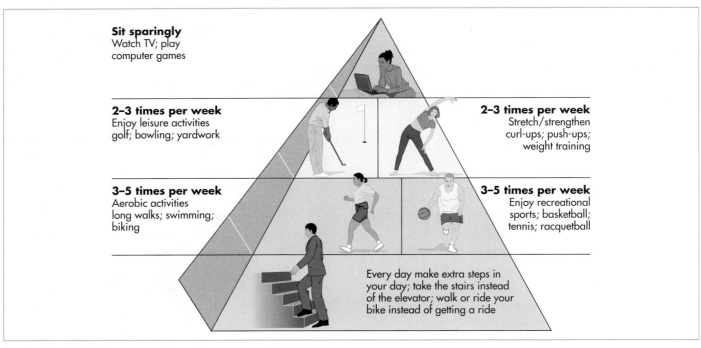

FIGURE 19-4 ■

The activity pyramid.

The Muscular System

Again, proper exercise and diet will help develop and maintain properly functioning muscles. Although many types of muscle-training programs are available, you need to investigate which type is best for you, depending on your needs or desired outcomes. **FIGURE 19-4** ■ presents the Activity Pyramid as a possible guide.

Avoid muscle-enhancing drugs; many are dangerous and have serious side effects. Again, careful critical investigation is the best rule to follow.

The Integumentary System

Proper diet and hydration is important for the functioning of the integumentary system. This is why it is important to drink plenty of water each day. Be careful when consuming alcohol, which is a diuretic and can cause a net water loss. Smoking also affects this system by causing premature aging of the skin.

Although sun exposure is important for the production of vitamin D in your body, limiting the amount of sun exposure to prevent skin cancer is equally important. Although most forms of skin cancer are treatable, some can be lethal. The effect of the sun is cumulative, and severe sunburns as a child can have severe consequences in adulthood. There are several ways to prevent excessive sun exposure. First, minimize your time in the sun between 10 a.m. and 4 p.m. because this is when the sun's rays are most intense. Wear long-sleeved shirts when possible, as well as brimmed hats, sunglasses (preferably wraparounds), and of course, apply SPF sunscreen daily, even if it's cloudy or in the winter.

The Cardiovascular System

A heart-healthy diet low in saturated fats (remember, we all need some fat for proper function), high in fiber, and rich in fruit and vegetables will help maintain an optimal cardiovascular system. Diet alone is not sufficient for a healthy heart, however. The proper level and regularity of exercise also helps condition the heart for maximum functioning. This can be as simple as brisk walking for 30 minutes a day, three to four times a week. Of course, the level of your exercise program depends on many individualized factors. As always, consult your doctor before beginning any exercise program.

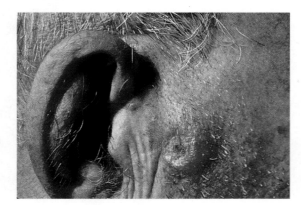

Squamous cell cancer.

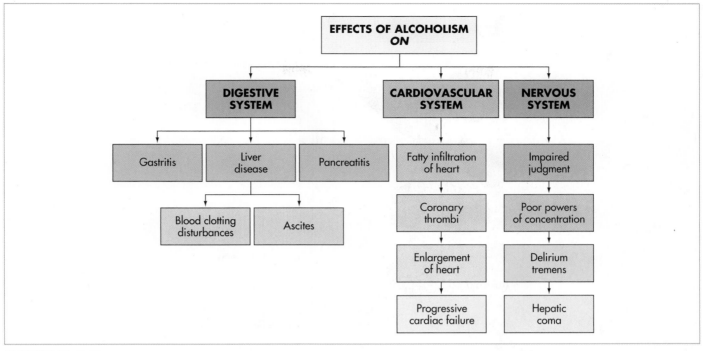

FIGURE 19–5 ■

The effects of alcoholism on the body systems.

Smoking, alcohol, and other drugs can adversely affect the cardiovascular and other systems. For an illustration of the effects of chronic alcoholism on the cardiovascular, digestive, and nervous system, please see **FIGURE 19–5** ■.

The Respiratory System

Smoking is the number-one preventable cause of respiratory diseases. Smoking can damage lung tissue and cause chronic diseases such as chronic bronchitis and emphysema, and can worsen asthma. (See **FIGURE 19–6** ■, which shows the constricted airway in an asthma attack.) In addition, smoking increases the occurrence of lung infections and colds as well as sinus infections. Approximately 80 percent of all lung cancers can be traced to smoking. Smoking also affects the heart by reducing the availability of oxygen to the heart muscle. Smoking, along with alcohol consumption, leads to an increase in stomach and mouth cancers. What we breathe in, depending on where we live or work, can also affect the health of the respiratory system. Both outdoor and indoor pollution can lead to a number of respiratory problems.

Occupational hazards can occur when workers are exposed to dust or vapors. For example, coal miners exposed to coal dust without proper protection and ventilation can develop black lung. The lung's initial response to an inhaled irritant is to close down or restrict the airway, thereby minimizing the inhalation of the substance. This can lead to severe breathing difficulties.

The Gastrointestinal System

A proper diet is critical for growth, development, and health in general. Lack of a proper diet, which leads to under-nourishment, can affect all the systems, as can be seen in **FIGURE 19–7** ■. Although most experts agree that the best source of vitamins and minerals comes from natural food sources, the responsible use of supplemental vitamins and minerals can play an important role in health. However, like everything in life, there can be too much of a good thing when it comes to taking nutritional supplements. For example, excessive dosages of fat-soluble vitamins (A, D, E, and K) can actually harm the body because they can build up to toxic levels. See **TABLE 19–1** ■ for a list of some of the vitamins and the systems they assist.

The Endocrine System

Again, proper diet and exercise assist the endocrine system. One of the areas of concern in professional and even high school sports is the use of performance-enhancement substances. For example, anabolic steroids are used to increase strength and endurance rapidly and to build muscle mass. Anabolic steroids are closely related to the male hormone testosterone. However, these steroids have *serious* side effects that include kidney damage, liver damage, increased risk of heart disease, irritability, and aggressive behavior. Women taking steroids can develop facial hair and deeper voices.

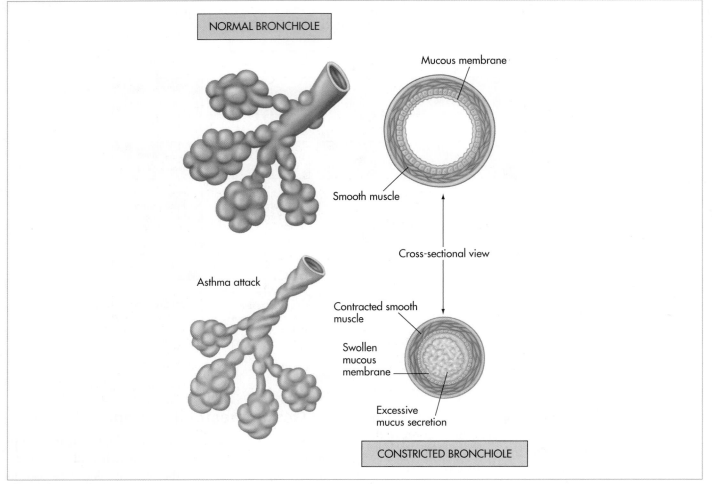

FIGURE 19–6 ■

The normal and constricted airway.

TABLE 19–1 VITAMINS AND THE BODY SYSTEMS

VITAMIN	DESCRIPTION
Vitamin A	Proper night vision; proper development of bones and teeth; mucous membrane and epithelial cell integrity; helps resist infection
Vitamin B	B_2 promotes healthy muscular growth; B_{12} is needed for healthy blood cell development and to prevent pernicious anemia; B_1 and B_{12} promote healthy function of nervous tissue; B_1 aids in carbohydrate metabolism, normal digestion, and appetite; niacin is necessary for fat synthesis and cellular respiration
Vitamin C	Aids in absorption of iron; promotes healing of fractures, development of teeth and bone matrix, and wound healing; ensures capillary integrity; bolsters immune system
Vitamin D	Promotes strong bones and teeth, regulates skeletal calcium reabsorption; aids in absorption of calcium and phosphorus from the intestinal tract; D_3 helps regulate release of parathyroid hormone
Vitamin E	Promotes muscle growth; E_1 necessary for hemolytic resistance of red blood cell membranes; helps prevent anemia for proper reproductive system functioning; current research shows that consumption from *natural* sources may reduce the risk of Parkinson's disease; further investigation is needed
Vitamin K	Needed for proper blood clotting

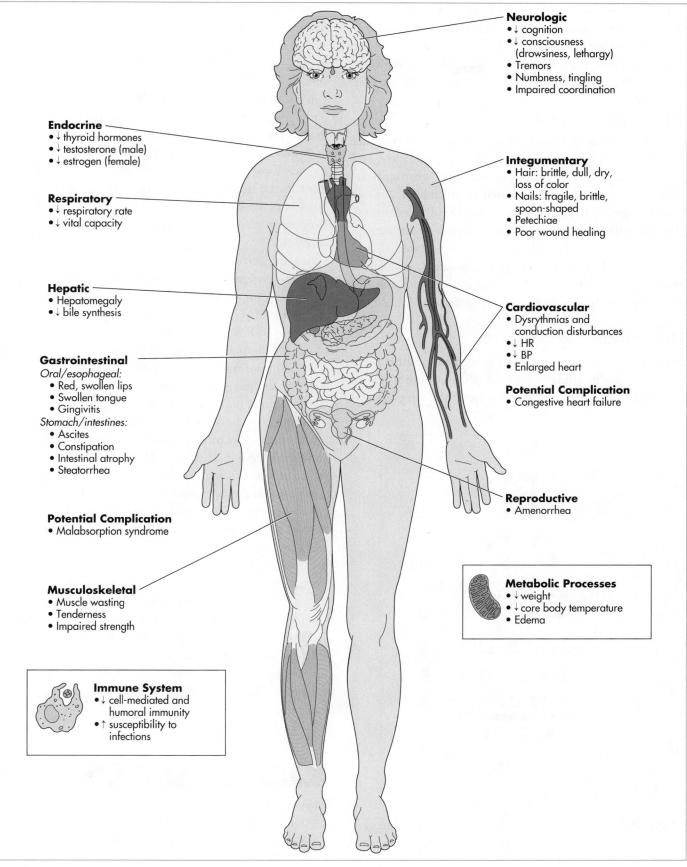

Neurologic
- ↓ cognition
- ↓ consciousness (drowsiness, lethargy)
- Tremors
- Numbness, tingling
- Impaired coordination

Endocrine
- ↓ thyroid hormones
- ↓ testosterone (male)
- ↓ estrogen (female)

Respiratory
- ↓ respiratory rate
- ↓ vital capacity

Hepatic
- Hepatomegaly
- ↓ bile synthesis

Gastrointestinal
Oral/esophageal:
- Red, swollen lips
- Swollen tongue
- Gingivitis
Stomach/intestines:
- Ascites
- Constipation
- Intestinal atrophy
- Steatorrhea

Potential Complication
- Malabsorption syndrome

Musculoskeletal
- Muscle wasting
- Tenderness
- Impaired strength

Integumentary
- Hair: brittle, dull, dry, loss of color
- Nails: fragile, brittle, spoon-shaped
- Petechiae
- Poor wound healing

Cardiovascular
- Dysrythmias and conduction disturbances
- ↓ HR
- ↓ BP
- Enlarged heart

Potential Complication
- Congestive heart failure

Reproductive
- Amenorrhea

Metabolic Processes
- ↓ weight
- ↓ core body temperature
- Edema

Immune System
- ↓ cell-mediated and humoral immunity
- ↑ susceptibility to infections

FIGURE 19–7 ■

The effects of undernourishment on the body systems.

In men, these substances diminish sperm production and lead to uncontrollable aggressive behavior. Some of these effects can be permanent even after ceasing the use of the drugs. The use of anabolic steroids is banned and is tested for in sports. See Chapter 12 for more information on steroids.

The Sensory System

Care of the sensory system includes proper diet, wearing hearing and sight protective devices when necessary, and periodic examination of the eyes and ears. Wearing hearing protection during activities that produce high levels of noise will greatly extend the functional life of your hearing. Damage to the ear is cumulative, so there is no better time to start than right now. In addition, protective eyewear should be worn any time the risk of eye injury can occur, such as in certain occupations, hobbies, and sports. FIGURE 19–8 ■ shows the Snellen eye chart for determining visual acuity.

The Immune System

Proper diet, rest, and exercise are needed for optimal functioning of the immune system. In addition, other factors can assist your immune system. One of the simplest and most effective ways to protect not only yourself but also your patients is hand washing. Always wash your hands before and after working with each of your patients. Being a staff member in a hospital or health care institution does not prevent you from carrying infectious organisms—in addition, you could be susceptible to becoming infected by hospital pathogens. Correct washing of your hands goes a long way in stopping the spread of infection.

Another way to protect yourself and others from the spread of pathogens via body fluids is to follow the Standard Precautions Guidelines (see FIGURE 19–9 ■). These guidelines are standard precautions that are to be followed for every patient with whom every health care professional interacts.

Having current immunizations is important to assist the immune system in being prepared for certain pathogens. Immunization schedules are recommended by the Centers for Disease Control and Prevention (CDC), the American Academy of Pediatrics (AAP), and the American Academy of Family Physicians (AAFP). Many individuals mistakenly believe immunizations occur only in childhood. Influenza vaccines are just one example of an immunization that is particularly important for the geriatric population.

Another important issue is the inappropriate use of antibiotics. Most infections can be handled by the body's immune system in a few days. The overuse of antibiotics has led to several critical health issues. First, many viral infections are mistakenly treated with antibacterial agents, which do nothing to the virus and cause harm to normal bacteria such as those in our intestinal system. Second, overuse does not allow the immune system of a child to properly develop and respond to future infections and can cause related disorders, such as asthma. Finally, many patients do not properly take their antibiotics. For example, they do not take the full dose for the full length of time but discontinue when they "feel better." However, often there are still surviving bacteria that are left that represent a stronger, drug-resistant strain, and they are now free to reproduce stronger drug-resistant offspring. This has led to small epidemics of drug-resistant infections.

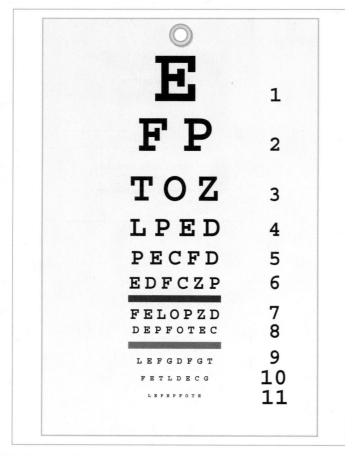

FIGURE 19–8 ■
The Snellen eye chart.

APPLIED SCIENCE

Antibiotics

The term *antibiotics* means "against life" and technically includes medications that inhibit or destroy any microorganism, including bacteria, viruses, and fungi. However, antibiotics in medicine have become associated only with antibacterial agents.

Standard Precautions Guidelines

Procedure	Wash Hands	Gloves	Gown	Mask	Eyewear
Talking to patient					
Adjusting IV fluid rate or noninvasive equipment	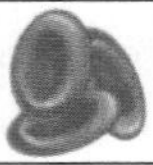 ✓				
Assess patient without touching blood, body, fluids, mucous membranes	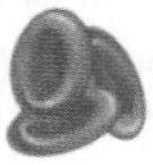 ✓				
Assess patient including contact with blood, body fluids, mucous membranes	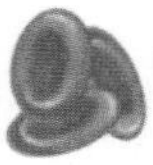 ✓	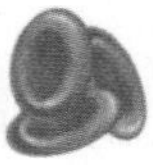 ✓			
Drawing blood	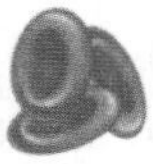 ✓	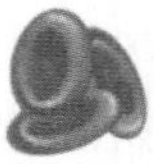 ✓			
Inserting venous access	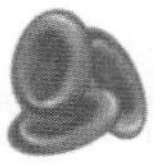 ✓	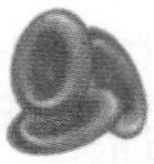 ✓			
Suctioning	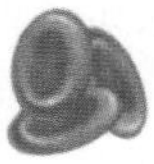 ✓	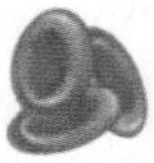 ✓	If splattering is likely	If splattering is likely	If splattering is likely
Handling soiled waste, linen, other materials	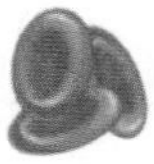 ✓	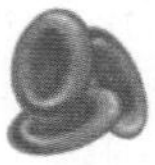 ✓	If they are extensively soiled or splattering is likely	If they are extensively soiled or splattering is likely	If they are extensively soiled or splattering is likely
Intubation	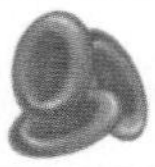 ✓	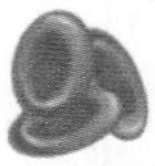 ✓	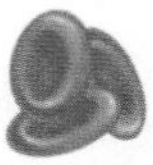 ✓	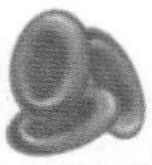 ✓	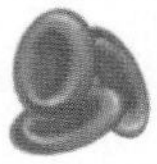 ✓
Inserting arterial access	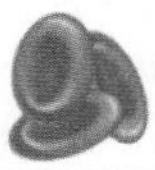 ✓	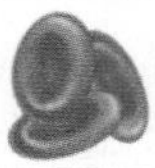 ✓	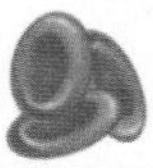 ✓	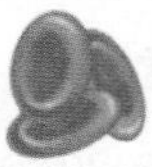 ✓	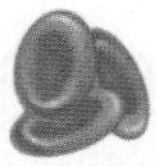 ✓
Endoscopy	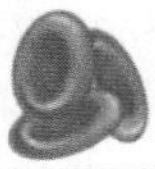 ✓	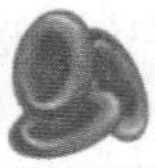 ✓	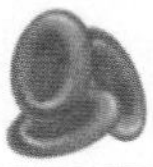 ✓	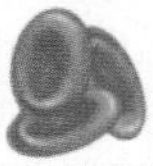 ✓	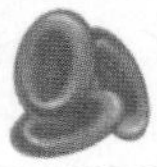 ✓
Operating and other procedures producing extensive splattering of blood or body fluids	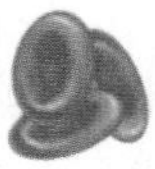 ✓	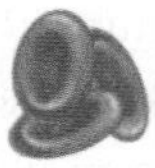 ✓	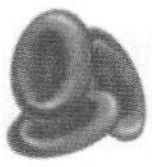 ✓	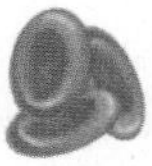 ✓	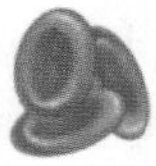 ✓

FIGURE 19–9 ■

Standard precaution guidelines. Additional guidelines/protocols may be utilized depending on the pathogen type and route of transmission as in the case of the *Ebola* virus.

Clinical Application

AGE- AND ACTIVITY-RELATED DIETS AND NUTRITIONAL NEEDS

At some time in our educational careers, we have seen the old food pyramid, which told us what portion of our diet should be dairy, what portion should be vegetables, and so forth. One of the problems with this pyramid was that it was designed to fit *everyone*. Unfortunately, not everyone is the same sex, height, shape, or age, nor has the same level of activity. In 2011, the USDA unveiled http://myplate.gov, which is meant to be a teaching tool for young children but also serves for adults to give a general recommendation for the amounts of various food groups to consume with each meal (see **FIGURE 19–10** ■).

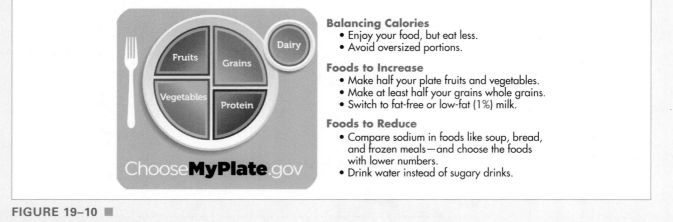

Balancing Calories
• Enjoy your food, but eat less.
• Avoid oversized portions.

Foods to Increase
• Make half your plate fruits and vegetables.
• Make at least half your grains whole grains.
• Switch to fat-free or low-fat (1%) milk.

Foods to Reduce
• Compare sodium in foods like soup, bread, and frozen meals—and choose the foods with lower numbers.
• Drink water instead of sugary drinks.

FIGURE 19–10 ■
MyPlate. (Source: U.S. Department of Agriculture.)

The Reproductive System

Don't smoke! Smoking mothers tend to have babies of lower birth weights, premature births, and a higher rate of SIDS (sudden infant death syndrome). And while we're talking about babies and children, don't forget about the hazards of secondhand smoke in the home. In homes that have at least one smoking parent, kids have slower than normal lung development and are predisposed to increased incidences of bronchitis, asthma, and ear infections (otitis media).

Diet

As the old saying goes, when you are pregnant you are eating for two. This doesn't mean that mom should pig out at every chance she gets. What it means is that diets should be followed that provide important vitamins, minerals, and nutrients for the developing fetus and to maintain the health of the mother. Think about it. If the diet is lacking in calcium, where does the fetus get calcium for bone development? It has to take it from the bones and teeth of the mother, thus decreasing the integrity of her systems. The congenital condition of **spina bifida** can be prevented by a dietary supplement of a member of the vitamin B complex, folic acid. The elimination of alcohol during pregnancy is also important to ensure the best chances of normal spinal cord and nervous system development.

Sexually Transmitted Diseases

Sexually transmitted diseases (STDs) are a growing problem and can have serious effects on the reproductive system and lethal effects on the body. Sometimes called *sexually transmitted infections (STIs)*, these are various types of pathogenic organisms that can be transmitted through unprotected sex (including oral sex). See TABLE 19–2 ■ for a list of STDs.

TABLE 19–2 SEXUALLY TRANSMITTED DISEASES

DISEASE	ORGANISM	SYMPTOMS
Herpes	Herpes simplex virus 2	Male: fluid-filled vesicles on penis
		Female: blisters in and around vagina
Gonorrhea	Neisseria gonorrhoeae	Male: purulent discharge from urethra, dysuria, and urinary frequency
		Female: purulent vaginal discharge, dysuria, urinary frequency, abnormal menstrual bleeding, abdominal tenderness; can lead to sterility
Chlamydia	Chlamydia trachomatis	May be asymptomatic
		Male: mucopurulent discharge from penis, burning and itching in genital area, dysuria, swollen testes; can lead to sterility
		Female: mucopurulent discharge from vagina, inflamed bladder, pelvic pain, inflamed cervix; can lead to sterility
Syphilis	Treponema pallidum	Systemic disease that can lead to lesions, lymph node enlargement, nervous system degradation, chancre sores
Genital warts	Human papilloma virus (HPV)	Cauliflowerlike growths on penis and vagina, some strains have been implicated in the development of cervical cancer

FOCUS ON PROFESSIONS

The **physician assistant (PA)** is trained in the diagnosis and treatment of all the body systems. To learn more about this profession, visit the websites of national associations, including the American Academy of Physician Assistants (AAPA) and the Association of Family Practice Physician Assistants (AFPPA).

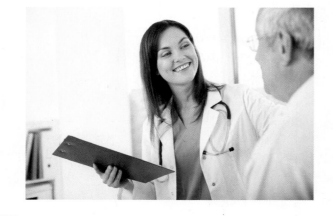

CANCER PREVENTION AND TREATMENT

All the body systems can be ravaged by cancer. Cancer is the runaway reproduction and spreading of abnormal cells and is a very complicated disorder. Each type of cancer, named for the location or the type of cells that are running amok (for example, colon cancer, prostate cancer, squamous cell carcinoma), has its own unique characteristics. However, in the past few years, medical science has learned a number of things about cancer that have made great improvements in cancer prevention and treatment.

Any number of triggers can make a cell cancerous, including genes, radiation, sunlight exposure, smoking, fatty foods, viruses, and chemical exposure. Some of these triggers, such as genes or some viruses, are difficult to avoid. But others, such as smoking, sunlight, radiation exposure, and fatty foods, can be pretty easily avoided by eating right, avoiding smoking, and wearing sunscreen. Many types of cancer can be prevented or managed with a healthy diet and exercise. Even genetic susceptibility to cancer does not make cancer unavoidable. Testing, such as mammograms (for breast cancer), colonoscopy (for colon cancer), and Pap Tests (for cervical cancer), can improve survival by catching cancers early, before they have spread, or even allowing the removal of abnormal cells before they become cancerous.

Treatments for cancer typically involve removal of the cancerous cells, if possible, and some form of treatment to kill any cells remaining in the body. *Chemotherapy* is the treatment of cancer with chemicals that kill rapidly dividing cells. *Radiation* uses energy waves to shrink tumors. Biological agents or immunotherapy targets the cancer by manipulating the immune system to hunt down and kill the cancer cells. New treatments are constantly under development to treat cancers that are difficult to fight. Research has made great strides in the treatment of cancer.

One of the deadliest forms of skin cancer is *melanoma*. It is formed by the runaway reproduction of melanocytes, the pigment-forming cells of the skin. People at the highest risk of melanoma are those with fair skin and light-colored eyes or hair, who have been exposed to lots of sun during their lifetime. However, new evidence indicates that even people who tan easily may develop melanoma if they get excessive sun exposure. Melanoma risk is higher for those living near the equator, but people in the northern parts of the United States are not without risk. Exposure to sunlight, particularly sunburns, is the key risk factor for melanoma. Genetic factors are involved in some cases of melanoma.

Melanoma can be easily prevented by decreasing exposure to ultraviolet (UV) light. Aside from staying indoors all the time, which isn't very practical, SPF sunscreen, limited sun exposure, and wearing protective clothing are the best ways to protect your skin from melanoma. Individuals at risk should have a skin screening on a regular basis.

Standard treatment for melanoma in early stages (stage I, no spread) has been the "watch and wait" approach. The melanoma is removed, and the patient is monitored for several years. Patients with more advanced melanomas often have lymph nodes sampled and removed to prevent further spread. This more extensive surgery was deemed unnecessary for patients in very early-stage disease. However, many studies have shown that even patients with no obvious spread of their cancer benefit from having lymph nodes sampled and removed if they contain cancer cells. Patients who had the procedure, called a *sentinel lymph node mapping and biopsy*, were 26 percent less likely to have their cancer return within 5 years than patients who only had the tumor removed. See **FIGURE 19–11** ■ for the possible causes and warning signs of cancer.

TEST YOUR KNOWLEDGE 19–3

Choose the best answer:

1. This vitamin is needed for proper blood clotting:
   a. A.
   b. B.
   c. C.
   d. K.

2. The abuse of this substance can have side effects such as facial hair and deeper voices in women, kidney and liver damage, and aggressive behavior.
   a. antidepressants
   b. aspirin
   c. anabolic steroids
   d. chocolate

3. The _____ eye chart is used to determine normal vision.
   a. Snellen
   b. Seymour
   c. See Clear
   d. Optical

4. The guidelines that help prevent the spread of disease by contact with body fluids are the
   a. barrier reef.
   b. splash guard.
   c. standard precautions.
   d. body shield.

5. Cancer is
   a. an abnormal growth of cells.
   b. an infection.
   c. a mainly genetic disease.
   d. caused mainly by behavior.

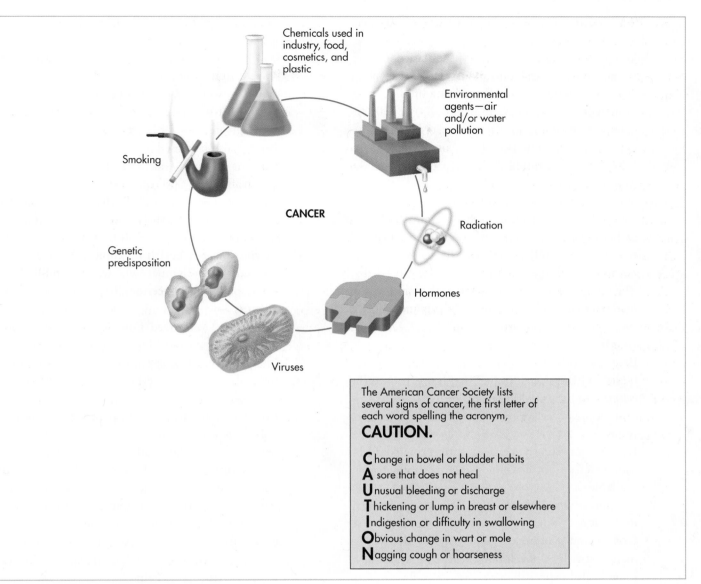

FIGURE 19–11 ■

Possible causes and warning signs of cancer.

MORE AMAZING FACTS

Remember those amazing facts we promised you at the beginning of the chapter? True to our word, here is a list of a few to amaze your friends and family.

- Senior citizens are more prone to food poisoning not only because of decreases in their senses of smell and taste but also because their digestive juices are not as acidic as they used to be and so cannot always efficiently destroy all the food-borne pathogens they ingest.
- Nerve impulses can travel up to 426 feet per second.
- Approximately 480,000 people die in the United States annually because of smoking-related diseases.

That is about equivalent to a jumbo jet full of passengers crashing *each day with no survivors*.

- On average, a healthy kidney filters about *180 quarts of fluid* every day. What makes this amazing is that the kidney is only about 4 inches long, 2 inches wide, and 1 inch thick.
- Hair grows about a quarter inch each month and grows faster during the day than at night. Hair also grows faster in the summer than in the winter.
- You use a little over half a pint of oxygen each minute when you are at rest.
- Everyone has one nare (nostril) that is larger than the other. If you don't believe it, take a look at people next time you go out to the mall or out to eat.

- Talk about a busy worker! Your heart beats over *36 million* times a year.
- You possess over *16,000 miles* of capillaries.
- Because viruses are continuously mutating, your immunity to influenza will not last a lifetime.
- More hair facts: You have from 110,000 to 150,000 hairs just on your head. Each strand of hair can support approximately 100 grams of weight, so, at least in theory, a full head of hair could support the weight of two African elephants.
- Vitamins, natural or in pill form, which is best? Research appears to indicate that vitamins and minerals from natural food sources are better utilized than synthetic pills. But the pills are better than nothing if your diet can't provide what is needed.
- The horns of a bull are composed of the same type of material that makes up your fingernails and toenails.
- You have about a quarter million sweat glands on your feet.
- Based on current research on the life span of fibroblasts and their doubling ability, humans have the *potential* to live to 120 years of age.
- Your eyes can see approximately 7 *million* shades of color.
- Due to its naturally sterile nature, urine could be used to clean out a wound when no antiseptic is available.
- The ability to roll your tongue into a tube is inherited, not everyone can do it (or cares to do it).
- Cavities and poor oral hygiene can contribute to an increased risk of developing heart disease. In fact, some health experts believe that daily flossing can add 6.4 years to your life. That's because bacteria that grow in the mouth of an individual with poor oral hygiene can escape into the bloodstream and travel throughout the body, causing problems. As a result, in worst-case scenarios, that individual may be at a 4 times greater risk for stroke and at a 14 times greater risk for heart attack. The risk for diabetes is also increased.
- Current research indicates that stomach cancer, which affects 33,000 Americans annually, may originate from bone marrow cells that enter the stomach to repair damage to the stomach lining.
- Walking uphill or downhill may make a difference in your desired health outcomes. A recent study showed that individuals who walked uphill cleared fats (especially triglycerides) from their blood faster, whereas downhill hiking reduced blood sugars more readily and improved glucose tolerance. Hiking either way removed LDL, or bad cholesterol. This information may be applicable for exercise regimens for diabetics who may have trouble with aerobic exercises.
- Congenital insensitivity to pain with **anhidrosis** (CIPA) is a rare genetic disorder that affects the development of the small nerve fibers that transmit the sensations of pain, heat, and cold to the brain. There are only 84 cases known in the United States. Patients with this untreatable condition receive bruises without knowing they are hurt. Because these patients can't sense extreme cold or heat, they don't sweat. Biting through their tongue while eating is a distinct possibility.

SUMMARY: Points of Interest

- Forensic science is the application of science to law. Natural sciences (including anatomy and physiology) and social sciences are used when solving crimes.
- Not only is forensic science used to solve current mysteries but it has also been used to solve ancient mysteries.
- The uniqueness of fingerprints were written about as early as the 1600s.
- DNA fingerprinting is a form of identifying individuals from small samples of body fluid or tissues.
- The geriatric population is the fastest-growing population in the United States.
- The hallmark sign of aging is the decreased ability to maintain homeostasis.
- Our bodies don't age evenly, and certain systems age more rapidly than others.
- The loss of mental capacities is not directly related to aging until age 75, when it is still minimal unless disease is present.

- Due to changes in the gastrointestinal, renal, and hepatic systems, older patients respond differently to many medications than middle-aged or young patients.
- Polypharmacy is the use of many drugs at the same time and often is the result of seeing many specialists at the same time.
- The most important personal choice you will make is a healthy lifestyle.

- To maintain a healthy lifestyle, it is important to eat properly, exercise, manage stress, and avoid bad habits.
- Some cancers, such as skin and lung cancer, can be highly preventable. Limiting the amount and intensity of sunlight exposure and not smoking are two ways that can help prevent cancer.

CASE STUDY

Riga and Mortis Smith are suspects in the murder of their rich aunt. They are identical twins. Tissue samples taken from under the fingernails of the aunt reveal the DNA of the murderer. The police know that Riga and Mortis are identical twins and that only one of them can be the murderer because one has a rock-solid alibi with reliable witnesses—but the witnesses do not know which twin it was.

a. Will the DNA testing prove who the real murderer is?

_____

_____

b. What other crime-solving forensics can tell for sure who the real murderer is?

_____

_____

REVIEW QUESTIONS

Multiple Choice

1. The pelvic angle of the female is
   a. less than 90 degrees.
   b. 100 degrees or greater.
   c. 75 degrees.
   d. greater than 180 degrees.

2. From ages 20 to 70, there is up to a _____ percent loss of lean body mass.
   a. 10
   b. 20
   c. 30
   d. 50

3. This vitamin is needed for strong bones and teeth and calcium absorption:
   a. A.
   b. B.
   c. C.
   d. D.

4. The overuse of this classification of drugs has caused drug-resistant strains of bacteria:
   a. steroids.
   b. antibiotics.
   c. diuretics.
   d. pain killers.

5. The congenital condition of spina bifida can be prevented by the addition of what vitamin during pregnancy?
   a. A
   b. folic acid
   c. niacin
   d. K

Fill in the Blank

1. Current nutritional guide published by the U.S. Dept. of Agriculture is called _____.

2. The fat soluble vitamins are _____, _____, _____, and _____.

3. Cauliflowerlike growths on the penis and vagina are _____ _____.

4. The test for cervical cancer is called the _____ _____.

Short Answer

1. Discuss various ways to prevent skin cancer.

_____

_____

_____

_____

2. List and discuss way to prevent STDs.

_____

_____

_____

_____

3. Discuss ways to protect yourself and your patient from the spread of infection.

_____

_____

_____

4. Discuss ways that forensic science can be used in solving crimes.

_____

_____

_____

Visit our new **MyHealthProfessions Lab** to accompany *Anatomy & Physiology for Health Professions.* Here you'll find a rich collection of quizzes, case studies, and animations for deeper understanding and application.

The Study Success Companion

THE KEY TO YOUR SUCCESSFUL JOURNEY

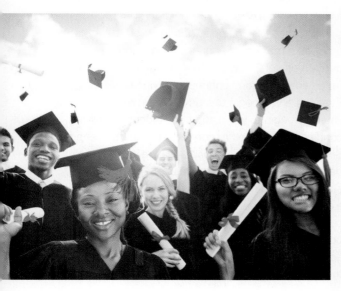

WHY USE THIS STUDY SUCCESS COMPANION?

On any journey, a well-written travel guide can make the experience positive, less stressful, and more productive. This is the main reason for including this guide along with your textbook.

Anatomy, physiology, and pathology can be tough topics to navigate, and it might feel like a very long and arduous journey. It is also a fascinating journey, though, for the human body is the vehicle in which we will all travel through life.

This guide provides effective study strategies, along with a simple and effective stress management system to help you through the rough parts of this journey and even throughout the rest of your life. In addition, this guide helps with "need-to-know" concepts, such as the metric system, that are usually not covered in an Anatomy and Physiologycourse due to time constraints. Knowing the metric system is critical because it is the mathematical language of anatomy and physiology and of medicine in general.

This *Study Success Companion* covers the following areas:

- Study skills
- Stress management
- The metric system

"The difference between ordinary and extraordinary is that little extra."

—Author unknown

STUDY SKILLS

Although you might have had courses on study skills, it can never hurt to review the fundamentals. We have chosen the top three general study skills we feel are critical, not just for this course, but for all the current and future courses you will ever take. The top three choices are:

1. Select a Good Time and Place to Study

As with any trip, there is *no* substitute for good planning and preparation. Successful preparation includes developing a daily schedule that includes proper study time. Don't be discouraged if your first few schedules don't work well; just don't forget to build in some flexibility. Be sure to schedule relaxation and recreational time, as these are important. Studies show that you learn more in three 30-minute sessions than in one marathon 2-hour session. Therefore, studying notes over shorter periods of time at more frequent intervals is more effective than long cramming sessions. We suggest using 30 to 45 minutes as your *maximum* study time without a break. A good way to check if you are studying efficiently is to periodically ask yourself questions about what you have just read. If you can't answer these questions, you probably are losing interest and need to take a short break and become more focused.

The time of day you choose to study is very important. It may not be the same time for everyone. Some people are "morning people"; others are not. The message for now is to schedule study times when you are most alert and focused.

The place you choose to study is also very important. Ideally, it should be the same place each time so that you "connect" this place to studying and consequently become focused. It should have minimal or no distractions and good lighting. The table or desk should have the needed study tools such as pen, paper, calculator, computer, and so on.

Clinical Application

CLASSICAL CONDITIONING

Throughout the text you will notice instances of the mind-body connection. The psychological term *classical conditioning* illustrates this concept and actually has an impact on study skills. The term came from an experiment performed on dogs by the Russian scientist, Ivan Pavlov. In this experiment, a bell was rung and dogs were then fed meat. The meat stimulated the dogs to salivate in anticipation of beginning the digestive process. Repeatedly, experimenters would ring a bell and feed the dogs. The dogs soon learned to connect the ringing of the bell to the arrival of meat. Eventually, the scientists only had to ring a bell and the dogs would salivate like crazy, even if they didn't receive meat.

So what's the purpose of telling you this story other than making you hungry or grossing you out? When you study in bed and then go to sleep repeatedly, you soon connect studying to sleeping. Every time you begin to study (even in mid-afternoon), you may begin to yawn and feel unfocused. You are conditioning yourself to connect studying to sleeping. Simply avoid studying in bed because you will not be as focused and therefore less effective. Besides, studying in bed may interfere with your ability to get a good night's sleep. Classical conditioning can also be used to your advantage in health care. Repeated, positive interactions and therapies with clients will "classically condition" them to feel good each time they see their health professional.

TEST YOUR KNOWLEDGE 1

Assess your current place of study by answering the following questions. Be critical and honest when you circle the response that best answers the question.

1. Do you have a dedicated study area?
   a. Sometimes
   b. Always
   c. Rarely

2. Is it quiet where you study?
   a. Sometimes
   b. Always
   c. Rarely

3. Are the conditions and lighting comfortable?
   a. Sometimes
   b. Always
   c. Rarely

4. Do you have all the tools (pencils, paper, electronic tools, etc.) you need to study at this place?
   a. Sometimes
   b. Always
   c. Rarely

Are you getting the most out of your study time?

How well did you do? For now, it doesn't matter so long as you were honest. Remember, this is an assessment of where you are now. Your eventual goal should be to have all your responses be "Always." If they are now—great! If not, you need to develop an action plan to make all the responses "Always" in the near future.

2. Use Good Study Habits

Take good, accurate, legible notes. Remember that the purpose of taking notes is to get key points from textbooks and lectures and not to write down every word that is said or written. Instead of highlighting the chapter, outline your chapters so you can make the connection from your brain to the pencil. This is what you'll need to do on the test. Outlining may *initially* take longer than highlighting, but you will learn the material better. Outlining will actually save you studying time in the long run. Review your lecture and outline notes frequently.

Also, make diagrams and pictures to help visualize concepts within your outline. The more you can "see it," the better you can understand relationships or how it all fits together. Use the website visualizations such as animations, videos, and interactive exercises to help reinforce the concepts in your mind's eye.

Anatomy and physiology are great subjects to study with a friend or study group. An excellent method to help truly learn the material is to explain concepts to each other. Each time you explain something, the oral recitation reinforces your understanding. *You'll soon learn that there is no better way to learn something than to teach it to someone else.*

APPLIED SCIENCE

How We Learn

A quick generalization of learning theory is as follows:
We learn:

10% of what we read
20% of what we hear
30% of what we see
50% of what we both see and hear
70% of what is discussed with others
80% of what we experience
95% of what we TEACH to someone else

Although some may argue the percentages, the general concepts are true to what the research on learning has shown. The more senses you can get involved in the learning process, the more internalized the learning becomes. Therefore, the text illustrations and website animations and videos enhance the learning process. Lab experiences and interactive games and exercises will also increase learning. Group or study discussions are highly beneficial and if you have to teach the group your concept, you will really learn what it is all about.

Other good study habits include taking personal responsibility for your success. Go to class and read the assigned readings *prior* to class. This will also help you to begin to develop professional responsibility skills that are crucial in health care. Because you will have properly prepared, these good study habits will greatly reduce your test anxiety. (However, it is normal to have some anxiety about taking an exam no matter how well you have prepared.)

Clinical Application

AIDING YOUR MEMORY

To succeed, it is important to truly "learn" the material and use critical thinking and problem-solving skills. One who knows how to obtain information and understand it, is much better off than someone who merely memorizes for short-term storage.

Say, for example, you memorize the steps to cardiopulmonary resuscitation (CPR) but you truly don't understand *why* you need to establish an open airway, or even *how* to actually do it. You may be able to repeat the steps on a paper-and-pencil test and receive a good grade, but what if, in six months, you are in a situation where you need to perform CPR on an individual in need? You don't want to say, "I had that six months ago and I really didn't learn the material."

Although the purpose of education is to encourage thinking skills rather than memorization, memory is vital. Memory is used as an index of success because most of the techniques used to measure learning rely on it. Therefore, a good memory is an asset that you should definitely develop. Try to memorize only when you are well rested, and use memorization techniques such as mnemonics. *Mnemonics* are words, rhymes, or formulas that aid your memory. Acronyms are one type of mnemonic. An *acronym* is a word made from the first letters of other words. For example, the ABCs of CPR remind you that **A** = establish **A**irway, **B** = rescue **B**reathing, and **C** = establish **C**irculation. This helps you to better remember the steps and their proper order in a critical situation.

You can also use rhymes or formulas to assist your memory. For example, "Spring forward, Fall back" helps us to adjust our clocks accordingly for Daylight Savings Time. You can also make up silly stories to help remember facts. In fact, the sillier the story, the easier it often is to remember.

Here are some other hints on test taking that may help further reduce the anxiety and increase your performance. First, know what type of test you are taking. With an objective exam (multiple choice, true/false) be sure you understand all directions first. With objective exams, usually your first idea about the answer is your best. If it is an essay exam (short answer), survey the questions, plan your time, and allot time to questions in proportion to their value.

Second, some people develop their own test-taking strategies. For example, they may do all the easy questions first and then return to the more difficult ones. Make sure you mark the questions you skipped or you may forget to return to them. And third, do not destroy your old exams—keep them and learn from them!

3. Take Care of Yourself

Learning requires a healthy mind, body, and attitude. It is important to exercise your brain to stay mentally fit, but it is also important to stay physically fit. A poor physical condition can distract the mind and minimize your mental focus. Eating right, exercising several times a week, and staying free of drugs will make you feel better and enhance your ability to learn. There may be times you must study when sick or tired. Begin these study sessions with slow rhythmic breathing. This can help you relax and, in turn, your concentration may improve. Remember to get sufficient rest, especially before exams. Learning to manage your stress level is so important to both your mental and physical fitness that the next section is devoted to this topic. Taking time for hobbies, music, or doing things you like to do is important to help refresh your mind.

TEST YOUR KNOWLEDGE 2

A portion of Chapter 19 is devoted to proper exercise, nutrition, and healthy living habits. Circle the answer to the following general questions and make an action plan for each "yes" answer.

1. Do you feel tired during the day when studying?
   a. Yes
   b. No

2. Do you feel stressed out when you start your study session?
   a. Yes
   b. No

3. Do you skip your exercise sessions during the week?
   a. Yes
   b. No

4. Do you eat a diet that is heavy in fats and "junk food"?
   a. Yes
   b. No

STRESS MANAGEMENT

Managing your stress is critical to your academic and personal success. Let's learn more about the concept of stress in order to better manage the stress in a positive manner.

Stress Misconceptions

The major misconception about stress is that all stress is bad for you. This is certainly not true. As you are reading this text, your body is probably in a room that is between 20 and 25 degrees Celsius. This may feel comfortable to you, but it is actually causing stress within your body. In order to survive, the body must react to this stress and make needed physiologic changes to maintain a core temperature of around 36 degrees Celsius and therefore it is continually working at a level we are not consciously aware of to adapt to an externally stressful environment. This response is vital and needed for our survival.

Here is another example of good stress: In Chapter 9, "The Nervous System," you learn about the sympathetic system and the fight-or-flight response. Picture for a moment the first time you are called on to do CPR on a cardiac arrest victim. This is going to be a stressful event in your life and may stimulate your sympathetic nervous system. Even though you practiced and trained hard, you are still uncertain of how it will be in a real life-and-death situation. This is normal. Your physical and psychological symptoms may include:

- Increased adrenalin levels for more energy to perform better
- Faster heart rate (*tachycardia*) to supply more oxygen to muscles
- Increased blood pressure to get more blood flow to the brain
- Pupil dilation to bring in more light to see better

Systems of Measurement

There are two major systems of measurement in our world today. The United States Customary System (USCS) is used in the United States and Myanmar (formerly Burma), and the System International (SI) is used everywhere else and especially in health care. The SI system is also known as the *metric system*, or the *international system*. The metric system is also the system used by drug manufacturers.

The USCS system is based on the British Imperial System and uses several different designations for the basic units of length, weight, and volume. We commonly call this the *English system*. For example, in the English system volumes can be expressed as ounces, pints, quarts, gallons, pecks, bushels, or cubic feet. Distance can be expressed in inches, feet, yards, and miles. Weights are measured in ounces, pounds, and tons. This may be the system you are most familiar with, but it is not the system of choice that is used throughout the world, nor within the medical profession. The reason is the English system is very cumbersome to use because it has no common base. It is very difficult to know the relationship between each of these units because they are not based, in an orderly fashion, according to the powers of 10 as in the metric system. For example, how many pecks are in a gallon? Just what is a peck? How many inches are in a mile? These all require extensive calculations and memorization of certain equivalent values, whereas in the metric system you simply move the decimal point the appropriate power of 10.

Most scientific and medical measurements utilize what is commonly referred to as the metric system. The metric system utilizes three basic units of measure for lengths, volume, and mass and these are the *meter, liter*, and *gram*, respectively. Although the term *mass* is commonly used for weight, weight is actually the force exerted on a body by gravity. In space, or zero gravity, all objects have mass but are indeed weightless. Since current health care is confined to earthly gravitational forces, we will use the term *weight*. TABLE 3 ■ gives you the metric designation for the three basic units of measure, along with an approximate English system comparison.

TABLE 3 METRIC AND ENGLISH SYSTEM COMPARISON

TYPE	UNIT	ENGLISH SYSTEM COMPARISON (APPROXIMATE SIZE)
Length	Meter	Slightly more than a yard
Volume	Liter	Slightly more than 1 quart
Mass/weight	Gram	About 1/40 of an ounce

Again, notice that there are only three basic types of measures (meter, liter, and gram) and the metric system has only one base unit per measure. Because the metric system is a base 10 system, prefixes are used to indicate different powers of 10. Conversion within the metric system is done by simply moving the decimal point in the appropriate direction by the power of 10 according to the prefix before the unit of measure. For example, the prefix *kilo* means 1000 ×, or 10^3. Therefore, one kilogram is equal to 1,000 grams. See TABLE 4 ■ for the common prefixes and their respective powers of 10.

It can be seen from Table 4 that a kilometer would be 1,000, or 10^3, meters. A centigram would be (.01) one-hundredth, or 10^{-2}, of a gram. Working with the metric system is easy because to change from one prefix to another you simply move the decimal point to the correct place. In other words, to convert within the system, simply move the decimal point for each power of 10 as indicated in the prefix.

Example Calculation 1

In drug dosage calculations you often need to convert between grams and milligrams and liters and milliliters. A common conversion requirement might be something like this: 500 milliliters is equal to how many liters? We know from Table 2 that 500 milliliters (mL) would be equal to 0.5 liter because we would simply move the decimal point three spaces (powers of 10) to the left for the equivalent value since we are starting with milliliters and going to the base unit of liters.

TABLE 4 COMMON PREFIXES OF THE METRIC SYSTEM

THOUSANDS	HUNDREDS	TENS	BASE UNITS	TENTH	HUNDREDTH	THOUSANDTH
Kilo	Hecto	Deca	Liter, meter, or gram	Deci	Centi	Milli
(K)	(H)	(Da)	(L) (m) (g)	(d)	(c)	(m)
10^3	10^2	10^1	10^0 or 1	10^{-1}	10^{-2}	10^{-3}

Metric Prefixes

Deci is associated with *decade*, meaning 10 years; *centi* is associated with *cents*, or a hundred cents in a dollar; and *milli* is associated with a *millipede* with a thousand legs. (Biological note: A millipede doesn't actually have a thousand legs, it just looks like it.)

Example Calculation 2

How many grams are equal to 50 kilograms? Start at kilograms on Table 4 and move to the unit you want to convert to—in this case, grams. You would need to move the decimal point three places (powers of 10) to the right to give an equivalent answer of 50,000 grams.

This knowledge of the metric system will prove invaluable to you as you work within the medical profession and even if you travel outside the United States. That is, of course, unless you go to Myanmar.

One final note before leaving this part of the discussion on the metric system: It has been determined that one cubic centimeter (cc) would hold the approximate volume of one milliliter (mL). Therefore, 1 cc = 1 mL. See **FIGURE 2** ▦. You may hear someone say you have 500 cc of an intravenous (IV) solution on hand, while someone else may say you have 500 mL of solution; either way they are both saying the same thing. Efforts are being made to standardize between cubic centimeters and milliliters, making milliliters the preferred choice. However, you will see and hear both used in health care settings.

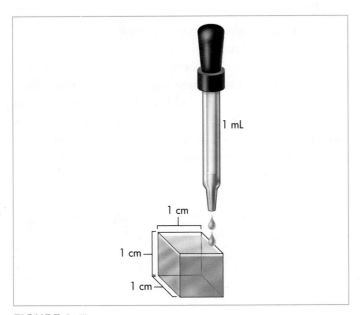

FIGURE 2 ▦

1 cc = 1 mL.

You will also note in the health care setting that decimals are always preceded by a zero if they are less than 1. For example, if you need one-half of a milligram, then it is written 0.5 mg. On the other hand, zeros are never used after whole numbers. For example, if you need five milligrams, then it is written 5 mg. This is part of the effort to reduce the number of medication errors.

Being able to convert temperatures from Fahrenheit to Celsius and from Celsius to Fahrenheit is another important conversion to know. The formulas to use are:

Fahrenheit to Celsius: $(F - 32) \times 5/9$
Celsius to Fahrenheit: $(C \times 9/5) + 32$

Check Your Work

Always check your answer to see if it makes sense. For example, a common mistake is moving the decimal point in the wrong direction. If you had done that in example calculation 1, you may have erroneously said that 500 milliliters is equal to 500,000 liters. If you visualize this you would know that 500 comparatively very small units (milliliters) in no way can equal 500,000 comparatively larger units (liters).

TEST YOUR KNOWLEDGE 3

Choose the best answer:

1. The metric system is based on the exponential power of:
   a. 100
   b. 10
   c. 2
   d. 15

2. Which of the following is *not* a basic unit of measure in the metric system?
   a. liter
   b. gram
   c. pound
   d. meter

Complete the following:

3. A cubic centimeter (cc) is equal to _____.

4. 500 grams is equal to how many kilograms?

   _____

5. 200 meters is equal to how many centimeters?

   _____

Conversion of Units

You should now be able to work comfortably within the metric system, but what if you need to take an English unit and convert it to a metric unit? For example, in the introduction of this Study Success Companion, we said that a certain drug order read to give a patient 5 milligrams per kilogram of body weight. You would need to know the relationship between pounds in the English system and kilograms in the metric system to properly treat this patient.

The following is a method for changing units or converting between the English and metric systems. This method, sometimes referred to as the *Factor-Label Method*, or *Fraction Method*, allows your starting units to cancel or divide out until you reach your desired unit. There are two basic steps:

Step One: Write down your starting value with units over 1. This places it in the form of a fraction, but since the number 1 is in the denominator, it does not change the numerical value.

Step Two: Place the starting unit in the denominator of the next fraction to divide or cancel out and place the desired unit in the numerator along with the corresponding equivalent values. Since the values are equivalent, this is the same as multiplication by 1, which does not change the value of the quantity. This allows you to treat the units as in the multiplication of fractions and "cancel" the units. Notice that by carefully placing the units so that canceling is possible, the units can be converted.

The following section shows an example of this conversion.

Example Calculation 3

How many inches are there in one mile?
First, put down what value is given as a fraction over 1.

$$\frac{1 \text{ mile}}{1}$$

Next, put miles in the denominator and the desired unit in the numerator with equivalent values. You know that 1 mile = 5,280 feet so:

$$1 \text{ mile} \times \frac{5,280 \text{ ft}}{1 \text{ mile}}$$

You've cancelled out miles, but need to go to inches. Just carry the process out until you reach your desired unit.

$$1 \text{ mile} \times \frac{5,280 \text{ ft}}{1 \text{ mile}} \times \frac{12 \text{ inches}}{1 \text{ ft}} = 63,360 \text{ inches}$$

Example Calculation 4

How many seconds are there in 8 hours?

$$\text{Step One: } \frac{8 \text{ hours}}{1}$$

$$\text{Step Two: } \frac{8 \text{ hours}}{1} \times \frac{60 \text{ minutes}}{1 \text{ hour}} \times \frac{60 \text{ seconds}}{1 \text{ minute}} \times 28,800 \text{ seconds}$$

TEST YOUR KNOWLEDGE 4

Complete the following:

1. How many days in 3 years? _____

2. How many inches in 4.5 yards? _____

3. How many quarts in 10.5 gallons? _____

Clinical Application

BODY SURFACE AREA

A 6-foot man who weighs 240 pounds may require a different dosage than a 6-foot man weighing 150 pounds. This is especially true with highly toxic agents such as those used in cancer chemotherapy. A method to determine the total body surface area (BSA) combines both height and weight in a single measurement to determine the true overall body size. Comparisons like this are called *nomograms*. See **FIGURE 3** ■ for a nomogram

used in determining BSA. Simply mark the patient's corresponding height and weight on the respective scale and either draw a straight line or use a ruler to find the intersection point to get the body surface area. Due to the poor eating habits of most Americans, the importance of BSA in relationship to the development of a form of diabetes is very important. Often, that form of diabetes may improve with simple weight loss.

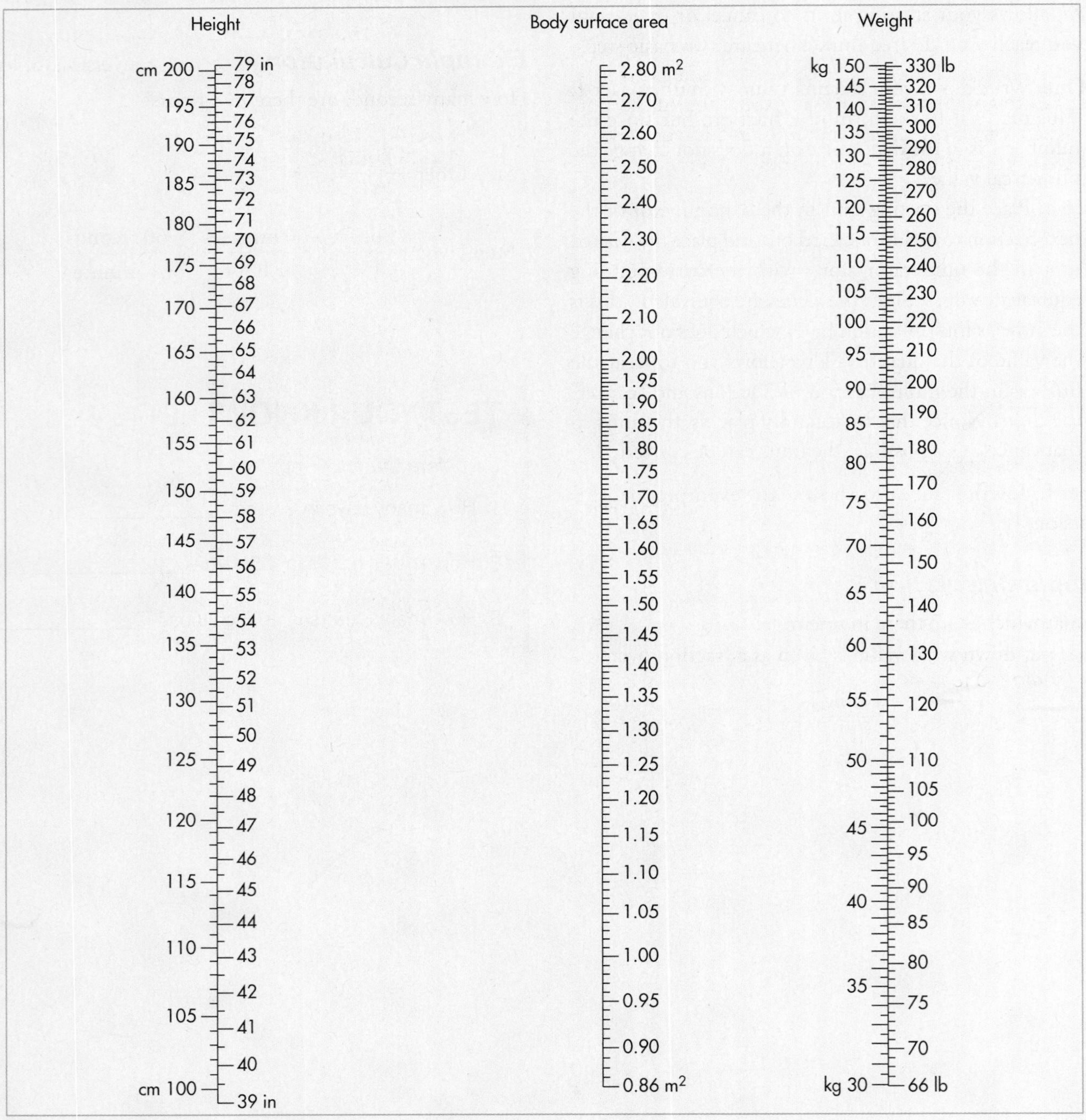

Height	Body surface area	Weight
cm 200 — 79 in 78 195 — 77 76 190 — 75 74 185 — 73 72 180 — 71 70 175 — 69 68 170 — 67 66 165 — 65 64 160 — 63 62 155 — 61 60 150 — 59 58 145 — 57 56 140 — 55 54 135 — 53 52 130 — 51 50 125 — 49 48 120 — 47 46 115 — 45 44 110 — 43 42 105 — 41 40 cm 100 — 39 in	2.80 m² 2.70 2.60 2.50 2.40 2.30 2.20 2.10 2.00 1.95 1.90 1.85 1.80 1.75 1.70 1.65 1.60 1.55 1.50 1.45 1.40 1.35 1.30 1.25 1.20 1.15 1.10 1.05 1.00 0.95 0.90 0.86 m²	kg 150 — 330 lb 145 — 320 140 — 310 135 — 300 130 — 290 — 280 125 — 270 120 — 260 115 — 250 110 — 240 105 — 230 100 — 220 95 — 210 90 — 200 — 190 85 — 180 80 — 170 75 — 160 70 — 150 65 — 140 60 — 130 55 — 120 50 — 110 — 105 45 — 100 — 95 — 90 40 — 85 — 80 35 — 75 — 70 kg 30 — 66 lb

FIGURE 3 ■

Nomogram for determining Body Surface Area (BSA).

Using the Factor Label Method for Conversion between Systems

One can attempt to memorize the hundreds of conversions between the English and metric systems, but that would be nearly impossible. All that is needed is to memorize one conversion in each of the three units of measure. This will allow a "bridging of the systems." These conversions are:

1 inch = 2.54 cm	Used for units of lengths
2.2 lbs = 1 kg	Used for units of mass or weights
1.06 qt = 1 L	Used for units of volume

Example Calculation 5

If a patient weighs 150 pounds, how many kilograms does he or she weigh? First, you must change pounds to kilograms; therefore, write the given weight as a fraction over 1. Then place the unit you want to cancel (pounds) in the denominator and the unit you want to convert to (kilograms) in the numerator of the next fraction.

$$\frac{150 \ \cancel{\text{pounds}}}{1} \times \frac{1 \ \text{kilogram}}{2.2 \ \cancel{\text{pounds}}} = 68.18 \ \text{kilograms}$$

Example Calculation 6

The conversion will not always be as direct as in the previous example, but it is no problem if you simply follow the system. For example, one foot is equal to how many centimeters? There is an equivalency somewhere for feet and centimeters, but you don't need to know that when using the Factor-Label Method and the conversion for distance.

Now, answer the question of how many centimeters are there in one foot. Remember, your unit conversion for length is 1 inch = 2.54 cm.

$$\frac{1 \ \cancel{\text{foot}}}{1} \times \frac{12 \ \cancel{\text{inches}}}{1 \ \cancel{\text{foot}}} \times \frac{2.54 \ \text{cm}}{1 \ \cancel{\text{inch}}} = 30.48 \ \text{cm}$$

TEST YOUR KNOWLEDGE 5

Choose the best answer:

1. The body surface nomogram compares what two units of measure?
   a. weight and sex
   b. height and sex
   c. surface area and length
   d. height and weight

Complete the following:

2. A quart of blood is equal to how many milliliters (mL)? _____

3. If a patient voids (passes) 3.2 liters of urine in a day, what is the amount in milliliters? _____

4. Convert 175 lbs to kilograms. _____

APPENDICES

Answers to Test Your Knowledge

Chapter 1

Page 3, 1–1
1. G
2. M
3. M
4. G
5. M

Page 7, 1–2
1. blueness of the extremities
2. one who studies the kidneys
3. enlarged cells
4. skin inflammation
5. removal of appendix
6. gastrectomy
7. osteopathy
8. electrocardiogram, EKG or ECG
9. arthritis
10. neurologist
11. NPO
12. PRN

Page 11, 1–3
1. a. vital sign
   b. not a vital sign
   c. vital sign
   d. not a vital sign
   e. not a vital sign
   f. vital sign
   g. vital sign
2. c
3. a
4. b
5. d
6. a

Chapter 2

Page 23, 2–1
1. person should be standing face forward, palms out as in Figure 2–1
2. a. prone
   b. Fowler's
   c. Fowler's
   d. supine

3. a. inferior
   b. anterior
   c. cephalic or cranial
   d. dorsal
   e. proximal
   f. internal
   g. deep
   h. central
   i. lateral
4. superficial
5. proximal; distal
6. superior
7. peripheral or pedal
8. central cyanosis

Page 26, 2–2
1. transverse or horizontal
2. anterior or ventral; posterior or dorsal
3. midsagittal
4. a. pericardial or thoracic
   b. spinal or vertebral
   c. abdominal or peritoneal
   d. thoracic or pleural
   e. pelvic
   f. cranial
5. nervous
6. magnetic

Page 32, 2–3
1. oral or buccal
2. axillary
3. umbilical
4. lumbar
5. patellar
6. liver or spleen
7. sternal

Chapter 3

Page 42, 3–1
1. atom
2. ions
3. electrolytes
4. solute; solvent
5. acidic; decrease

6. diluents

7. 1%

Page 45, 3–2

1. Biological

2. amino acids

3. lipids

4. a. hydrophilic

   b. hydrophobic

   c. hydrophobic

5. energy

Page 48, 3–3

1. b

2. a

3. c

4. removed

5. ATP

Chapter 4

Page 60, 4–1

1. diffusion

2. lower; higher

3. filtration

4. diffusion

5. facilitated diffusion

6. a. active

   b. passive

   c. passive

   d. active

   e. passive

   f. active

Page 64, 4–2

1. a. nucleus

   b. endoplasmic reticulum

   c. mitochondria

   d. Golgi bodies or Golgi apparatus

   e. flagella

   f. nucleus

   g. lysosomes

   h. cilia

Page 67, 4–3

1. b

2. a

3. c

4. d

5. d

Chapter 5

Page 80, 5–1

1. c

2. b

3. a

4. c

5. b

6. d

7. c

page 84, 5–2

1. b

2. b

3. a

4. d

5. b

6. c

7. d

Page 97, 5–3

1. respiratory

2. urinary

3. skeletal

4. nervous and sensory system

5. immune/lymphatic

6. cardiovascular

7. digestive or gastrointestinal

8. integumentary

9. reproductive

Chapter 6

Page 105, 6–1

1.

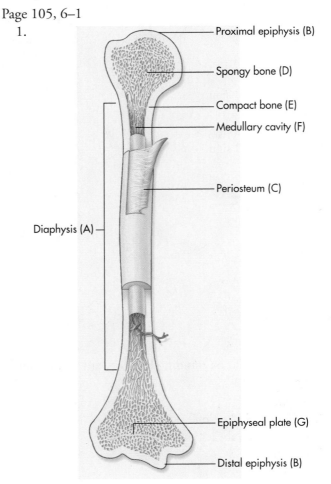

Proximal epiphysis (B)

Spongy bone (D)

Compact bone (E)

Medullary cavity (F)

Periosteum (C)

Diaphysis (A)

Epiphyseal plate (G)

Distal epiphysis (B)

2. Found in the skull, clavicle, vertebrae of the spinal column, sternum, ribs, pelvis, and the epiphysis of the long bones and is needed for the production of red blood cells.

3. Provides support and allows for movement, protects organs, produces red blood cells, and acts as storage for minerals and fats.

4. b
5. a
6. b

Page 109, 6–2
1. a
2. d
3. b
4. c
5. d
6. a
7. a. comminuted
   b. green stick
   c. compound

Page 113, 6–3
1. d
2. b
3. d
4. b
5. a
6. a
7. c

page 121, 6–4
1. d
2. c
3. c
4. d
5. b
6. b
7. d

Chapter 7

Page 128, 7–1
1. c
2. d
3. b
4. d
5. d

Page 133, 7–2
1. rotation
2. flexion or adduction
3. extension or abduction

4. agonist or primary mover
5. point of origin
6. kinesiology

Page 137, 7–3
1. actin
2. calcium and ATP
3. sarcomere
4. acetylcholine (ACh)
5. myosin; actin
6. acetylcholine (ACh)

Page 139, 7–4
1. hamstrings
2. quadriceps; pelvis; patella and tibia
3. sternocleidomastoid
4. gastrocnemius
5. biceps brachii; triceps brachii
6. hamstrings
7. vastus lateralis

Chapter 8

Page 153, 8–1
1. a. epidermis
   b. dermis (corium)
   c. subcutaneous fascia (hypodermis)
2. (any four)
   a. Protects from invasion of pathogens
   b. Keeps you from drying out
   c. Storage unit for fatty tissue
   d. Produces vitamin D
   e. Helps regulate body temperature
   f. Helps to provide sensory input
3. d
4. c
5. c
6. b

Page 160, 8–2
1. b
2. c
3. b
4. d
5. c

Chapter 9

Page 172, 9–1
1. b
2. b
3. c

4. b
5. b

Page 176, 9–2

1. c
2. b
3. b
4. a
5. b

Page 179, 9–3

1. c
2. d
3. c
4. c
5. b

page 186, 9–4

1. b
2. b
3. b
4. c
5. a

Chapter 10

Page 194, 10–1

1. d
2. c
3. d
4. c
5. c
6. b

Page 199, 10–2

1. c
2. c
3. b
4. c
5. 1. hypoglossal   e. control tongue muscles
   2. trigeminal   d. chewing
   3. vestibulocochlear b. balance
   4. olfactory   c. smell
   5. optic   a. vision

Page 203, 10–3

1. a
2. a
3. b
4. c
5. b

page 206, 10–4

1. a
2. b
3. b

4. b
5. d

Chapter 11

Page 218, 11–1

1. a
2. c
3. d
4. b
5. b
6. c

Page 223, 11–2

1. c
2. c
3. pinna
4. cerumen
5. hammer
6. incus
7. stapes
8. vertigo

Chapter 12

Page 235, 12–1

1. c
2. c
3. c
4. c
5. b
6. b

page 240, 12–2

1. c
2. a
3. b
4. a
5. a

page 243, 12–3

1. c
2. c
3. b
4. a

page 248, 12–4

1. c
2. d
3. c
4. d
5. a. type I
  b. Type II
  c. Type II

Chapter 13

Page 258, 13–1
1. d
2. d
3. d
4. left ventricle
5. right
6. tricuspid

Page 264, 13–2
1. b
2. b
3. c
4. b
5. systole; diastole
6. coronary

Page 268, 13–3
1. a
2. b
3. b
4. albumin
5. mononuclear agranulocytes
6. albumin, fibrinogen

Page 272, 13–4
1. a
2. a
3. b
4. c
5. agglutination
6. vitamin K

page 277, 13–5
1. c
2. d
3. d
4. a. tunica interna
   b. tunica media
   c. tunica externa
5. tunica media
6. inotropism

Chapter 14

Page 292, 14–1
1. d
2. a
3. c
4. c
5. d
6. olfaction; phonation

Page 296, 14–2
1. d
2. d

3. c
4. d
5. b
6. b
7. c

Page 301, 14–3
1. d
2. b
3. a
4. d
5. a
6. a
7. hemoglobin

Page 308, 14–4
1. b
2. d
3. d
4. d
5. c
6. hemopoiesis or hematopoiesis

Chapter 15

Page 319, 15–1
1. d
2. d
3. c
4. b
5. b
6. d
7. b

Page 320, 15–2
1. b
2. d
3. c
4. c

Page 325, 15–3
1. d
2. c
3. d
4. d
5. c
6. d

Page 330, 15–4
1. a
2. b
3. c
4. b

Page 335, 15–5
1. c
2. c

3. a
4. c
5. a

Chapter 16

Page 346, 16–1
1. c
2. a
3. b
4. d
5. crown; neck; root

Page 352, 16–2
1. c
2. b
3. c
4. c
5. parasympathetic/
autonomic

Page 357, 16–3
1. b
2. c
3. d
4. a
5. c

Page 360, 16–4
1. b
2. c
3. b
4. d
5. b

Chapter 17

Page 375, 17–1
1. b
2. d
3. b
4. c
5. c

Page 380, 17–2
1. a
2. b
3. a
4. d
5. b

Page 385, 17–3
1. c
2. a
3. b

4. c
5. b

Chapter 18

Page 394, 18–1
1. c
2. b
3. d
4. c
5. b

Page 398, 18–2
1. d
2. b
3. c
4. b
5. b

Page 402, 18–3
1. b
2. c
3. b
4. c
5. b

Page 405, 18–4
1. c
2. c
3. b
4. b
5. d

Page 407, 18–5
1. b
2. d
3. a
4. b

Page 410, 18–6
1. b
2. a
3. d
4. b

Chapter 19

Page 423, 19–1
1. c
2. d
3. b
4. d
5. b

Page 426, 19–2
1. d
2. c

3. b
4. a

Page 436, 19–3
  1. d
  2. c
  3. a
  4. c
  5. a

Study Success Companion

Page SS-15, 3
  1. b
  2. c

3. 1 milliliter
4. 0.5 kilogram
5. 20,000 centimeters

Page SS-16, 4
  1. 1095 days
  2. 162 inches
  3. 42 quarts

Page SS-16, 5
  1. d
  2. 943 milliliters
  3. 3200 milliliters
  4. 79.55 kilograms

Medical Terminology, Word Parts, and Singular and Plural Endings

Word Parts Arranged Alphabetically and Defined

The medical word parts that have been presented in this textbook are summarized with their definitions for quick reference. Prefixes are listed first, followed by combining forms and suffixes.

PREFIX	DEFINITION
a-	without, absence of
ab	away from
ad-	toward
an-	without, absence of
ana-	up, toward, apart
ante-	before
anti-	against, opposing
bi-	two
brady-	slow
di-	two
dia-	around, passing through
dys-	bad, abnormal
en-	within, upon, on, over
endo-	within, inner, absorbing
epi-	upon
eu-	normal, good
ex-	outside, away from
exo-	outside, away from
hemi-	one-half
homo-	same
hydro-	water
hyper-	excessive
hypo-	under, below normal
im-	not
inter-	between
intra-	within
macro-	large
meta-	after, change
micro-	small
mono-	single
multi-	many
myo-	muscle

PREFIX	DEFINITION
neo-	new
nulli-	none
ortho-	straight, normal
pan-	all, entire
para-	near, alongside; departure from normal
per-	through
peri-	around, about, surrounding
poly-	many
post-	after
pre-	before
pro-	forward, preceding
quad-	four
re-	again
sub-	beneath
sym-	together, joined
syn-	together, joined
tachy-	rapid, fast
tetra-	four
trans-	through, across, beyond
uni-	one

COMBINING FORM	DEFINITION
abdomin/o	abdomen, abdominal cavity
acou/o	hearing
acoust/o	hearing
acr/o	extremity, extreme
aden/o	gland
adren/o	adrenal gland
aer/o	air or gas
albumin/o	albumin
alveol/o	alveolus (air sac)

COMBINING FORM	DEFINITION
amni/o	amnion, amniotic fluid
amnion/o	amnion, amniotic fluid
andr/o	male
angi/o	blood vessel
ankyl/o	crooked
anter/o	front
aort/o	aorta
appendic/o	to hang onto, appendix
aque/o	water
arter/o	artery
arteri/o	artery
arthr/o	joint
astheni/o	weakness
atel/o	imperfect, incomplete
ather/o	fat
atri/o	atrium
aud/o	hearing
audi/o	hearing
aur/i	ear
aut/o	self
azot/o	urea, nitrogen
bacter/o	bacteria
balan/o	glans penis
bi/o	life
bil/i	bile
blast/o	germ, bud
blephar/o	eyelid
bronch/i	bronchus (airway)
bronch/o	bronchus (airway)
burs/o	purse or sac; bursa
calc/i	calcium
cancer/o	cancer
carcin/o	cancer
card/o	heart
cardi/o	heart
carp/o	wrist
cartil/o	gristle, cartilage
caud/o	tail
cec/o	blind intestine, cecum
cel/o	hernia, protrusion
celi/o	abdomen, abdominal cavity
cephal/o	head
cerebell/o	cerebellum (little brain)

COMBINING FORM	DEFINITION
cerebr/o	cerebrum (brain)
cerumin/o	wax
cervic/o	cervix, neck
cheil/o	lip
chir/o	hand
chol/e	bile, gall
chondr/o	cartilage
chori/o	membrane, chorion
chromat/o	color
clon/o	spasm
col/o	colon
colp/o	vagina
conjunctiv/o	to bind together, conjunctiva
cor/o	pupil
core/o	pupil
corne/o	horny, cornea
coron/o	crown, circle
cortic/o	outer covering, cortex
cost/o	rib
cran/o	skull, cranium
crani/o	skull, cranium
crin/o	to secrete
crypt/o	hidden
cutane/o	skin
cyan/o	blue
cyst/o	bladder, sac
cyt/o	cell
dacry/o	tear
dent/i	teeth
derm/o	skin
dermat/o	skin
diaphragmat/o	diaphragm
dipl/o	double
dips/o	thirst
dist/o	away
diverticul/o	small blind pouch, diverticulum
dors/o	back
duct/o	to lead or to convey
duoden/o	twelve, duodenum
dur/o	hard
ech/o	sound
electr/o	electricity
embol/o	throwing in or release of

COMBINING FORM	DEFINITION
embry/o	embryo
encephal/o	brain
endocrin/o	endocrine
enter/o	small intestine
epididym/o	epididymis
epiglott/o	epiglottis
episi/o	vulva
eryth/o	red
erythr/o	red
esophag/o	gullet, esophagus
esthesi/o	sensation
eti/o	cause (of disease)
fasci/o	fascia
femor/o	thigh
fet/i	fetus
fet/o	fetus
fibr/o	fiber
fibul/o	clasp of buckle, fibula
fovea/o	small pit
gangli/o	ganglion
gastr/o	stomach
gen/o	formation, cause, produce
ger/o	old age
geront/o	old age
gingiv/o	gums
gli/o	glue, neuroglia
glomerul/o	little ball, glomerulus
gloss/o	tongue
gluc/o	glucose, sugar
glut/o	buttock
glyc/o	glycogen, sugar
glycos/o	sugar
gravid/o	pregnancy
gravidar/o	pregnancy
gyn/o	woman
gynec/o	woman
halat/o	breath
hem/o	blood
hemat/o	blood
hepat/o	liver
hern/o	protrusion, hernia
herni/o	protrusion, hernia
heter/o	other

COMBINING FORM	DEFINITION
hidr/o	sweat
hist/o	tissue
hom/o	sameness, unchanging
hormon/o	to set in motion
hydr/o	water
hymen/o	hymen
hyster/o	uterus
idi/o	person, self
ile/o	ileum of small intestine, to roll
ili/o	flank, groin, ilium of the pelvis
immun/o	exempt; immunity
infect/o	to enter, invade
infer/o	below
inguin/o	groin
ir/o	rainbow, iris
irid/o	rainbow, iris
ischi/o	haunch, hip joint, ischium
jejnun/o	empty, jejunum
kal/i	potassium
kerat/o	hard, horny; cornea
ket/o	ketone bodies
keton/o	ketone bodies
kinesi/o	motion
kyph/o	hump
labyrinth/o	labyrinth, internal ear
lacrim/o	tear
lact/o	milk
lamin/o	thin, lamina, layer
lapar/o	abdomen, abdominal cavity
laryng/o	larynx
later/o	side
leuk/o	white
lingu/o	tongue
lip/o	fat, lipid
lith/o	stone
lob/o	lobe
lord/o	bent forward
lumb/o	loin, lower back
lymph/o	clear water or fluid
lys/o	dissolution
mal/o	bad
mamm/o	breast
mast/o	breast

COMBINING FORM	DEFINITION
meat/o	opening
medi/o	middle
megal/o	abnormally large
melan/o	dark, black
men/o	month, menstruation
mening/o	meninges, membrane
menisc/o	crescent-shaped moon, meniscus membrane
menstru/o	month, menstruation
ment/o	mind
metr/o	uterus
mon/o	one
muc/o	mucus
my/o	muscle
myc/o	fungus
myel/o	bone marrow; spinal cord; medulla; myelin
myelon/o	bone marrow; spinal cord; medulla; myelin
myring/o	membrane; eardrum
myx/o	mucus
nas/o	nose
nat/o	birth
natr/o	sodium
necr/o	death
nephr/o	kidney
neur/o	sinew or cord, nerve, fascia
noct/i	night
nucl/o	kernel, nucleus
nyct/o	night, nocturnal
nyctal/o	night, nocturnal
obstetr/o	midwife, prenatal development
ocul/o	eye
olig/o	few in number
omphal/o	umbilicus (navel)
onc/o	tumor
onych/o	nail
oophor/o	ovary
opt/o	eye, vision
opthalm/o	eye
or/o	mouth
orch/o	testis or testicle
orchi/o	testis or testicle

COMBINING FORM	DEFINITION
orchid/o	testis or testicle
orth/o	straight
oste/o	bone
ot/o	ear
ov/i	egg
ov/o	egg
ovari/o	ovary
ox/o	oxygen
palat/o	roof of mouth, palate
pancreat/o	sweetbread, pancreas
par/o	parturition or labor
parathyroid/o	parathyroid
pariet/o	wall
part/o	labor
patell/o	small pan, patella
path/o	disease
pector/o	chest
ped/o	child
pediatr/o	child
pelv/l	basin, pelvis
pen/o	penis
peps/o	digestion
perine/o	perineum
peritone/o	to stretch over, peritoneum
phag/o	eat, swallow
phalang/o	row of soldiers, fingers
pharyng/o	pharynx (throat)
phas/o	speech
phleb/o	vein
phot/o	light
physi/o	nature
plegi/o	paralysis
pleur/o	pleura
pneum/o	lung or air
pneumat/o	lung or air
pod/o	foot
polyp/o	polyp
poster/o	back
presby/o	old age
prim/i	first
proct/o	anus
prostat/o	prostate gland
proxim/o	near

COMBINING FORM	DEFINITION
pseud/o	false
psych/o	mind
pub/o	grown up
pulmon/o	lung
py/o	pus
pyel/o	pelvis (renal)
pylor/o	pylorus
quad/o	four
quadr/i	four
rachi/o	spine
radi/o	spoke of a wheel, radius
rect/o	straight, erect, rectum
ren/o	kidney
retin/o	net, retina
rhabd/o	rod
rhin/o	nose
sacr/o	sacred, sacrum
salping/o	tube: eustachian tube; fallopian tube
sarc/o	flesh, muscle
scler/o	thick, hard; sclera
scoli/o	curved
seb/o	sebum, oil
semin/o	seed
sept/o	wall, partition
sigm/o	the letter *s*, sigmoid colon
sinus/o	cavity
somat/o	body
somn/o	sleep
son/o	sound
sperm/o	seed
spermat/o	seed
sphygm/o	pulse
spin/o	spine or thorn
spir/o	breathe
splen/o	spleen
spondyl/o	vertebra
staped/o	stapes
staphyl/o	grapelike clusters (bacterium)
stasis/o	standing still
sten/o	narrowness, constriction
stern/o	chest, sternum
steth/o	chest

COMBINING FORM	DEFINITION
stomat/o	mouth
strept/o	twisted or gnarled (bacterium)
super/o	above
synov/o	binding eggs; synovial
synovi/o	binding eggs; synovial
taxi/o	reaction to a stimulus
ten/o	to stretch out; tendon
tend/o	to stretch out; tendon
tendin/o	to stretch out; tendon
test/o	testis, testicle
testicul/o	small testis, testicle
thalam/o	thalamus
therm/o	heat
thorac/o	thorax (chest)
thromb/o	clot
thym/o	wartlike, thymus gland
thyr/o	shield, thyroid
tom/o	cut, section
ton/o	tone, tension, pressure
toxic/o	poison
trache/o	trachea
trich/o	hair
tubercul/o	little mass of swelling
tympan/o	eardrum
umbilic/o	navel
ur/o	urine
ureter/o	ureter
urethr/o	urethra
urin/o	urine
uter/o	womb, uterus
uvul/o	grape, uvula
vagin/o	sheath, vagina
valvul/o	little valve
varic/o	dilated vein
vas/o	blood vessel; duct
vascul/o	little blood vessel
ven/o	vein
ventr/o	front, belly
ventricul/o	little belly or cavity, ventricle
vertebr/o	joint, vertebra
vesic/o	bladder, sac
vesicul/o	vesicle (seminal vesicle)

COMBINING FORM	DEFINITION
vitr/o	glassy
vitre/o	glassy
vulv/o	vulva
xanth/o	yellow
xer/o	dry

SUFFIX	DEFINITION
-a	singular
-ac	pertaining to
-ad	toward
-al	pertaining to
-algesia	pain
-algia	pain
-apheresis	removal
-ar	pertaining to
-ary	pertaining to
-asthenia	weakness
-atresia	closure; absence of a normal body opening
-capnia	carbon dioxide
-cele	hernia, swelling, protrusion
-centesis	surgical puncture
-clasia	break apart
-clast	break apart
-crit	separate
-cusis	hearing condition
-cyte	cell
-desis	surgical fixation, fusion
-drome	run, running
-dynia	pain
-eal	pertaining to
-ectasis	expansion, dilation
-ectomy	excision
-elle	small
-emesis	vomiting
-emetic	vomiting
-emia	blood (condition of)
-gen	formation, cause, produce
-genesis	origin, cause
-genic	pertaining to formation, causing, producing
-gram	recording
-graph	instrument for recording

SUFFIX	DEFINITION
-graphy	recording process
-hemia	blood (condition of)
-ia	diseased state (condition of)
-ial	pertaining to
-iasis	condition of
-iatry	treatment, specialty
-ic	pertaining to
-ion	pertaining to
-ior	pertaining to
-is	pertaining to
-ism	condition or disease
-ist	one who practices
-itis	inflammation
-lepsy	seizure
-logist	one who studies
-logy	study of
-lytic, -lysis	to loosen, dissolve
-malacia	softening
-meter	measuring instrument
-metry	measurement
-oid	resemblance to
-oma	abnormal swelling, tumor
-opia	vision
-opsy	view of
-osis	process or condition that is usually abnormal
-otomy	cutting into, excision
-ous	pertaining to
-oxia	oxygen
-paresis	paralysis (minor)
-pathy	disease
-penia	abnormal reduction in number, deficiency
-pepsia	digestion
-pexy	surgical fixation, suspension
-phagia	eating or swallowing
-phasia	speaking
-phil	loving, affinity for
-philia	loving, affinity for
-phobia	fear
-phonia	sound or voice
-phylaxis	protection
-physis	growth

SUFFIX	DEFINITION
-plasia	shape, formation
-plasm	something shaped
-plasty	surgical repair
-plegia	paralysis (major)
-pnea	breathing
-poiesis	formation
-practic	one who practices
-ptosis	falling downward (condition of)
-ptysis	spit out a fluid
-rrhagia	bleeding, hemorrhage
-rrhaphy	suturing
-rrhea	excessive discharge
-rrhexis	rupture
-salpinx	trumpet, fallopian tube
-sarcoma	malignant tumor
-sclerosis	hardening
-scope	viewing instrument

SUFFIX	DEFINITION
-scopy	process of viewing
-sis	state of
-some	body
-spasm	sudden, involuntary muscle contraction
-stasis	standing still
-stenosis	narrowing, constriction
-stomy	surgical creation of an opening
-tic	pertaining to
-tocia	birth, labor
-tome	cutting instrument
-tomy	incision
-tripsy	surgical crushing
-trophy	nourishment, development
-um	pertaining to
-uria	urine, urination
-y	process of

Endings in Medical Terminology

1. **Plural endings.** The following list provides a summary of plural endings that are in common use with medical terms. Examples are provided to demonstrate how these endings are applied.

ENDINGS SINGULAR	PLURAL	EXAMPLES SINGULAR	PLURAL
-a	-ae	fistula	fistulae
-ax	-aces	hemothorax	hemothoraces
-ex	-ices	cortex	cortices
-is	-es	mastoiditis	mastoidites
-ix	-ices	cicatrix	cicatrices
-ma	-mata	fibroma	fibromata
-on	-a	contusion	contusia
-um	-a	bacterium	bacteria
-us	-i	fungus	fungi
-y	-ies	episiotomy	episiotomies

2. **Adjective endings.** The following list provides a summary of suffixes that mean "pertaining to" and form an adjective (a description of a noun) when combined with a root.

ENDING	EXAMPLE	DEFINITION
-ac	cardiac	pertaining to the heart
-al	endotracheal	pertaining to within the trachea
-ar	submandibular	pertaining to below the mandible
-ary	pulmonary	pertaining to a lung
-eal	esophageal	pertaining to the esophagus

ENDING	EXAMPLE	DEFINITION
-ic	leukemic	pertaining to leukemia
-ous	fibrous	pertaining to fiber
-tic	cyanotic	pertaining to cyanotic (blue)

3. Diminutive endings. The endings listed provide the meaning of "small" to the word of origin.

ENDING	EXAMPLE	DEFINITION
-icle	ossicle	small bone
-ole	bronchiole	small bronchus (airway)
-ula	macula	small macule (spot)
-ule	pustule	small pimple

4. Diagnostic endings. The endings in this list summarize the suffixes that are in common use to indicate measurements, treatments, and procedures.

ENDING	MEANING	EXAMPLE	DEFINITION
-gram	record	bronchogram	recording of bronchus image
-graph	recording instrument	sonograph	ultrasound instrument
-graphy	process of recording	echocardiography	procedure of heart recording
-iatrics	treatment	pediatrics	treatment of children
-iatry	treatment	psychiatry	treatment of the mind
-ist	one who specializes	optometrist	specialist in eye measurement
-logist	one who studies	audiologist	one who studies hearing
-logy	study of	oncology	study of cancer
-meter	instrument of measure	spirometer	instrument measuring breathing
-metry	process of measuring	spirometry	process of measuring breathing
-scope	instrument for exam	endoscope	instrument for examination within
-scopy	examination	endoscopy	examination within

Clinical Abbreviations

Listed here are the currently *acceptable abbreviations* to use; however, different health care facilities may use others as well. The Joint Commission, which accredits and certifies over 15,000 health care organizations and programs in the United States, has created a list of abbreviations that *should not* be used because in handwritten documents or forms they may cause confusion or problems. Visit the Joint Commission website to view their Official "Do Not Use" List of Abbreviations. It is important that health care employees follow their facility policy regarding the use of medical abbreviations. With the advent and further use of electronic health records (EHR) the need for handwritten documentation, and therefore errors, should be reduced.

ABBREVIATION	MEANING	ABBREVIATION	MEANING
ABGs	arterial blood gases	ANS	autonomic nervous system
ac	before meals	ante	before
ACAT	automated computerized axial tomography	AP	anteroposterior
Acc	accommodation	APAP	acetaminophen (Tylenol)
ACL	anterior cruciate ligament	aq	aqueous (water)
ACTH	adrenocorticotropic hormone	ARC	AIDS-related complex
AD	right ear, Alzheimer's disease	ARD	acute respiratory disease
ad lib	as desired	ARDS	adult respiratory distress syndrome
ADD	attention deficit disorder	ARF	acute respiratory failure, acute renal failure
ADH	antidiuretic hormone		
ADHD	attention deficit hyperactivity disorder	ARMD	age-related macular degeneration
ADL	activities of daily living	AROM	active range of motion
AE	above elbow	AS	aortic stenosis, arteriosclerosis, left ear
AF	atrial fibrillation		
AGN	acute glomerulonephritis	ASA	aspirin
AHF	antihemophilic factor	ASCVD	arteriosclerotic cardiovascular disease
AI	artificial insemination		
AIDS	acquired immunodeficiency syndrome	ASD	atrial septal defect
		ASHD	arteriosclerotic heart disease
AK	above knee	ASL	American Sign Language
ALL	acute lymphocytic leukemia	AST	aspartate transaminase
ALS	amyotrophic lateral sclerosis	Astigm.	astigmatism
ALT	alanine transaminase	ATN	acute tubular necrosis
am, AM	morning	AU	both ears
AMI	acute myocardial infarction	AuD	doctor of audiology
AML	acute myelogenous leukemia	AV, A-V	atrioventricular
amt	amount	Ba	barium
Angio	angiography	BaE	barium enema

ABBREVIATION	MEANING
basos	basophil
BBB	bundle branch block (L for left; R for right)
BC	bone conduction
BCC	basal cell carcinoma
BDT	bone density testing
BE	barium enema, below elbow
bid	twice a day
BK	below knee
BM	bowel movement
BMR	basal metabolic rate
BMT	bone marrow transplant
BNO	bladder neck obstruction
BP	blood pressure
BPD	bipolar disorder
BPH	benign prostatic hypertrophy
bpm	beats per minute
Bronch	bronchoscopy
BS	bowel sounds
BSE	breast self-examination
BSN	bachelor of science in nursing
BUN	blood urea nitrogen
BX, bx	biopsy
$\bar{c}$	with
C	100
C1, C2, etc.	first cervical vertebra, second cervical vertebra, etc.
Ca^{2+}	calcium
CA	cancer, chronological age
CABG	coronary artery bypass graft
CAD	coronary artery disease
cap(s)	capsule(s)
CAPD	continuous ambulatory peritoneal dialysis
CAT	computerized axial tomography
cath	catheterization
CBC	complete blood count
CBD	common bile duct
CC	clean catch urine specimen, cardiac catheterization, chief complaint, chief concern
CCS	certified coding specialist
CCU	cardiac care unit, coronary care unit

ABBREVIATION	MEANING
CD4	protein on T-cell helper lymphocyte
CDH	congenital dislocation of the hip
c.gl.	correction with glasses
CGL	chronic granulocytic leukemia
chemo	chemotherapy
CHF	congestive heart failure
chol	cholesterol
Ci	Curie
CIS	carcinoma in situ
Cl^-	chloride
CLL	chronic lymphocytic leukemia
CLS	clinical laboratory scientist
CLT	clinical laboratory technician
CMA	certified medical assistant
CML	chronic myelogenous leukemia
CNA	certified nurse aide
CNIM	certification in neurophysiologic intraoperative monitoring
CNS	central nervous system
CO_2	carbon dioxide
CoA	coarctation of the aorta
COLD	chronic obstructive lung disease
COPD	chronic obstructive pulmonary disease
COTA	certified occupational therapy assistant
CP	cerebral palsy, chest pain
CPD	cephalopelvic disproportion
CPK	creatine phosphokinase
CPR	cardiopulmonary resuscitation
CRF	chronic renal failure
crit	hematocrit
CRT	certified respiratory therapist
C & S	culture and sensitivity test
CS, C-section	Cesarean section
CSD	congenital septal defect
CSF	cerebrospinal fluid
CT	computerized tomography, cytotechnologist
CTA	clear to auscultation
CTS	carpal tunnel syndrome

ABBREVIATION	MEANING
CUC	chronic ulcerative colitis
CV	cardiovascular
CVA	cerebrovascular accident
CVD	cerebrovascular disease
CVS	chorionic villus biopsy
Cx	cervix
CXR	chest x-ray
cyl lens	cylindrical lens
cysto	cystoscopic exam
D	diopter (lens strength)
D & C	dilation and curettage
D/C, d/c	discontinue
dB	decibel
DC	doctor of chiropractic
DDM	doctor of dental medicine
DDS	doctor of dental surgery
DEA	Drug Enforcement Agency
decub	lying down, decubitus ulcer
Derm, derm	dermatology
DI	diabetes insipidus, diagnostic imaging
diff	differential
dil	dilute
disc	discontinue
disp	dispense
DJD	degenerative joint disease
DM	diabetes mellitus
DO	doctor of osteopathy
DOB	date of birth
DOE	dyspnea on exertion
DPT	diphtheria, pertussis, tetanus; doctor of physical therapy
dr	dram
DRE	digital rectal exam
DSA	digital subtraction angiography
DSM-IV	*Diagnostic and Statistical Manual for Mental Disorders, Fourth Edition*
DTR	deep tendon reflex; dietetic technician, registered
DUB	dysfunctional uterine bleeding
DVA	distance visual acuity
DVT	deep vein thrombosis
Dx	diagnosis

ABBREVIATION	MEANING
E. coli	*Escherichia coli*
EBV	Epstein-Barr virus
ECC	endocervical curettage, extracorporeal circulation
ECCE	extracapsular cataract extraction
ECG	electrocardiogram
Echo	echocardiogram
ECT	electroconvulsive therapy
ED	erectile dysfunction, emergency department
EDC	estimated date of confinement
EEG	electroencephalogram, electroencephalography
EENT	eyes, ears, nose, throat
EGD	esophagogastroduodenoscopy
EHR	electronic health record
EKG	electrocardiogram
ELISA	enzyme-linked immunosorbent assay
elix	elixir
EM	emmetropia (normal vision)
EMB	endometrial biopsy
EMG	electromyogram
EMT-B	emergency medical technician-basic
EMT-I	emergency medical technician-intermediate
EMT-P	emergency medical technician-paramedic
emul	emulsion
Endo	endoscopy
ENT	ear, nose, throat
EOM	extraocular movement
eosins, eos	eosinophil
ER	emergency room
ERCP	endoscopic retrograde cholangiopancreatography
ERT	estrogen replacement therapy
ERV	expiratory reserve volume
ESR	erythrocyte sedimentation rate
ESRD	end-stage renal disease
e-stim	electrical stimulation
ESWL	extracorporeal shock-wave lithotripsy

ABBREVIATION	MEANING
et	and
ET	endotracheal
EUA	exam under anesthesia
FBS	fasting blood sugar
FDA	Federal Drug Administration
Fe	iron
FEF	forced expiratory flow
FEKG	fetal electrocardiogram
FEV	forced expiratory volume
FHR	fetal heart rate
FHT	fetal heart tone
fl	fluid
FOBT	fecal occult blood test
FRC	functional residual capacity
FS	frozen section
FSH	follicle-stimulating hormone
FTND	full-term normal delivery
FVC	forced vital capacity
Fx, FX	fracture
G_1	first pregnancy
Ga	gallium
GA	general anesthesia
GB	gallbladder
GC	gonorrhea
GERD	gastroesophageal reflux disease
GH	growth hormone
GI	gastrointestinal
gm	gram
GOT	glutamic oxaloacetic transaminase
gr	grain
grav I	first pregnancy
gt	drop
gtt	drops
GTT	glucose tolerance test
GU	genitourinary
GVHD	graft vs. host disease
GYN, gyn	gynecology
H_2O	water
HA	headache
HAV	hepatitis A virus
Hb	hemoglobin
HBOT	hyperbaric oxygen therapy

ABBREVIATION	MEANING
HBV	hepatitis B virus
HCG, hCG	human chorionic gonadotropin
HCO_3^-	bicarbonate
HCT, Hct	hematocrit
HCV	hepatitis C virus
HD	Hodgkin's disease
HDL	high-density lipoproteins
HDN	hemolytic disease of the newborn
HEENT	head, ears, eyes, nose, throat
HF	heart failure
Hgb, HGB	hemoglobin
HIV	human immunodeficiency virus
HMD	hyaline membrane disease
HNP	herniated nucleus pulposus
HPV	human papilloma virus
HRT	hormone replacement therapy
hs	hour of sleep
HSG	hysterosalpingography
HSV	*Herpes simplex* virus
HTN	hypertension
HZ	hertz
IBD	inflammatory bowel disease
IBS	irritable bowel syndrome
IC	inspiratory capacity
ICCE	intracapsular cataract cryoextraction
ICP	intracranial pressure
ICU	intensive care unit
I & D	incision and drainage
ID	intradermal
IDDM	insulin-dependent diabetes mellitus
Ig	immunoglobins (IgA, IgD, IgE, IgG, IgM)
i	one
ii	two
iii	three
IM	intramuscular
inj	injection
I & O	intake and output
IOL	intraocular lens
IOP	intraocular pressure
IPD	intermittent peritoneal dialysis

ABBREVIATION	MEANING
IPPB	intermittent positive pressure breathing
IRDS	infant respiratory distress syndrome
IRV	inspiratory reserve volume
IUD	intrauterine device
IV	intravenous
IVC	intravenous cholangiogram
IVF	*in vitro* fertilization
IVP	intravenous pyelogram
JRA	juvenile rheumatoid arthritis
JVP	jugular venous pulse
K+	potassium
kg	kilogram
KS	Kaposi's sarcoma
KUB	kidney, ureter, bladder
L	left, liter
L1, L2, etc.	first lumbar vertebra, second lumbar vertebra, etc.
LASIK	laser-assisted in-situ keratomileusis
LAT, lat	lateral
LAVH	laparoscopic-assisted vaginal hysterectomy
LBW	low birth weight
LDH	lactate dehydrogenase
LDL	low-density lipoproteins
LE	lower extremity
LGI	lower gastrointestinal series
LH	luteinizing hormone
liq	liquid
LL	left lateral
LLE	left lower extremity
LLL	left lower lobe
LLQ	left lower quadrant
LMP	last menstrual period
LP	lumbar puncture
LPN	licensed practical nurse
LUE	left upper extremity
LUL	left upper lobe
LUQ	left upper quadrant
LVAD	left ventricular assist device
LVH	left ventricular hypertrophy
lymphs	lymphocyte

ABBREVIATION	MEANING
LVN	licensed vocational nurse
mA	milliampere
MA	mental age
MAO	monoamine oxidase
MARs	Medication Administration Records
mcg	microgram
mCi	millicurie
MCV	mean corpuscular volume
MD	doctor of medicine, muscular dystrophy
mEq	milliequivalent
mets	metastases
mg	milligram
MH	marital history
MI	myocardial infarction, mitral insufficiency
mL	milliliter
MLT	medical laboratory technician
mm	millimeter
MM	malignant melanoma
mm Hg	millimeters of mercury
MMPI	Minnesota Multiphasic Personality Inventory
Mono	mononucleosis
monos	monocyte
MR	mitral regurgitation
MRA	magnetic resonance angiography
MRI	magnetic resonance imaging
MRSA	Methicillin-Resistant *Staphylococcus Aureus*
MS	mitral stenosis, multiple sclerosis, musculoskeletal
MSH	melanocyte-stimulating hormone
MSN	master of science in nursing
MT	medical technologist
MTX	methotrexate
MUA	manipulation under anesthesia
MV	minute volume
MVP	mitral valve prolapse
n & v	nausea and vomiting
Na+	sodium
NB	newborn

ABBREVIATION	MEANING
NG	nasogastric (tube)
NGU	nongonococcal urethritis
NHL	non-Hodgkin's lymphoma
NIDDM	non-insulin-dependent diabetes mellitus
NK	natural killer cells
NMR	nuclear magnetic resonance
no sub	no substitute
noc	night
non rep	do not repeat
NP	nurse practitioner
NPDL	modular, poorly differentiated lymphocytes
NPH	neutral protamine Hagedorn (insulin)
npo	nothing by mouth
NS	normal saline
NSAID	nonsteroidal anti-inflammatory drug
NSR	normal sinus rhythm
O_2	oxygen
OA	osteoarthritis
OB	obstetrics
OCD	obsessive-compulsive disorder
OCPs	oral contraceptive pills
OD	overdose, right eye, doctor of optometry
oint.	ointment
OM	otitis media
O & P	ova and parasites
Ophth.	ophthalmology
OR	operating room
ORIF	open reduction-internal fixation
Orth, ortho	orthopedics
OS	left eye
OT	occupational therapy
OTC	over the counter
Oto	otology
OTR	occupational therapist
OU	each eye
oz	ounce
$\overline{p}$	after
P	pulse
PI	first delivery

ABBREVIATION	MEANING
PA	posteroanterior, physician assistant, pernicious anemia
PAC	premature atrial contraction
PAP	Papanicolaou test, pulmonary arterial pressure
para I	first delivery
PARR	postanesthetic recovery room
PBI	protein-bound iodine
pc	after meals
PCA	patient-controlled administration
PCP	*Pneumocystis carinii* pneumonia
PCV	packed cell volume
PDA	patent ductus arteriosus
PDR	*Physician's Desk Reference*
PE tube	polyethylene tube placed in the eardrum
PEG	pneumoencephalogram, percutaneous endoscopic gastrostomy
per	with
PERRLA	pupils equal, round, react to light and accommodation
PET	positron emission tomography
PFT	pulmonary function test
pH	acidity or alkalinity
PharmD	doctor of pharmacy
PID	pelvic inflammatory disease
PKU	phenylketonuria
PM, pm	evening
PMN	polymorphonuclear neutrophil
PMP	previous menstrual period
PMS	premenstrual syndrome
PND	paroxysmal nocturnal dyspnea, postnasal drip
PNS	peripheral nervous system
po	phone order, by mouth
polys	polymorphonuclear neutrophil
PORP	partial ossicular replacement prosthesis
pp	postprandial (after meals)
PPD	purified protein derivative (tuberculin test)
preop, pre-op	preoperative
prep	preparation, prepared
PRK	photo refractive keratectomy

ABBREVIATION	MEANING
PRL	prolactin
prn	as needed
Pro-time	prothrombin time
PROM	passive range of motion
prot	protocol
PSA	prostate specific antigen
pt	pint
PT	prothrombin time, physical therapy, physical therapist
PTA	physical therapy assistant
PTC	percutaneous transhepatic cholangiography
PTCA	percutaneous transluminal coronary angioplasty
PTH	parathyroid hormone
PUD	peptic ulcer disease
PVC	premature ventricular contraction
q	every
qam	every morning
qh	every hour
qhs	during hours of sleep
qs	quantity sufficient
R	respiration, right, roentgen
Ra	radium
RA	rheumatoid arthritis
rad	radiation absorbed dose
RAI	radioactive iodine
RAIU	radioactive iodine uptake
RBC	red blood cell
RD	respiratory disease, registered dietitian
RDA	recommended daily allowance
RDH	registered dental hygienist
RDS	respiratory distress syndrome
REEGT	registered electroencephalography technologist
REM	rapid eye movement
REPT	registered evoked potential technologist
Rh⁻	Rh-negative
Rh⁺	Rh-positive
RHIA	registered health information administrator

ABBREVIATION	MEANING
RHIT	registered health information technician
RIA	radioimmunoassay
RL	right lateral
RLE	right lower extremity
RLL	right lower lobe
RLQ	right lower quadrant
RML	right mediolateral, right middle lobe
RN	registered nurse
ROM	range of motion
RP	retrograde pyelogram
RPh	registered pharmacist
RPR	rapid plasma reagin (test for syphilis)
RPSGT	registered polysomnographic technologist
RRT	registered radiologic technologist, registered respiratory therapist
RUE	right upper extremity
RUL	right upper lobe
RUQ	right upper quadrant
RV	reserve volume
Rx	take
$\bar{s}$	without
S1	first heart sound
S2	second heart sound
SA, S-A	sinoatrial
SAD	seasonal affective disorder
SAH	subarachnoid hemorrhage
SBFT	small bowel follow-through
SC, sc	subcutaneous
SCC	squamous cell carcinoma
SCI	spinal cord injury
SCIDS	severe combined immunodeficiency syndrome
Sed-rate	erythrocyte sedimentation rate
SEE-2	Signing Exact English
SG	skin graft, specific gravity
s.gl.	without correction or glasses
SGOT	serum glutamic oxaloacetic transaminase
SIDS	sudden infant death syndrome

ABBREVIATION	MEANING
Sig	label as follows/directions
SK	streptokinase
sl	under the tongue
SLE	systemic lupus erythematosus
SMAC	sequential multiple analyzer computer
SMD	senile macular degeneration
SOB	shortness of breath
sol	solution
SOM	serous otitis media
SPP	suprapubic prostatectomy
SR	erythrocyte sedimentation rate
ss	one-half
st	stage
ST	skin test, esotropia
stat, STAT	at once, immediately
STD	skin test done, sexually transmitted disease
STSG	split-thickness skin graft
subcu	subcutaneous
subq	subcutaneous
supp.	suppository
suppos	suppository
susp	suspension
syr	syrup
T	tablespoon
t	teaspoon
T & A	tonsillectomy and adenoidectomy
T1, T2, etc.	first thoracic vertebra, second thoracic vertebra, etc.
T_3	triiodothyronine
T_4	thyroxine
T_7	free thyroxine index
tab	tablet
TAH-BSO	total abdominal hysterectomy-bilateral salpingo-oophorectomy
TB	tuberculosis
tbsp	tablespoon
TENS	transcutaneous electrical nerve stimulation
TFT	thyroid function test

ABBREVIATION	MEANING
THA	total hip arthroplasty
THR	total hip replacement
TIA	transient ischemic attack
tid	three times a day
tinc	tincture
TKA	total knee arthroplasty
TKR	total knee replacement
TLC	total lung capacity
TMJ	temporomandibular joint
TNM	tumor, nodes, metastases
TO	telephone order
top	apply topically
TORP	total ossicular replacement prothesis
tPA	tissue-type plasminogen activator
TPN	total parenteral nutrition
TPR	temperature, pulse, and respiration
tr	tincture
TSH	thyroid-stimulating hormone
tsp	teaspoon
TSS	toxic shock syndrome
TUR	transurethral resection
TURP	transurethral resection of prostate
TX, Tx	traction, treatment
U/A, UA	urinalysis
UC	uterine contractions, urine culture
UE	upper extremity
UGI	upper gastrointestinal, upper gastrointestinal series
ung	ointment
URI	upper respiratory infection
US	ultrasound
UTI	urinary tract infection
UV	ultraviolet
VA	visual acuity
VC	vital capacity
VCUG	voiding cystourethrography
VD	venereal disease
VF	visual field

ABBREVIATION	MEANING
VFib	ventricular fibrillation
VLDL	very low density lipoproteins
VO	verbal order
VRE	Vancomycin-resistant entero-coccus
VS	vital signs

ABBREVIATION	MEANING
VSD	ventricular septal defect
V_T	tidal volume
VT	ventricular tachycardia
WBC	white blood cell
wt	weight
X	times

Laboratory Reference Values

Abbreviations Used in Reporting Laboratory Values

ABBREVIATION	MEANING
cm^3	cubic centimeter
cu μ	cubic microns
dL	deciliter
fL	femtoliter
g	gram
g/dL	grams per deciliter
kg	kilogram
L	liter
mol (M)	mole
mEq	milliequivalent
mg	milligram
mg/dL	milligram per deciliter
mm	millimeter
mmol	millimole
mm^3	cubic millimeter
mm Hg	millimeter of mercury
ng	nanogram
ng/dL	nanogram per deciliter
ng/mL	nanogram per milliliter
pg	picogram
U/L	units per liter
uIU/mL	units International Unit per milliliter

Hematology Tests: Normal Ranges*

Erythrocytes–Red blood cells (RBC)	Females 4.2–5.4 million/mm^3
	Males 4.6–6.2 million/mm^3
	Children 4.5–5.1 million/mm^3
Hemoglobin (HGB, Hgb)	Females 12.0–14.0 g/dL
	Males 14.0–16.0 g/dL
Hematocrit (HCT)	37.0–54%
	Females 37–47%
	Males 40–54%
Leukocytes–White Blood Cells	4500–11,000/mm^3 blood cells (WBC)

Differential (WBCs)	Neutrophils 54–62%
	Lymphocytes 20–40%
	Monocytes 2–10%
	Eosinophils 1–2%
	Basophils 0–1%
Thrombocytes–Platelets	200,000–400,000/mm^3

*These values may vary between hospital laboratories.

Hematology Tests: Coagulation Tests

Bleeding time	2.75–8.0 min
Prothrombin time (PT)	12–14 sec
Partial Thromboplastin Time (PTT)	30–45 sec

Blood Chemistries: Normal Ranges

A/G ratio	0.7–2.0 g/dL
Alanine aminotransferase	5–30 U/L (ALT, SGPT)
Albumin	3.5–5.5 g/dL
Alkaline phosphatase (ALP)	20–90 U/L
Anion gap	10–17 mEq/L
Aspartate aminotransferase	10–30 U/L (AST, SGOT)
Bilirubin	0.3–1.1 mg/dL
Blood urea nitrogen (BUN)	8–20 mg/dL
Calcium (Ca)	9.0–11.0 mg/dL
Chloride (Cl)	100–108 mmol/L
Cholesterol	<200 mg/dL
High-density lipoprotein (HDL)	>60 mg/dL
Low-density lipoprotein (LDL)	<100 mg/dL
Creatine phosphokinase (CPK)	Females 30–135 U/L
	Males 55–170 U/L
Creatinine	0.9–1.5 mg/dL
Free T$_4$	0.8–1.8 ng/dL
Globulin	1.4–4.8 g/dL
Glucose (fasting)	70–115 mg/dL
Lactate dehydrogenase (LDH)	100–190 U/L
Phosphate (PO$_4$)	3.0–4.5 mg/dL
Potassium (K)	3.5–5.0 mEq/L
Prostate specific antigen	0.0–4.0 ng/mL (PSA) Male
Sodium (Na)	136–145 mEq/L
Testosterone	241–827 ng/dL
Thyroid stimulating	0.5–6.0 uIU/mL hormone (TSH)
Thyroxine (T$_4$)	4.4–9.9 mcg/dL

Blood Chemistries: Normal Ranges (continued)

Triglycerides	<150 mg/dL
Uric acid	Females 1.5–7.0 mg/dL
	Males 2.5–8.0 mg/dL

Urinalysis: Normal Ranges

Color	yellow to amber
Turbidity (appearance)	Clear to slightly hazy
Specific gravity	1.003–1.030
Reaction (pH)	5.0–7.0
Odor	Faintly aromatic
Output	1–1.5 liters per day
Protein	Negative
Glucose	Negative
Ketones	Negative
Bilirubin	Negative
Blood	Negative
Urobilinogen	0.1–1.0
Nitrite	Negative
Leukocytes	Negative

Normal Values of Arterial Blood Gases*

pH	7.35–7.45
PaO_2	80–100 mm Hg
$PaCO_2$	35–45 mm Hg
HCO_3^-	22–26 mEq/L
O_2 saturation	95–98%

*Some normal values will vary according to the kind of test carried out in the laboratory.

Common Blood Chemistries and Examples of Disorders They Indicate

TEST	ABBREVIATION	NORMAL RANGE	EXAMPLES OF POSSIBLE DIAGNOSIS	
			RESULTS INCREASED	RESULTS DECREASED
Alkaline phosphate	ALP	30–115 mU/mL	Liver disease, bone disease, mononucleosis	Malnutrition hypothyroidism, chronic nephritis
Blood urea nitrogen	BUN	8–25 mg/dL	Kidney disease, dehydration, GI bleeding	Liver failure, malnutrition
Calcium	Ca	8.5–10.5 mg/dL	Hypercalcemia, bone metastases, Hodgkin's disease	Hypocalcemia, renal failure, pancreatitis
Chloride	Cl	96–11 mEq/L	Dehydration, eclampsia, anemia	Ulcerative colitis, burns, heat exhaustion

TEST	ABBREVIATION	NORMAL RANGE	EXAMPLES OF POSSIBLE DIAGNOSIS	
			RESULTS INCREASED	RESULTS DECREASED
Cholesterol	CHOL	120–200 mg/dL	Atherosclerosis, nephrosis, obstructive jaundice	Malabsorption, liver disease, hyperthyroidism
Creatinine	Creat	0.4–1.5 mg/dL	Chronic nephritis, muscle disease, obstruction of urinary tract	Muscular dystrophy
Globulin	Glob	1.0–3.5 g/dL	Brucellosis, rheumatoid arthritis, hepatic carcinoma	Severe burns
Glucose fasting blood sugar	FBS	70–110 mg/100 mL	Diabetes mellitus	Excess insulin
Two-hour postprandial	2-hr PPBS	140 mg/dL	Cushing syndrome, brain damage	Addison's disease, CA of pancreas
Lactic acid	LDH	100–225 mU/mL	Acute MI, acute leukemia, hepatic disease	
Potassium	K	3.5–5.5 mEq/L	Renal failure, acidosis, cell damage	Malabsorption, severe burn, diarrhea
Serum glutamic-oxaloacetic	SGOT	0–41 mU/mL	MI, liver disease, pancreatitis	Uncontrolled diabetes mellitus with acidosis
Serum glutamic pyruvic transaminase	SGPT	0–45 mU/mL	Active cirrhosis, pancreatitis, obstructive jaundice	
Sodium	Na	135–145 mEq/L	Diabetes insipidus, coma, Cushing syndrome	Severe diarrhea, severe nephritis, vomiting
Free thyroxine	T4	1–2.3 mg/dL	Thyroiditis, hyperthyroidism, Graves' disease	Goiter, myxedema, hypothyroidism
Total bilirubin	TB	0.1–1.2 mg/dL	Liver disease, hemolytic anemia, lupus erythremia	
Triglycerides	TRIG	40–170 mg/dL	Liver disease, atherosclerosis, pancreatitis	Malnutrition
Uric acid	UA	2.2–9.0 mg/dL	Renal failure, gout, leukemia, eclampsia	

Vitamins and Minerals: Sources, Function, and Effects of Deficiency and Toxicity

NUTRIENT	PRINCIPAL SOURCES	FUNCTIONS	EFFECTS OF DEFICIENCY AND TOXICITY
Vitamin A (retinol)	Fish liver oils, liver, egg yolk, butter, cream, vitamin A-fortified margarine; as carotenoids: dark green, leafy vegetables; yellow fruits; red palm oil	Photoreceptor mechanism of retina, integrity of skin	**Deficiency**: night blindness, keratomalacia, increased morbidity and mortality in young children **Toxicity**: headache, peeling of skin
Vitamin D (cholecalciferol, ergocalciferol)	Ultraviolet irradiation of the skin (main source); fortified milk (main dietary source), fish liver oils, butter, egg yolk, liver	Calcium and phosphorus absorption; resorption, mineralization, and maturation of bone	**Deficiency**: rickets (sometimes with tetany), osteomalacia **Toxicity**: anorexia, renal failure
Vitamin E group (α-tocopherol and other tocopherols)	Vegetable oil, wheat germ, leafy vegetables, egg yolk, margarine, legumes	Intracellular antioxidant, scavenger of free radicals in biologic membranes	**Deficiency**: RBC hemolysis or rupture of red blood cells, neurologic damage **Toxicity**: interference with enzymes
Vitamin K group (phylloquinone and menaquinones)	Leafy vegetables, pork, liver, vegetable oils, intestinal flora after newborn period	Formation of coagulation factors, and bone proteins	**Deficiency**: hemorrhage from deficiency of coagulation factors
Thiamine (vitamin B_1)	Dried yeast, whole grains, meat (especially pork, liver), enriched cereal products, nuts, legumes, potatoes	Carbohydrate metabolism, central and peripheral nerve cell function, heart function	**Deficiency**: beriberi (peripheral nerve degeneration), heart failure, Wernicke Korsakoff syndrome
Riboflavin (vitamin B_2)	Milk, cheese, liver, meat, eggs, enriched cereal products	Many aspects of energy and protein metabolism, integrity of mucous membranes	**Deficiency**: dry lips, mouth sores, dermatitis
Niacin (nicotinic acid, niacinamide)	Dried yeast, liver, meat, fish, legumes, whole-grain enriched cereal products	Carbohydrate metabolism	**Deficiency**: pellagra (dermatitis, swelling of the tongue, gastrointestinal and nervous system disturbance)
Vitamin B6 group (pyridoxine, pyridoxal, pyridoxamine)	Dried yeast, liver, organ meats, whole-grain cereals, fish, legumes	Many aspects of protein metabolism	**Deficiency**: convulsions, nervous system disturbance **Toxicity**: peripheral degeneration of nervous tissue
Folic acid	Fresh green leafy vegetables, fruits, organ meats, liver, dried yeast	Maturation of red blood cells	**Deficiency**: anemia, neural tube defects

NUTRIENT	PRINCIPAL SOURCES	FUNCTIONS	EFFECTS OF DEFICIENCY AND TOXICITY
Vitamin B$_{12}$ (cobalamins)	Liver, meats (especially beef, pork, organ meats), eggs, milk and milk products	Maturation of red blood cells, neural function, DNA synthesis	**Deficiency**: pernicious anemia, megaloblastic anemia
Biotin	Liver, kidney, egg yolk, yeast, cauliflower, nuts, legumes	Amino acid and fatty acid metabolism	**Deficiency**: dermatitis, swelling of the tongue
Vitamin C (ascorbic acid)	Citrus fruits, tomatoes, potatoes, cabbage, green peppers	Essential to bone tissue, collagen formation, vascular function, tissue oxygenation, and wound healing	**Deficiency**: scurvy (hemorrhages, loose teeth, gingivitis, bone disease)
Sodium	Wide distribution—beef, pork, sardines, cheese, green olives, corn bread, potato chips, sauerkraut	Acid-base balance, fluid balance, blood acidity, muscle contractility, nerve transmission	**Deficiency**: confusion, coma **Toxicity**: confusion, coma
Chloride	Wide distribution—mainly animal products but some vegetables; similar to sodium	Acid-base balance, fluid balance, blood acidity, kidney function	**Deficiency**: failure to thrive in infants hypertension **Toxicity**: increase in extracellular volume
Potassium	Wide distribution—whole and skim milk, bananas, prunes, raisins, meats	Muscle activity, nerve transmission, intracellular acid-base balance and water retention	**Deficiency**: paralysis, cardiac disturbances **Toxicity**: paralysis, cardiac disturbances
Calcium	Milk and milk products, meat, fish, eggs, cereal products, beans, fruits, vegetables	Bone and tooth formation, blood coagulation, neuro-muscular irritability, muscle contractility, myocardial conduction	**Deficiency**: long term: osteoporosis tetany, neuromuscular hyperexcitability **Toxicity**: gastrointestinal paralysis, kidney failure, psychosis
Phosphorus	Milk, cheese, meat, poultry, fish, cereals, nuts, legumes	Bone and tooth formation, acid-base balance, component of nucleic acids, energy production	**Deficiency**: irritability, weakness, blood cell disorders, gastrointestinal tract and kidney dysfunction **Toxicity**: accumulation in kidney disease
Magnesium	Green leaves, nuts, cereal grains, seafood	Bone and tooth formation, nerve conduction, muscle contraction, enzyme activation	**Deficiency**: neuromuscular irritability **Toxicity**: hypotension, respiratory failure, cardiac disturbances
Iron	Wide distribution (except dairy products)—soybean flour, beef, kidney, liver, beans, clams, peaches; heme iron in meat well absorbed (10–30%); non-heme iron in vegetables poorly absorbed (1–10%)	Hemoglobin and myoglobin formation, cytochrome enzymes, iron-sulfur proteins	**Deficiency**: anemia, decreased work performance, impaired learning ability **Toxicity**: nausea, vomiting, diarrhea, gastrointestinal damage; fatal in children
Iodine	Seafood, iodized salt, eggs, dairy products, drinking water in varying amounts	Synthesis of thyroid hormones	**Deficiency**: hypothyroid, impaired fetal growth and brain development **Toxicity**: hyperthyroidism

NUTRIENT	PRINCIPAL SOURCES	FUNCTIONS	EFFECTS OF DEFICIENCY AND TOXICITY
Fluorine	Seafood, vegetables, grains, tea, coffee, fluoridated water (sodium fluoride 1.0–2.0 ppm)	Bone and tooth formation	**Deficiency**: predisposition to dental caries, osteoporosis **Toxicity**: mottling and pitting of permanent teeth
Zinc	Meat, liver, eggs, oysters, peanuts, whole grains	Component of enzymes; skin integrity, wound healing, growth	**Deficiency**: growth retardation, small reproductive gland (testes) acrodermatitis enteropathica cause zinc deficiency
Copper	Organ meats, oysters, nuts, dried legumes, whole-grain cereals	Enzyme component, red blood cell synthesis, bone formation	**Deficiency**: anemia in malnourished children **Toxicity**: nausea, vomiting, diarrhea, brain damage
Chromium	Brewer's yeast, liver, processed meats, whole-grain cereals, spices	Promotion of glucose tolerance	**Deficiency**: impaired glucose tolerance in malnourished children, some diabetics, and some elderly persons
Selenium	Wide distribution—meats and other animal products	Functions as an antioxidant with vitamin E	**Deficiency**: rare; muscle weakness **Toxicity**: loss of hair and nails, nausea, dermatitis, polyneuritis
Manganese	Whole-grain cereals, green leafy vegetables, nuts, tea	Component of enzymes	**Primary Deficiency**: rare **Toxicity**: Rare due to occupational exposure
Molybdenum	Milk, beans, breads, cereals	Component of coenzyme	**Deficiency**: tachycardia, headache, nausea, disorientation

Sources: Data adapted from *Merck Manual*, Merck & Company, Incorporated, Whitehouse Station, NJ. 1999; *Taber's Cyclopedic Medical Dictionary*, 22nd ed. Philadelphia, PA: F. A. Davis, 2013; Roberta Pavy Ramont, Dee Maldonado Niedringhaus, and Mary Ann Towle, *Comprehensive Nursing Care*, 2nd ed. Upper Saddle River, NJ.: Pearson, 2012.

abdominopelvic cavity *(ab DOM ih no PELL vik KAV ih tee)* Continuous cavity within the abdomen and pelvis that contains the largest organs of the gastrointestinal system.

abduction *(ahb DUK shun)* Moving a body part away from the midline of the body.

abruptio placentia *(ah BRUP tee oh plah SEN shah)* The sudden, premature detachment of the placenta from the normal site of uterine implantation. It may be a partial or complete detachment.

absorption *(ab SORP shun)* Process by which digested food nutrients move through villi of the small intestine into the bloodstream or substances move from the kidney tubules into the bloodstream.

accessory muscles Muscles in the neck, chest, and abdomen that can be used to increase ventilation.

acetylcholine *(ah seet ul KOH leen)* Neurotransmitter between neurons in the brain and spinal cord, also between a neuron and a voluntary skeletal muscle (the neuromuscular junction).

acetylcholinesterase An enzyme that breaks down acetylcholine. Also referred to as AChE.

actin *(ak TIN)* The thin filament protein in muscle fibers needed for contraction.

action potential The change of the electrical charge of a nerve or muscle fiber when stimulated. Action potentials are all or none.

active transport The movement of cellular material that requires energy.

acute condition A disease process that exhibits a rapid onset of signs and symptoms.

adaptation The adjustment of an organism to changing environments.

adaptive (acquired) immunity The immune system's ability to "learn" to fight specific pathogens. This is why you get chickenpox only once and why immunizations work.

Addison's disease A relatively rare disease in which the patient exhibits a gradual and progressive failure of the adrenal glands with an insufficient production of steroid hormones.

adduction *(add DUK shun)* Moving a body part toward the midline of the body.

adenoid *(AD eh noid)* Lymphoid tissue in the superior part of the nasopharynx. Also known as the pharyngeal tonsil.

adenosine diphosphate (ADP) *(ah DEN oh sin die FOSS fate)* The compound that can be converted to ATP for energy storage. When ATP is broken down to ADP, energy is released that can be used for cellular energy.

adenosine triphosphate (ATP) *(ah DEN oh sin try FOSS fate)* Energy storage molecule used to power muscle contraction and other cellular reactions.

adrenal *(ah DREE nal)* Referring to the adrenal gland.

adrenal cortex *(ah DREE nal KOR teks)* The outermost part of the adrenal gland. It produces and secretes three groups of hormones: mineralocorticoids (aldosterone), glucocorticoids (cortisol), and some androgens (male hormones).

adrenal medulla *(ah DREE nal meh DULL lah)* The innermost part of the adrenal gland. It produces and secretes the hormones epinephrine and norepinephrine.

adventitia *(ADD ven TISH ah)* The outermost covering of a structure or organ.

afferent arterioles *(AFF er ent ahr TEE ree ohlz)* Small arteries traveling toward an organ.

agglutinate *(ah GLUE tin ate)* To clump.

agonist *(AG on ist)* The muscle that contracts while another muscle relaxes at the same time to cause movement; the primary mover.

albumin *(al BYOO men)* The most abundant plasma protein.

aldosterone *(al DOSS ter ohn)* Most abundant and biologically active of the mineralocorticoid hormones secreted by the adrenal cortex. It regulates the balance of electrolytes, keeping sodium (and water) in the blood while excreting potassium in the urine.

alimentary tract *(AL ah MEN tar ee)* Alternate name for the gastrointestinal system.

alveolar capillary membrane *(al VEE oh lahr)* The gas exchange region of the lung.

alveoli *(al VEE oh lye)* Hollow spheres of cells in the lungs where oxygen and carbon dioxide are exchanged.

amblyopia *(AM blee OH pee ah)* To prevent double vision, the brain ignores visual images from a misaligned eye (strabismus). Also known as lazy eye.

amenorrhea *(ah MEN oh REE ah)* The absence of or lack of menstruation.

amino acids The building blocks of proteins.

amnion A membranous sac that encases the fetus.

ampulla The widened area of the oviduct.

anabolic steroids A class of steroids that causes unnaturally large and rapid increases of muscle mass to enhance performance with potentially serious side effects.

anabolism *(ah NAB oh lizm)* Assembly of new molecules in the body.

analgesic nephropathy The overuse of analgesics leading to kidney damage. The severity of the damage may be enhanced with the abuse of alcohol.

anaphase The stage of mitosis and meiosis during which chromosomes move to opposite sides of the cell.

anaphylaxis Inflammation that becomes systemic, spreading throughout the whole body.

anastomosis *(ah NASS toh MOE sis)* The natural connection between two vessels. The suturing of one blood vessel to another.

anatomical position *(an ah TOM ih kal)* This is a standard position in which the body is standing erect, the head is up with the eyes looking forward, the arms are by the sides with the palms facing forward, and the legs are straight with the toes pointing forward.

anatomy *(ah NAT o mee)* The study of the structures of the human body.

anastomoses *(ah NASS toh MOE sees)* The plural form of anastomosis.

anemia *(ah NEE mee ah)* Any condition in which the number of erythrocytes in the blood is decreased.

anesthesia *(an ess THEE zee ah)* Condition in which sensation of any type, including touch, pressure, proprioception, or pain, has been prevented.

aneurysm *(AN yoo rizm)* Area of dilation and weakness in the wall of an artery. This can be congenital or where arteriosclerosis has damaged the artery. With each heartbeat, the weakened artery wall balloons outward. Aneurysms can rupture without warning. A dissecting aneurysm is one that is enlarging by tunneling between the layers of artery wall.

angiotensin-converting enzyme (ACE) *(AN jee oh TEN sin)* An enzyme made by the lungs that converts angiotensin I to angiotensin II.

angiotensinogen *(AN jee oh ten SIN oh jen)* A protein made by the liver that is converted into angiotensin I by renin.

anhidrosis *(an HIGH droe sis)* A genetic- or disease-related condition of diminished or lack of ability to sweat. This condition may be temporary or permanent and general or localized.

antagonists Something that does the opposite of the agonist, specifically a muscle which does the opposite of the prime mover.

antebrachial The area of the forearm.

antecubital The area in front of the elbow.

anterior The front of the body.

anterior commissure *(KAH mih sure)* A nerve pathway in the anterior part of the brain that allows communication between the right and left halves of the cerebrum.

antibody *(AN tee BOD ee)* Proteins secreted by B lymphocytes (plasma cells) that attack infected cells.

antibody-mediated immunity Immunity that results from a formation of antibodies in response to antigens.

antidiuretic hormone (ADH) *(AN tih dye yoo RET ick)* Hormone secreted by the posterior pituitary gland. It stimulates the kidneys to move water back into the blood to increase the volume of blood.

antigen presenting cells (APCs) Cells that engulf antigens and display them as markers.

antigens *(AN tih jenz)* Substance that causes a formation of antibodies. Cell surface markers that help the immune system identify cells.

antiseptic A substance capable of destroying microorganisms.

anus *(AY nus)* External opening of rectum. The external anal sphincter is under voluntary control. The perianal area is around the anus.

anvil One of the three small bones in the ear.

aorta The main trunk of the body's arterial portion of the cardiovascular system.

apex The rounded top of each lung and the gently rounded inferior tip of the heart.

apocrine glands *(APP oh krin)* Sweat glands found in the pubic and axillary regions that open into the hair follicles.

aponeurosis *(APP oh new ROH sis)* A flat, fibrous sheet of connective tissue that attaches muscle to bone or other tissues, or may sometimes act as a fascia.

appendicitis *(ah PEN dih SIGH tis)* Inflammation and infection of the appendix.

appendicular skeleton *(app en DIK yoo lahr)* The bones of the shoulders, arms, hips, and legs.

appendix *(ah PEN dicks)* Long, thin pouch on the exterior wall of the cecum. It contains lymphatic tissue.

aqueous humor *(AY kwee us)* Clear, watery fluid produced in the eye. It circulates through the posterior and anterior chambers and takes nutrients and oxygen to the cornea and lens.

arachnoid mater *(ah RACK noyd MAY ter)* The middle layer of the meninges, named for its weblike appearance. The space under the arachnoid mater (subarachnoid space) contains cerebrospinal fluid.

areola The darkened area that surrounds the nipple of each breast.

arrhythmia An irregular heartbeat or the loss of a heart rhythm.

arteries Blood vessels that carry blood away from the heart.

arterioles *(ahr TEE ree ohlz)* Smallest branch of an artery.

arteriosclerosis *(ar TEE ree oh skleh ROH sis)* Progressive degenerative changes that produce a narrowed, hardened artery.

arthritis *(ahr THRYE tis)* Inflammation of the joints.

articulation *(ahr TICK you LAY shun)* A joint where two bones come together and join or articulate.

artificial active immunity Vaccination. Intentional exposure to pathogens so patient makes own antibodies.

artificial passive immunity Injection of antibodies to help patient fight infection.

asexual reproduction Reproduction in which sex cells are not utilized.

association neurons Neurons that mediate the impulses between sensory and motor neurons.

asthma *(AZ mah)* Sudden onset of hyperreactivity of the bronchi and bronchioles with bronchospasm (contraction of the smooth muscle). Inflammation and swelling severely narrow the lumen of the airways.

astrocyte *(ASS troh site)* Star-shaped cell that provides structural support for neurons, connects them to capillaries, and forms the blood–brain barrier.

ataxia *(ah TAK see uh)* Lack of coordination of the muscles during movement, particularly the gait. Caused by diseases of the brain or spinal cord, cerebral palsy, or an adverse reaction to a drug.

atelectasis *(ah tell LEK tah sis)* Incomplete expansion or collapse of part or all of a lung due to mucus, tumor, or a foreign body that blocks the bronchus. The lung is said to be atelectatic. Also known as collapsed lung.

atherosclerosis *(ath er oh skleh ROH sis)* Hardening of the arteries as a result of plaque buildup in the lumen of the arteries.

atom The smallest part of an element consisting of a nucleus (composed of protons and neutrons) and surrounding electrons.

atrial natriuretic hormone (ANH) *(AY tree al NAY tree your ET ick)* Hormone released by the atria when blood pressure rises. Causes increased excretion of water by the kidney, thereby decreasing blood pressure.

atrioventricular (AV) node *(AY tree oh vehn TRIK yoo lahr)* Small formation of tissue located between the right atrium and right ventricle. The AV node is part of the conduction system of the heart and receives electrical impulses from the SA node.

atrioventricular (AV) valve The valve situated between the atrium and the ventricle.

atrium (atria) *(AY tree um, AY tree ah)* Two upper chambers of the heart. Intra-atrial structures are located within the atria.

atrophy *(AT roh fee)* Loss of muscle bulk in one or more muscles. It can be caused by malnutrition, decreased usage, or can occur in any part of the body that is paralyzed and the muscles receive no electrical impulse from the nerves.

auditory canal One of two canals that lead to the ear.

auricle *(AW rih kul)* The visible external ear. Also known as the pinna.

autocrine Cell signaling that occurs when a cell sends out a signal that affects the cell itself.

autonomic nervous system Division of the peripheral nervous system that carries nerve impulses to the heart, involuntary smooth muscles, and glands. It includes the parasympathetic nervous system (active during sleep and light activity) and the sympathetic nervous system (active during increased activity, danger, and stress).

autoregulation The ability to control blood flow as in cases of minor blood fluctuations in the kidney where the delicate filters must be protected.

autorhythmicity *(AW toh rith MIH sih tee)* The heart's ability to generate its own stimulus.

AV bundle Section of the conduction system of the heart after the AV node. It splits into the right and left bundle branches. Also called the bundle of His.

avascular *(ay VAS cue lair)* Containing no blood vessels.

axial skeleton *(AK see al SKELL eh ton)* The bones of the head, chest, and back.

axillary Pertains to the area of the armpit.

axon *(AK son)* Part of the neuron that is a single, elongated branch at the opposite end from the dendrites. It receives an electrical impulse and releases neurotransmitters into the synapse. Axons are covered by an insulating layer of myelin.

axon terminal The endpoint of an axon that an impulse reaches and then connects with a receiving cell. The space between the axon terminal and the receiving cell is called the synapse.

B lymphocytes *(B LIMF oh sights)* White blood cells that make antibodies to destroy specific pathogens.

bacilli *(bah SILL eye)* The plural form of bacillus. Rod-shaped bacteria.

bacteria *(back TEER ee ah)* Asexually reproducing pro-karyotic cells capable of creating an infection.

basal nuclei *(BAY zal NOO klee eye)* Clusters of cells (nuclei) deep in the diencephalon, midbrain, and cerebrum, which help fine-tune voluntary movements.

base The inferior region of each lung. The superior region of the heart.

basophils *(BAY soh filz)* Least numerous of the leukocytes. It is classified as a granulocyte because granules in its cyto-plasm stain dark blue to purple with basic dye. It releases histamine and heparin at the site of tissue damage.

benign *(bee NINE)* Nonmalignant.

benign prostatic hyperplasia (BPH) *(bee NINE pross TAT ik high PER play zhe uh)* A noncancerous enlargement of the prostate. This condition is the leading cause of lower urinary tract symptoms in men.

bicuspid A two-leafed or cusped structure.

blood platelets Blood cells responsible for clotting. Also known as thrombocytes.

body The midportion and largest region of the stomach.

bolus *(BOW lus)* A mass of masticated food.

botulism A potentially fatal condition caused by the toxin released by the organism, *Clostridium botulinum* that blocks the release of acetylcholine at the neuromuscular junction.

brachial artery Major artery that carries blood to the upper arm.

brain stem Most inferior part of the brain that joins with the spinal cord. It is composed of the midbrain, pons, and medulla oblongata.

breast cancer Cancer of the breast; one of the leading causes of death in women between the ages of 32 and 52.

Broca's area The region in the left hemisphere of the brain responsible for the speaking movements of the lips, tongue, and vocal cords (motor speech area).

bronchi *(BRONG kye)* Tubular air passages that branch off the trachea to the right and left and enter each lung. They carry inhaled and exhaled air to and from the lungs.

bronchioles *(BRONG kee ohlz)* Small tubular air passage-ways that branch off the bronchi. They carry inhaled and exhaled air to and from the alveoli.

bronchospasm Constriction of the airways of the lungs.

buccal *(BUCK uhl)* Pertaining to cheek or mouth region.

buccal (oral) cavity The space within the mouth.

bulbourethral gland *(BUHL boh yoo REE thral)* A part of the male reproductive system that provides mucus and an alkaline substance for the semen before it is ejaculated.

bundle of His *(HISS)* Section of the conduction system of the heart after the AV node. It splits into the right and left bundle branches. Also called the AV bundle.

bursa *(BURR sah)* Fluid-filled sac that decreases friction where a tendon rubs against a bone near a synovial joint.

calcium A metallic element needed for strong bones and teeth, blood clotting, proper nerve and muscle function, acid–base balance, and enzyme activation.

calcium ion channels Pathways that allow calcium ions to pass through.

callus A mass of tissue that forms around a break in a bone and is converted into bone in healing.

calyx cup-shaped area within the kidney around the tips of the pyramids to collect the urine that continually drains through the pyramids. Plural: calyces.

cancellous bone *(CAN cell us)* Spongy bone found in the epiphyses of long bones. Its spaces are filled with red bone marrow that makes blood cells.

canine teeth Long, pointed teeth located between the inci-sors and the premolars. The canines sink deeply into food to hold it. There are four canines, two in the maxilla and two in the mandible. Also known as cuspids (because they have one large, pointed cusp) or eyeteeth.

capillaries *(KAP ih lair eez)* Smallest blood vessels in the body. Connecting blood vessels between arterioles and venules. The exchange of oxygen, carbon dioxide, nutrients and waste takes place in the capillaries.

capillary bed A network of capillaries.

capsid *(CAP sid)* The protein covering around a virus particle.

carbohydrates A group of organic chemicals that includes sugars, starches, and glycogen that are necessary nutrients for the body. Carbohydrates are a basic source of energy.

cardiac Pertaining to the heart.

cardiac muscle Specialized, striated muscle that is found only in the heart. It makes up the walls of the heart and causes it to contract.

cardiac region Area of the stomach (closest to the heart) that surrounds the lower esophageal sphincter.

cardiology The study of the structure, function, and pathology of the cardiac (cardiovascular) system.

cardiopulmonary Pertaining to the heart and lungs.

cardiovascular system Body system that includes the heart, arteries, veins, and capillaries. It distributes blood throughout the body.

carina *(kuh RINE uh)* A structure with a projecting central ridge such as occurs at the bifurcation of the mainstem bronchi in the lung.

carotene *(CARE oh teen)* A yellow pigment found in plant and animal tissue. The precursor of vitamin A.

carpal tunnel syndrome (CTS) A painful or tingling sensation to portions of the palm, thumb, index, middle, and ring fingers mainly due to repetitive motion's effect on the median nerve distribution of the hand. It also may affect the arm and shoulder.

carpals The eight small bones of the wrist joint.

cartilage *(KAR tih lij)* Smooth, firm, but flexible connective tissue.

cartilaginous joints Joints that are held together by cartilage discs.

catabolism *(kah TA boh lizm)* Breaking down of molecules in the body.

cataract *(KAT ah rakt)* Clouding of the lens. Protein molecules in the lens begin to clump together. Caused by aging, sun exposure, eye trauma, smoking, and some medications.

cauda equina *(KAW dah EE Kwine ah)* Part of the spinal cord that consists of spinal nerves L2 through the coccygeal (Co) nerve.

caudal *(KAWD uhl)* Toward the tailbone, feet, or lower part of the body.

cecum *(SEE kum)* First part of the large intestine. A short, pouchlike area. The appendix is attached to its external wall.

cell cycle The total life of an eukaryotic cell consisting of two phases: interphase and the mitotic phase.

cell division Another term for cellular reproduction.

cell-mediated immunity Destruction of pathogens by T lymphocytes. T lymphocytes directly attack infected cells, destroying them.

cell membrane Semipermeable barrier that surrounds a cell and holds in the cytoplasm. It allows water and some nutrients to enter and waste products to leave the cell.

cellular reproduction The process of making a new cell.

cellular respiration The process by which oxygen is utilized to break down glucose and other nutrients for the energy needed for cellular activity. This process occurs at the cellular level.

cementum *(see MEN tum)* Continuous layer of bonelike connective tissue that covers the dentin layer of the tooth and roots below the gum line. It begins at the gum line where the enamel stops. It anchors one side of the periodontal ligaments.

central Refers to locations near the center of the body (torso and head).

central canal Hollow, fluid-filled space in the center of the spinal cord.

central nervous system (CNS) Division of the nervous system that includes the brain and the spinal cord.

centrioles *(SEN tree olz)* Organelles that play a role in mitosis.

centrosomes *(SEN troh soamz)* Region of cytoplasm usually near the nucleus that contains one to two centrioles.

cephalic *(seh FAHL ik)* Toward the head of the body.

cerebellum *(ser eh BELL um)* Small rounded section that is the most posterior part of the brain. Monitors muscle tone and position and coordinates new muscle movements.

cerebral palsy (CP) A general term for the nonprogressive motor-impairment conditions caused by lesions or abnormalities of the brain that occur during the early stages of development.

cerebral vascular accident (CVA) (stroke) A sudden loss of neurological function due to a decrease of blood flow to regions of the brain caused either by hemorrhage or blockage.

cerebrospinal fluid (CSF) *(SER ee broh SPY nal)* The fluid cushion that protects the brain and spinal cord from shock.

cerebrum *(ser EE brum)* The largest and most visible part of the brain. Its surface contains gyri and sulci and is divided into two hemispheres.

cerumen *(seh ROO men)* Sticky wax that traps dirt in the external auditory canal.

ceruminous glands *(seh ROO men us)* Gland that produces the waxlike substance in the ear.

cervical Pertaining to the region of the neck or to the distal portion of the uterus (cervix).

cervix *(SER viks)* The neck or the part of an organ that resembles the shape of a neck.

chemical synapse *(SIN aps)* Site of communication between neurons and other excitable cells. Neurotransmitters are released from the neuron (presynaptic cell), which travel to a muscle or gland cell (the postsynaptic cell), allowing communication between the two cells.

chief complaint (CC) The reason a patient seeks medical help; also called chief concern.

Chlamydia trachomatis *(klah MID ee ah tray KOH mah tis)* A species of a bacterial genus that is an intracellular parasite and causes genital infections in men and women. It is a sexually transmitted disease.

cholecystitis *(KOH lee sis TYE tiss)* Acute or chronic inflammation of the gallbladder because of gallstones.

cholecystokinin (CCK) *(KOH lee SIS toe KINE in)* Hormone released by the duodenum when it receives food from the stomach. It causes the gallbladder to release bile and the pancreas to release its digestive enzymes.

cholelithiasis *(KOH lee lih THY ah sis)* One or more gallstones in the gallbladder. Choledocholithiasis occurs when a gallstone becomes lodged in the common bile duct.

cholesterol Lipid-containing compound that is a component of bile (from the liver), sex hormones, neurotransmitters, and cell membranes.

chondrosarcoma *(KON droe sar KOE ma)* Cancer of the cartilage.

choroid *(KOH royd)* Spongy membrane of blood vessels that begins at the iris and continues around the eye. In the posterior cavity, it is the middle layer between the sclera and the retina.

chromatin *(CROW ma tin)* Genetic material found in the nucleus of a cell.

chronic bronchitis *(brong KYE tis)* Chronic inflammation or infection of the bronchi. Inflammation of the bronchi is due to pollution or smoking.

chronic conditions Symptoms that gradually develop from a disease process that may have been there for some time.

chronic obstructive pulmonary disease (COPD) A general term for a grouping of diseases (including chronic bronchitis and emphysema) that affects the efficiency of breathing, leading to difficulty of breathing on exertion.

chronic renal failure An ongoing, progressive kidney disease.

chyle *(KILE)* A substance similar to milk formed from digested and absorbed fats.

chyme *(KIME)* Mixed food and digestive juices in the stomach and small intestine.

cilia *(SILL ee ah)* Small hairs that flow in waves to move foreign particles away from the lungs toward the nose and the throat, where they can be expelled. Also found inside the fallopian tubes to propel an ovum toward the uterus.

ciliary muscles *(SILL ee AIR ee)* Smooth muscle that alters the lens of the eye to accommodate for near vision.

circulation The movement of blood to and from the heart.

circumduction The movement of a limb in a circle. Making arm circles is an example of circumduction.

clavicle Collarbone.

clitoris *(KLIT oh ris)* A small erectile body of the female genitalia.

closed fracture A fracture that has not broken through the skin.

clot A thrombus or coagulated blood.

coagulation The formation of a blood clot by platelets and clotting factors.

cochlea *(KOCH lee ah)* Structure of the inner ear that is associated with the sense of hearing. It relays information to the brain via the cochlear branch of the vestibulocochlear nerve.

collecting duct Common passageway that collects fluid from many nephrons. The final step of reabsorption takes place there, and the fluid is known as urine.

colon The longest part of the large intestine. It has four parts: the ascending colon, the transverse colon, the descending colon, and the S-shaped sigmoid colon.

columnar A column-shaped structure.

comminuted fracture A fracture in which the bone is broken into many pieces, shattered.

commissures *(KAHM ih shoorz)* Transverse bands of nerve fibers; carry information from one side of the nervous system to the other.

common bile duct   Duct that carries bile from both the liver and the gallbladder.

compact bone   Hard or dense bone forming the superficial layer of all bones.

complement cascade   A series of chemical reactions triggered by infection that leads to the destruction of a pathogen.

compound (open) fracture   Injury in which the broken bone pierces the skin, leaving an open wound.

conchae   *(KONG kay)* Shelflike structures inside the nasal cavity.

concussion   A mild blunt force brain injury.

cones   Light-sensitive cells in the retina that detect colored light. There are three types of cones, each of which responds to either red, green, or blue light.

congenital   A condition that was present at birth.

congenital hypothyroidism   A condition in which babies do not produce enough thyroid hormone; can cause developmental disabilities.

congestive heart failure (CHF)   Inability of the heart to pump sufficient amounts of blood. Caused by chronic coronary artery disease or hypertension.

conjunctiva   *(KON junk tih vah)* Delicate, transparent mucous membrane that covers the inside of the eyelids and the anterior surface of the eye. It produces clear, watery mucus.

conjunctivitis   *(KON JUNK tih VYE tis)* Inflamed, reddened, and swollen conjunctivae with dilated blood vessels on the sclerae. Caused by a foreign substance in the eye or an infection.

constipation   A decrease in an individual's frequency of defecation usually with a difficult or incomplete passage of stool (may be excessively hard stool).

contraception   Prevention of pregnancy.

corium   *(CORE ee um)* Layer of skin immediately under the epidermis. Also known as the true skin or dermis.

cornea   *(KOR nee ah)* Transparent layer over the anterior part of the eye. It is a continuation of the white sclera.

coronal plane   *(kor ROHN al)* Also called frontal plane; an imaginary vertical plane that divides the entire body into anterior and posterior sections. The coronal plane is named for the coronal suture where the frontal and parietal skull bones meet.

coronary arteries   Blood vessels that supply oxygen rich blood to the tissues of the heart.

corpus callosum   *(KOR pus kah LOH sum)* Thick white band of nerve fibers that connects the two hemispheres of the cerebrum and allows them to communicate and coordinate their activities.

corpus luteum   *(KOR pus LOU tee um)* Small endocrine structure that secretes progesterone and estrogen.

cortex   Outer layer of an organ including kidney, cerebrum, and adrenal gland. Layer of hair shaft between cuticle and medulla.

corticobulbar tract   *(KOR ti coe BUL bar)* Spinal cord tract that carries impulses to the brain stem from the motor cortex. Carries orders for voluntary movements.

corticospinal tract   *(KOR ti coe SPY nal)* Pertains to the tract between the cerebral cortex and spinal cord. Carries orders for voluntary movements.

countercurrent circulation   Exchange of substances between two streams on either side of a membrane. Helps control concentration of fluids as in the nephron loop.

covalent bond   *(coh VAY lent)* A molecular bond in which valence electrons are shared.

cramp   Spasmodic muscle contraction.

cranial   *(KRAY nee uhl)* Pertaining to the skull.

cranial cavity   Houses the brain.

cranial nerves   Twelve pairs of nerves that originate in the brain. Carry sensory nerve impulses to the brain from the nose, eyes, ears, and tongue for the senses of smell, vision, hearing, and taste. Carry sensory nerve impulses to the brain from the skin of the face. Carry motor nerve impulses from the brain to the muscles of the face, mouth, throat, eye, and salivary glands.

cross-sectioning   Making slices of a sample for examination purposes.

crown   White part of the tooth that is visible above the gum line.

crural   *(CRUR al)* Pertains to the leg.

cryptorchidism   *(kript OR kid izm)* A condition in which testicles fail to descend into the scrotum.

cuboidal   *(cue BOYD al)* A cube-shaped structure.

Cushing's syndrome   A condition that is the result of excessive exposure to glucocorticoid hormones, including signs of "moon face," "buffalo hump," immunosuppression, poor wound healing, thinning of skin, and muscular weakness.

cuspids   Canine teeth.

cutaneous membranes   *(cue TAY nee us)* Membranes of the skin.

cuticle Layer of dead skin that arises from the epidermis around the proximal end of the nail. It keeps microorganisms from the nail root.

cyanosis *(sigh ah NOH sis)* Bluish-gray discoloration of the skin from abnormally low levels of oxygen in the tissues.

cystic duct Duct that carries bile to and from the gallbladder.

cytokines *(SIGH toe kines)* Chemicals released by injured body tissues that summon leukocytes and cause them to move to the area.

cytokinesis *(SIGH toe kih NEE sus)* The separation of the cell's cytoplasm into two parts following the division of the cell's nucleus.

cytoplasm *(SIGH toe plazm)* Gel-like intracellular substance. Organelles are embedded in it.

cytoskeleton *(SIGH toe SKELL eh ton)* Protein rods that make up the structure of cell parts including cilia, flagella, and myofilaments.

cytotoxic T cells *(sigh toe TOX ick)* Type of T lymphocyte that matures in the thymus. Cytotoxic T cells destroy all types of pathogens as well as body cells infected with viruses.

deciduous teeth *(dee SID you us)* Teeth that erupt during childhood from age 6 months to 2 years. Also called the milk teeth, baby teeth, or primary teeth.

decubitus *(dee KYOO bih tus)* Lying-down position; on the back. Often used to refer to pressure sores caused by being in one position for too long.

deep Away from the body's surface.

defecation *(def eh CAY shun)* Process by which undigested food fiber and water are removed from the body in the form of a bowel movement.

dehydration Loss of water.

dehydration synthesis reactions Linking together small molecules to form large ones by removing water to form bonds.

denaturation The process by which proteins lose their structure by application of an external stress or compound such as strong acid or base, radiation, organic solvent, or heat.

dendrite *(DEN drite)* Multiple branches at the end of a neuron that carry information to the cell body.

dendritic cells *(DEN drit ick)* One of several types of antigen presenting cells that stimulate adaptive immunity.

dentin Hard layer of tooth just beneath the enamel layer.

deoxyribonucleic acid (DNA) *(dee AWK see RYE bow NEW klee ick)* Sequenced pairs of nucleotides that form a double helix. A segment of DNA makes up a gene.

depolarization Changing of the permeability of the cell membrane of any excitable cell, such as a cardiac muscle or a neuron, that leads to a decrease in charge across the cell membrane.

dermatology The study of skin; medical specialty treating the skin.

dermis *(DER mis)* Layer of skin under the epidermis. It is composed of collagen and elastin fibers. It contains arteries, veins, nerves, sebaceous glands, sweat glands, and hair follicles.

diabetes insipidus *(in SIP eh dus)* A condition with excessive urination due to either inadequate antidiuretic hormone or an inability of the kidney to respond to the available antidiuretic hormone.

diabetes mellitus *(mel EYE tiss)* A condition characterized by abnormally high blood glucose (hyperglycemia). Type 1 diabetes (formerly called insulin-dependent diabetes mellitus [IDDM] or juvenile onset diabetes) is caused by the destruction of the insulin-producing cells of the pancreas. Type 2 (formerly called noninsulin-dependent diabetes mellitus [NIDDM] or late onset diabetes) is caused by insensitivity of the body's tissues to insulin.

diabetic nephropathy *(neh FROP ah thee)* A type of kidney damage caused by prolonged high blood glucose.

diagnose To determine the cause of a patient's signs and symptoms.

diagnosis *(dye ig NOH sis)* A determination of the cause of the patient's symptoms and signs.

diaphragm *(DYE ah fram)* Muscular sheet that divides the thoracic cavity from the abdominal cavity. Most important ventilation muscle.

diaphysis *(dye AFF ih sis)* The straight shaft of a long bone.

diarrhea The passage of watery or unformed stools.

diastole *(dye ASS toe lee)* Resting period between contractions. It is when the heart fills with blood.

diencephalon *(dye in SEFF ah lon)* Central part of the brain that contains that thalamus and hypothalamus.

differentiation Process by which embryonic cells assume different shapes and functions in different parts of the body.

diffusion The process of movement of a substance from high concentration to low concentration.

digestion Process of mechanically and chemically breaking food down into nutrients that can be used by the body.

digital   Pertaining to the fingers or toes.

diluent   *(DILL you ent)* Substance used to thin a fluid or dilute a solution.

disaccharide   *(die SACK eh ride)* A carbohydrate that is composed of two monosaccharides.

disease   A condition in which the body fails to function normally; literally means "not [dis] at ease."

distal   *(DISS tuhl)* Moving from the body toward the end of a limb (arm or leg).

distal tubule   Tubule of the nephron that begins at the loop of Henle (nephron loop). It empties into the collecting duct. Reabsorption and secretion take place there.

dorsal   *(DOR suhl)* Pertaining to the posterior of the body.

dorsal column tract   Spinal cord pathway that carries fine touch sensation from the spinal cord to the brain.

dorsal recumbent position   Body position in which the patient is lying on her or his back with knees flexed and feet flat on the table or bed. This position is used for some surgical procedures and examinations of the vagina and rectum.

dorsal root ganglion   *(GANG lee on)* A collection of sensory neurons on the dorsal roots of the spinal cord.

dorsiflexion   Movement of foot that points toes up.

duodenum   *(DOO oh DEE num)* First part of the small intestine. It secretes cholecystokinin and secretin, hormones that stimulate the gallbladder and pancreas to release bile and digestive enzymes.

dura mater   *(DOO rah MAY ter)* Tough, outermost layer of the meninges. The dura mater lies just under the bones of the cranium and vertebrae.

dysmenorrhea   *(DIS men oh REE ah)* Difficult menstruation.

dysrhythmia   Abnormal or disordered heart rhythm.

eardrum   Membrane that divides the external ear from the middle ear. Also known as the tympanic membrane.

eccrine glands   *(EKK rin)* Sweat glands that cover the entire skin surface.

ectopic pregnancy   An abnormal placement of an embryo implantation in the uterine tubes.

efferent arteriole   *(EFF er ent ahr TEE ree ohlz)* Small blood vessels that carry blood away from the glomeruli of the kidney.

eggs   A type of special cell called a gamete that are produced by females.

ejaculation   The expulsion of semen (sperm and assorted chemicals) from the urethra.

ejaculatory duct   The passageway for sperm and chemicals that leads to the urethra.

electrical synapses   Occur when cells do not need chemicals to transmit information from one cell to another, but instead transfer information freely using special connections called gap junctions.

electrolyte   Chemical element that carries a positive or negative charge and conducts electricity when dissolved in a solution: Examples include: sodium (Na^+), potassium (K^+), chloride (Cl^-), calcium (Ca^{++}), and bicarbonate (HCO_3^-). Electrolytes are carried in the plasma. Excess amounts in the blood are removed by the kidneys.

electromyography (EMG)   *(ee LEK troh my OG rah fee)* Diagnostic procedure to diagnose muscle disease or nerve damage. A needle electrode inserted into a muscle records electrical activity as the muscle contracts and relaxes. The electrical activity is displayed as waveforms on an oscilloscope screen and permanently recorded on paper as an electromyogram.

electrons   A negatively charged particle that revolves around the nucleus of an atom.

element   The smallest complete particle of a substance that cannot be separated by ordinary means.

embolus   *(EM boh lus)* Mass of undissolved matter present in the blood or lymphatic vessels that was brought there by the blood or lymph current.

emphysema   *(em fih SEE mah)* Chronic pulmonary disease resulting in destruction of air spaces distal to the terminal bronchiole.

empyema   *(em pye EE mah)* Localized collection of purulent material (pus) in the thoracic cavity from an infection in the lungs. Also known as pyothorax.

emulsification   *(ee MULL sih fih KAY shun)* Process performed by bile of breaking down large fat droplets into smaller droplets with more surface area.

enamel   Glossy, thick white layer that covers the crown of the tooth. Enamel is the hardest substance in the body.

endemic   Native to a particular location or population.

endocardium   *(EHN doh KAR dee um)* Innermost layer of the heart. It covers the inside of the heart chambers and valves.

endochondral ossification   *(EHN doh KON drall)* The process in which shaped cartilage is replaced with bone.

endocrine system   *(EHN doh krin)* Body system that includes the testes, ovaries, pancreas, adrenal glands, thymus, thyroid gland, parathyroid glands, pituitary gland,

and pineal gland. It produces and releases hormones into the blood to direct the activities of other body organs.

endocrinology The study of the endocrine system and its related functions and disorders.

endocytosis *(en doh sigh TOE sis)* Ingestion of substances by a cell. Substances are taken into the cells after being surrounded by vesicles.

endolymph *(EN doh limf)* Fluid within the labyrinth of the ear.

endometrium *(EHN doh MEE tree um)* Inner lining of the uterus.

endomysium *(EHN doh mice ee uhm)* A connective tissue sheath that encases each muscle fiber.

endoplasmic reticulum *(en doh PLAZ mick ree TIH cue lum)* Organelle that consists of a network of channels that transport materials within the cell. Also the site of protein, fat, and glycogen synthesis.

endosteum The membrane that lines the marrow cavity of a bone.

end-stage renal failure The level of kidney failure that can only be remedied by a kidney transplant.

English system The weights and measures system that is commonly used in the United States.

enzyme Molecules that speed up the rate of chemical reactions in cells. Enzymes are particularly important in the breakdown and synthesis of biological molecules.

eosinophils *(EE oh SIN oh filz)* Type of leukocyte. It is classified as a granulocyte because it has granules in the cytoplasm. The nucleus has two lobes. Eosinophils are involved in allergic reactions and defense against parasites.

ependymal cells *(eh PEN deh mal)* Specialized cells that line the walls of the ventricles and spinal canal and produce cerebrospinal fluid.

epicardium The serous membrane on the surface of the myocardium.

epidemic Widespread disease.

epidermis *(ep ih DER mis)* Thin, outermost layer of skin. The most superficial part of the epidermis consists of dead cells filled with keratin. The deepest part (basal layer) contains constantly dividing cells and melanocytes.

epididymis *(ep ih DID ih mis)* The comma-shaped duct on the posterior and lateral part of the testes connecting the testes to the vas deferens.

epidural space *(ep ih DOO ral)* Area between the dura mater and the vertebral body.

epigastric region Region overlying the stomach; superior medial portion of abdominal cavity.

epiglottis *(ep ih GLOT iss)* Lidlike structure that seals off the larynx, so that swallowed food goes into the esophagus.

epimysium *(ep ih MY see um)* Connective tissue, continuous with the tendon, that surrounds a muscle.

epinephrine *(ep ih NEFF rin)* Hormone secreted by the adrenal medulla in response to stimulation by nerves of the sympathetic nervous system.

epiphyseal plate *(ep ih FEEZ ee al)* The growth plate.

epiphysis *(eh PIFF ih sis)* The widened ends of a long bone. Each end contains the epiphysial plate where bone growth takes place.

epithelial cells *(ep ih THEE lee al)* Cells that make up epithelial tissue—a tissue that covers surfaces and lines cavities.

epithelial tissue Layers of cells that form the epidermis of the skin as well as the surface layer of mucous and serous membranes.

equilibrium Balance.

erectile dysfunction disorder (EDD) Occurs when the penis cannot attain full erection or maintain an erection.

erection The expansion and stiffening of the penis due to increased blood flow to that area.

erythrocyte *(eh RITH roh sight)* A red blood cell. Erythrocytes contain hemoglobin and carry oxygen and carbon dioxide to and from the lungs and cells of the body.

erythropoiesis *(eh RITH roh poy EE sis)* Formation of red blood cells.

erythropoietin *(eh RITH roh poy EE tin)* In the body, a hormone secreted by the kidneys when the number of red blood cells decreases. It stimulates the bone marrow to make more red blood cells. As a drug, erythropoietin does the same.

esophagus *(eh SOFF ah gus)* Flexible, muscular tube that moves food from the pharynx to the stomach.

estrogen Any natural or artificial substance that causes the development of female sex characteristics.

etiology *(ee tee ALL oh jee)* The cause or origin of a disease.

eukaryotic cell *(you CARE ee AH tic)* A cell type that makes up the human body. The cell includes a nucleus (usually with several chromosomes) and cellular organelles.

eustachian tube *(yoo STAY she an)* Tube that connects the middle ear to the nasopharynx and equalizes the air pressure in the middle ear.

exacerbation Made worse, or increased severity of a disease.

excitable cell   A cell that carries a small electrical charge when stimulated. Each time charged particles flow across a cell membrane, a tiny electrical current is generated. A neuron is an example.

excretion   Removal of waste matter from body.

exocytosis   *(EX oh sigh TOH sis)* Secretion. The expulsion of material from a cell using vesicles.

extension   Straightening a joint to increase the angle between two bones or two body parts.

extensor muscle   Muscle that produces extension when it contracts.

external   Near or on the outside surface of the body or an organ.

external auditory meatus   *(AW dih toh ree mee AYE tus)* Opening at the entrance to the external auditory canal where sound waves enter the ear.

external ear   The outer region of the ear— including the part we can see.

external respiration   Gas exchange in the lungs that occurs between the blood and the air in the external atmosphere.

external urethral sphincter   *(yoo REE thral SFINK ter)* One of two valves, which allows voluntary control of urination.

facilitated diffusion   Also known as carrier mediated passive transport; the movement of substances into cells via carrier proteins.

fallopian tubes   (oviducts, uterine tubes) Accessory genitalia, these are the passageways for the eggs to get to the uterus.

fascicles   Bundles of muscle fibers (cells).

femoral artery   Major artery that carries blood to the upper leg.

femur   The thigh bone that extends from the hip to the knee.

fertilization   The union and combination of genetic material of the egg and sperm creating a zygote.

fibrin   Insoluble fiber strands that are formed by the activation of clotting factors. Fibrin traps erythrocytes, and this forms a blood clot.

fibrinogen   *(fye BRIN oh jenn)* Blood clotting factor.

fibroblasts   Any cell from which connective tissue is created.

fibromyalgia   *(FIE broh my AL jee uh)* Pain located at specific, small trigger points along the neck, back, and hips. The trigger points are very tender to the touch and feel firm.

fibrous joints   Joints held together by short strands of connective tissue that are either immobile or slightly mobile. The sutures in your skull are fibrous joints.

fibrous pericardium   *(pear eh CAR dee um)* The a tough membrane surrounding the heart.

fibula   *(FIB you lah)* The smaller, lateral bone in the lower leg.

filtration   Process in which water and substances in the blood are pushed through the pores of the glomerulus. The resulting fluid is known as filtrate.

fimbria   *(FIM bree ah)* Ciliated, fringe-shaped structures at the ends of the fallopian tubes.

first-degree burn   Burn that has damaged only the outer layer of skin, the epidermis; considered a partial thickness burn.

fissure   *(FISH er)* Deep division on the surface of the brain and spinal cord.

flaccid   *(FLAH sid)* Limp or without muscle tone.

flagella   *(flah JELL ah)* Hairlike processes on bacteria or protozoa that cause movement.

flexion   *(FLEK shun)* Bending of a joint to decrease the angle between two bones or two body parts. Opposite of extension.

flexor muscle   Muscle that produces flexion when it contracts.

flora   *(FLOOR ah)* Plant life occurring in a specific environment. Often used to refer to bacteria, even though they are not plants. Example: the intestinal flora.

follicle   *(FALL ih kul)* 1. Mass of cells with a hollow center. It holds an oocyte before puberty and a maturing ovum after puberty. The follicle ruptures at the time of ovulation and becomes the corpus luteum. 2. Also a site where a hair is formed. The follicle is located in the dermis.

follicle-stimulating hormone (FSH)   Secreted by the anterior lobe of the pituitary gland, it stimulates the maturation of ovarian follicles in women. In men, it is important for spermatogenesis.

follicular phase   *(fall LICK you lar)* The time from the beginning of the menstrual cycle until ovulation within the female menstrual cycle. Happens at the same time as the proliferative phase.

forensic science   *(for IN sik)* The application of science and medicine to law.

formed elements   The cellular parts of blood that include red and white blood cells and platelets.

fornix   *(FOR niks)* 1. Tract of nerves that joins all the parts of the limbic system. 2. Area of the superior part of the vagina that lies behind and around the cervix.

fourth-degree burns   Burns that penetrate to the bone or other underlying structures such as muscles and tendons; also full thickness burns.

Fowler's position A semi-sitting position with the torso at a 45- to 60-degree angle.

frenulum *(FREN you lum)* Structure that attaches the lower side of the tongue to the gum.

frontal lobe Lobe of the cerebrum that predicts future events and consequences. Exerts conscious control over the skeletal muscles.

frontal plane An imaginary plane parallel with the long axis of the body that divides the body into an anterior and posterior section. Also known as the coronal plane.

full thickness burns Burns that affect all three of the skin layers; called third-degree burns.

fundus *(FUN dus)* A larger part, base, or body of a hollow organ such as the dome-shaped top of the bladder, uterus above the fallopian tubes, or rounded, most superior part of the stomach.

fungus *(FUN gus)* A plantlike organism that includes molds and yeasts. Plural: fungi.

furuncle *(FOO rung kle)* A boil.

gamete *(GAM eet)* A mature male or female reproductive cell (spermatozoon or ovum).

ganglia *(GANG lee ah)* Masses of nervous tissue composed of mostly nerve cell bodies located outside the brain and spinal cord. Singular: ganglion.

gap junctions Special connections or pathways for intercellular communications.

gastrin *(GAS trin)* Hormone produced by the stomach that stimulates the release of hydrochloric acid and pepsinogen in the stomach.

gastroenterology The study of the alimentary canal.

gastrointestinal (GI) system Body system that includes the oral cavity, pharynx, esophagus, stomach, small and large intestines, and the accessory organs of the liver, gallbladder, and pancreas. Its function is to digest food and remove undigested food from the body. Also known as the gastrointestinal tract and digestive system or tract.

gene An area on a chromosome that contains all the DNA information needed to produce one type of protein molecule.

genitalia *(jen ih TAIL ee uh)* Reproductive organs.

genitourinary system *(JEN eh toe YUR ih nair ee)* Combination of two closely related body systems: the male genitalia and the urinary system. Also known as the urogenital system.

geriatric *(JAIR ee AT rik)* Relating to the older patient population.

gestation period *(jes TAY shun)* The period of time during which the developing baby grows within the uterus; approximately 40 weeks.

gingiva *(JIN jih vuh)* Referring to the gums.

glans penis Tip of the penis.

glaucoma *(glaw KOH mah)* Increased intraocular pressure (IOP) because aqueous humor cannot circulate freely. In open-angle glaucoma, the angle where the edges of the iris and cornea touch is normal and open, but the trabecular meshwork is blocked. Open-angle glaucoma is painless but destroys peripheral vision, leaving the patient with tunnel vision. In closed-angle glaucoma, the angle is too small and blocks the aqueous humor. Closed-angle glaucoma causes severe pain, blurred vision, and photophobia. Glaucoma can progress to blindness.

glia *(GLEE ah)* Nonnervous or supporting tissue found in the brain and spinal cord; made of glial cells.

glial cells *(GLEE all)* Cells that include astrocytes, oligodendrocytes, ependymal cells, microglia cells, Schwann cells, and satellite cells.

globulins *(GLOB you linz)* Plasma proteins that form antibodies that protect us from infection.

glomerular capsule *(glow MARE you lar)* A double-layered membrane that surrounds the glomerulus within the nephron of the kidney.

glomerular filtrate *(glow MARE you lar FILL trate)* The filtered fluid within the glomerulus.

glomerular filtration Occurs when fluid and molecules pass from the glomerular capillaries into the glomerular capsule, across a filter composed of the wall of the capillaries and the podocytes of the glomerular capsule.

glomerulonephritis *(glow MARE you loh neh FRY tiss)* An inflammatory disease of the glomerular capsular membranes of the kidneys.

glomerulosclerosis *(glow MARE you lo sklee ROW sis)* Scarring of the glomerulus.

glomerulus *(gloh MARE yoo lus)* Network of intertwining capillaries within Bowman's capsule in the nephron. Filtration takes place in the glomerulus.

glottis *(GLOT iss)* V-shaped structure of mucous membranes and vocal cords within the larynx.

glucose A simple sugar found in foods and also the sugar in the blood.

gluteal *(GLOO tee uhl)* Pertains to buttocks.

glycerol *(GLIS er oll)* Another term for glycerin, which is found in fats.

glycogen *(GLIE koh jen)* The form that glucose (sugar) takes when it is stored in the liver and skeletal muscles; a polysaccharide.

Golgi apparatus *(GOAL jee app uh rat us)* Organelle of the cell that packages cellular material for transport.

gonad *(GO nad)* A generic term for the male testes and female ovaries.

gonadotropin-releasing hormone *(GON ah doh TROH pin)* Released from the hypothalamus, this substance causes an increase in the secretion of LH and FSH from the pituitary gland.

graafian follicle *(GRAPH fee in)* A mature follicle in its sac.

graded potential Change in the charge across a cell membrane that is proportional to the size of the stimulus.

granulosa cells Helper cells that surround the primary oocyte.

Graves' disease A distinct form of hyperthyroid disease that includes an enlarged thyroid gland and various ocular findings such as proptosis (abnormal protrusion of the eyeball), stare, and lid lag.

greenstick fracture Incomplete fracture of a bone in which the bone is bent and cracks.

gross anatomy A term synonymous with macroscopic anatomy.

Guillain-Barré syndrome (GBS) *(GEY yan bar RAY)* A neuromuscular disease that usually leads to ascending flaccid paralysis.

gustatory sense *(GUS ta tore ee)* Sense of taste.

gynecology The study and treatment of female health issues, especially related to reproduction and female reproductive organs.

gyri *(JIE rie)* Convolutions of the cerebral hemispheres of the brain.

hairline fracture Cracks in bone.

hammer One of the three small bones of the ear, also known as the malleus.

Hashimoto's disease An autoimmune disease involving inflammation and then destruction and fibrosis of the thyroid gland, which leads to hypothyroidism.

haversian systems *(haa VER zhin)* The organizational unit of compact bone, with osteocytes surrounding a central canal. Also called an osteon.

helper T cells Stimulate the production of B cells. Also known as a CD4 cells.

hematology The study of blood and blood diseases.

hematopoiesis *(HE mah tow poy EE sis)* Formation of blood cells. Also called hemopoiesis.

hemisphere One-half of the cerebrum, either the right hemisphere or the left hemisphere.

hemoglobin *(HEE moh GLOH binn)* Substance in an erythrocyte that binds to oxygen and carbon dioxide. Its globin chains give it a round shape. When it is bound to oxygen, it forms the compound oxyhemoglobin.

hemolytic uremic syndrome An acute condition consisting of acute nephropathy, thrombocytopenia, and microangiopathic hemolytic anemia. This condition is often caused by the consumption of raw meat containing *E. coli*.

hemophilia *(HEE moh FILL ee ah)* Inherited genetic abnormality of a gene on the X chromosome that causes an absence or deficiency of a specific clotting factor. When injured, hemophiliac patients cannot easily form a blood clot and will continue to bleed for long periods of time.

hemopoiesis *(HEE moh poy EE sus)* Formation of blood cells. Also called hematopoiesis.

hemostasis *(HEE moh STAY sis)* The cessation of bleeding after the formation of a blood clot.

hemothorax *(HEE moh THOH raks)* Presence of blood in the thoracic cavity, usually from trauma.

heparin Substance that inhibits coagulation of blood.

hepatic duct *(heh pah TIC)* Duct that carries bile from the liver.

hernia A weakness in the muscles of the abdominal wall that allows loops of intestine to balloon outward.

herpes simplex virus 2 *(HER peez)* The virus that causes repeated painful vesicular eruptions on the genitals, mucosal surfaces, and the skin.

hilum *(HIGH lim)* 1. Indentation on the medial side of each lung where the bronchus, pulmonary artery, pulmonary vein, and nerves enter the lung. 2. Indentation in the medial side of each kidney where the renal artery enters and renal vein and the ureter leave.

histamine *(HIS tah meen)* Released by basophils. Increases capillary permeability.

homeostasis *(hoh mee oh STAY sis)* State of equilibrium of the internal environment of the body, including fluid balance, acid–base balance, temperature, metabolism, and so forth, to keep all the body systems functioning optimally.

horizontal plane Another name for the transverse plane.

hormonal control The control of hormone levels by other hormones released by other glands in the body.

hormone *(HOR mohn)* Chemical messenger of the endocrine system that is released by a gland or organ and travels through the blood.

human chorionic gonadotropin *(KOH ree ON ick GON uh doh TROH pin)* A hormone secreted to stimulate the corpus luteum, which secretes progesterone and a small amount of estrogen to maintain the uterine lining.

human papilloma virus *(pap ih LOW ma)* A virus directly linked as a cause of cervical cancer.

humerus The bone of the upper arm extending from the shoulder to the elbow.

humoral control Glandular secretion controlled by body fluids such as the secretion of insulin due to changing levels of blood glucose.

Huntington's disease A genetic disease that exhibits a progressive loss of neurons from basal nuclei and the cerebral cortex leading to involuntary movement, emotional and behavioral disturbances, and dementia.

hydrocele *(HIGH droh seel)* The accumulation of serous fluid in a saclike cavity. A common form is caused by the inflammation of the epididymis or testis.

hydrocephalus *(high droh SEF uh lus)* Condition of excess CSF that can be caused by blockage of the narrow passages between the ventricles due to trauma, birth defects or tumors, or decreased reabsorption of cerebrospinal fluid (CSF) due to subarachnoid bleeding.

hydrogen bond Weak bond between polar molecules due to attraction between hydrogen and a negatively charged atom.

hydrolysis reactions A reaction in which a large molecule is split into small molecules by the addition of water.

hydrophilic Water loving, or a substance that readily mixes with water.

hydrophobic Water fearing, or a substance that does not readily mix with water.

hydrothorax Fluid in the pleural space, a pleural effusion.

hymen A perforated membrane that covers the external opening of the vagina.

hyperopia *(HIGH per OH pee ah)* Farsightedness. Light rays from a far object focus correctly on the retina, creating a sharp image. However, light rays from a near object come into focus posterior to the retina, creating a blurred image.

hyperpolarized The charge across the cell membrane is more negative than resting.

hypertrophy *(high PER troh fee)* Greater than normal growth.

hypochondriac region *(high poh KAHN dree ack)* The part of the abdomen beneath the ribs. There are left and right hypochondriac regions.

hypodermis The fatty tissue layer below the dermis of the skin.

hypogastric region The region inferior to the umbilical region of the abdomen, between the right and left inguinal regions.

hypothalamus *(high poh THAL ah mus)* Endocrine gland located in the brain just below the thalamus. It produces (but does not secrete) antidiuretic hormone (ADH) and oxytocin. The hypothalamus is in the center of the brain just below the thalamus and coordinates the activities of the pons and medulla oblongata. It also controls heart rate, blood pressure, respiratory rate, body temperature, sensations of hunger and thirst, and the circadian rhythm. It also produces hormones as part of the endocrine system. In addition, the hypothalamus helps control emotions (pleasure, excitement, fear, anger, sexual arousal) and bodily responses to emotions; regulates the sex drive; contains the feeding and satiety centers; and functions as part of the "fight-or-flight" response of the sympathetic nervous system.

ileum *(ILL ee um)* The third part of the small intestine which connects to the large intestine.

iliac region The right and left most inferior regions of the abdomen; also called the inguinal region. The groin.

ilium *(ILL ee um)* Most superior hip bone. Bony landmarks include the iliac crest and the anterior–superior iliac spine (ASIS). Posteriorly, each ilium joins one side of the sacrum.

immune system A series of cells, chemicals, and barriers that protect the body from invasion by pathogens. Some of the weapons are active, some are passive, some are inborn, and others are acquired. Together they form a system that is remarkably good at keeping the body free of infection.

immunology The study of diseases and conditions of the immune system.

impulse conduction When an action potential is formed and travels down the axon from the cell body to the terminal.

incisors *(in SIZE erz)* Chisel-shaped teeth in the middle of the dental arch that cut and tear food on their incisal surface. There are eight incisors, four in the maxilla and four in the mandible.

incontinence *(in KAHN tih nens)* A condition of involuntary urination or defecation.

incus *(ING kus)* Second bone of the middle ear. It is attached to the malleus on one end and the stapes on the other end. Also known as the anvil.

infarct *(in FARKT)* Cellular death due to lack of blood flow (perfusion).

inferior Pertaining to the lower half of the body or a position below an organ or structure.

inferior vena cava The vena cava is one of the largest veins in the body. The inferior vena cava receives blood from the abdomen, pelvis, and lower extremities and takes it to the heart.

inflammation Tissue reaction to injury that includes swelling and reddening due to increased blood flow to the area.

infundibulum *(IN fun DIB you lum)* Any funnel-shaped organ or cavity; first part of uterine tube. Another name for pituitary stalk.

ingestion Process of taking in material (particularly food).

inguinal region *(ING gweh nal)* The groin. Also called iliac region.

innate (inborn) immunity *(ih NATE)* The first line of defense against pathogens that you are born with. Does not remember specific pathogens.

inner ear Intricate communicating passage of the ear essential for maintaining equilibrium; also called the labyrinth.

inotropism *(EYE no TROPE iz em)* An influence on the force of muscular contraction.

insula *(IN soo la)* The deep lobes of the cerebral hemispheres.

integumentary system The protective covering of the body; includes the skin, hair, and nails.

intercalated discs *(in TER kuh LATE ed)* Structures that connect heart tissue cells to facilitate a smooth contraction.

interferon *(in ter FEAR on)* Substance released by macrophages that have engulfed a virus. Interferon stimulates body cells to produce an antiviral substance that keeps a virus from entering a cell and reproducing.

interleukin *(in ter LOO kin)* Released by macrophages, it stimulates B cell and T lymphocytes and activates NK cells. It also produces the fever associated with inflammation and infection.

internal Structures deep within the body or an organ.

internal medicine A special branch of medicine that studies the function, interrelatedness, and treatment of the various body systems.

internal respiration Occurs when oxygenated blood is transported internally via the cardiovascular system to the cells and tissues where gas exchange occurs and oxygen moves into the cells as carbon dioxide is removed.

internal urethral sphincter *(you REE thrahl SFINK ter)* Located at the junction of the bladder and the urethra, it is one of the muscular rings that controls urination.

interneurons *(in ter NURE ons)* Neurons that facilitate communication between neurons. Also called association neurons.

interphase The part of the cell cycle in which the cell is performing normal functions and is stockpiling needed materials and preparing for cell division.

intramembranous ossification Formation of bone from the center out in a soft tissue membrane. Skull bones are formed this way.

inversion A movement in which the plantar surface of the foot faces the midline of the body.

ions Charged atoms or molecules.

ionic bond The bond that holds compounds together by the strong electrical attractions between the opposite charges of the ions involved.

iris *(EYE ris)* Colored ring of tissue whose muscles contract or relax to change the size of the pupil in the center of the iris.

ischemia *(iss KEE mee ah)* Tissue injury due to a decrease in blood flow.

ischium *(ISS kee um)* The lower posterior portion of the hip bone.

isthmus *(ISS muss)* The narrower portion of the uterus and uterine tubes. Generally refers to a narrow portion of an organ.

jejunum *(jee JOO num)* Second part of the small intestine.

joint Area where two bones come together (articulation).

juxtaglomerular apparatus This structure is responsible for initiating the renin-angiotensin mechanism that elevates blood pressure and increases sodium retention.

keloid An excessive mass of scar tissue that has a raised, firm, irregular shape.

keratin *(KAIR eh tin)* Hard protein found in the cells of the outermost part of the epidermis and in the nails.

keratinization *(KAIR eh tin eye ZAY shun)* The process of forming a horny growth such as fingernails.

kidney Organ of the urinary system that filters blood and produces urine, controlling fluid and ionic balance.

kinesiology *(keh NEE see ALL oh gee)* The study of muscles and body movements.

labia *(LAY bee ah)* An outer pair of vertical fleshy lips covered with pubic hair (the labia majora) and a smaller, thinner, inner pair of lips (the labia minora) that partially cover the clitoris and urethral and vaginal openings. Part of the external female genitalia. The soft external structure forming the boundary of the mouth to the oral cavity (labium oris).

labia majora *(LAY bee ah mah JOR ah)* Two prominences that surround the vulva comprised of rounded fat deposits that meet and protect the rest of the external genitalia. The labia majora meet anteriorly to form the mons pubis.

labia minora *(LAY bee ah mih NOR ah)* Lateral border of the vaginal vestibule that meets to form the prepuce.

labor The actual process whereby the fetus is delivered from the uterus through the vagina and into the outside world.

labyrinth *(LAB ih rinth)* Intricate communicating passage of the inner ear essential for maintaining equilibrium.

labyrinthitis *(LAB ih rinn THYE tiss)* Bacterial or viral infection of the semicircular canals of the inner ear, causing severe vertigo.

lacrimal apparatus *(LAK rim al app ah RAT tus)* Structures involved with the secretion and production of tears.

lacrimal gland Part of the lacrimal apparatus of the eye; produces the tears needed for constant cleansing and lubrication, which are spread over the eye surfaces by blinking.

lactating Producing milk.

lacteal *(LACK tee al)* 1. Pertaining to milk. 2. Part of the villi of the small intestine, containing lymph vessels for absorption of lipids.

lacunae *(luh KOO nay)* An empty space or hollow region.

lamina propria *(LAM eh nah pro PREE ah)* The middle layer of the bronchial wall that contains smooth muscle, lymph, and nerve tracts.

large intestine Organ of absorption between the small intestine and the anal opening to the outside of the body. The large intestine includes the cecum, appendix, colon, rectum, and anus. Also known as the large bowel.

laryngitis *(lar in JIGH tis)* Hoarseness or complete loss of the voice, difficulty swallowing, and cough due to swelling and inflammation of the larynx.

laryngopharynx *(la RING goh FAIR inks)* Relates to both the larynx and pharynx.

larynx *(LAIR inks)* Triangular-shaped structure in the anterior neck (visible as the laryngeal prominence or Adam's apple) that contains the vocal cords and is a passageway for inhaled and exhaled air. Also known as the voice box.

lateral *(LAT er al)* Pertaining to the side of the body or the side of an organ or structure.

left-side heart failure A potentially life-threatening condition. The healthy right pump pushes blood through the vasculature of the lungs on its way to the left-side pump. If the left side can't keep up with the blood being delivered to it, the blood backs up into the lungs, increasing the pressure in those blood vessels.

lens Clear, hard, disk in the eye. The muscles and ligaments of the ciliary body change its shape to focus light rays on the retina.

lesion *(LEE zhun)* General category for any area of visible damage on the skin, whether it is from disease or injury.

leukemia *(loo KEE mee uh)* Cancer of leukocytes (white blood cells), including mature lymphocytes, immature lymphoblasts, as well as myeloblasts and myelocytes that mature into neutrophils, eosinophils, or basophils. The malignant leukocytes crowd out the production of other cells in the bone marrow. Leukemia is named according to the type of leukocyte that is the most prevalent and whether the onset of symptoms is acute or chronic. Types of leukemia include acute myelogenous leukemia (AML), chronic myelogenous leukemia (CML), acute lymphocytic leukemia (ALL), and chronic lymphocytic leukemia (CLL).

leukocytes *(LOO koh sights)* White blood cells. There are five different types of mature leukocytes: neutrophils, eosinophils, basophils, lymphocytes, and monocytes.

leukocytosis Increase in the number of white blood cells above normal.

leukopenia Abnormal decrease of white blood cells.

ligament Fibrous bands that hold two bone ends together in a synovial joint.

limbic system *(LIM bick)* Processes memories and controls emotions, mood, motivation, and behavior. Links the conscious to the unconscious mind. Limbic system consists of the thalamus, hypothalamus, hippocampus, amygdaloid bodies, and fornix.

lingual *(LING gwal)* Pertaining to the tongue.

lingula *(LING gu lah)* A general term for a tongue-shaped process of a body structure.

lipids Fats.

lipocyte Cell in the subcutaneous layer that stores fat.

lithotomy position *(lith OT ah mee)* A common position for surgical procedures and medical examination of the pelvis, lower abdomen, and reproductive organs. In the lithotomy position, the patient is placed on her or his back with feet elevated (usually in stirrups). This is also the traditional position for childbirth in Western nations.

lithotripsy *(LITH oh trip see)* Medical or surgical procedure that uses sound waves to break up a kidney stone.

lobes 1. Large divisions of the lung, visible on the outer surface. 2. Large area of the hemisphere of the cerebrum. Each lobe is named for the bone of the skull that is next to it: frontal lobe, parietal lobe, temporal lobe, and occipital lobe.

longitudinal fissure Divides the cerebrum into right and left hemispheres.

lower esophageal sphincter (LES) Ringed muscle leading into the stomach.

lumbar region Two of the nine regions of the abdominopelvic area. The right and left lumbar regions are inferior to the right and left hypochondriac regions. Also refers to the lower back, spinal cord, and spinal column.

lumen Open region in the center of a large tube—for example, the center of the tubes in the digestive and respiratory systems and the blood vessels.

lunula *(LOO nyoo lah)* Whitish half-moon visible under the proximal portion of the nail plate. It is the visible tip of the nail root.

luteal phase *(LOO tee al faze)* (secretory phase) The time between ovulation and menses.

luteinizing hormone (LH) *(LOO tee ah NIZE ing)* One of the four hormones responsible for female reproduction.

lymph *(LIMF)* Fluid that flows through the lymphatic system.

lymph nodes *(LIMF nohdz)* Small, encapsulated pieces of lymphoid tissue located along the lymphatic vessels. Lymph nodes filter and destroy invading microorganisms and cancerous cells present in the lymph.

lymphatic fluid *(lim FAT ik)* Clear and colorless fluid of the lymphatic system.

lymphatic system Body system that includes lymphatic vessels, lymph nodes, lymph fluid, and lymphoid tissues (tonsils and adenoids, appendix, Peyer's patches), lymphoid organs (spleen and thymus), and the blood cells, lymphocytes, and macrophages.

lymphatic trunk The main stem of a lymphatic vessel.

lymphatic vessels Vessels that begin as capillaries carrying lymph, continue through lymph nodes, and empty into lymphatic trunks. Can also be used as a general term for any vessel carrying lymph.

lymphocyte *(LIMF oh sight)* A white blood cell responsible for much of the body's immune protection.

lymphocyte activation Stimulation of lymphocytes, "waking them up" to fight a pathogen.

lymphocyte proliferation Reproduction of activated lymphocytes so there are many copies.

lysis *(LYE sis)* Destruction or breakdown.

lysosome *(LIE so soam)* Organelle that consists of a small sac with digestive enzymes in it. These destroy pathogens that invade the cell.

macrophages *(MAC roh fage ez)* Antigen presenting cells that take fragments of the pathogen they have eaten and present them to a B cell (lymphocyte). This stimulates the B cell to become a plasma cell and make antibodies against that specific pathogen. Macrophages also activate helper T cells in this way. Macrophages also produce special immune response chemicals: interferon, interleukin, and tumor necrosis factor.

macroscopic anatomy *(MAK roh SCAH pick)* Study of large structures of the body.

major calyx, minor calyces *(KAY licks, KAY leh seez)* Tubes in the kidney that carry urine from the nephrons to the renal pelvis.

malignant *(muh LIG nant)* Cancerous, able to spread to distant parts of the body.

malleus *(MALL ee us)* First bone of the middle ear. It is attached to the tympanic membrane on one end and to the incus on the other end. Also known as the hammer.

mammary glands *(MAM ah ree)* Milk-secreting glands found in female breasts.

margination Forming a margin or walling off of an area.

mast cells Connective tissue cells that are important in cellular defense and contain heparin and histamine.

mastication *(MASS tih CAY shun)* Process of chewing, during which the teeth and tongue together tear, crush, and grind food. This is part of the process of mechanical digestion.

mastitis *(mass TYE tis)* An infection or inflammation of the breast.

matrix The intercellular material of a connective tissue.

medial *(MEE dee al)* Pertaining to the middle of the body or the middle of an organ or structure.

median plane Divides the body into right and left halves; also called the midsagittal plane.

mediastinum *(mee dee ah STY num)* Central area within the thoracic cavity. It contains the trachea, esophagus, heart, and other structures.

medulla *(meh DULL ah)* The middle of a structure. Examples: medulla oblongata, renal medulla, adrenal medulla.

medulla oblongata *(meh DULL ah OB long GAH ta)* Most inferior part of the brain stem that joins to the spinal cord. It relays nerve impulses from the cerebrum to the cerebellum. It contains the respiratory center. Cranial nerves IX through XII originate there.

medullary cavity *(MED uh lair ee)* The hollow center of a long bone. Also called the marrow cavity.

meibomian glands *(my BOH me an)* Oil glands inside eyelids. Also called tarsal glands.

meiosis *(my OH sis)* The division of cells in order for reproduction to occur. Known as reduction division because the cells lose half their chromosomes. Makes gametes.

melanin *(MELL an in)* Dark brown or black pigment that gives color to the skin and hair.

melanocytes *(mell AN oh sights)* Cells that produce melanin.

melanoma A malignant pigmented mole or tumor. Cancer of the melanocytes.

melatonin *(MELL ah TOH nin)* Hormone secreted by the pineal body. It maintains the 24-hour wake–sleep cycle known as the circadian rhythm.

membrane A thin soft pliable layer of tissue that can line a cavity or cover an organ or structure.

memory B cells Antibody-producing cells that are produced when a pathogen is encountered the first time. Memory B cells are stored until the pathogen comes again. They are responsible for secondary response.

memory T cells Memory cells responsible for cell-mediated immunity. They are produced when a pathogen is encountered the first time. Memory T cells are stored until the pathogen comes again. They are responsible for secondary response.

menarche *(men AR kee)* The first menstrual cycle.

Ménière's disease *(MAIN ee AIRZ)* Recurring and progressive disease that includes progressive deafness, ringing ears, dizziness, and the feeling of fullness in the ears.

meninges *(men IN jeez)* Three separate membranes that envelope and protect the entire brain and spinal cord. The meninges include the dura mater, arachnoid mater, and pia mater.

meningitis *(men in JYE tiss)* Inflammation of the meninges of the brain or spinal cord by a bacterial or viral infection.

Initial symptoms include fever, headache, nuchal rigidity (stiff neck) lethargy, vomiting, irritability, and photophobia.

menopause The cessation of menstruation as characterized by symptoms such as hot flashes, dizziness, headaches, and emotional changes.

menses *(MEN seez)* The time during the monthly flow of bloody fluid from the endometrium.

menstruation *(MEN stroo AY shun)* The cyclic hormonal shedding of the uterine endometrium.

mesentery *(MEZ in TARE ee)* Membranous sheet of peritoneum that supports the jejunum and ileum.

mesometrium *(MEZ oh ME tree um)* Attaches the uterus to the lateral pelvic walls. Part of broad ligament.

mesosalpinx *(MEZ oh sal pinks)* Suspends the uterine tubes.

mesovarium A ligament that suspends the ovary. Part of broad ligament.

metabolism *(meh TAB oh lizm)* Process of using oxygen and glucose to produce energy for cells. Metabolism also produces by-products like carbon dioxide and other waste products. The ongoing cycle of anabolism and catabolism.

metacarpals Long bones of the hand between the carpals and phalanges.

metaphase Phase of cell division during which chromosomes line up in the center of the cell.

metastasis *(meh TASS tuh sis)* Process by which cancerous cells break off from a tumor and move through the blood vessels or lymphatic vessels to other sites in the body.

metatarsals Long bones of the feet between tarsals and phalanges.

metric system Sytem of measurement based on the power of 10.

microglia *(my crow GLEE ah)* Cells that move, engulf, and destroy pathogens anywhere in the central nervous system.

microscopic anatomy *(MY kroh SCAH pick ah NAH tom ee)* Study of structures that require the aid of magnification.

midbrain An area that connects the pons and the cerebellum with the hemispheres of the cerebrum.

middle ear A space within the ear that contains the three smallest bones (ossicles) of the body; also called the tympanic cavity.

midsagittal plane *(mid SAJ ih tuhl)* An imaginary vertical plane that divides the entire body into right and left sides and creates a midline. The midsagittal plane is named for the sagittal suture of the skull. Also called the median plane.

mitochondria *(MITE oh KAHN dree uh)* The organelle of the cell which makes ATP, cellular energy.

mitosis *(my TOE sis)* The process of cells sorting the chromosomes so that each new cell gets all the correct numbers of copies of genetic material.

mitotic phase The phase devoted to actual cell division.

mitral Pertains to the bicuspid or mitral valve of the heart.

mixed nerve A nerve that carries both sensory and motor information.

molar Largest tooth, located posterior to the premolar. It crushes and grinds food on its large, flat occlusal surface.

molecule A combination of atoms (the same type or different types) held strongly together enough to be considered a unit.

monocyte A type of white blood cell that is a mononuclear agranulocyte. Monocytes are found in higher-than-normal amounts when a chronic (long-term) infection occurs in the body. Like neutrophils, monocytes destroy invaders through phagocytosis.

mononuclear phagocyte system Includes macrophages, monocytes, and several other types of phagocytic cells found in organs and tissues. Also includes the spleen, lymph nodes, liver, lungs, adipose tissue, and mucosa. Osteoclasts, which destroy bone, for example, are part of the system, as are the macrophages in the alveoli of the lungs. Also called the reticuloendothelial system.

monosaccharide *(mon oh SACK eh ride)* A simple sugar such as glucose.

mons pubis Formed by the labia majora.

morbidity Long-term disability.

mortality Death, usually referring to the death rate in a population or from a particular disease.

motor neuron Neuron that innervates muscle tissue.

motor system The system responsible for movement.

mucosa Any mucous membrane, an epithelial membrane lining body cavities with openings to the outside. Mucous membranes produce mucus. The digestive system, reproductive system, urinary system, and respiratory system all are lined with mucous membranes.

mucous Pertaining to mucus producing structures.

mucus A viscid fluid secreted by glands and mucous membranes.

muscle Many muscle fascicles grouped together and surrounded by fascia.

muscular dystrophy *(MUS kyoo lahr DIS troh fee)* Genetic disease due to a mutation of the gene that makes the muscle protein dystrophin. Without dystrophin, the muscles weaken and then atrophy. Symptoms appear in early childhood as weakness first in the lower extremities and then in the upper extremities. The most common and most severe form is Duchenne's muscular dystrophy; Becker's muscular dystrophy is a milder form.

muscularis externa *(mus koo LAR ris)* The outside muscular layer of an organ or tubule.

myalgia *(my AL jee uh)* Pain in one or more muscles due to injury or muscle disease. Polymyalgia is pain in several muscle groups.

myasthenia gravis *(my as THEE nee ah GRAV iss)* Abnormal and rapid fatigue of the muscles, particularly evident in the muscles of the face; there is ptosis of the eyelids. Symptoms worsen during the day and can be relieved by rest. The body produces antibodies against its own acetylcholine receptors located on muscle fibers. The antibodies destroy many of the receptors. There are normal levels of acetylcholine, but too few receptors remain to produce sustained muscle contractions.

mycelia *(my SEE lee ah)* A mass of fibers from fungi/molds.

myelin *(MY eh lin)* Fatty sheath around the axon of a neuron. It acts as an insulator to increase the speed of impulse conduction. Myelin around the axons of the brain and spinal cord is produced by oligodendrocytes. Myelin around axons of the cranial and spinal nerves is produced by Schwann cells. An axon with myelin is said to be myelinated.

myocardium *(my oh CAR dee um)* The middle layer of the walls of the heart composed of cardiac muscle.

myofibril *(my oh FIE bril)* Thin filament (actin) and thick filament (myosin) within the muscle fiber that give it its characteristic striated appearance. The interaction between actin and myosin causes muscle contraction.

myometrium *(MY oh MEE tree um)* The muscle layer of the uterus.

myopia *(my OH pee ah)* Nearsightedness. Light rays from a near object focus correctly on the retina, creating a sharp image. However, light rays from a far object come into focus anterior to the retina, creating a blurred image.

myosin *(MY oh sin)* The thick protein filament found in muscle fibers.

nares *(NAIR eez)* The paired external openings of the nasal cavity.

nasal Pertaining to the nose.

nasal cavity Hollow area inside the nose that is lined with mucosa or mucous membrane.

nasopharynx *(NAY zoh FAIR inks)* Uppermost portion of the throat where the posterior nares unite. The nasopharynx contains the opening for the eustachian tubes and the adenoids.

natural active immunity Antibodies developed due to exposure to a pathogen.

natural killer (NK) cell Type of lymphocyte that matures in the red marrow and is the body's first cellular defense against invading microorganisms. Without the help of antibodies or complement, an NK cell recognizes a pathogen by the antigens on its cell wall and releases chemicals that penetrate and destroy it. Part of innate immunity.

natural passive immunity Immunity due to the passage of antibodies from mother to child across the placenta or in breast milk.

neck Transitional area between the root and crown where the tooth becomes narrower. The neck of the tooth is located just above and below the gum line. Can refer to the narrow part of any bone or structure.

necrosis *(neh KROH sis)* Gray-to-black discoloration of the skin in areas where the tissue has died.

negative feedback loop Physiological process that works against the trend. Most often brings a variable back to set point. For example, as blood pressure rises, heart rate may decrease to bring blood pressure back to "normal."

negative selection The destruction of lymphocytes that destroy "self" antigens. These lymphocytes must be deleted to prevent autoimmunity.

Neisseria gonorrhoeae *(nye SEE ree ah gon ah REE ah)* A gram-negative organism responsible for the STD gonorrhea.

nephrology The study of the structure and function of the kidneys and the related diseases and treatments.

nephron *(NEFF rahn)* Microscopic functional unit of the kidney.

nephron loop Structure within the kidney responsible for countercurrent circulation. Includes the descending and ascending loop. Also called the loop of Henle.

nephropathy *(neff ROPP ah thee)* General word for any disease process involving the kidney.

nerves Bundles of individual axons.

nervous system Body system that includes the brain, spinal cord, and nerves. It receives signals from parts of the body and interprets them as pain, touch, temperature, body position, taste, sight, smell, and hearing; coordinates body movement; and maintains and interprets memory and emotion.

neural control Control of hormone levels in the body by the nervous system.

neuroglia (glial cells) *(noo ROG lee uh)* Cells that hold neurons in place and perform specialized tasks. Includes astrocytes, ependymal cells, microglia, oligodendrocytes, satellite cells, and Schwann cells.

neurology The study of the nervous system and its diseases and treatments.

neuromuscular Pertaining to the nervous and muscular system.

neuromuscular junction Area on a single muscle fiber where a neuron connects; a type of chemical synapse.

neuron *(NOO ron)* An individual nerve cell. The functional part of the nervous system.

neuron body Where metabolism occurs in the neuron.

neurosurgery Branch of medicine that surgically treats disorders of the nervous system.

neurotransmitter *(noo roh TRANS mit ter)* Chemical messenger that travels across the synapse between a neuron and another neuron, muscle fiber, or gland.

neutrons A neutral subatomic particle found in the nucleus of an atom.

neutrophil *(NOO troh fil)* A type of leukocyte that performs nonspecific phagocytosis.

nociceptors *(NO see SEP torz)* Branches of nerve fibers, or free nerve endings, that are receptive to pain.

nodal cells (pacemaker cells) Special cardiac cells that create a rhythmic electrical impulse.

nodes of Ranvier *(ron vee AYE)* Places on a myelinated nerve fiber without myelin that facilitate impulse conduction.

norepinephrine *(nor EP ih neff rin)* 1. Neurotransmitter for the sympathetic nervous system. It goes between neurons and an involuntary muscle, organ, or gland. Controls the fight-or-flight response. 2. Hormone secreted by the adrenal medulla in response to stimulation by nerves of the sympathetic nervous system.

normal flora Organisms within or on our bodies that are either normally harmless or are essential.

nuclei Plural form of nucleus, a central point around which matter is gathered/collected, a central structure such as the nucleus of a cell or nucleus of an atom. Also deep gray matter areas surrounded by white matter in the nervous system.

nucleic acids   Chemicals (such as DNA or RNA) that carry genetic information.

nucleolus   Round, central region within the nucleus. It makes ribosomes.

obstetrics   Medical specialty that deals with pregnancy and childbirth.

occipital lobe   *(awk SIP eh tal)* Lobe of the cerebrum that receives sensory information from the eyes. Contains the visual cortex for the sense of sight.

olfaction   The sense of smell.

oligodendrocytes   *(AH li go DEN droe sites)* Neuroglial cells that produce myelin in the CNS.

oocyte   *(OH oh site)* An immature stage of an ovum.

oogenesis   *(OH oh JEN eh sis)* The process by which eggs are produced.

ophthalmologist   *(off thal MALL oh jist)* A doctor who specializes in the eyes.

ophthalmology   *(off thal MALL oh jee)* The study of the structure and function of the eye and other sight-related structures and related diseases and treatments.

oral   Pertaining to the mouth.

oral (buccal) cavity   The space within the mouth.

orbit   Bony socket in the skull that surrounds all but the anterior part of the eyeball.

orbital cavity   The region that contains the eyeball.

organ   A part of the body, composed of tissues, that has one or more specialized functions.

organelles   *(OR guh NELLZ)* Small structures in the cytoplasm that have various specialized functions. Organelles include mitochondria, ribosomes, the endoplasmic reticulum, the Golgi apparatus, and lysosomes.

organic molecules   Carbon-based molecules necessary for life.

oropharynx   *(OR oh FAIR inks)* Middle portion of the throat just behind the oral cavity. It begins at the level of the soft palate and ends at the epiglottis.

orthopedics   The branch of medicine that deals with bone, joint, cartilage, ligament, and tendon structure and function, and their related diseases and treatments.

osmosis   *(ahss MOE sis)* The passage of the solvent through a semipermeable membrane to equalize concentrations.

osmotic pressure   The pressure that develops when two solutions of varying concentrations are separated by a semipermeable membrane.

osseous tissue   *(AH see us)* Bone, a type of connective tissue.

ossicles   *(AHS ih kulz)* Three tiny bones in the middle ear that function in the process of hearing: malleus, incus, and stapes.

ossification   *(OSS ih fih KAY shun)* Process by which tissue is changed into bone from infancy through puberty. Also known as osteogenesis.

osteoarthritis   *(OSS tee oh ahr THRYE tiss)* Chronic inflammatory disease of the joints, particularly the large weight-bearing joints of the knees and hips, although it often occurs in the joints that move repeatedly like the shoulders, neck, and hands.

osteoblasts   Cells that form new bone.

osteoclasts   Cells that break down old or damaged areas of bone.

osteocytes   *(OSS tee oh sites)* Mature bone cells that live in the matrix.

osteogenesis   Process by which tissue is changed into bone from infancy through puberty. Also known as ossification.

osteomalacia   *(OSS tee oh mah LAY she ah)* Abnormal softening of the bones due to a deficiency of vitamin D.

osteons   *(OSS tee ons)* The microscopic units of compact bone.

osteoporosis   *(OSS tee oh por OS sis)* Condition of increased bone porosity that weakens the bones, usually seen in the elderly.

osteoprogenitor cells   Nonspecialized cells found in the periosteum, endosteum, and central canal of compact bones.

otitis media   *(oh TYE tis MEE dee ah)* Acute or chronic bacterial infection of the middle ear.

otolaryngology   The study of the structure and function of the ear, nose, and larynx and their related diseases and treatments. Also known as otorhinolaryngology.

otorhinolaryngology   The study of the structure and function of the ear, nose, and larynx and their related diseases and treatments. Also known as otolaryngology.

oval window   Opening in the temporal bone between the middle ear and the vestibule of the inner ear. The opening is covered by the end of the stapes.

ovarian cycle   *(oh VAIR ee an)* The monthly maturation and release of eggs from the uterus.

ovary   *(OH vah ree)* The almond-shaped gland that produces the ovum and the three hormones progesterone, estrogen, and inhibin. Female gonads. Plural: ovaries.

oviducts Another term for fallopian tubes and uterine tubes.

ovulation Release of ovum from ovary. Occurs when the pituitary stops producing FSH and starts producing luteinizing hormone. At day 14, the follicle ruptures and the ovum is released.

oxytocin *(AHK see TOH sin)* Hormone secreted by the posterior pituitary gland. It stimulates the uterus to contract and begin labor. It stimulates the "let-down reflex" to get milk flowing for breast-feeding.

pacemaker cells Cells or group of cells that automatically generate electrical impulses.

palate *(PAL at)* Roof of the mouth.

palatine tonsils *(PAL ah tine TAHN silz)* Lymphoid tissue on either side of the throat where the soft palate arches downward in the oropharynx.

pancreas *(PAN kree ass)* A digestive and endocrine organ located in the abdominal cavity that produces digestive enzymes (amylase, lipase, protease, peptidase) and releases them into the duodenum. It also contains the islets of Langerhans (alpha, beta, and delta cells) that produce and secrete the hormones glucagon, insulin, and somatostatin.

pancreatitis *(PAN kree ah TYE tiss)* Inflammation or infection of the pancreas.

pandemic Infection spreading to several countries or around the world.

paracrine *(PAIR ah kreen)* Cell signaling. A cell sends out a signal that affects nearby cells that are different from the signaling cell.

paralysis Temporary or permanent loss of muscle function that may be flaccid or rigid in nature.

parasympathetic nervous system Division of the autonomic nervous system that uses the neurotransmitter acetylcholine and carries nerve impulses to the heart, involuntary smooth muscles, and glands. Sometimes referred to as "resting and digesting."

parathyroid glands *(PAIR ah THIGH royd)* Endocrine glands, four of them, on the posterior lobes of the thyroid gland. They produce and secrete parathyroid hormone.

parathyroid hormone (PTH) A hormone that increases blood calcium.

parietal lobe *(pah RYE eh tal)* Lobe of the cerebrum that receives sensory information about temperature, touch, pressure, vibration, and pain from the skin and internal organs.

parietal pleura *(pah RYE eh tal PLOO rah)* One of the two layers of the pleura. It lines the thoracic cavity.

parotid salivary gland *(pah ROT id SAHL ih vair ee)* Gland that secretes saliva that helps to lubricate food so that it is easier to chew and swallow.

partial thickness burn Burn that has damaged only the outer layer of skin, the epidermis or part of the dermis; considered a first-degree or second-degree burn.

passive transport The general term for the transportation of cellular material without the use of energy.

patellar *(puh TELL ahr)* Pertaining to the kneecap.

patellar tendon (knee-jerk) reflex Leg extension caused by the stretching of the quadriceps muscle or patellar tendon. Often elicited by the doctor striking the knee with a reflex hammer.

pathogen *(PATH oh jenn)* Microorganism that causes a disease. Pathogens include bacteria, viruses, protozoa, and other microorganisms, such as cells like fungi or yeast.

pathology *(path ALL oh jee)* The study of disease.

pectoral Concerning the chest.

pedal Pertaining to the foot or feet.

pelvic Pertaining to a pelvis.

penis The male organ of urination and intercourse.

pepsin Digestive enzyme produced by the stomach that breaks down food protein into smaller protein molecules.

peptic ulcer disease (PUD) A condition in which there is a breakdown of the mucosal membrane of the esophagus, stomach, or small intestine. Stress is considered a factor as is the organism *Helicobacter pylori*.

perforating canals Canals running between the periosteum and the central canals in compact bone. They contain blood vessels. Also called Volkmann's canals.

perforin *(PER fuh rin)* Chemical secreted by cytotoxic T cells that makes holes in the cell membranes of pathogens or infected cells, killing them.

perfusion Blood flow to a particular region.

pericardial cavity A potential space between the layers of the pericardium.

perilymph *(PER ih limf)* Pale lymph fluid found in the labyrinth of the inner ear.

perimetrium *(pair ee MEE tree um)* The serous layer of the uterus.

perimysium Connective tissue inside muscle that surrounds bundles of muscle fibers (fascicles).

perineum The area between the vagina and the anus.

periodontal *(PAIR ee oh DON tal)* Literally means "around the teeth" and may refer to the area of the gum.

periosteum *(pair ee OSS tee um)* Thick, fibrous membrane that goes around and covers the outside of a bone.

peripheral Referring to "away from center" or the extremities.

peripheral nervous system (PNS) Division of the nervous system that includes the cranial nerves and the spinal nerves.

peripheral neuropathy A condition in which the peripheral nerves produce pain and dysfunction. This condition is often caused by diabetes.

peripheral resistance A resistance to blood flow in the peripheral blood vessels, which may be a result of peripheral vasoconstriction.

peripheral vascular disease (PVD) Any disease of the arteries of the extremities.

peristalsis *(pair ih STALL sis)* Contractions of the smooth muscle of the gastrointestinal tract that propel food through it. Can also be the process of smooth muscle contractions that propel urine through the ureter.

peritubular capillaries *(per ee TUBE you ler)* Capillaries surrounding the renal tubules.

pH A value that indicates how acidic or alkaline a substance is.

phagocytosis *(fag oh sigh TOH sis)* The process by which a phagocyte destroys a foreign cell or cellular debris; a type of endocytosis.

phalanges *(fah LAN jeez)* The plural form of phalanx, which relates to any digits of the hands and feet.

pharyngitis *(fair in JIGH tis)* Bacterial or viral infection of the throat. When the bacteria group A beta-hemolytic streptococcus causes the infection, it is known as strep throat.

pharyngoesophageal sphincter *(fah RING goh ee SOFF uh JEE al SFINK ter)* A muscular ring located at the beginning of the esophagus acting as a door to allow food into the esophagus.

pharynx *(FAIR inks)* The throat; contains the passageways for food and for inhaled and exhaled air.

pheochromocytoma *(fee oh KROH mo sie TOH ma)* A neuroendocrine tumor that creates a surgically correctible form of hypertension.

phonation Producing sounds.

phospholipid *(FOS foh LIP id)* The primary substance in the lipid portion of a cell membrane. The molecules have a hydrophilic "head" and hydrophobic "tails."

photopigments Chemicals in the retinal cells that have light sensitivity.

physiology *(fiz ee ALL oh jee)* The study of the function of the body's structures.

pia mater *(PEE ah MAY ter)* Thin, delicate innermost layer of the meninges that covers the surface of the brain and spinal cord. It contains many small blood vessels.

pineal body *(PIN ee al)* or **gland** A part of the diencephalon that is responsible for the secretion of melatonin.

pinna *(PIN ah)* The auricle of the exterior ear that collects sound waves.

pinocytosis *(pie no sigh TOE sis)* Process in which a cell absorbs fluid material. A type of endocytosis.

pituitary gland *(pih TOO ih tair ee)* Endocrine gland in the brain that is connected by a stalk of tissue to the hypothalamus. It is known as the master gland of the body and consists of the anterior and the posterior pituitary gland. Also known as the hypophysis.

placenta A spongy structure lining the uterus that nourishes the developing fetus and is attached to the fetus via an umbilical cord.

plantar Referring to the sole of the foot.

plaque *(plack)* An area on the skin or mucous membranes composed of lipids and/or calcium. Plaque can build up in blood vessels, creating a partial or total blockage.

plasma *(PLAZ mah)* Clear, straw-colored fluid portion of the blood that carries blood cells and contains dissolved substances like proteins, glucose, minerals, electrolytes, clotting factors, complement proteins, hormones, bilirubin, urea, and creatinine.

plasma cells A type of B cell that produces antibodies to non–self-antigens.

plasma proteins *(PLAZ mah)* Protein molecules in the plasma.

platelet Cell fragment that is flat and does not have a nucleus. It is active in the blood clotting process. Also known as a thrombocyte.

pleural cavities *(PLOO ruhl)* The space between the parietal and visceral layers of the pleura surrounding the lungs.

pleural effusion *(PLOO ruhl eh FYOO zhun)* Accumulation of fluid within the pleural space that may be due to inflammation or infection of the pleura and lungs.

pleural fluid A slippery liquid contained within the microscopic intrapleural space (pleural cavity) of the lungs.

plexus *(PLECK sus)* A network of nerves or vessels.

plicae circulares *(PLY kay sir cue LAIR es)* One of the transverse folds in the small intestine.

pneumocyte *(NEW moh site)* Flat, pancakelike cells that are interspersed with simple cuboidal cells to make up the walls of the alveoli, the air sacs in the lungs.

pneumonia Usually an infectious lung disease characterized by fever, excessive secretions, shortness of breath, lethargy, and cough.

pneumothorax *(NEW moh THOH raks)* Large volume of air that forms in the pleural space and progressively separates the two pleural membranes.

podocytes Special epithelial cells found in the inner layer of the glomerular (Bowman's) capsule that act as the filter for blood from the glomerulus into the glomerular capsule.

point of insertion The end of a muscle that is attached to the moving bone, with the muscle action moving the insertion toward the origin.

point of origin The end of a muscle that is attached to a stationary bone.

polar covalent bond A covalent bond in which the electrons are shared unequally.

polarized cell A cell that has a separation of charge across its cell membrane.

polycythemia *(PALL ee sigh THEE mee ah)* Increased number of erythrocytes due to uncontrolled production by the red marrow. The cause is unknown. The viscosity of the blood increases; it becomes viscous (thick), and the total blood volume is increased.

polysaccharides Made when many monosaccharides are linked together.

pons Area of the brain stem that relays nerve impulses from the body to the cerebellum and back to the body. Area where nerve tracts cross from one side of the body to the opposite side of the cerebrum. Cranial nerves V through VIII originate there.

positive feedback Vicious cycle. During positive feedback, physiological processes send body chemistry or other attributes moving further and further away from equilibrium (set point). The trend will continue until something breaks the cycle.

positive selection During lymphocyte development, only those lymphocytes that can actually react to antigens will survive.

postcentral gyrus Ridge on the surface of the cerebrum posterior to the central sulcus in each hemisphere. The postcentral gyrus contains the primary somatic sensory area for your sense of touch.

posterior The back of the body. Dorsal.

postpartum depression A condition that can occur up to 6 months following childbirth and affects 10 to 20% of women who have recently delivered. In severe cases, the welfare of the child and/or mother may be a concern.

precapillary sphincters *(SFINK terz)* Smooth muscle structures that control the blood flow to the capillaries from the terminal arterioles.

precentral gyrus Ridge on the surface of the cerebrum anterior to the central sulcus in each hemisphere. The postcentral gyrus contains the primary motor cortex for voluntary movements.

premenstrual syndrome (PMS) A collection of physical and psychological changes that occurs before menstruation in many women.

presbyopia *(PREZ bee OH pee ah)* Loss of flexibility of the lens with blurry near vision and loss of accommodation.

primary mover (agonist) A muscle or muscle group that causes movement.

primary oocytes *(OH oh sites)* Produced by the oogonia during mitosis.

primary polycythemia A condition in which chronic low levels of oxygen (due to bone marrow cancer) cause the body to produce more than normal amounts of erythrocytes to transport more efficiently the decreased oxygen available.

primary response The body's initial response to a pathogen. Antibodies destroy pathogens using several methods, including inactivating the antigen, causing antigens to clump together, activating complement cascade, causing the release of chemicals to stimulate the immune system, and enhancing phagocytosis.

primordial follicles *(pry MORE dee all FALL ih kulz)* Follicles that stay dormant until puberty. Once signaled by hormones, they develop into primary follicles.

prions *(PREE ons)* An infectious abnormal protein.

proctology *(prock TALL oh gee)* A medical specialization that deals with the treatment of diseases related to the colon, rectum, and anus.

progesterone *(proh JESS ter ohn)* A steroid hormone that creates changes in the endometrium to facilitate implantation of the blastocyte.

prognosis *(prog NOH sis)* The predicted outcome of a disease.

prokaryotic *(pro CARE ee AAH tick)* Pertaining to a cell that has no nucleus or many organelles. Bacteria are prokaryotic cells.

prolactin *(proh LACK tin)* Hormone secreted by the anterior pituitary gland. It stimulates milk glands of the breasts to develop during puberty and to produce milk during pregnancy.

proliferative phase The time between the end of menses and ovulation within the female menstrual cycle. Also called follicular phase.

prone position Lying with the anterior section of the body down.

prophase The first stage of mitosis in which the nucleus disappears, the chromosomes become visible, the centrioles move toward the sides of the cell, and the spindle fibers form.

prostaglandins Molecules that are short-range hormones that are formed rapidly and act in the immediate area.

prostate cancer A slow-growing cancer originating in the prostate gland. Can be treated effectively if detected early.

prostate gland A chestnut-size gland that secretes a slightly alkaline fluid that forms part of the seminal fluid.

proteins A class of compounds that are synthesized by all living organisms with many different functions. They are made of long chains of amino acids.

prothrombin *(pro THROM bin)* Blood-clotting factor that is activated just before the thrombus is formed.

proton A positively charged subatomic particle found in the nucleus of an atom.

protozoa *(proh toh ZOH uh)* Unicellular organisms.

proximal *(PROK sim al)* Referring to "near" a reference point.

proximal tubule The part of the renal tubule closest to the glomerulus. Many substances are secreted or absorbed in this part of the renal tubule.

pseudostratified Type of epithelial tissue that looks stratified but is only a single layer of cells. The cells are different sizes, which makes the tissue look stratified under the microscope.

ptyalin *(TYE ah lin)* A salivary enzyme that changes starch and glycogen to maltose and glucose.

pubis *(PEW bis)* The region above the genitalia where pubic hair grows.

pudendal cleft *(pew DEN dall)* The opening between the two labia majora.

pulmonary artery *(PULL moh nair ee)* Artery that carries blood from the heart to the lungs. The pulmonary artery is the only artery in the body that carries blood that has low levels of oxygen.

pulmonary trunk The great vessel that leaves the right ventricle of the heart and branches into the right and left pulmonary arteries.

pulmonary veins The blood vessels that bring oxygenated blood from the lungs to the left atrium of the heart.

pulmonology The study of the diseases and treatments of the lungs.

pulp Internal portion of connective tissue within the tooth.

pupil Round opening in the iris that allows light rays to enter the internal eye.

pustule *(PUS tyool)* A small elevation of skin filled with lymph or pus.

pyloric sphincter *(pye LOR ik SFINK ter)* Muscular ring that keeps food in the stomach from entering the duodenum.

pylorus *(pye LOR us)* Narrowing canal of the stomach just before it joins the duodenum. It contains the pyloric sphincter.

radius The shorter bone on the thumb side of the forearm. The radius rotates partially around the ulna.

rapid eye movement (REM) The dream stage of sleep.

reabsorption Process by which water and substances in the filtrate move out of the renal tubule and into the blood in a nearby capillary.

rectum Final part of the large intestine. It is a short, straight segment that lies between the sigmoid colon and the outside of the body.

red blood cells (RBCs) Contain hemoglobin and carry oxygen and carbon dioxide to and from the lungs and cells of the body. Also called erythrocytes.

red marrow Tissue in the interior of bones that makes blood cells. Also called red bone marrow.

reduction division The division of cells in order for reproduction to occur. Meiosis is called reduction division because the daughter cells produced at the end of meiosis have half as many chromosomes as the original mother cell.

reflex Involuntary muscle reaction that is controlled by the spinal cord. In response to pain, the spinal cord immediately sends a command to the muscles of the body to move. All of this takes place without conscious thought or processing by the brain. The entire circuit is also known as a reflex arc.

refractory period Short period of time when an excitable cell is resting and unresponsive to electrical impulses.

regenerate The regrowth of an injured or missing cell or tissue.

regenerative medicine Branch of medicine which studies the possibility of growing human tissue and organs to replace those damaged by disease or injury.

regulatory T cells Type of T cell that shuts down or decreases immune response.

relapse Repeated reactivation of the symptoms of a chronic disease.

remission Period during which a chronic disease has no obvious symptoms.

renal artery *(REE nal AHR ter ee)* Major artery that carries blood to the kidney.

renal capsule A fibrous layer of connective tissue that covers the kidney.

renal columns Extensions of cortical tissue that separate adjacent renal pyramids.

renal corpuscle *(REE nal KOR pus el)* The filtration apparatus of the kidney, consists of the glomerulus and the glomerular capsule.

renal cortex *(REE nal CORE tex)* The tissue layer of the kidney just beneath the renal capsule.

renal hilum *(REE nal HIGH lum)* The indentation that gives the kidney its bean-shaped appearance.

renal medulla *(REE nal meh DULL lah)* The middle region of the kidney.

renal nephron *(NEFF rahn)* Fundamental functional unit of the kidney; consists of the renal corpuscle and renal tubule.

renal pelvis *(REE nal PELL vis)* Funnel-shaped part of the kidney that collects urine.

renal pyramids Triangle-shaped structures of the renal medulla that are composed of collecting tubules for the urine formed in the kidney.

renal tubule The part of the nephron, a series of tubes, in which secretion and reabsorption take place. Consists of proximal tubule, nephron loop, distal tubule, and collecting duct.

renal vein Major blood vessels that carry blood away from the kidneys.

renin-angiotensin-aldosterone *(RIN en-an gee oh TEN sen-al DOSS ter ohn)* A complex hormone system that regulates blood volume and blood pressure. The system is triggered when blood flow to the kidney decreases.

repolarization The opposite of depolarization. The cell returns to resting potential.

reticular formation A diffuse network of nuclei in the brain stem.

reticuloendothelial system Includes macrophages, monocytes, and several other types of phagocytic cells found in organs and tissues. Also includes the spleen, lymph nodes, liver, lungs, adipose tissue, and mucosa. Osteoclasts, which destroy bone, for example, are part of the system, as are the macrophages in the alveoli of the lungs. Also called the mononuclear phagocyte system.

respiration *(ress pir RAY shun)* The process of gas exchange at the lungs or tissue sites. Oxygen and carbon dioxide are exchanged in the alveoli during external respiration and at the cellular level during internal respiration.

resting cell A cell that is not firing an impulse.

reticulospinal tract *(ree TICK you low spine al)* A neural pathway that carries motor information from the reticular formation to the spinal cord, which helps coordinate movements.

retina *(RET eh nah)* Membrane lining the posterior cavity of the eye. It contains rods and cones. Landmarks include the optic disk and macula.

Rh factor A blood group discovered on the surface of erythrocytes of rhesus monkeys and found to a variable degree in humans. Can be Rh-negative or Rh-positive.

Rh-negative A blood type in which the Rh antigen is not found in the surface of a red blood cell.

Rh-positive A blood type in which the Rh antigen is found in the surface of a red blood cell.

rheumatology *(ROO mah TALL oh jee)* A specialization of medicine in which the study and treatment of connective tissue and joints is conducted.

rhinoplasty *(RYE noh plass tee)* Surgical procedure that uses plastic surgery to change the size or shape of the nose.

ribonucleic acid (RNA) *(rye bow new KLEE ick)* Molecule contained in ribosomes and necessary for making proteins.

ribosome *(RYE bow soamz)* Granular organelle located throughout the cytoplasm and on the endoplasmic reticulum. Ribosomes contain RNA and proteins and are the site of protein synthesis.

right-side heart failure Formerly known as *cor pulmonale*, this is a potentially serious condition in which the right-side pump can't move blood as efficiently as it should.

rigor mortis *(RIG or MORE tis)* A stiffness that occurs in dead bodies as a result of retained calcium and decreased ATP.

rima glottidis *(RIE mah GLOT ti diss)* The space between the vocal cords.

rods Light-sensitive cells in the retina. They detect shades of black and white and function in daytime and nighttime vision.

root Part of the tooth that is hidden below the gum line. The premolars have one or more roots. The molars have multiple roots.

rotation   Spin a body part on its axis.

rubrospinal tract   A neural pathway that carries motor information from the midbrain to the spinal cord, which helps coordinate movements.

rugae   *(ROO gay)* 1. Deep folds in the gastric mucosa. 2. Folds in the mucosa of the bladder that disappear as the bladder fills with urine and expands.

saltatory conduction   Conduction along the nodes of Ranvier in a myelinated axon. Impulse jumps from node to node.

sagittal   Cuts to slice the organ into smaller sections for closer examination.

sarcolemma   The cell membrane of a muscle cell.

sarcomeres   *(SAR koh meerz)* Portion of striated muscle fibril that lies between the two adjacent z-lines. It is the sarcomere which gets shorter when the muscle contracts.

sarcoplasmic reticulum   A specialized series of interconnecting tubules and sacs that surround each myofibril.

satellite cells   Neuroglia cells that enclose the cell bodies of neurons in the spinal ganglia.

saturated fat   Lipid that has no double bonds, so hydrogen cannot be added. These fats are thought to be unhealthy.

scapula   Shoulder blade.

scar   During tissue repair, tissue is replaced with connective tissue high in collagen fibers rather than with the original tissue. Typically scar tissue does not function in the same way as the original tissue.

Schwann cell   *(SHWAN)* Cell that forms the myelin sheaths around axons in the peripheral nervous system.

sclera   *(SKLAIR ah)* White, tough, fibrous connective tissue that forms the outer layer around most of the eye. Also known as the white of the eye.

scrotum   *(SKRO tuhm)* A pouchlike structure that contains the testes and a portion of the spermatic cord.

sebaceous glands   *(see BAY shus)* An exocrine gland of the skin that secretes sebum. Sebaceous glands are located in the dermis. Their ducts join with a hair, and sebum coats the hair shaft as it moves toward the surface of the skin. Also known as oil glands.

sebum   *(SEE bum)* Oily substance secreted by sebaceous glands.

second-degree burns   Burns that involve the entire depth of the epidermis and a portion of the dermis, but are still considered *partial thickness* burns.

secondary polycythemia   *(PALL ee sigh THEE mee ah)* A condition in which chronic low levels of oxygen (due to lung disease or living in high altitudes) cause the body to produce more than normal amounts of erythrocytes to transport more efficiently the decreased oxygen available.

secondary response   Increased immune response mediated by memory cells when meeting a pathogen that it recognizes.

secretion   *(sih CREE shun)* The movement of a chemical out of a cell or gland.

segmentation   Division into similar parts.

self-recognition vs. non–self-recognition   The ability of the immune system to distinguish between the body's cells and cells that do not belong in the body.

semen   *(SEE men)* A sperm-containing, thick fluid produced by males.

semicircular canals   Three canals in the inner ear that are oriented in different planes (horizontally, vertically, obliquely) that help the body keep its balance. It relays information to the brain via the vestibular branch of the vestibulocochlear nerve.

semilunar valves   Valves within the heart that are located between the ventricles and large arteries that carry blood away from the heart.

seminal vesicles   *(SEM ih nal VESS ih kulz)* Secrete fluid that makes up much of the volume of semen.

seminiferous tubules   *(SEM ih NIF er us TOO byoolz)* Structures composed of epithelium and areolar tissue that contain sperm stem cells and sperm helper cells. Sperm develop here.

sensations   Measurements of conditions that occur inside and outside the body.

sensory association area   Area of the cerebral cortex located in the parietal lobe just posterior to somatic sensory cortex that allows *understanding* and *interpretation* of somatic sensory information.

sensory neurons   A neuron that conducts sensory impulses towards the spinal cord or brain.

sensory system   Includes the peripheral nervous system's "input devices."

septum   *(SEHP tum)* 1. Wall of cartilage and bone that divides the nasal cavity into right and left sides. 2. Partitioning wall that divides the right atrium from the left atrium (interatrial septum) and the right ventricle from the left ventricle (interventricular septum).

serosa   *(seh ROSE ah)* A serous membrane.

serous membrane *(SEER us)* Double-layered membrane lining a body cavity. The parietal layer lines the wall of the cavity, and the visceral layer covers the organs in the cavity. There is a potential, fluid-filled cavity between the layers.

serous pericardium Cardiac epithelial membranes with a potential space between them.

sertoli cells *(sir TOW lee)* Sperm helper cells, also called nurse cells.

set point The normal physiologic range (such as blood pressure or body temperature) needed to maintain homeostasis.

sexually transmitted diseases (STDs) Infectious diseases often transmitted via sexual contact. Also known as sexually transmitted infections or STIs.

shin splints Inflammatory condition of the connective muscles surrounding the tibia; medical name is medial tibial stress syndrome.

sickle cell anemia An inherited blood disorder producing abnormally shaped (sickle shape) and functioning red blood cells.

signs An objective, measurable indicator of disease or malfunction of the body.

simple fracture A bone fracture that does little damage to surrounding tissues and does not cause an open wound in the skin.

sinoatrial node (SA) *(sigh noh AY tree al)* Pacemaker of the heart. Small knot of tissue located in the posterior wall of the right atrium in a shallow channel near the entrance of the superior vena cava. The SA node dictates the heart rate at 70 to 80 beats per minute when the body is at rest. It generates the electrical impulse for the entire conduction system of the heart.

sinus Hollow cavity within a bone of the cranium. Often refers to any cavity in a structure.

skeletal muscle *(SKELL eh tal)* One of three types of muscles in the body, but the only muscle that is under voluntary, conscious control. Under the microscope, skeletal muscle has a striated appearance.

smooth muscle One of three types of body muscles that is involuntarily controlled and found in the lining of the airways, blood vessels, and uterus. It is not striated.

solute The substance dissolved in water or a solution.

solution The liquid containing a dissolved substance.

solvent A liquid that reacts with a solute bringing it into solution, dissolving.

somatic nervous system *(so MAT ick)* Division of the peripheral nervous system that uses the neurotransmitter acetylcholine and carries nerve impulses to the voluntary skeletal muscles.

somatic sensation The sense of touch.

somatic sensory system The system that receives and interprets your sense of touch.

spasm Involuntary contraction of a muscle.

sperm (spermatozoa) The male gamete.

spermatids *(SPER mah tidz)* Cells that result from the division of secondary spermatocytes.

spermatocytes *(sper MAT oh sites)* Cells form the spermatogonium that divide to form spermatids.

spermatogenesis Sperm production.

spermatogonia *(SPER mat oh GO nee uh)* Large unspecialized germ cells that form primary spermatocytes by mitosis.

spermatozoa *(sper MAT oh ZOE ah)* The plural form of spermatozoon, the mature male sex cell. Sperm.

sphincter *(SFINK ter)* Muscular ring around a tube; a valve.

sphygmomanometer *(SFIG moh man AAHM et ter)* Instrument used to measure blood pressure; BP cuff.

spina bifida *(SPY nah BIFF ih dah)* A congenital defect in which the vertebral arches fail to form properly, leading to varying levels of disability due to the exposure of the spinal cord.

spinal cavity *(SPY nal)* A continuation of the cranial cavity as it travels down the midline of the back. The spinal cavity lies within and is protected by the bones (vertebrae) of the spinal column. The spinal cavity contains the spinal cord, the spinal nerves, and spinal fluid. Also called the vertebral cavity.

spinal cord Part of the central nervous system. Continuous with the medulla oblongata of the brain and extending down the back in the spinal cavity. Ends at L2 and separates into individual nerves (cauda equina).

spinal nerves Thirty-one pairs of nerves. Each pair comes out from the spinal cord between two vertebrae. An individual spinal nerve consists of dorsal nerve roots and ventral nerve roots.

spinal roots Axon bundles attached to each spinal cord segment. The dorsal roots are sensory, and the ventral roots are motor. The dorsal and ventral roots join to form the spinal nerves.

spinocerebellar tract *(SPY no ser eh BELL ar)* Sensory pathway from the spinal cord to the cerebellum.

spinothalamic tract *(SPY no THAL uh mick)* Sensory pathway from the spinal cord to the thalamus and eventually the primary somatic sensory cortex. Contains pain and crude touch information.

spiral fracture A fracture in which the bone is twisted apart.

spleen Lymphoid organ located in the abdominal cavity near the stomach. The spleen destroys old erythrocytes, breaking their hemoglobin into heme and globins. It also acts as a storage area for whole blood. Its white pulp is lymphoid tissue that contains B and T lymphocytes.

spongy bone Also called cancellous; forms connecting structures that partially enclose many intercommunicating spaces within bone.

spores A protective barrier to allow for future reproduction in a hostile environment.

sprain Overstretching or tearing of a ligament.

squamous cells *(SKWAY mus)* A flat, scaly epithelial cell.

stapes *(STAY peez)* Third bone of the middle ear. It is attached to the incus on one end and the oval window on the other end. Also known as the stirrup.

startle reflex Involuntary response to sudden onset of stimuli.

sternal Pertaining to the sternum.

sternum *(STER num)* Medial bone of the anterior thorax to which the clavicle and ribs are attached. Also known as the breastbone.

steroids Ringed lipids that function as extremely powerful hormones.

strain Overstretching of a muscle, often due to physical overexertion. This causes inflammation, pain, swelling, and bruising as the capillaries in the muscle tear. There can be small tears in the muscle itself. Also known as a pulled muscle.

stratified *(STRAT ih fied)* Having more than one layer.

stratum basale *(STRAY tum BAY sell)* The stem cell layer of the epidermis.

stratum corneum *(STRAY tum core NEE um)* The outermost horny layer of the epidermis.

stratum germinativum *(STRAY tum JER meh NAY tee vum)* The region of cell birth within the skin. Same as stratum basale.

striated muscle *(STRY ate ed)* Muscle with lines on the surface of the muscle fibers when viewed under a microscope. Both skeletal and cardiac muscle are striated. Smooth muscle is not.

stroke A sudden neurological disfunction caused by a vascular injury (decreased or absent blood flow) to a portion of the brain. The blood flow blockage can be caused by a clot or by hemorrhage.

stroke volume The volume of blood ejected from the ventricles during each heartbeat.

subarachnoid space *(SUB ah RACK noyd)* Space beneath the arachnoid layer of the meninges. It is filled with cerebrospinal fluid.

subcutaneous fascia *(sub cue TAY nee us FASH ee uh)* Connective tissue layer beneath the skin.

subdural hematoma An abnormal collection of blood in the space between the archnoid and dura mater.

subdural space *(sub DOO ral)* The space between the arachnoid and dura mater.

sublingual salivary glands *(sub LING gwall SAHL ih vair ee)* Smallest of salivary glands found between the tongue and the mandible, one on each side.

submandibular salivary glands *(SUB man dib you lar SAHL ih vair ee)* Salivary glands beneath the mandible or jaw.

submucosa Layer of connective tissue under a mucous membrane.

substrates An underlying layer or a foundation. Also the term for molecules which are reactants in an enzyme catalyzed reaction.

sulcus *(SULL cus)* Shallow groove on the surface of the CNS. Plural: sulci.

superficial Relating to or located near the surface.

superior Pertaining to the upper half of the body or a position above an organ or structure. In humans, toward the head.

superior vena cava One of the largest veins that drain venous blood from the upper portions of the body to the heart.

supine position *(sue PINE)* Position of lying on the posterior part of the body. Also known as the dorsal supine position.

surfactant *(sir FAC tant)* Protein-fat compound that reduces surface tension and keeps the walls of the alveolus from collapsing inward with each inhalation.

sympathetic nervous system Division of the autonomic nervous system that uses the neurotransmitter norepinephrine and carries nerve impulses to the heart, involuntary muscles, and glands during times of increased activity, danger, or stress.

symptom A change in the body or any of its functions as perceived by the patient. It is a subjective consideration by the patient.

synapse *(SIN aps)* Space between the axon of one neuron and the dendrites of the next neuron or between a neuron and muscle.

syndrome *(SIN drohm)* A set of symptoms and signs associated with and characteristic of one particular disease.

syndrome of inappropriate antidiuretic hormone secretion (SIADH) A condition characterized by severe hyponatremia (low blood sodium), usually due to overproduction of ADH. It leads to fluid retention and very dilute plasma.

synergistic A cooperating action of certain muscles.

synovial fluids *(sin OH vee al)* Clear lubricating fluid that is secreted by the synovial membrane.

synovial joints Joints that possess a joint cavity lined with a synovial membrane that is filled with synovial fluid.

synovial membrane *(sin OH vee al)* The membrane lining a capsule of the synovial joint.

systems An organized grouping of organs that perform specific functions.

systole *(SIS toh lee)* Combined contractions of the atria and the ventricles.

T lymphocytes *(T LIMF oh sights)* White blood cells involved in adaptive immunity. There are four types of T lymphocytes: helper T cells, cytotoxic T cells, memory T cells, and regulatory T cells.

tachycardia *(TACK ee CAR dee ah)* A more rapid than normal heart rate (greater than 100 beats per minute in an adult).

tactile corpuscles *(TACK tile KOR pus ulz)* Elongated bodies found in nerve ends that act as receptors for slight pressure or touch.

tarsal glands Oil glands under the eyelid. Also called meibomian glands.

tarsals The bones of the ankle forming the proximal portion of the foot.

taste buds Sensory end organs that provide us with a sense of taste.

telophase Phase of cell division when the chromosomes are at opposite ends of the cell.

temporal lobe Lobe in the cerebrum that receives sensory information from the auditory cortex for hearing and the olfactory cortex for smelling.

tendon Cordlike white band of nonelastic fibrous connective tissue that attaches a muscle to a bone.

tendonitis Inflammation of any tendon from injury or overuse.

terminal disease A disease that results in death regardless of treatment.

testes *(TESS teez)* Small, egg-shaped glands in the scrotum. Also known as the testicles. They contain interstitial cells that secrete testosterone and also contain the seminiferous tubules that produce spermatozoa. The male gonads.

testicles *(TESS tih kulz)* See testes.

testicular cancer *(tess TICK you lahr)* A cancer that starts in the testes.

testosterone *(tess TOSS ter ohn)* The steroid hormone responsible for the growth and development of male (masculine) characteristics.

tetanus *(TET ah nus)* An acute infectious disease caused by a bacterium that can lead to severe spasms and rigid paralysis of voluntary muscles.

thalamus *(THAL ah mus)* Relay station in the brain that receives sensory nerve impulses from many parts of the nervous system and sends them on for processing. Also part of the motor coordination system.

thallium *(THAL ee um)* As a radioisotope, it is used by nuclear medicine to assess myocardial perfusion and viability.

third-degree burns Burns that affect all three of the skin layers and are therefore called full thickness burns.

thoracic cage *(tho RASS ik)* The portion of the skeleton that include the ribs, sternum, and thoracic vertebrae that house and protect the lungs, heart, and great vessels.

thoracic cavity Hollow space within the thorax that is filled with the lungs and structures in the mediastinum.

thoracic duct The main lymph duct of the body.

thoracic surgery Cutting open the thoracic cavity to repair structures inside.

thrombin *(THROM bin)* An enzyme that reacts with fibrinogen, converting it to fibrin, which forms a clot.

thrombocyte *(THROM boh sight)* Cell fragment that is flat and does not have a nucleus. It is active in the blood-clotting process. Thrombocytes are also known as blood platelets.

thrombocytopenia *(THROM boh SIGH toh PEE nee ah)* Deficiency in the number of thrombocytes. This can be due to exposure to radiation or toxic chemicals or drugs that damage the stem cells in the bone marrow.

thrombus *(THROM bus)* A blood clot.

thymosin A hormone produced by the thymus gland that helps with the maturation of white blood cells during childhood to fight infections.

thymus *(THIGH mus)* Lymphoid organ in the thoracic cavity.

thymus gland An endocrine gland that releases hormones known as thymosins. The thymosins cause lymphoblasts in the thymus to mature into T lymphocytes.

thyroid gland *(THIGH royd)* Endocrine gland in the neck that produces and secretes the hormones T3, T4, and calcitonin. Its two lobes and narrow connecting bridge (isthmus) give it a shieldlike shape.

thyroid hormones The hormones thyroxine (T_4), triiodothyronine (T_3), and calcitonin, which are secreted by the thyroid gland. T_4 and T_3 contain iodine and control cell metabolism and growth. Calcitonin decreases blood calcium by stimulating bone-building cells.

tibia *(TIBB e uh)* The larger and medial leg bone located between the knee and the ankle.

tinnitus *(tinn EYE tus)* Perceived internal sounds (buzzing, ringing, hissing, or roaring) that are heard constantly or intermittently in one or both ears, even in a quiet environment.

tissues Collection of similar cells that perform a particular function.

tongue Large muscle that fills the oral cavity and assists with eating and talking. It contains taste buds and receptors for the sense of taste.

tonsils Masses of lymphocyte-producing lymphatic tissues located in the posterior of the pharynx. The three sets of tonsils include the palatine tonsils, located on either side of the oropharynx; the pharyngeal tonsils (adenoids), located at the posterior nasopharynx; and the lingual tonsils, located at the base of the tongue.

tonus *(TONE us)* A partial steady contraction of a muscle; firmness.

trabecular *(tra BECK you la)* The structure of spongy bone, beam-like bony supports. Plural: trabeculae.

trachea *(TRAY kee ah)* Rigid tubular air pipe between the larynx and the bronchi that is a passageway for inhaled and exhaled air.

transdermal patches Adhesive patches containing medicine that are placed on the skin where medication is slowly absorbed into the bloodstream.

transient ischemic attack A ministroke.

transitional *(tran ZISH un al)* Moving from one state to another. A type of stratified epithelium with atypical cells.

transverse fissure *(tranz VERS)* Divides the cerebrum from the cerebellum.

transverse plane Plane that divides the body into top and bottom sections, superior and inferior.

traumatic brain injury (TBI) Occurs when force is applied to the skull and causes brain damage.

Trendelenburg position *(tren DELL in berg)* A patient position in which the head is lower than the torso and legs. This is usually accomplished by elevating the foot of the patient's bed.

Treponema pallidum *(TREP oh NEE mah PAL ih dum)* The organism that causes syphilis.

tricuspid Pertains to having three cusps or points, as in the tricuspid valve of the right heart.

true capillaries The actual vessels where exchange is made between the blood and the cells.

T-tubules Spread excitation into the inside of the muscle fiber.

tubal ligation Method of female sterilization in which the fallopian tubes are cut, clipped, or tied off, preventing the egg from traveling from the ovary to the uterus.

tuberculosis (TB) *(too BER kew LOH sis)* Lung infection caused by the bacterium mycobacterium tuberculosis and spread by airborne droplets expelled by coughing.

tubular reabsorption Movement of substances out of the renal tubule and back into the blood. The substances will be retained in the body.

tubular secretion Movement of substances from the blood into the renal tubule. These substances will leave the body in the urine.

tumor necrosis factor (TNF) *(neh KROH sis)* Released by macrophages, it destroys endotoxins produced by certain bacteria. It also destroys cancer cells.

tunica externa *(TOO nik ah ex TERN ah)* The outer layer of an blood vessel.

tunica interna *(TOO nik ah in TERN ah)* The inner lining of an blood vessel.

tunica media *(TOO nik ah mee DEE ah)* The middle muscular layer of an blood vessel.

tunica vaginalis *(TOO nik ah VAJ in AL is)* A serous membrane that surrounds the testis.

turbinates Three long projections (superior, middle, inferior) of the ethmoid bone that jut into the nasal cavity: superior, middle, and inferior. They break up the stream of air as they enter the nose. Also known as the nasal conchae.

turgor The ability of skin to return back to normal after being stretched.

tympanic cavity A space within the ear that contains the three smallest bones (ossicles) of the body; also called the middle ear.

tympanic membrane *(tihm PAN ik)* Membrane that divides the external ear from the middle ear. Also known as the eardrum.

ulna The larger bone of the forearm, on the opposite side of the thumb. It extends from the elbow to the wrist.

umami *(you MAH me)* A fifth taste sensation triggered by glutamates, also called the "savory" taste sensation.

umbilical region Abdominal region containing the navel (umbilicus, belly button).

universal donor A person who has type O blood, which can be transfused to any individual of the ABO blood groups.

universal recipient A person who has type AB blood and can receive blood from all the ABO blood groups.

unsaturated fat Lipid that contains many double bonds so hydrogen can be added. Thought to be more healthy than saturated fats.

upper respiratory infection (URI) Bacterial or viral infection of the nose that can spread to the throat and ears. The nose is a part of the respiratory system as well as the ENT system. Also known as a common cold or head cold.

ureter *(yoo REE ter)* Tube that connects the pelvis of the kidney to the bladder.

urethra *(yoo REE thrah)* Tube that connects the bladder to the outside of the body.

urinary bladder Holding receptacle for urine before it is expelled (voided) from the body.

urology The branch of medicine that studies the urinary system of both sexes.

uterine cycle Consists of the monthly buildup, degeneration, and shedding of the uterine lining.

uterine tubes Provides a passageway for eggs to get to the uterus. Also called oviducts and Fallopian tubes.

uterus *(YOO ter us)* The reproductive organ that contains and nourishes the embryo and the fetus once the fertilized egg is implanted until the time the fetus is born.

uvula *(YEW view lah)* Fleshy structure attached to the soft palate which covers the opening to the nasopharynx during swallowing.

vagina *(vah JYE nah)* (birth canal) A structure that accepts the penis during intercourse and allows for the passage of menstrual fluid as well as providing a passageway for the baby during childbirth.

vaginitis *(vaj ih NYE tis)* Infection/inflammation of the vagina.

vagus nerve *(VAY gus)* Cranial nerve X. Sensation and movement of the throat. Sensory and motor for thoracic and abdominal organs.

valvular insufficiency A pathologic condition in which the valve(s) of the heart do not function correctly, affecting the amount of blood being ejected.

valvular stenosis A constriction or narrowing of a heart valve.

vas deferens *(VAS DEFF er enz)* A tube running from the scrotum to the penis, it joins with the seminal vesicles to form the ejaculatory duct.

vascular shunt In a capillary bed, it is the main vessel connecting the arteriole to the venule.

vasculature Network of blood vessels in a particular organ.

vasectomy Method of male sterilization in which the vas deferens is tied off, preventing the sperm from traveling out of the penis during sexual intercourse.

vasoconstrict *(VAY zoh con STRICT)* A blood vessel becomes narrower due to muscle contraction.

vasoconstriction *(VAY zoh con STRIK shun)* Constriction of the smooth muscle in the artery wall causes the artery to become smaller in diameter.

vasodilate *(VAY zoh DIE late)* Opposite of vasoconstrict.

vasodilation *(VAY zoh die LAY shun)* Relaxation of the smooth muscle in the artery wall causes the artery to become larger in diameter.

vein Blood vessel that carries blood away from the cells and back to the heart. Veins have one-way valves that keep blood from flowing backwards, away from the heart.

ventilation *(ven tih LAY shun)* The bulk movement of gas into and out of the lungs.

ventral Pertaining to the anterior of the body particularly the abdomen.

ventral root A root of the spinal cord that carries motor information.

ventricles *(VEN trih kulz)* 1. Two lower chambers of the heart. Intraventricular structures are located in the ventricles. 2. Four hollow chambers within the brain that contain cerebrospinal fluid. The two lateral ventricles are within the right and left hemispheres of the cerebrum. The third ventricle is small and connects the lateral ventricles to the fourth ventricle, which is at the level of the pons and medulla oblongata.

venules *(VEHN yulz)* Smallest branch of a vein.

vertebrae *(VER teh bray)* One of 33 irregularly shaped bony segments of the spinal column.

vertebral cavity *See* Spinal cavity.

vertigo Sensation of being off balance when the body is not moving. Caused by upper respiratory infection, middle- or inner-ear infection, head trauma, or degenerative changes of the semicircular canals.

vesicle *(VESS ih kuhl)* A small bladder or blister; a membrane-bound storage sac inside a cell.

vestibular reflex Reflex that maintains balance.

vestibule *(VES tih byool)* A space into which the urethra (anterior) and vagina (posterior) empty.

vestibule chamber A small cavity or space at the beginning of a canal.

vestibulocochlear nerve *(VES tih byool KOHK lee are)* The eighth cranial nerve responsible for hearing and balance. Sometimes called the acoustic nerve.

vibrissae *(vie BRISS ee)* Coarse hairs in the nose that act as the first line of defense for the respiratory system.

villi *(VILL eye)* Microscopic projections of the mucosa within the lumen of the small intestine.

virus A microorganism that depends on other cells for its metabolic and reproductive needs.

visceral *(VISS er al)* Pertaining to organs.

visceral muscle Also called smooth muscle; the type of muscle found in all the organs (except the heart) of the body, such as the stomach and other digestive organs, the uterus, the blood vessels, and bronchial airways. Its ability to contract and return to a relaxed state plays a vital role in many of the body's internal workings.

visceral pleura *(VISS er al PLOO rah)* One of the two membranes of the pleura. It covers the surface of the lung.

vital signs Medical procedure during a physical examination in which the temperature, pulse, and respirations (TPR), as well as the blood pressure, are measured.

vitreous humor *(VIT ree us)* Clear, gel-like substance that fills the posterior cavity of the eye.

vocal cords Connective tissue bands in the larynx that vibrate and produce sounds for speaking and singing.

vulva *(VULL vah)* The area of the female external genitalia posterior to the mons veneris.

Wernicke's area The region in the cerebral hemisphere of the brain. Processes language information such as word sounds, recall, recognition, and interpretation.

white blood cells (WBCs) Leukocytes; responsible for the immune response.

withdrawal reflex Automatic response that causes pulling away from unpleasant stimuli, such as pain.

yellow marrow Adipose tissue inside bones.

Z lines Lines visible on the surface of skeletal muscle that mark the ends of each sarcomere.

zygote *(ZIGH goht)* The cell produced by the union of two gametes. It is a fertilized ovum.

PHOTO CREDITS

All Chapter Openers (Map and Pushpin), Sergign/Fotolia; **p. 1**, Mopic/Shutterstock; **p. 3a**, Sebastian Kaulitzki/Shutterstock; **p. 3b**, Photo courtesy CDC; **p. 8**, Goodluz/Shutterstock; **p. 23**, Wavebreakmedia/Shutterstock; **p. 25**, A., Santibhavank P/Shutterstock; **p. 25**, B., CGinspiration/Shutterstock; **p. 25**, C., Santibhavank P/Shutterstock; **p. 51**, Naeblys/Shutterstock; **p. 61**, Wavebreakmedia/Shutterstock; **p. 69**, Peeradach Rattanakoses/Shutterstock; **p. 70**, Photo courtesy CDC; **p. 71**, Ralph C. Eagle Jr./Science Source; **p. 74**, Alxhar/Fotolia; **p. 78**, Jose Luis Calvo/Shutterstock; **p. 100**, Adimas/Fotolia; **p. 103a**, Andrew Syred/Science Source; **p. 103b**, Susumu Nishinaga/Photo Researchers/Science Source; **p. 107a**, Wang song/Shutterstock; **p. 107b**, itsmejust/Shutterstock; **p. 107c**, English/Custom Medical Stock Photo; **p. 108**, Tyler Olson/Shutterstock; **p. 114**, Puwadol Jaturawutthichai/Shutterstock; **p. 125**, Microcozm/Fotolia; **p. 127**, Jose Luis Calvo/Shutterstock; **p. 137**, @erics/Fotolia; **p. 143**, Jose Luis Calvo/Shutterstock; **p. 148**, krishnacreations/Fotolia; **p. 154A**, CMSP / Custom Medical Stock Photo; **p. 154B**, JPD/Custom Medical Stock Photo; **p. 155**, Cavan Images/Getty Images; **p. 156A**, Suzanne Tucker/Shutterstock; **p. 156B**, Suzanne Tucker/Shutterstock; **p. 157**, Image Point Fr/Shutterstock; **p. 164A**, Rob Byron/Shutterstock; **p. 164B**, CLS Design/Shutterstock; **p. 164C**, Olavs/Shutterstock; **p. 164D**, Bahadir Yeniceri/Shutterstock; **p. 164E**, Australis Photography/Shutterstock; **p. 164F**, Joseph S.L. Tan Matt/Shutterstock; **p. 164G**, Naiyyer/Shutterstock; **p. 167**, StudioSmart/Shutterstock; **p. 172B**, Ktsdesign/Shutterstock; **p. 190**, shumpc/Fotolia; **p. 210**, Federico Marsicano/Shutterstock; **p. 213**, Purestock/Getty Images; **p. 219**, Stefan Kiefer/imagebroker/Corbis; **p. 228A**, Levent Konuk/Shutterstockes; **p. 228C**, Pavel L Photo and Video/Shutterstock; **p. 228D**, Photo courtesy CDC; **p. 231**, Designua/Shutterstock; **p. 246**, Ariel Skelley/Getty Images; **p. 250A**, CMSP/Custom Medical Stock Photo; **p. 251C**, Photo courtesy CDC; **p. 251D**, Bettina Cirone/Photo Researchers/Science Source; **p. 254**, Sebastian Kaulitzki/Shutterstock; **p. 263**, David Joel/MacNeal Hospital/Getty Images; **p. 267B**, Ggw1962/Shutterstock; **p. 285**, Naeblys/Fotolia; **p. 287A**, Ed Reschke/Getty Images; **p. 287B**, BSIP/UIG/Getty Images; **p. 289**, 3660 Group Inc./Getty Images; **p. 293A**, Dr. Gladden Willis/Getty Images; **p. 303**, Michal Heron/Pearson Education. Inc.; **p. 314**, Maya2008/Shutterstock; **p. 318**, Morsa Images; **p. 322B**, Sebastian Kaulitzki/Shutterstock; **p. 340**, Henrik Sorensen/Getty Images; **p. 346**, Nejron Photo/Shutterstock; **p. 354A**, Science Photo Library/STEVE GSCHMEISSNER/Getty Images; **p. 361A**, CNRI/Science Source; **p. 368**, Lightspring/Shutterstock; **p. 379**, Arthur Glauberman/Science Source; **p. 380**, Monkey Business Images/Shutterstock; **p. 390**, Giovanni Cancemi/Fotolia; **p. 393A & B**, CNRI/Photo Researchers/Science Source; **p. 393 (Figure 18-2)**, Eleonora_os/Shutterstock; **p. 411**, Claude Edelmann/Science Source; **p. 413**, Gelpi/Fotolia; **p. 419**, Liam Norris/Cultura/Getty Images; **p. 420**, Kyrien/Shutterstock; **p. 422**, Tony Graham /DK Images; **p. 425**, Guy Drayton/Dorling Kindersly; **p. 426**, Auremar/Fotolia; **p. 428**, National Cancer Institute; **p. 435**, Pressmaster/Shutterstock; **p. 441**, Rawpixel/Shutterstock.

Note: Page numbers with *f* indicate figures; those with *t* indicate tables.